Handbook of Gastrointestinal Medicine

Editor: Donald Maxmilian

FOSTER ACADEMICS
www.fosteracademics.com

www.fosteracademics.com

FOSTER ACADEMICS

Cataloging-in-Publication Data

Handbook of gastrointestinal medicine / edited by Donald Maxmilian.
p. cm.
Includes bibliographical references and index.
ISBN 978-1-63242-659-8
1. Gastrointestinal system--Diseases. 2. Gastrointestinal system--Diseases--Diagnosis.
3. Gastrointestinal system--Diseases--Treatment. 4. Gastroenterology. I. Maxmilian, Donald.
RC801 .H36 2019
616.33--dc23

Foster Academics,
118-35 Queens Blvd., Suite 400,
Forest Hills, NY 11375, USA

ISBN 978-1-63242-659-8 (Hardback)

Printed and bound in China.

Contents

Preface XI

Chapter 1 **A Lethal Complication of Endoscopic Therapy: Duodenal Intramural Hematoma** 1
Turan Calhan, Abdurrahman Sahin, Resul Kahraman, Barış Soydaş, Ali Tosun and Egemen Cebeci

Chapter 2 **Recurrent Hepatocellular Carcinoma in Patient with Crohn's Disease: Incidental or Expected Outcome of Azathioprine?** 5
Youssef Botros, Mary Mathews, Hiren Patel, Nihar Shah, Walid Baddoura and Andrew de la Torre

Chapter 3 **Esophageal Cicatricial Pemphigoid as an Isolated Involvement Treated with Mycophenolate Mofetil** 9
Sandra Sánchez Prudencio, Daniel Domingo Senra, Daniel Martín Rodríguez, Belén Botella Mateu, Carlos Esteban Jiménez-Zarza, Felipe de la Morena López, José Jiménez Reyes, Manuel Nevado Santos and Beatriz de Cuenca Morón

Chapter 4 **Lanreotide Autogel in the Treatment of Persistent Diarrhea following a Total Colectomy** 13
Patrick Schoeters and Karl De Pooter

Chapter 5 **Severe Gastroparesis following Radiofrequency Catheter Ablation for Atrial Fibrillation: Suggestion for Diagnosis, Treatment and Device for Gastroparesis after RFCA** 18
Dong Seok Lee and Sang Jin Lee

Chapter 6 **Self-Expandable Metal Stent Placement for Closure of a Leak after Total Gastrectomy for Gastric Cancer: Report on Three Cases** 24
Dario Raimondo, Emanuele Sinagra, Tiziana Facella, Francesca Rossi, Marco Messina, Massimiliano Spada, Guido Martorana, Pier Enrico Marchesa, Rosario Squatrito, Giovanni Tomasello, Attilio Ignazio Lo Monte, Giancarlo Pompei and Ennio La Rocca

Chapter 7 **Psoas Muscle Infiltration Masquerading Distant Adenocarcinoma** 29
Kamel A. Gharaibeh, Arnaldo Lopez-Ruiz and Tauqeer Yousuf

Chapter 8 **Portal Vein Thrombosis due to Prothrombin Gene Mutation following Sleeve Gastrectomy** 34
Murad Baba, Jordan Fakhoury and Amer Syed

Chapter 9 **Diagnosis and Treatment of Esophageal Granular Cell Tumor: A Case Report** 38
Ramin Niknam, Kamran Bagheri Lankarani and Bita Geramizadeh

Chapter 10 **Amyand's Hernia: Rare Presentation of a Common Ailment** ... **42**
Sanjeev Singhal, Anu Singhal, Sanjay Singh Negi, Rahul Tugnait, Pankaj Kumar Arora, Bishwanath Tiwari, Pawan Malik, Lav Gupta, Amit Bimal, Abhishek Gupta, Rahul Gupta, Pushkar Chouhan and Chandra Kant Singh

Chapter 11 **Epigenetic Alterations in a Gastric Leiomyoma** ... **48**
M. T. Branham, M. Pellicer, E. Campoy, M. Palma, A. Correa and M. Roqué

Chapter 12 **Acute Pancreatitis Secondary to Hemobilia after Percutaneous Liver Biopsy: A Rare Complication of a Common Procedure, Presenting in an Atypical Fashion** ... **53**
Ramy Mansour and Justin Miller

Chapter 13 **Ulcerating Ileocolitis in Severe Amatoxin Poisoning** ... **57**
Matthias Peter Hilty, Marcel Halama, Anne-Katrin Zimmermann, Marco Maggiorini and Andreas Geier

Chapter 14 **Left Colon Diverticulitis Presenting as Perforated Lumbar Abscess: A Case Report** ... **61**
Daniel Paramythiotis, Konstantinia Kofina, Vassileios N. Papadopoulos and Antonios Michalopoulos

Chapter 15 **Clinical Outcome of a Portosplenomesenteric Venous Thrombosis in Necrotizing Acute Pancreatitis with Protein C and S Deficiency Treated by Anticoagulation Therapy Alone** ... **65**
Firmin Ankouane, Mathurin Kowo, Bernadette Ngo Nonga, Eric Magny, Edith Hell Medjo and Elie Claude Ndjitoyap Ndam

Chapter 16 **Resolution of Fundic Gland Polyposis following Laparoscopic Magnetic Sphincter Augmentation and Subsequent Cessation of Proton Pump Inhibitors** ... **71**
Joel R. Brockmeyer, Erin E. Connolly, Richard J. Wittchow and Shanu N. Kothari

Chapter 17 **Infected Renal Cyst as a Complication of Dropped Gallstones during Laparoscopic Cholecystectomy** ... **75**
Chelsea Kennedy-Snodgrass, Vivian Keenan and Douglas S. Katz

Chapter 18 **The Traumatic Tube: Bleeding Rectal Ulcer Caused by Flexi-Seal Device** ... **80**
Abhinav Tiwari, Himani Sharma, Khola Qamar, Yaseen Alastal, Thomas Sodeman and Ali Nawras

Chapter 19 **A Case of Segmental Arterial Mediolysis Presenting as Mucosal Gastric Hematoma** ... **84**
Shunsuke Sakuraba, Hajime Orita, Shuhei Ueda, Satoshi Tokuda, Tomoaki Ito, Tomoyuki Kushida, Mutsumi Sakurada, Hiroshi Maekawa, Ryo Wada and Koichi Sato

Chapter 20 **Fenofibrate: A Nonlithogenic Means of Recurrent Drug-Induced Pancreatitis** ... **88**
Thamer Kassim, Joy-Marie Hermes, Abdullah Abdussalam, Ahmed Aly and Subhash Chandra

Chapter 21 **When the Benign Pneumatosis Intestinalis Becomes no Longer Benign: A Rare Case of Bowel Perforation in a Patient with Systemic Sclerosis** ... **93**
Jian Guan, Alvina Munaf, Alric V. Simmonds and Irteza Inayat

Chapter 22 **Cannabinoid Hyperemesis Syndrome: A Case Report of Cyclic Severe Hyperemesis and Abdominal Pain with Long-Term Cannabis use** 97
Julia Hermes-Laufer, Lola Del Puppo, Ihsan Inan, François-Xavier Troillet and Omar Kherad

Chapter 23 **Esophageal Lichen Planus: Understanding a Potentially Severe Stricturing Disease** 101
Bharat Rao, Abhishek Gulati, Blair Jobe and Shyam Thakkar

Chapter 24 **Gastrointestinal Involvement of Testicular Germ Cell Tumor: A Case Report** 105
Oluwaseun Shogbesan, Abdullateef Abdulkareem, Asad Jehangir, Sunila Byreddy, Sharon Swierczynski and Anthony Donato

Chapter 25 **Primary Mucosal Melanoma of the Stomach** 110
O. Phillips, A. Higdon, R. Colaco and H. Fish

Chapter 26 **A Case of Complete Remission from Advanced Gastric Adenocarcinoma with Synchronous Liver Metastasis in Response to EOX Chemotherapy** 115
Zhi-jun Yan, Jia-xin Wang, You-yi Liu, Zhen-hui Li, Li-juan Zhang, Ping Gan, Xiao Han, Li-kun Luan and You-guo Dai

Chapter 27 **Colonoscopic Splenic Injury: A Simplified Radiologic Approach** 122
Tara Chen, Qiu Tong and Alexander Kurchin

Chapter 28 **Salivary Gland Heterotopia in the Gastroesophageal Junction: A Case Series** 126
Lina Abdul Karim, Dong Hyang Kwon and Metin Ozdemirli

Chapter 29 **Hemorrhage from Extra-Antral Gastric Antral Vascular Ectasia in a Patient with Duodenal Heterotopic Gastric Mucosa** 131
John Gubatan, Nathan Raines, Hasan Khosravi, Tracy L. Challies and Tyler M. Berzin

Chapter 30 **A Calcium Enterolith in a Patient with Crohn's Disease and its In Vitro Dissolubility in Citric Acid** 136
Masaya Iwamuro, Haruo Urata, Sakiko Hiraoka, Masayasu Ohmori, Yoshitaka Kondo, Yoshiro Kawahara and Hiroyuki Okada

Chapter 31 **Deep Venous Thrombosis and Bilateral Pulmonary Embolism Revealing Silent Celiac Disease: Case Report** 142
Igor Dumic, Scott Martin, Nadim Salfiti, Robert Watson and Tamara Alempijevic

Chapter 32 **Yogi Detox Tea: A Potential Cause of Acute Liver Failure** 150
Keerthana Kesavarapu, Mitchell Kang, Jaewook James Shin and Kenneth Rothstein

Chapter 33 **A Severe Case of Tuberculosis Radiologically and Endoscopically Mimicking Colorectal Cancer with Peritoneal Carcinomatosis** 154
Timo Rath, Raja Atreya, Walter Geißdörfer, Roland Lang, Andreas Nägel and Markus F. Neurath

Chapter 34 **Medical Treatment of Postendoscopic Submucosal Dissection Phlegmonous Gastritis in an Elderly Diabetic Woman with Myelodysplastic Syndrome** 158
Ko Matsuura, Shinsuke Hiramatsu, Rika Taketani, Kohei Ishibashi, Masanao Uraoka, Shinichi Baba, Akihiro Nakamura, Hiroshi Takihara, Chie Ueda and Taro Inoue

Chapter 35 **Association between Oesophageal Diverticula and Leiomyomas: A Report of Two Cases** 163
Muhammad Chowdhry, Christina Spyratou, Bruno Lorenzi, Sritharan Kadirkamanathan and Alexandros Charalabopoulos

Chapter 36 **Atypical Aortoesophageal Fistula with Atypical and Delayed Presentation and Negative Imaging Studies** 167
Seifeldin Hakim, Mihajlo Gjeorgjievski, Lohit Garg, Molly Orosey and Tusar Desai

Chapter 37 **Pancreaticopleural Fistula: A Review of Imaging Diagnosis and Early Endoscopic Intervention** 172
Ali Kord Valeshabad, Jennifer Acostamadiedo, Lekui Xiao, Winnie Mar and Karen L. Xie

Chapter 38 **Seronegative Intestinal Villous Atrophy: A Diagnostic Challenge** 178
Cláudio Martins, Cristina Teixeira, Suzane Ribeiro, Daniel Trabulo, Cláudia Cardoso, João Mangualde, Ricardo Freire, Ana Luísa Alves, Élia Gamito, Isabelle Cremers and Ana Paula Oliveira

Chapter 39 **Two Cases of Leiomyoma in the Colon Masquerading as Other Types of Colonic Pedunculated Polyps** 182
Ailee Ikeda, Masaya Iwamuro, Takehiro Tanaka, Toshihiro Inokuchi, Asuka Nakarai, Yuusaku Sugihara, Keita Harada, Sakiko Hiraoka, Yoshiro Kawahara and Hiroyuki Okada

Chapter 40 **A Case Report and Literature Review of *Clostridium difficile* Negative Antibiotic Associated Hemorrhagic Colitis Caused by *Klebsiella oxytoca*** 187
Aaron Fisher and Alexandra Halalau

Chapter 41 **Polypoid Dysplasia in Barrett's Esophagus: Diagnosis, Management and Very Different Outcomes in Two Consecutive Cases** 191
Megan Murphy, Christina Tofani, Kunjal Gandhi and Anthony Infantolino

Chapter 42 **Two Cases of White Globe Appearance in Autoimmune Atrophic Gastritis** 195
Masaya Iwamuro, Takehiro Tanaka, Hiromitsu Kanzaki, Seiji Kawano, Yoshiro Kawahara and Hiroyuki Okada

Chapter 43 **Thromboelastometry Identified Alteration of Clot Stabilization and Factor XIII Supplementation Need in a Patient with Decompensated Liver Disease Undergoing Liver Biopsy** 200
Tomaz Crochemore and Felicio Aragão Savioli

Chapter 44 **An Unusual Case of Gastrointestinal Bleeding from Isolated Gallbladder Varices in a Patient with Pancreatic Cancer Complicated by Portal Biliopathy** 204
Mahir Gachabayov, Kubach Kubachev, Elbrus Abdullaev, Nonna Zarkua, Abakar Abdullaev and Artur Fokin

Chapter 45 **A Rare Clinical Presentation of Cholangiocarcinoma** 208
Elisa Gravito-Soares, Marta Gravito-Soares, Pedro Figueiredo and Luis Tomé

Chapter 46 **Hydrogen Peroxide Induced Colitis: A Case Report** ... 212
Dushyant Pawar, Anna Calara, Roy Jacob, Nancy Beck and Alan N. Peiris

Chapter 47 **A Mysterious DRESS Case: Autoimmune Enteropathy Associated with DRESS Syndrome** ... 218
Abimbola Adike, Vaishnavi Boppana, Dora Lam-Himlin, Melissa Stanton, Steven Nelson and Kevin C. Ruff

Chapter 48 **Metastatic Renal Cell Cancer to Thyroid Diagnosed by Endoscopic Ultrasound Guided Fine Needle Aspiration Technique** ... 223
Yousef Abdel-Aziz, Tariq Hammad, Mohamad Nawras, Hayder Abdulwahid and Ali Nawras

Chapter 49 **Moderate Hypertriglyceridemia Causing Recurrent Pancreatitis: A Case Report** ... 227
Vijay Gayam, Amrendra Kumar Mandal, Pavani Garlapati, Mazin Khalid, Arshpal Gill and Khalid Mowyad

Chapter 50 **Rare Case of an Epithelial Cyst in an Intrapancreatic Accessory Spleen Treated by Robot-Assisted Spleen Preserving Distal Pancreatectomy** ... 231
Willemijn P. M. van Dijck, Vincent P. Groot, Lodewijk A. A. Brosens, Jeroen Hagendoorn, Inne H. M. Borel Rinkes, Maarten S. van Leeuwen and I. Quintus Molenaar

Chapter 51 **A Case of Thermal Esophageal Injury Induced by Sodium Picosulfate with Magnesium Citrate** ... 237
Dong-Hyuk Yang, Byoung Wook Bang, Kye Sook Kwon, Hyung Kil Kim and Yong Woon Shin

Chapter 52 **Combined Approach of Cryoablation and Stent-In-Stent Technique for Removal of an Embedded Esophageal Stent** ... 242
Madhuri Chandnani, Jonah Cohen and Tyler M.Berzin

Chapter 53 **Pyogenic Liver Abscess with no Predisposing Risk Factors** ... 246
Matthew Chadwick, Leonid Shamban and Michael Neumann

Chapter 54 **Gastrointestinal Bleeding Secondary to Portal Hypertensive Duodenopathy in a Patient with Decompensated Liver Cirrhosis** ... 250
Rohini Krishna, Samuel O. Igbinedion, Richie Diaz, Nazneen Hussain and Moheb Boktor

Chapter 55 **A Rare Encounter with an Expanding Pseudocyst of the Spleen** ... 254
Ashish Lal Shrestha and Pradita Shrestha

Permissions

List of Contributors

Index

Preface

The world is advancing at a fast pace like never before. Therefore, the need is to keep up with the latest developments. This book was an idea that came to fruition when the specialists in the area realized the need to coordinate together and document essential themes in the subject. That's when I was requested to be the editor. Editing this book has been an honour as it brings together diverse authors researching on different streams of the field. The book collates essential materials contributed by veterans in the area which can be utilized by students and researchers alike.

The branch of medicine that studies the digestive system and its disorders is referred to as gastroenterology. Diseases related to the gastrointestinal tract, namely the stomach, oesophagus, small intestine, large intestine and rectum, and the organs responsible for digestion, which includes the liver, gallbladder and pancreas are known as gastrointestinal diseases. Some oral diseases associated with the gastrointestinal tract include gastroesophageal reflux disease, Gardner's syndrome, Peutz-Jeghers syndrome, atrophic glossitis, angular cheilitis and sideropenic dysphagia. Some other diseases associated with the gastrointestinal tract include oesophageal diseases, such as Barrett's oesophagus, gastric diseases such as atrophic gastritis, intestinal diseases such as enterocolitis and liver diseases such as fatty liver. This book aims to shed light on some of the unexplored aspects of gastrointestinal medicine. It will also provide interesting topics for research which interested readers can take up. This book includes contributions of experts and doctors which will provide innovative insights to readers.

Each chapter is a sole-standing publication that reflects each author´s interpretation. Thus, the book displays a multi-facetted picture of our current understanding of application, resources and aspects of the field. I would like to thank the contributors of this book and my family for their endless support.

Editor

A Lethal Complication of Endoscopic Therapy: Duodenal Intramural Hematoma

Turan Calhan,[1] Abdurrahman Sahin,[2] Resul Kahraman,[2] Barış Soydaş,[1] Ali Tosun,[3] and Egemen Cebeci[4]

[1] *Department of Gastroenterology, Mehmet Akif İnan Training and Research Hospital, Şanlıurfa, Turkey*
[2] *Department of Gastroenterology, Umraniye Training and Research Hospital, Istanbul, Turkey*
[3] *Department of Radiology, Mehmet Akif İnan Training and Research Hospital, Şanlıurfa, Turkey*
[4] *Department of Nephrology, Okmeydanı Training and Research Hospital, Istanbul, Turkey*

Correspondence should be addressed to Turan Calhan; trncalhan@hotmail.com

Academic Editor: Hideto Kawaratani

Duodenal intramural hematoma (DIH) usually occurs in childhood and young adults following blunt abdominal trauma. It may also develop in the presence of coagulation disorders and may rarely be an iatrogenic outcome of endoscopic procedures. Management of DIH is usually a conservative approach. A case of intramural duodenal hematoma that developed following endoscopic epinephrine sclerotherapy and/or argon plasma coagulation and that was nonresponsive to conservative therapy in a patient with chronic renal failure who died from sepsis is being discussed in this report. Clinicians should be aware of such possible complications after endoscopic hemostasis in patients with coagulation disorders.

1. Introduction

Endoscopic hemostatic procedures such as local injection of epinephrine, polidocanol, and fibrin tissue adhesive onto the mucosa, argon plasma coagulation (APC), and hemoclipping are commonly used for the treatment of bleeding ulcers, instead of the open surgical approaches used in the past [1]. Although the risks are usually considered to be minimal, there are reports describing that duodenal intramural hematomas may develop as a complication after diagnostic or therapeutic endoscopy, especially in patients susceptible to hemorrhage, such as those with chronic renal disease [2]. Herein we discuss a case of duodenal intramural hematoma (DIH), complicated by acute pancreatitis, obstructive jaundice, and sepsis, which developed after endoscopic epinephrine sclerotherapy and/or APC and which was nonresponsive to conservative therapy in a patient with chronic renal failure secondary to hypertensive nephrosclerosis.

2. Case Presentation

A 65-year-old male patient was admitted to the clinic with weakness and dark stool persisting for the last 3-4 days. He had hypertension (HT) and chronic renal failure (CRF) and no habit of smoking or alcohol consumption. He had no history of using anticoagulants or antiaggregant drugs. On physical examination, the patient appeared pale and tired. His skin turgor and tone were decreased. Blood pressure was 90/60 mmHg, pulse rate 120 beats/min, and body temperature 36.4°C. Lung examination was normal. Abdominal examination demonstrated mild epigastric tenderness and melena was identified by rectal examination. Initial laboratory values were as follows: glucose: 107 mg/dL, urea: 361 mg/dL, creatinine: 7.1 mg/dL, sodium: 139 mEq/L, potassium: 3.86 mEq/L, leukocyte: 21.300/mm^3, hemoglobin: 7.8 g/dL, platelets: 100.000/mm^3, prothrombin time: 12 sec, and INR: 1.05. Serum transaminase, bilirubin, and amylase-lipase values were within normal ranges. Crystalloid and

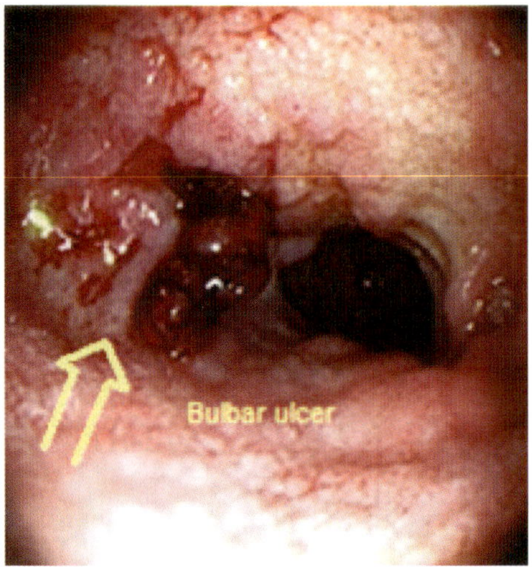

FIGURE 1: Bleeding ulcer covered with fresh red clot at the anterior wall of the bulb duodenal segment II opening. There was oozing bleeding at the ulcer when the clot was eliminated (prior to endoscopic procedure).

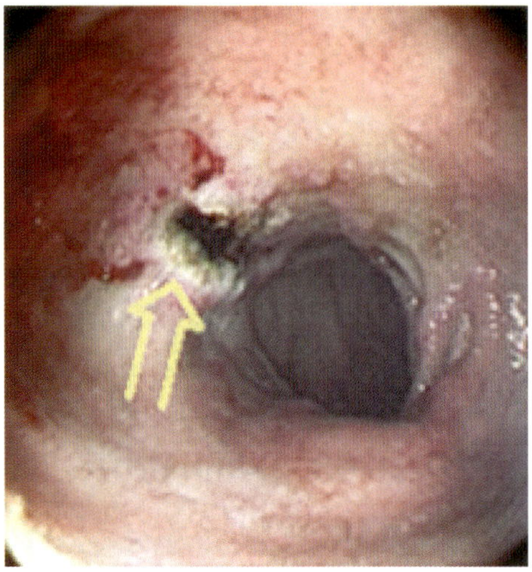

FIGURE 2: The image following endoscopic epinephrine sclerotherapy plus endoscopic argon plasma coagulation (arrow) procedure for bleeding bulbar ulcer shows complete cessation of bleeding.

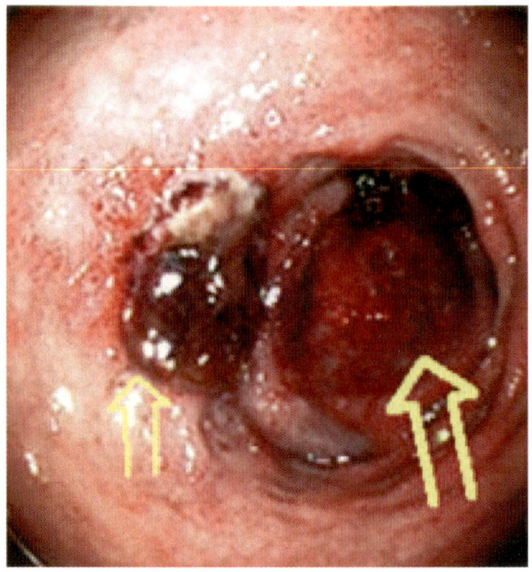

FIGURE 3: Intramural duodenal hematoma at the posterior duodenal wall not causing complete luminal obstruction (large arrow), which developed 36 hours after endoscopic procedure. The ulcer appears stable following endoscopic treatment (small arrow).

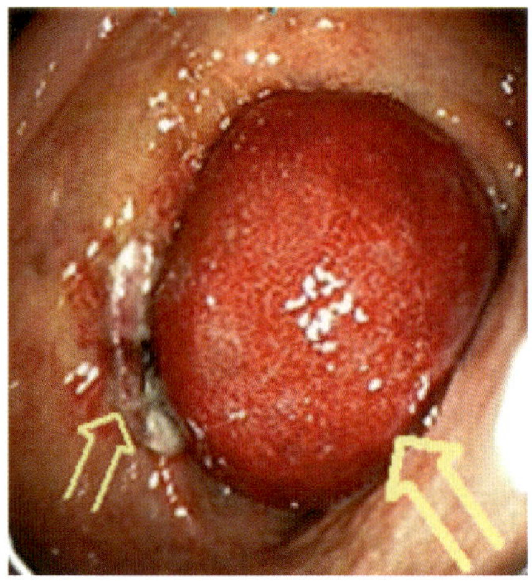

FIGURE 4: Giant intramural duodenal hematoma causing complete luminal obstruction 60 hours after the endoscopic procedure (large arrow). Bulbar ulcer appears stable (small arrow).

colloid fluid replacement were promptly given intravenously, parenteral proton-pump inhibitor was initiated, and four units of erythrocyte suspension was administered. Following hemodynamic stabilization, the patient underwent upper gastrointestinal endoscopy (UGIE). A 9 mm sized ulcer, covered with fresh red clot, was observed at the anterior wall of the bulb. The clot was removed and oozing bleeding was seen at the base of the ulcer; epinephrine was then injected into the areas adjacent to the ulcer. A vascular lesion at the ulcer base was coagulated with argon plasma coagulation (APC) during the same session (Figures 1 and 2). Although there had been no evidence of clinical bleeding (no hematemesis or melena), hemoglobin and hematocrit values declined approximately 36 hours later from this intervention, and a second UGIE was carried out. On endoscopic examination, there was no bleeding from the ulcer. However, the posterior wall mucosa of the second part of the duodenum, at approximately 2 cm distal to the ulcer, was erythematous with no obstruction (Figure 3). Postoperatively the patient developed nausea, vomiting, abdominal pain, and jaundice after the second endoscopic assessment. Serum total bilirubin and direct bilirubin values increased up to 23 mg/dL and 19 mg/dL, respectively. Plasma amylase level was 1389 U/L, and lipase level was 991 U/L. At the third day of admission, a final UGIE was performed to investigate the possible presence of a hematoma. The ulcer was stable but the mucosa of the second part of the duodenum was erythematous and was also significantly protruded towards the lumen, resulting in complete obstruction (Figure 4). Upper abdominal magnetic resonance imaging (MRI) and computerized tomography

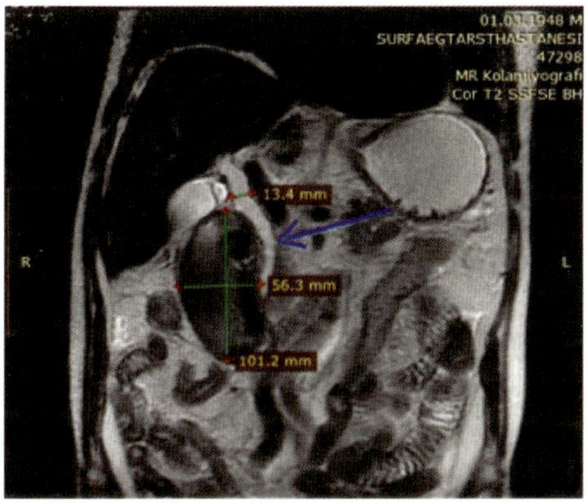

FIGURE 5: Coronal T2A magnetic resonance imaging. The image shows a hematoma with a diameter of approximately 10.1 × 5.6 cm. Bile ducts are dilated (common bile duct (CBD) diameter 13.4 mm). Distally, pressure caused by the hematoma on the CBD and reduced CBD diameter is apparent (blue arrow).

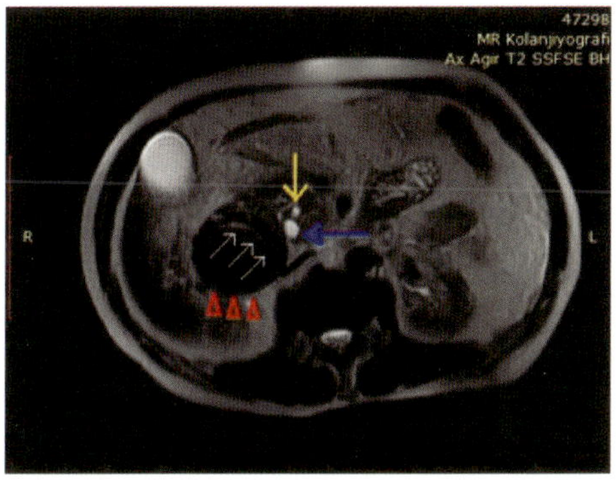

FIGURE 6: T2A magnetic resonance imaging from the axial plane. Intramural duodenal hematoma adjacent to the pancreas head (red arrow heads). Duodenal lumen appears to be pushed forward due to the hematoma with significant narrowing of its lumen (white arrows). Common bile duct (blue arrow) and pancreatic duct (yellow arrow) are dilated due to pressure caused by the hematoma.

(CT) demonstrated a mass with size 5.6 × 10.1 cm at the section corresponding to the second and third parts of the duodenum, consistent with an intramural hematoma causing complete obstruction of the lumen. The lesion compressed the bile ducts and the pancreatic duct resulting in dilation of the common bile duct and main pancreatic duct (Figures 5, 6, and 7). Decompression with a nasogastric tube was performed and a conservative treatment modality was attempted (total parenteral nutrition, intravenous fluid, and careful observation). However, the patient did not respond to conservative treatment and his overall condition deteriorated rapidly with signs of sepsis developing. In response, ultrasonography-guided percutaneous hematoma drainage was performed. The patient's clinical parameters did not improve although the hematoma was drained. The patient died because of sepsis, septic shock, and multiorgan failure.

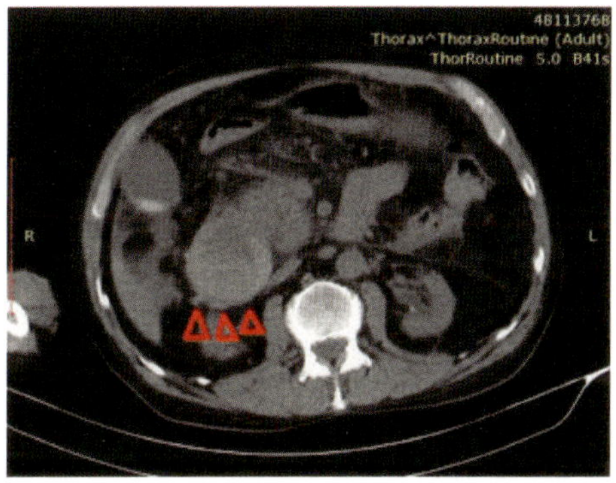

FIGURE 7: Computerized tomography image from the same axial plane as magnetic resonance imaging (Figure 6), showing intramural hematoma (red arrow heads).

3. Discussion

Duodenal intramural hematoma is an unusual condition in adults [3]. Blunt abdominal trauma is involved in the etiology of most of the cases (more than 80%) [4]. Nontraumatic DIHs usually result from anticoagulant treatment, blood dyscrasia, pancreatic diseases, intestinal arterial aneurysm rupture, and endoscopic procedures on the duodenal mucosa [5]. DIHs following endoscopic intervention (e.g., biopsy, sclerotherapy, and APC) are extremely rare [6, 7]. DIHs usually occur at the posterior wall of the duodenum fixed with the retroperitoneum in front of the vertebral colon, a region that is rich in submucosal vascular structure [4]. It has been reported that hematomas may particularly develop more often in the presence of conditions that predispose to bleeding, including hepatic cirrhosis and renal failure [1, 8]. Treatment of DIHs is usually conservative and recovery with conservative treatment has been shown especially in childhood and in cases with gastric outlet obstruction [9]. When conservative treatment is not effective, surgical drainage choices of ultrasound- or CT-guided drainage (laparotomy, laparoscopic drainage) are used [10]. Additionally, endoscopic incision and drainage techniques are used in the treatment as a more comfortable method [11]. There have been reports in the literature of DIH cases following both APC and endoscopic epinephrine sclerotherapy [1, 12]. Epinephrine sclerotherapy followed by APC during a single session was performed to our patient. The patient had CRF and unexplained thrombocytopenia (100.000/mm^3) as risk factors. The etiology of hemorrhagic diathesis in CRF is multifactorial. Several factors, including platelet dysfunction, anemia, and inadequate renal excretion of drugs, are involved [13]. We believe that DIH was caused rather by sclerotherapy in the current case. However, it is likely that APC could have caused or contributed to the condition.

Following the observation of endoscopic findings suggestive of DIH, imaging methods were performed to confirm the diagnosis. Although abdominal ultrasonography was performed initially, chosen for its noninvasive nature and convenience, it was suboptimal due to abdominal gas and demonstrated an abdominal mass with indefinite margins.

Abdominal CT was performed to determine the location of the mass, to rule out possible perforation and to view the size of the mass. Simultaneous MR cholangiography was also undertaken to demonstrate the dilatation of the bile ducts. After establishing the DIH diagnosis with imaging techniques, nasogastric decompression was performed and conservative treatment (total parenteral nutrition, intravenous fluid, and careful observation) was attempted. However, a giant hematoma leading to icterus and sepsis, complete duodenal obstruction, and acute pancreatitis developed at 60 hours. He was considered unresponsive to conservative treatment and ultrasonography-guided percutaneous hematoma drainage was performed. The patient unfortunately died on the next day due to sepsis, septic shock, and multiorgan failure.

There have been reports in the literature describing failure with conservative treatment in cases of DIH that developed following endoscopic sclerotherapy complicated with jaundice and acute pancreatitis [2], even including fatal outcome [14]. Conservative treatment may be followed for patients without complete duodenal obstruction and/or complications. However, in cases involving complete intestinal obstruction and/or pressure on adjacent organs, we believe that the hematoma should be identified as early as possible and evacuated dynamically both internally and externally to avoid fatal outcomes (acute pancreatitis, obstructive jaundice, aspiration pneumonia, and sepsis/septic shock). As a minimally invasive treatment choice, ultrasound- or CT-guided drainage, laparotomy, laparoscopic drainage, and endoscopic incision and drainage should be considered earlier for such cases.

In conclusion, it should be kept in mind that endoscopic hemostatic procedures in the presence of conditions predisposing patients to bleeding (e.g., chronic renal failure and hepatic cirrhosis) may lead to complications, and any deterioration should prompt a reassessment, utilizing imaging methods as necessary. Intramural hematoma should be considered in differential diagnosis for patients with no clinical evidence of bleeding (no hematemesis or melena) but with reduced hematocrit levels after endoscopic intervention. Clinicians should not insist on maintaining the treatment when complications such as complete luminal obstruction, acute pancreatitis secondary to pressure on the adjacent organs, and obstructive jaundice develop and should consider other treatment choices earlier.

References

[1] K. Sugai, E. Kajiwara, Y. Mochizuki et al., "Intramural duodenal hematoma after endoscopic therapy for a bleeding duodenal ulcer in a patient with liver cirrhosis," *Internal Medicine*, vol. 44, no. 9, pp. 954–957, 2005.

[2] B. Rohrer, J. Schreiner, P. Lehnert, H. Waldner, and W. Heldwein, "Gastrointestinal intramural hematoma, a complication of endoscopic injection methods for bleeding peptic ulcers: a case series," *Endoscopy*, vol. 26, no. 7, pp. 617–621, 1994.

[3] R. A. Parrish, H. T. Edmondson, and W. H. Moretz, "Duodenal and biliary obstruction secondary to intramural hematoma," *The American Journal of Surgery*, vol. 108, no. 3, pp. 428–430, 1964.

[4] W. R. Jones, W. J. Hardin, J. T. Davis, and J. D. Hardy, "Intramural hematoma of the duodenum: a review of the literature and case report," *Annals of Surgery*, vol. 173, no. 4, pp. 534–544, 1971.

[5] A. Fingerhut, F. Rouffet, C. Eugene, J. P. Fendler, D. Hillion, and R. Ronat, "Nontraumatic intramural hematoma of the duodenum. Report of 4 cases and review of the literature," *Digestion*, vol. 26, no. 4, pp. 231–235, 1983.

[6] M. R. Lukman, A. Y. Jasmi, and S. S. Niza, "Massive dissecting intramural duodenal hematoma following endoscopic haemostasis of a bleeding duodenal ulcer," *Asian Journal of Surgery*, vol. 29, no. 2, pp. 98–100, 2006.

[7] C. Grasshof, A. Wolf, F. Neuwirth, and C. Posovszky, "Intramural duodenal haematoma after endoscopic biopsy: case report and review of the literature," *Case Reports in Gastroenterology*, vol. 6, no. 1, pp. 5–14, 2012.

[8] S. Chung, C. W. Park, H. W. Chung, S. J. Shin, and Y. S. Chang, "Intramural duodenal hematoma and hemoperitoneum after endoscopic treatment in a patient with chronic renal failure on hemodialysis: a case report," *Cases Journal*, vol. 2, article 9083, 2009.

[9] R. J. Touloukian, "Protocol for the nonoperative treatment of obstructing intramural duodenal hematoma during childhood," *The American Journal of Surgery*, vol. 145, no. 3, pp. 330–334, 1983.

[10] G. J. Nolan, C. Bendinelli, and J. Gani, "Laparoscopic drainage of an intramural duodenal haematoma: a novel technique and review of the literature," *World Journal of Emergency Surgery*, vol. 6, no. 1, article 42, 2011.

[11] Y.-M. Pan, T.-T. Wang, J. Wu, and B. Hu, "Endoscopic drainage for duodenal hematoma following endoscopic retrograde cholangiopancreatography: a case report," *World Journal of Gastroenterology*, vol. 19, no. 13, pp. 2118–2121, 2013.

[12] B. Keum, H. J. Chun, Y. S. Seo et al., "Gastric intramural hematoma caused by argon plasma coagulation: treated with endoscopic incision and drainage (with videos)," *Gastrointestinal Endoscopy*, vol. 75, no. 4, pp. 918–919, 2012.

[13] D. Kaw and D. Malhotra, "Platelet dysfunction and end-stage renal disease," *Seminars in Dialysis*, vol. 19, no. 4, pp. 317–322, 2006.

[14] F. Sadry and H. Hauser, "Fatal pancreatitis secondary to iatrogenic intramural duodenal hematoma: a case report and review of the literature," *Gastrointestinal Radiology*, vol. 15, no. 4, pp. 296–298, 1990.

2

Recurrent Hepatocellular Carcinoma in Patient with Crohn's Disease: Incidental or Expected Outcome of Azathioprine?

Youssef Botros,[1] Mary Mathews,[1] Hiren Patel,[2] Nihar Shah,[3] Walid Baddoura,[2] and Andrew de la Torre[4]

[1]*Department of Internal Medicine, St. Joseph's Regional Medical Center, New York Medical College, Paterson, NJ 07503, USA*
[2]*Department of Gastroenterology, St. Joseph's Regional Medical Center, New York Medical College, Paterson, NJ 07503, USA*
[3]*Department of Gastroenterology, Joan C. Edwards School of Medicine, Marshall University, Huntington, WV 25755, USA*
[4]*Department of General and Hepatobiliary Surgery, St. Joseph's Regional Medical Center, Paterson, NJ 07503, USA*

Correspondence should be addressed to Youssef Botros; dr_youssefatef@yahoo.com

Academic Editor: Hideto Kawaratani

Hepatocellular carcinoma (HCC) usually occurs in patients with underlying risk factors such as liver cirrhosis and chronic hepatitis B. Although patients with Crohn's disease (CD) are at an increased risk to develop malignancies such as colon cancer, the incidence of HCC in this population is extremely rare. We report a case of 62-year-old male with long history of CD treated with azathioprine (AZA) and aminosalicylic acid (ASA) who was incidentally diagnosed with HCC, for which left hepatectomy was done. Four years later during routine follow-up, patient had another hepatic lesion and underwent resection of the mass. The mechanism of occurrence of HCC in patient with CD is still controversial and may include immune mediated changes and medication related complications. AZA was reported in all case reports of CD that developed HCC. Through this report we hope to explore the complex pathophysiological mechanisms contributing to the development of HCC in the Crohn's disease patient population.

1. Introduction

Hepatocellular carcinoma (HCC) is the sixth most common neoplasm worldwide, with about 600,000 deaths annually [1]. HCC usually occurs in patients with underlying risk factor, for example, liver cirrhosis or chronic hepatitis B [2]. Patients with Crohn's disease (CD) are at increased risk of developing cancers, and colon cancer is considered the most important cause of excess mortality among these patients [3]. The incidence of HCC in the Crohn's disease patient population is extremely rare [4]. There are only few cases of HCC in patients with CD reported in literature with only one case reported of recurrent HCC [5]. We report a case of recurrent HCC in a CD patient without underlying liver disease who was treated with azathioprine (AZA) and aminosalicylic acid (ASA).

2. Case Presentation

We present a case of a 62-year-old male with 42-year history of small intestinal CD diagnosed at the age of 20, requiring two small bowel resection surgeries during this course of time. Our patient was solely on prednisone therapy for an extended period of time and switched to AZA (150 mg daily) for the last 21 years with relatively well controlled symptoms. During routine follow-up screening tests, he was incidentally found to have left lobe liver mass and was diagnosed with HCC for which he received left lobe hepatectomy at the age of 58. The AZA dose was reduced to 50 mg daily.

On subsequent follow-up, four years after the initial resection, he was found to have liver mass and was admitted to the hospital for further evaluation. On presentation to hospital, the patient appeared well without any evidence of jaundice

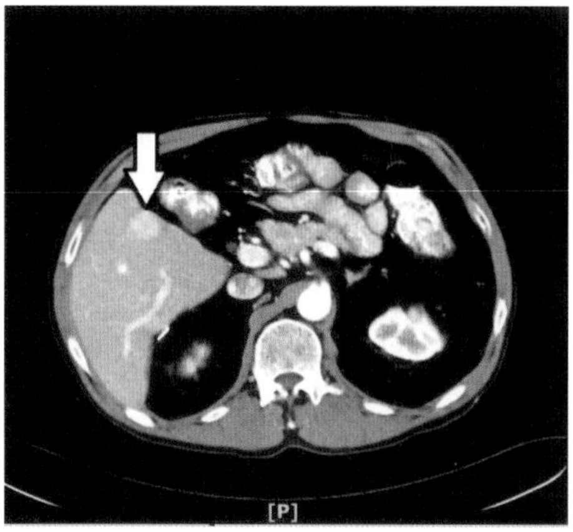

Figure 1: Arterial phase showing 2.2 × 1.6 × 2.1 lesion in segment V.

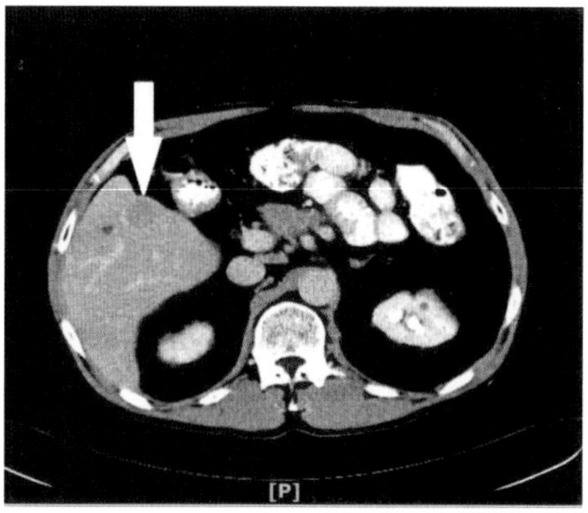

Figure 2: Hepatic lesion showing early wash out in venous phase.

or stigmata of chronic liver disease. Preoperative blood work including liver profile and viral hepatitis markers was entirely normal: AST 18 U/L (<37 U/L), ALT 16 (<60 U/L), albumin 3.5 g/dL (3.5–5 g/dL), bilirubin 0.8 mg/dL (0.3–1.2 mg/dL), and INR 1.0, alpha-fetoprotein 10.3 ng/mL (<6.1 ng/mL), prothrombin time 13.3 seconds, and platelet count 210/μL.

Triple phase contrast enhanced CT of abdomen showed solitary mass in the segment 5 of the right lobe measuring 2.2 × 1.6 × 2.1 cm, with arterial enhancement and early wash out in the venous phase, and no evidence of lymphadenopathy or extrahepatic metastasis (Figures 1 and 2).

The decision toward surgical excision of the tumor was made. Patient underwent laparoscopic resection of segment 5 with no postoperative complications. Microscopically, the resected mass showed moderately differentiated hepatocellular carcinoma without evidence of microvascular invasion (Figure 3).

There was no postoperative adverse events and AZA was discontinued and patient was kept on oral budesonide.

3. Discussion

The occurrence of HCC among patients with CD is extremely rare, with only about 12 cases reported in the literature [5–16]. Most of the patients with CD who developed HCC received AZA, with a few cases who did not receive AZA but were eventually found to have underlying liver disease [9, 15].

The exact mechanism for the occurrence of HCC in patients with CD without underlying liver disease is not well established. Is it a pathophysiological outcome of Crohn's disease itself? Or is it more related to the treatments of CD? The answers to these scientific queries require further investigations.

AZA use is associated with increased risk of many malignancies including squamous cell skin cancer in patients with rheumatological diseases and lymphoma among IBD patients [17, 18]. However, there are no retrospective studies in medical literature reporting any correlation between the use of AZA and occurrence of HCC in patients with CD.

There have been only two reported cases of hepatocellular carcinoma in patients receiving azathioprine for clinical conditions other than CD, one in patient with ulcerative colitis and the other case in renal transplant patient [19, 20].

The relation between long term use of AZA and development of HCC is still controversial, and the mechanism by which AZA can predispose to HCC is thought to be due to increase in the hepatic cells turnover. Arber et al. demonstrated this effect on animals by injecting rats with AZA and measuring the distance of labeled liver cells from the portal space and found increase in the hepatocytes' and littoral cells' streaming velocities in the AZA treated rats compared to the control group. This can possibly lead to aberrant cell growth via abnormal mechanisms [21]. AZA can also precipitate to cancers via decreasing the immunity against cancer cells and increasing the susceptibility to oncogenic viruses [10].

Other possible mechanisms for the occurrence of HCC in CD patients have been postulated; some endothelial-cell adhesion molecules and chemokines that are restricted to the gut under normal condition become abnormally expressed in the liver in IBD patients. This can lead to immune response mediated by mucosal T cells, against these antigens and subsequently hepatic damage [22].

Another reported pathophysiological mechanism is a correlation between the gut microbiota in patients with CD and occurrence of HCC. Fox et al. showed that gut microbiota can define the risk of HCC development in response to environmental factors including carcinogenic chemicals and hepatitis virus transgenes. Colonization of gut with harmful bacteria is thought to alter bowel mucosal integrity facilitating the passage of harmful bacteria to portal circulation. Also this change in gut microbiota can increase secretion of cytokines acting on the liver and upregulating the transcription of numerous cytokines and receptors that act as key regulator of hepatic injury carcinogenesis [23, 24].

In conclusion, there appears to be complex interplay of pathophysiological mechanisms in patients with CD, leading to the development of HCC while on AZA therapy.

Gastroenterologist should be aware of this rare association between using AZA in CD and development of HCC. We hope that this intriguing area receives robust scientific

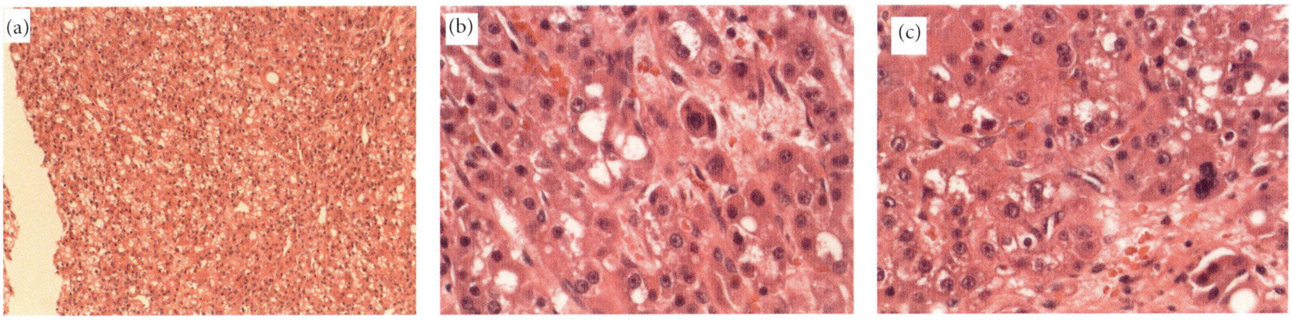

FIGURE 3: Moderately differentiated HCC, hematoxylin and eosin: low power (a) and high power (b and c).

inquiry in order to establish a strong correlation and find out if patients on AZA for CD should have screening for HCC.

Authors' Contribution

All authors played a role in preparing this paper.

References

[1] D. M. Parkin, F. Bray, J. Ferlay et al., "Global cancer statistics, 2002," *CA: A Cancer Journal for Clinicians*, vol. 55, pp. 74–108, 2005.

[2] M.-P. Bralet, J.-M. Régimbeau, P. Pineau et al., "Hepatocellular carcinoma occurring in nonfibrotic liver: epidemiologic and histopathologic analysis of 80 french cases," *Hepatology*, vol. 32, no. 2, pp. 200–204, 2000.

[3] J. Askling, P. W. Dickman, P. Karlén et al., "Family history as a risk factor for colorectal cancer in inflammatory bowel disease," *Gastroenterology*, vol. 120, no. 6, pp. 1356–1362, 2001.

[4] K. Hemminki, X. Li, J. Sundquist, and K. Sundquist, "Cancer risks in Crohn disease patients," *Annals of Oncology*, vol. 20, no. 3, pp. 574–580, 2009.

[5] S. S. Cattan, D. Wendum, O. Chazouilleres, J. Schmitz, and J.-P. Gendre, "Hepatocellular carcinoma and focal hepatic glycogenosis after prolonged azathioprine therapy," *Human Pathology*, vol. 31, no. 7, pp. 874–876, 2000.

[6] F. L. Lee, S. M. Murray, J. Prior, and D. R. Shreeve, "Primary liver cell cancer occurring in association with Crohn's disease treated with prednisolone and azathioprine," *Hepato-Gastroenterology*, vol. 30, no. 5, article 188, 1983.

[7] M. L. Borum, "Unusual development of hepatocellular carcinoma in a patient with Crohn's disease," *Digestive Diseases and Sciences*, vol. 46, no. 10, pp. 2199–2200, 2001.

[8] S. C. Chen, O. W. Cummings, M. P. Hartley, C. A. Filomena, and W. K. Cho, "Hepatocellular carcinoma occurring in a patient with Crohn's disease treated with both azathioprine and infliximab," *Digestive Diseases and Sciences*, vol. 51, no. 5, pp. 952–955, 2006.

[9] B. Demarchi, F. Bresso, D. Novero et al., "Hepatocellular carcinoma complicating primary sclerosing cholangitis in Crohn's disease. A case report," *Minerva Gastroenterologica e Dietologica*, vol. 53, no. 3, pp. 279–283, 2007.

[10] J. Samarasena and M. Borgaonkar, "Development of hepatocellular carcinoma in a patient with Crohn's disease treated with azathioprine," *Digestive Diseases and Sciences*, vol. 52, no. 10, pp. 2748–2750, 2007.

[11] H. Miura, T. Kawaguchi, M. Takazoe, S. Kitamura, and H. Yamada, "Hepatocellular carcinoma and Crohn's disease: a case report and review," *Internal Medicine*, vol. 48, no. 10, pp. 815–819, 2009.

[12] A. Murakami, Y. Tanaka, M. Ueda et al., "Hepatocellular carcinoma occurring in a young Crohn's disease patient," *Pathology International*, vol. 59, no. 7, pp. 492–496, 2009.

[13] M. Ishida, S. Naka, H. Shiomi et al., "Hepatocellular carcinoma occurring in a Crohn's disease patient," *World Journal of Gastroenterology*, vol. 16, no. 25, pp. 3215–3218, 2010.

[14] K. J. Fortinsky, A. Alali, K. Jeejeebhoy, S. Fischer, M. Sherman, and S. Fung, "Metastatic hepatocellular carcinoma in a patient with Crohn's disease treated with azathioprine and infliximab: a case report and literature review," *Case Reports in Gastrointestinal Medicine*, vol. 2014, Article ID 340836, 4 pages, 2014.

[15] H. Oya, Y. Sato, S. Yamamoto, T. Takeishi, T. Kobayashi, and K. Hatakeyama, "Living related donor liver transplantation for primary sclerosing cholangitis with hepatocellular carcinoma and Crohn's disease: a case report," *Transplantation Proceedings*, vol. 36, no. 8, pp. 2297–2298, 2004.

[16] S. H. Jang, J. H. Kim, J. W. Lee et al., "A case of hepatocellular carcinoma in a patient with Crohn's disease," *The Korean Journal of Medicine*, vol. 88, no. 4, pp. 424–429, 2015.

[17] J. M. P. A. van den Reek, P. P. M. van Lümig, M. Janssen et al., "Increased incidence of squamous cell carcinoma of the skin after long-term treatment with azathioprine in patients with auto-immune inflammatory rheumatic diseases," *Journal of the European Academy of Dermatology and Venereology*, vol. 28, no. 1, pp. 27–33, 2014.

[18] D. S. Kotlyar, J. D. Lewis, L. Beaugerie et al., "Risk of lymphoma in patients with inflammatory bowel disease treated with azathioprine and 6-mercaptopurine: a meta-analysis," *Clinical Gastroenterology and Hepatology*, vol. 13, no. 5, pp. 847.e4–858.e4, 2015.

[19] S. Gruber, L. P. Dehner, and R. L. Simmons, "De novo hepatocellular carcinoma without chronic liver disease but with 17 years of azathioprine immunosuppression," *Transplantation*, vol. 43, no. 4, pp. 597–600, 1987.

[20] S. Russmann, A. Zimmermann, S. Krähenbühl, B. Kern, and J. Reichen, "Veno-occlusive disease, nodular regenerative hyperplasia and hepatocellular carcinoma after azathioprine treatment in a patient with ulcerative colitis," *European Journal of Gastroenterology and Hepatology*, vol. 13, no. 3, pp. 287–290, 2001.

[21] N. Arber, G. Zajicek, J. Nordenberg, and Y. Sidi, "Azathioprine treatment increases hepatocyte turnover," *Gastroenterology*, vol. 101, no. 4, pp. 1083–1086, 1991.

[22] D. H. Adams and B. Eksteen, "Aberrant homing of mucosal T cells and extra-intestinal manifestations of inflammatory bowel disease," *Nature Reviews Immunology*, vol. 6, no. 3, pp. 244–251, 2006.

[23] J. G. Fox, Y. Feng, E. J. Theve et al., "Gut microbes define liver cancer risk in mice exposed to chemical and viral transgenic hepatocarcinogens," *Gut*, vol. 59, no. 1, pp. 88–97, 2010.

[24] S.-M. Zheng, D.-J. Cui, and Q. Ouyang, "Gut-liver axis plays a role in hepatocarcinogenesis of patients with Crohn's disease," *World Journal of Gastroenterology*, vol. 17, no. 26, pp. 3171–3172, 2011.

3

Esophageal Cicatricial Pemphigoid as an Isolated Involvement Treated with Mycophenolate Mofetil

Sandra Sánchez Prudencio,[1] Daniel Domingo Senra,[1] Daniel Martín Rodríguez,[1] Belén Botella Mateu,[1] Carlos Esteban Jiménez-Zarza,[1] Felipe de la Morena López,[1] José Jiménez Reyes,[2] Manuel Nevado Santos,[3] and Beatriz de Cuenca Morón[1]

[1] *Gastroenterology Department, Hospital Infanta Cristina, Avenida 9 de Junio, No. 2, 28981 Parla, Madrid, Spain*
[2] *Dermatology Department, Hospital Infanta Cristina, Avenida 9 de Junio, No. 2, 28981 Parla, Madrid, Spain*
[3] *Pathology Department, Hospital Infanta Cristina, Avenida 9 de Junio, No. 2, 28981 Parla, Madrid, Spain*

Correspondence should be addressed to Sandra Sánchez Prudencio; sandra.sanchez@salud.madrid.org

Academic Editor: Haruhiko Sugimura

Cicatricial pemphigoid (CP) is a rare blistering autoimmune disease. Esophageal involvement occurs in widespread disease and rarely appears as the only affected organ. We report a 67-year-old Caucasian female with esophageal dysphagia and weight loss. Several oral panendoscopies showed multiple exudative ulcerations with fibrin and webs in mid- and proximal esophagus and a peeling mucosa. There were no lesions in other organs. We established the diagnosis performing a direct immunofluorescence (DIF), demonstrating IgG3 and complement deposition along the basement membrane. As initial treatment the patient received prednisone 60 mg and 1 gr twice daily of mycophenolate mofetil (MMF) as a steroid-sparing agent due to its lower toxicity and its selective mechanism of action. Six months later there was a significant clinical improvement and the esophageal ulcerations had disappeared, developing cicatricial fibrous rings, although no stenosis was present. Four years later, the patient remains asymptomatic with a low maintenance dose of MMF.

1. Introduction

Cicatricial pemphigoid (CP), also known as mucous membrane pemphigoid, is a rare blistering autoimmune disease that primarily affects mucous membranes of the oropharynx, conjunctiva, and genitals and less frequently the skin [1, 2]. Esophageal involvement occurs in widespread disease and rarely appears as the only affected organ. In these cases the disease usually has an aggressive course, even with esophageal stenosis requiring dilations. So it is important that an aggressive treatment with corticotherapy and immunosuppressor drugs be prescribed from the beginning [3].

We report the second case of CP with only esophageal lesions and the first case treated with prednisone and mycophenolate mofetil (MMF) without disease symptoms during four years of evolution.

2. Case Report

We present a 67-year-old female with high blood pressure and previous ictus with no sequelae. She was being treated with antiaggregant (acetyl salicylic acid). She complained of two-year evolution of intermittent dysphagia for solids, not associated with chest pain or significant weight loss. A high resolution esophageal manometry and 24-hour pH-metry were found to be normal. An oral panendoscopy showed multiple exudative ulcerations with fibrin (Figure 1) and webs in mid- and proximal esophagus (Figure 2) and a peeling mucosa (Figure 3). Initially we suspected pill-induced esophagitis so that the acetyl salicylic acid (ASA) intake was stopped and antiacid was prescribed, but the patient did not improve. Several oral panendoscopies (OPE) were carried out with similar findings discarding peptic and viral

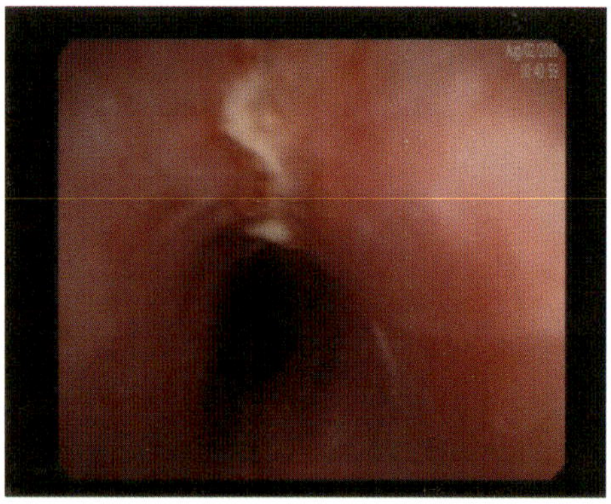

Figure 1: Esophageal ulcerations.

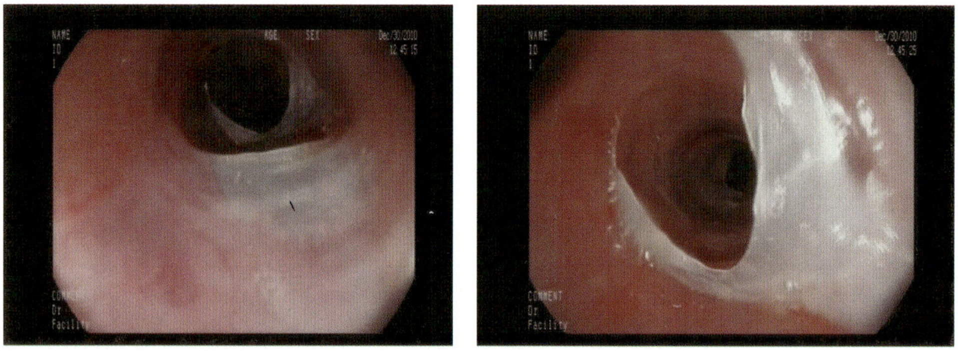

Figure 2: Esophageal webs in mid- and proximal esophagus.

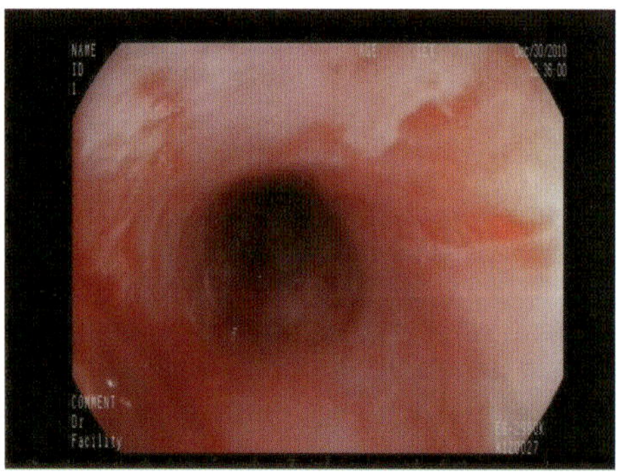

Figure 3: Peeling esophageal mucosa.

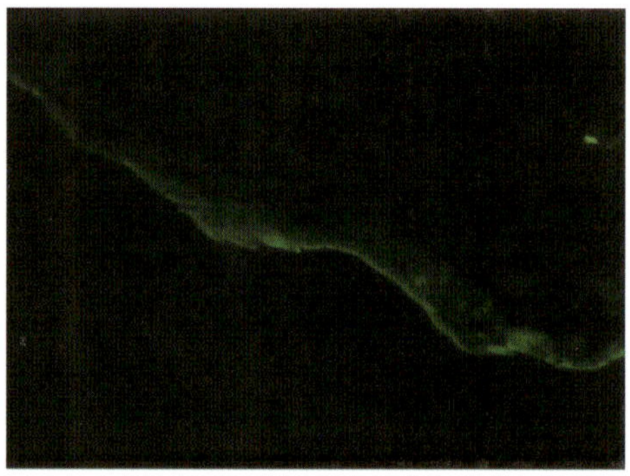

Figure 4: IgG deposition along the basement membrane.

esophagitis, candidiasis, and even HIV. An esophagogram did not show esophageal stenosis and a thoracic-cervical CT was also normal. We performed diagnosis of exclusion with the possibility of esophageal pemphigoid cause of esophageal ulcers. Therefore we performed a biopsy with direct immunofluorescence (DIF), demonstrating IgG and C3 complement deposition along the basement membrane (Figures 4-5). There were no ocular or skin lesions, only vulvar erythema with no pemphigoid signs on the biopsy. As initial treatment the patient received prednisone at 1 mg/kg daily (60 mg) and 2 gr daily of MMF as a steroid-sparing agent. Six months later there was a significant clinical improvement: the patient had no dysphagia and had gained weight. Moreover the esophageal ulcerations had disappeared, developing cicatricial fibrous rings, although no stenosis was present (Figure 6). This allowed us to use MMF maintenance dose of 500 mg daily. The control gastroscopies showed no evidence of reactivation of the disease. Four years later the patient continues asymptomatic, without other extraesophageal manifestations.

3. Discussion

CP is a chronic autoimmune disease and occurs in middle-aged patients and more commonly in women, with an incidence of 1/100000 annually. It presents like subepithelial

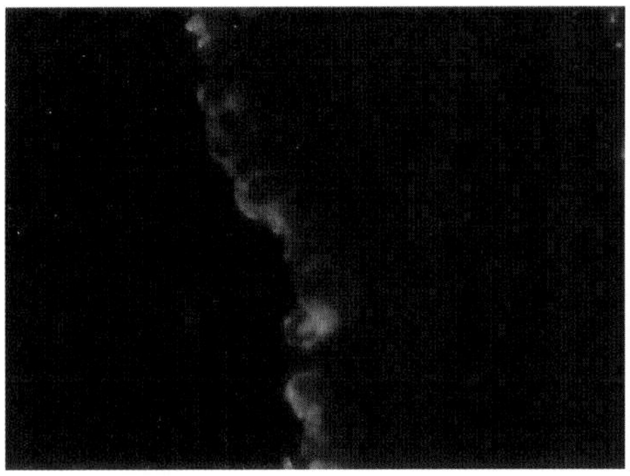

FIGURE 5: C3 deposition along the basement membrane.

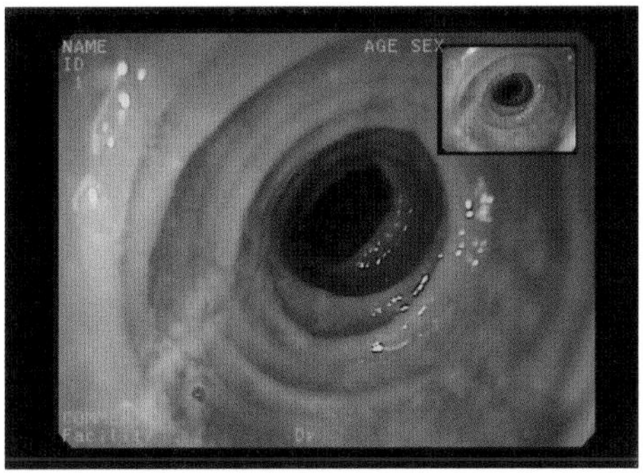

FIGURE 6: Six-month treatment later: cicatricial fibrous rings, no stenosis.

blisters basically in mucosa, which progress to scar and fibrosis. Oropharynx is the most common site, presenting as gingivitis or palate, tongue, and lip lesions. Also ocular lesions are frequent; in fact CP can be limited to the eyes, starting with an insidious form as a chronic conjunctivitis, but causing more serious illness like entropion, symblepharon, ankyloblepharon, or even blindness. Other locations are nasopharynx, larynx, esophagus, and genitals [1, 4]. Skin lesions are infrequent and they are usually mild. Esophageal involvement is rare, with an incidence of 3%, and normally appears in disseminated disease [5–8]. Interestingly, this may be present up to 10 years after the initial onset of the disease [9, 10]. In the first stage we can observe webs and ulcerations and in the last phase fibrotic rings that inevitably develop into stenosis. PC diagnosis requires a high index of suspicion, mainly if the oesophagus is the only affected organ [10]. In this case we needed several attempts until biopsy perilesional ulcer from esophagus was obtained for DIF. This is the most sensitive and specific test to CP diagnosis. In the vast majority of patients (80–100%) it displays a linear, continuous band along the basement membrane zone of IgG (predominantly IgG4), C3, and occasionally IgA. DIF using salt split improves its sensibility. The indirect immunofluorescence (IIF) shows circulating anti-basement membrane zone IgG antibodies (or IgA) at low titles [1, 11]. Some cases require other techniques for diagnosis such as the immunochemical test or immunoelectron microscopy. Histologic examinations show subepithelial blisters with an underlying superficial inflammatory infiltrate containing lymphocytes, histiocytes, and eosinophils, but these findings are nonspecific [12]. Esophageal PC management depends on clinical presentation and the severity of the symptoms. Oral systemic corticoids are the most commonly used in advanced illnesses, specifically prednisone 1 mg/kg, with good short term [5] results. However, systematic glucocorticoids are often associated with immunosuppressors like azathioprine or cyclophosphamide as steroid-sparing agents [7, 13, 14]. But these treatments can cause significant side effects such as marrow aplasia, infections, neoplasia, or hemorrhagic cystitis. MMF is an immunosuppressive drug that selectively inhibits T and B lymphocytes blocking the de novo purine synthesis. Doses of 2–2,5 gr/d represent a promising therapy due to their low toxicity and their selective mechanism of action. In fact, there are some reported clinical cases treated with MMF successfully [15]. Esophageal PC usually cause esophageal stenosis that needs repeated dilations [3, 4, 7, 16]. In most cases this technique achieves good results but it entails a high risk of perforation [3]. All patients require long term monitoring because PC is a chronic and recurrent disease. Our patient was initially treated with 60 mg/d of prednisone with descendent dosage and MMF 2 g/d (1 g/12 hours). Two months later we practiced an OPE, demonstrating improvement of the lesions and six months later there was complete recovery of ulcerations and she was asymptomatic for dysphagia and without any bullous lesions in other organs. After clinical and endoscopic improvement we maintained dose of 500 mg MMF daily indefinitely to prevent recurrence of disease and complications like esophageal strictures and to avoid possible PC involvement of other organs. There is only one reported case in the literature of isolated esophageal involvement [13], treated with cyclophosphamide instead of MMF with marked initial symptomatic response, but with short term follow-up. We decided not to use cyclophosphamide due to its potential adverse effects. MMF was administered based on the good response observed in several published clinical cases that primarily treated pemphigoid with ocular involvement with MMF. All of them reported good response and minimal adverse effects [17–19].

Esophageal PC is a rare condition and its natural history and prognosis are not completely known [1].

This is the second case with only esophageal affectation after four years of follow-up and the first treated with MMF with good evolution.

We recommend to make DIF of perilesional mucosa in patients with multiple esophageal erosions without clear etiology.

References

[1] D. Bruch-Gerharz, M. Hertl, and T. Ruzicka, "Mucous membrane pemphigoid: clinical aspects, immunopathological features and therapy," *European Journal of Dermatology*, vol. 17, no. 3, pp. 191–200, 2007.

[2] L. S. Chan, A. Razzaque Ahmed, G. J. Anhalt et al., "The first international consensus on mucous membrane pemphigoid: definition, diagnostic criteria, pathogenic factors, medical treatment and prognostic indicators," *Archives of Dermatology*, vol. 138, no. 3, pp. 370–379, 2002.

[3] C. Sacher and N. Hunzelmann, "Cicatricial pemphigoid (mucous membrane pemphigoid): current and emerging therapeutic approaches," *American Journal of Clinical Dermatology*, vol. 6, no. 2, pp. 93–103, 2005.

[4] L. S. Ostlere, R. B. Mallet, P. J. Howard, and C. A. Holden, "Oesophageal webs associated with cicatricial pemphigoid," *Clinical and Experimental Dermatology*, vol. 20, no. 2, pp. 176–178, 1995.

[5] S. F. Isenberg, "Esophageal presentation of cicatrical pemphigoid," *Otolaryngology: Head and Neck Surgery*, vol. 118, no. 6, pp. 845–847, 1998.

[6] A. Stallmach, S. Weg-Remens, C. Moser, H. Bonkoff, G. Feifel, and M. Zeitz, "Esophageal involvement in cicatricial pemphigoid," *Endoscopy*, vol. 30, no. 7, pp. 657–661, 1998.

[7] W.-K. Syn and M. M. Ahmed, "Esophageal involvement in cicatricial pemphigoid: a rare cause of dysphagia," *Diseases of the Esophagus*, vol. 17, no. 2, pp. 180–182, 2004.

[8] L. J. Warren, F. Wojnarowska, and J. D. Wilkinson, "Oesophageal involvement in cicatricial pemphigoid," *Australasian Journal of Dermatology*, vol. 38, no. 3, pp. 148–151, 1997.

[9] S.-J. Tang, "Esopagheal involvement in mucous membrane pemphigoid," *Gastroenterology*, vol. 136, pp. e6–e7, 2009.

[10] J.-H. Park, H.-J. Chun, Y.-T. Jeen et al., "Esophageal cicatricial pemphigoid," *Gastrointestinal Endoscopy*, vol. 55, no. 7, article 909, 2002.

[11] J. Setterfield, B. Bhogal, P. Shirlaw et al., "A comprehensive study of the clinical, immunopathological and immunogenetic findings in cicatricial pemphigoid," *British Journal of Dermatology*, vol. 135, article 13, 1996.

[12] A. R. Ahmed, B. S. Kurgis, and R. S. Rogers, "Cicatricial pemphigoid," *Journal of the American Academy of Dermatology*, vol. 24, no. 6, pp. 987–1001, 1991.

[13] H. Sallout, G. J. Anhalt, and F. H. Al-Kawas, "Mucous membrane pemphigoid presenting with isolated esophageal involvement: a case report," *Gastrointestinal Endoscopy*, vol. 52, no. 3, pp. 429–433, 2000.

[14] A. G. Pandya, K. J. Warren, and P. R. Bergstresser, "Cicatricial pemphigoid successfully treated with pulse intravenous cyclophosphamide," *Archives of Dermatology*, vol. 133, no. 2, pp. 245–247, 1997.

[15] M. Megahed, S. Schmiedeberg, J. Becker, and T. Ruzicka, "Treatment of cicatricial pemphigoid with mycophenolate mofetil as a steroid-sparing agent," *Journal of the American Academy of Dermatology*, vol. 45, no. 2, pp. 256–259, 2001.

[16] A. F. Watkinson, D. F. Vretenar, M. D. Morrison, and H. J. Burhenne, "Bening mucous membrane pemphigoid: treatment of esophageal stricture," *Canadian Association of Radiologists Journal*, vol. 45, no. 2, pp. 140–142, 1994.

[17] J. M. Nottage, K. M. Hammersmith, A. P. Murchison, A. F. Felipe, R. Penne, and I. Raber, "Treatment of mucous membrane pemphigoid with mycophenolate mofetil," *Cornea*, vol. 32, no. 6, pp. 810–815, 2013.

[18] E. Daniel, J. E. Thorne, C. W. Newcomb et al., "Mycophenolate mofetil for ocular inflammation," *American Journal of Ophthalmology*, vol. 149, no. 3, pp. 423–432, 2010.

[19] H.-H. Xu, V. P. Werth, E. Parisi, and T. P. Sollecito, "Mucous membrane pemphigoid," *Dental Clinics of North America*, vol. 57, no. 4, pp. 611–630, 2013.

4

Lanreotide Autogel in the Treatment of Persistent Diarrhea following a Total Colectomy

Patrick Schoeters[1] and Karl De Pooter[2]

[1]*Department of Gastroenterology, AZ Herentals, 2200 Herentals, Belgium*
[2]*Department of Gastrointestinal Surgery, AZ Herentals, 2200 Herentals, Belgium*

Correspondence should be addressed to Patrick Schoeters; patrick.schoeters@azherentals.be

Academic Editor: Anthony J. Lembo

Diarrhea is one of the most common complications following colectomy in patients with slow transit constipation (STC). Early postoperative diarrhea is usually treated with opioid agonists; however, to date, published data on the management of persistent diarrhea after colectomy for STC are scarce. Here, we report a case of severe diarrhea after a total colectomy with ileorectal anastomosis. One year after the surgery, the patient presented with persistent diarrhea. Treatment with a long-acting somatostatin analogue, lanreotide Autogel, was initiated. One month after the first injection of lanreotide Autogel the diarrhea was resolved. The patient's stool transit was markedly improved (type 4 or type 5 according to the Bristol Stool Chart compared to type 7 before the treatment), positively affecting the patient's quality of life (mean score of 2.1 on the Irritable Bowel Syndrome Quality of Life questionnaire compared to 3.9 before the treatment). This case report describes a successful use of lanreotide Autogel in a patient with persistent diarrhea after a total colectomy.

1. Introduction

Chronic constipation is one of the most common gastrointestinal conditions characterized by infrequent bowel movements, presence of hard stools, an excessive time to evacuate, straining, and sensation of incomplete bowel evacuation [1]. Recent Rome III Diagnostic Criteria for Functional Constipation defined constipation as <3 bowel movements per week and the occurrence of specific bowel symptoms, that is, straining, lumpy/hard stools, incomplete evacuation, sensation of anorectal obstruction, and manual maneuvers for defecation in >25% of defecations [2–4]. Slow transit constipation (STC) is a functional colonic disorder characterized by reduced frequency of high-amplitude propagated contractions and severe impairment of colonic motor activity that, in some cases, may lead to a true colonic inertia [5–8]. The reported rates of prevalence of chronic constipation vary by geographic region and disease definition from 1% to almost 40%; a recent meta-analysis based on 41 studies reported a pooled prevalence of 14% [7, 9–14]. Patients with STC represent 15–30% of all constipated patients; STC is most common in young women [8, 15]. Typical treatment options for patients with STC include dietary changes, enemas, laxatives, and pharmacologic therapy; other options such as biofeedback, sacral nerve stimulation, and surgery may be considered in patients with STC who are resistant to medical therapy [6, 8, 15–18]. Total colectomy with ileorectal anastomosis is the most widely used surgical procedure for patients with STC who do not respond to conventional treatments [15, 17, 19–22]. Diarrhea is one of the most common complications following colectomy and has been reported in up to 46% of patients who underwent colectomy [17, 19–21, 23–28]. During the adaptation phase following surgery, administration of fiber, motility agents (loperamide, diphenoxylate and atropine sulfate, or codeine), and binders (cholestyramine) may help in reducing bowel frequency [17, 23]. Although postoperative diarrhea is usually transient and can be controlled with medication, in some patients, failure of intestinal adaptation may lead to intractable diarrhea [17]. Here, we report the successful use of a long-acting somatostatin analogue, lanreotide, in the treatment of persistent diarrhea after a total colectomy.

2. Case Report

In July 2013, a 22-year-old woman presented with serious constipation. Between 2003 and 2005, she had been suffering from constipation and urine retention. In 2011, the patient had a car accident, after which she developed a whiplash and migraine, which was treated with valproate and carbamazepine. In 2012, she was diagnosed with reflux esophagitis grade A, treated with pantoprazole (40 mg/day), resolor (2 mg/day), otilonium bromide (40 mg 3x/day), mesalazine (1 g 3x/day), questran (4 g 3x/day), and loperamide (2 mg 3x/day). Upon admission to the hospital in July 2013, the patient was diagnosed with STC, confirmed by a radiopaque marker ingestion study which demonstrated a marked delay in the colonic transit time and by functional pelvic examination showing reasonably good sphincter pressures but incomplete relaxation of the pelvic floor. The patient was treated with prucalopride and pelvic floor training. However, the patient's symptoms progressed despite the medical treatment. Therefore, a decision of laparoscopic total colectomy with ileorectal anastomosis completed with biofeedback training of the pelvic floor was made. The patient underwent surgery under general anesthesia in July 2013. The procedure was successful and no complications during the surgery were recorded. Following the surgery, a smooth recovery with slow mobilization of the gastrointestinal transit was noted. The patient left the hospital in a good general condition with dietary advice 10 days following the surgery.

Six months after the surgery, the patient developed diarrhea (6–8 episodes/day), which was treated with otilonium bromide, cholestyramine, mesalazine, and loperamide. However, the treatment was unsuccessful. In May 2014, the patient presented to our hospital with continuous refractory diarrhea defined as >3 stools/day and nonresponsiveness to standard antidiarrheal therapy. Upon admission, the patient completed the Irritable Bowel Syndrome Quality of Life (IBS-QoL) questionnaire consisting of 34 questions describing the bowel problems experienced during the past 30 days [29, 30]. According to a 1–5 scale, where 1 indicates "not at all," 2 indicates "slightly," 3 indicates "moderately," 4 indicates "quite a bit," and 5 indicates "extremely/a great deal," the patient assigned a score of 4 or 5 to the majority of her bowel problems; the mean score at admission was 3.9 (Table 1). The patient's stool was classified as type 7 according to the Bristol Stool Chart [7]. Infectious or inflammatory nature of the diarrhea was excluded by gastroscopy and ileoscopy as well as negative coprocultures. The diarrhea was generally accompanied by mild bowel spasms, but no mucus or blood was seen in the stools. Endoscopy at ileorectal anastomosis revealed small erosion at the anastomosis. Treatment with a short-acting somatostatin analogue, octreotide, administered subcutaneously for 3 days at 0.1 mg/day was initiated. Following 3 octreotide administrations, a mild response to treatment was observed; however, due to practical considerations, the treatment was switched to the long-acting somatostatin analogue, lanreotide, administered subcutaneously every 28 days. Lanreotide Autogel was administered as monthly injections at 90 mg dose during 5 months. Following the 1st injection the patient's diarrhea had improved; however, after the 5th injection, the diarrhea had worsened again. Therefore, the lanreotide dose was increased to 120 mg. Following the 1st injection of lanreotide Autogel 120 mg, the diarrhea was resolved (2 stools/day) and the patient's stool was classified as type 4 or type 5 stool on the Bristol Stool Chart. Furthermore, the patient's QoL had also improved, as indicated by lower scores she assigned to her bowel problems in the IBS-QoL questionnaire after the treatment with lanreotide Autogel 120 mg (mean score 2.1, Table 1). Lanreotide Autogel 120 mg was administered during 5 months; the patient follow-up at 5 months after the 1st lanreotide Autogel 120 mg administration revealed no diarrhea recurrence. At the end of this report, the patient's treatment with lanreotide Autogel 120 mg was still ongoing.

3. Discussion

Chronic constipation is a frequently encountered disorder in clinical practice. Most constipated patients benefit from standard medical approaches. However, these therapies fail in some patients. Colectomy with an ileorectal anastomosis aiming at increasing bowel movement frequency is the most widely accepted operative technique for patients with STC refractory to conventional treatments. However, diarrhea is one of the most common postoperative complications after colectomy for STC affecting up to 46% of patients [17, 19–21, 23–28]. Diarrhea after colectomy might severely affect a patient's QoL, although it generally resolves after one year following the surgery [15, 24]. Treatment of early postoperative diarrhea with diphenoxylate/atropine and loperamide has been reported [28]. However, the published reports on the management of persistent postcolectomy diarrhea are scarce.

Here, we describe the successful use of a long-acting somatostatin analogue, lanreotide, in the management of persistent diarrhea following a total colectomy. Following the administration of lanreotide Autogel, the patient's diarrhea significantly improved and was ultimately resolved within 28 days after treatment initiation. Following the treatment, the patient's stool form was classified as type 4 or type 5 according to the Bristol Stool Chart, compared to type 7 before the lanreotide Autogel 120 mg administration, indicating that this treatment was effective. The use of somatostatin analogues, a short-acting octreotide and a long-acting lanreotide, in the control of diarrhea has been also previously reported in patients with carcinoid tumors [31–34], diabetes [35], and idiopathic refractory diarrhea [36]. Somatostatin plays a regulatory function in several organs and systems, including the gastrointestinal tract, where it inhibits the gastrointestinal motility and colonic fluid secretion [37]. Although the mechanism by which somatostatin analogues affect bowel function has not yet been fully elucidated, it is likely that somatostatin analogues act by inhibiting the intestine hormone secretion, lengthening the intestinal transit time, and increasing the water absorption [38]. In this report, the improved transit following the lanreotide Autogel administration positively impacted the patient's QoL. In the absence of a specific questionnaire that could be used to assess the QoL of patients with persistent diarrhea, we used the IBS-QoL questionnaire that

TABLE 1: Irritable Bowel Syndrome Quality of Life questionnaire score before and after the lanreotide Autogel treatment.

IBS-QoL question	Before lanreotide	After lanreotide
(Q1) I feel helpless because of my bowel problems.	5	2
(Q2) I am embarrassed by the smell caused by my bowel problems.	4	2
(Q3) I am bothered by how much time I spend on the toilet.	5	2
(Q4) I feel vulnerable to other illnesses because of my bowel problems.	3	2
(Q5) I feel fat/bloated because of my bowel problems.	5	2
(Q6) I feel like I'm losing control of my life because of my bowel problems.	5	2
(Q7) I feel my life is less enjoyable because of my bowel problems.	5	2
(Q8) I feel uncomfortable when I talk about my bowel problems.	5	3
(Q9) I feel depressed about my bowel problems.	4	2
(Q10) I feel isolated from others because of my bowel problems.	5	2
(Q11) I have to watch the amount of food I eat because of my bowel problems.	4	3
(Q12) Because of my bowel problems, sexual activity is difficult for me.	4	3
(Q13) I feel angry that I have bowel problems.	4	2
(Q14) I feel like I irritate others because of my bowel problems.	5	2
(Q15) I worry that my bowel problems will get worse.	5	2
(Q16) I feel irritable because of my bowel problems.	4	3
(Q17) I worry that people think I exaggerate my bowel problems.	3	2
(Q18) I feel I get less done because of my bowel problems.	4	2
(Q19) I have to avoid stressful situations because of my bowel problems.	4	2
(Q20) My bowel problems reduce my sexual desire.	3	2
(Q21) My bowel problems limit what I can wear.	3	1
(Q22) I have to avoid strenuous activity because of my bowel problems.	3	2
(Q23) I have to watch the kind of food I eat because of my bowel problems.	3	3
(Q24) Because of my bowel problems I have difficulty being around people I do not know well.	4	2
(Q25) I feel sluggish because of my bowel problems.	4	2
(Q26) I feel unclean because of my bowel problems.	4	3
(Q27) Long trips are difficult for me because of my bowel problems.	4	3
(Q28) I feel frustrated that I cannot eat when I want because of my bowel problems.	2	2
(Q29) It is important to be near a toilet because of my bowel problems.	5	3
(Q30) My life revolves around my bowel problems.	4	2
(Q31) I worry about losing control of my bowels.	4	2
(Q32) I fear I won't be able to have a bowel movement.	1	1
(Q33) My bowel problems are affecting my closest relationships.	2	1
(Q34) I feel that no one understands my bowel problems.	2	2
Mean score	**3.9**	**2.1**

IBS-QoL, Irritable Bowel Syndrome Quality of Life.
Before lanreotide, score before lanreotide Autogel treatment.
After lanreotide, score after lanreotide Autogel treatment.
Q, question.

has been widely used in IBS patients [29, 30]. This questionnaire has been also used in a recent multicenter, prospective study evaluating the effect of lanreotide Autogel 120 mg in 36 patients with idiopathic refractory diarrhea, which showed improved symptoms of diarrhea and QoL upon the treatment (Medard; ClinicalTrials.gov NCT00891371) [36]. These and our results suggest that lanreotide Autogel is effective in the management of persistent refractory diarrhea.

Disclosure

Lanreotide Autogel is a registered trademark of Ipsen NV.

Acknowledgments

The authors thank Urszula Miecielica (XPE Pharma and Science) who provided medical writing services on behalf of Ipsen. Medical writing services were funded by Ipsen NV.

References

[1] A. Koch, W. A. Voderholzer, A. G. Klauser, and S. Müller-Lissner, "Symptoms in chronic constipation," *Diseases of the Colon and Rectum*, vol. 40, no. 8, pp. 902–906, 1997.

[2] Rome Foundation, *Appendix A: Rome III Diagnostic Criteria for Functional Gastrointestinal Disorders*, Rome Foundation, 2014.

[3] G. F. Longstreth, W. G. Thompson, W. D. Chey, L. A. Houghton, F. Mearin, and R. C. Spiller, "Functional bowel disorders," *Gastroenterology*, vol. 130, no. 5, pp. 1480–1491, 2006.

[4] D. Q. Shih and L. Y. Kwan, "All roads lead to Rome: update on Rome III criteria and new treatment options," *Gastroenterology Report*, vol. 1, no. 2, pp. 56–65, 2007.

[5] C. N. Andrews and M. Storr, "The pathophysiology of chronic constipation," *Canadian Journal of Gastroenterology*, vol. 25, pp. 16B–21B, 2011.

[6] G. Bassotti and C. Blandizzi, "Understanding and treating refractory constipation," *World Journal of Gastrointestinal Pharmacology and Therapeutics*, vol. 5, no. 2, pp. 77–85, 2014.

[7] G. Bassotti, G. de Roberto, L. Sediari, and A. Morelli, "Toward a definition of colonic inertia," *World Journal of Gastroenterology*, vol. 10, no. 17, pp. 2465–2467, 2004.

[8] J. C. Frattini and J. J. Nogueras, "Slow transit constipation: a review of a colonic functional disorder," *Clinics in Colon and Rectal Surgery*, vol. 21, no. 2, pp. 146–152, 2008.

[9] G. L. McCrea, C. Miaskowski, N. A. Stotts, L. Macera, S. M. Paul, and M. G. Varma, "Gender differences in self-reported constipation characteristics, symptoms, and bowel and dietary habits among patients attending a specialty clinic for constipation," *Gender Medicine*, vol. 6, no. 1, pp. 259–271, 2009.

[10] C. S. J. Probert, P. M. Emmett, H. A. Cripps, and K. W. Heaton, "Evidence for the ambiguity of the term constipation: the role of irritable bowel syndrome," *Gut*, vol. 35, no. 10, pp. 1455–1458, 1994.

[11] M. I. P. Sanchez and P. Bercik, "Epidemiology and burden of chronic constipation," *Canadian Journal of Gastroenterology*, vol. 25, supplement B, pp. 11B–15B, 2011.

[12] A. Sonnenberg and T. R. Koch, "Physician visits in the United States for constipation: 1958 to 1986," *Digestive Diseases and Sciences*, vol. 34, no. 4, pp. 606–611, 1989.

[13] E. Surrenti, D. M. Rath, J. H. Pemberton, and M. Camilleri, "Audit of constipation in a tertiary referral gastroenterology practice," *The American Journal of Gastroenterology*, vol. 90, no. 9, pp. 1471–1475, 1995.

[14] N. C. Suares and A. C. Ford, "Prevalence of, and risk factors for, chronic idiopathic constipation in the community: systematic review and meta-analysis," *The American Journal of Gastroenterology*, vol. 106, no. 9, pp. 1582–1591, 2011.

[15] A. Lembo and M. Camilleri, "Chronic constipation," *The New England Journal of Medicine*, vol. 349, no. 14, pp. 1360–1368, 2003.

[16] A. Bove, M. Bellini, E. Battaglia et al., "Consensus statement AIGO/SICCR diagnosis and treatment of chronic constipation and obstructed defecation (part II: treatment)," *World Journal of Gastroenterology*, vol. 18, no. 36, pp. 4994–5013, 2012.

[17] J. A. McCoy and D. E. Beck, "Surgical management of colonic inertia," *Clinics in Colon and Rectal Surgery*, vol. 25, no. 1, pp. 20–23, 2012.

[18] J. Tack, S. Müller-Lissner, V. Stanghellini et al., "Diagnosis and treatment of chronic constipation—a European perspective," *Neurogastroenterology and Motility*, vol. 23, no. 8, pp. 697–710, 2011.

[19] E. C. Han, H.-K. Oh, H.-K. Ha et al., "Favorable surgical treatment outcomes for chronic constipation with features of colonic pseudo-obstruction," *World Journal of Gastroenterology*, vol. 18, no. 32, pp. 4441–4446, 2012.

[20] G. Sohn, S. Y. Chang, W. K. Chan et al., "Surgical outcomes after total colectomy with ileorectal anastomosis in patients with medically intractable slow transit constipation," *Journal of the Korean Society of Coloproctology*, vol. 27, no. 4, pp. 180–187, 2011.

[21] C. H. Knowles, M. Scott, and P. J. Lunniss, "Outcome of colectomy for slow transit constipation," *Annals of Surgery*, vol. 230, no. 5, pp. 627–638, 1999.

[22] A. E. Bharucha, J. H. Pemberton, and G. R. Locke III, "American gastroenterological association technical review on constipation," *Gastroenterology*, vol. 144, no. 1, pp. 218–238, 2013.

[23] D. E. Beck, "Surgical management of constipation," *Clinics in Colon and Rectal Surgery*, vol. 18, no. 2, pp. 81–84, 2005.

[24] G. P. FitzHarris, J. Garcia-Aguilar, S. C. Parker et al., "Quality of life after subtotal colectomy for slow-transit constipation: both quality and quantity count," *Diseases of the Colon and Rectum*, vol. 46, no. 4, pp. 433–440, 2003.

[25] M. Zutshi, T. L. Hull, R. Trzcinski, A. Arvelakis, and M. Xu, "Surgery for slow transit constipation: are we helping patients?" *International Journal of Colorectal Disease*, vol. 22, no. 3, pp. 265–269, 2007.

[26] A. J. Pikarsky, J. J. Singh, E. G. Weiss, J. J. Nogueras, and S. D. Wexner, "Long-term follow-up of patients undergoing colectomy for colonic inertia," *Diseases of the Colon and Rectum*, vol. 44, no. 2, pp. 179–183, 2001.

[27] R. M. Mollen, H. C. Kuijpers, and A. T. Claassen, "Colectomy for slow-transit constipation: preoperative functional evaluation is important but not a guarantee for a successful outcome," *Diseases of the Colon and Rectum*, vol. 44, no. 4, pp. 577–580, 2001.

[28] J. H. Pemberton, D. M. Rath, and D. M. Ilstrup, "Evaluation and surgical treatment of severe chronic constipation," *Annals of Surgery*, vol. 214, no. 4, pp. 403–413, 1991.

[29] D. A. Andrae, D. L. Patrick, D. A. Drossman, and P. S. Covington, "Evaluation of the Irritable Bowel Syndrome Quality of Life (IBS-QOL) questionnaire in diarrheal-predominant irritable bowel syndrome patients," *Health and Quality of Life Outcomes*, vol. 11, article 208, 2013.

[30] D. L. Patrick, D. A. Drossman, I. O. Frederick, J. DiCesare, and K. L. Puder, "Quality of life in persons with irritable bowel syndrome: development and validation of a new measure," *Digestive Diseases and Sciences*, vol. 43, no. 2, pp. 400–411, 1998.

[31] G. A. Kaltsas, G. M. Besser, and A. B. Grossman, "The diagnosis and medical management of advanced neuroendocrine tumors," *Endocrine Reviews*, vol. 25, no. 3, pp. 458–511, 2004.

[32] S. W. J. Lamberts, A.-J. van der Lely, W. W. de Herder, and L. J. Hofland, "Octreotide," *The New England Journal of Medicine*, vol. 334, no. 4, pp. 246–254, 1996.

[33] D. O'Toole, M. Ducreux, G. Bommelaer et al., "Treatment of carcinoid syndrome: a prospective crossover evaluation of lanreotide versus octreotide in terms of efficacy, patient acceptability, and tolerance," *Cancer*, vol. 88, no. 4, pp. 770–776, 2000.

[34] P. Ruszniewski, S. Ish-Shalom, M. Wymenga et al., "Rapid and sustained relief from the symptoms of carcinoid syndrome: results from an open 6-month study of the 28-day prolonged-release formulation of lanreotide," *Neuroendocrinology*, vol. 80, no. 4, pp. 244–251, 2004.

[35] T. J. Ulahannan and A. Amaratunga, "Successful treatment of diabetic autonomic diarrhoea with monthly subcutaneous lanreotide," *Practical Diabetes International*, vol. 26, no. 8, pp. 326–328, 2009.

[36] R. Bisschops, V. De Ruyter, G. Demolin et al., "Lanreotide autogel 120 mg as a treatment for chronic idiopathic refractory Diarrhea: a multicenter prospective trial," *Gastroenterology*, vol. 146, no. 5, supplement 1, p. S-72, 2014, Abstract 320.

[37] S. W. J. Lamberts, A. J. van der Lely, and L. J. Hofland, "New somatostatin analogs: will they fulfil old promises?" *European Journal of Endocrinology*, vol. 146, no. 5, pp. 701–705, 2002.

[38] K. E. Gyr and R. Meier, "Pharmacodynamic effects of Sandostatin in the gastrointestinal tract," *Digestion*, vol. 54, supplement 1, pp. 14–19, 1993.

Severe Gastroparesis following Radiofrequency Catheter Ablation for Atrial Fibrillation: Suggestion for Diagnosis, Treatment, and Device for Gastroparesis after RFCA

Dong Seok Lee[1] and Sang Jin Lee[1,2]

[1] *Department of Internal Medicine, Gangneung Asan Medical Center, University of Ulsan College of Medicine, Gangneung, Republic of Korea*
[2] *Department of Internal Medicine, Gangneung Asan Medical Center, Sacheon-myeon, Gangneung, Gangwon-do 210-711, Republic of Korea*

Correspondence should be addressed to Sang Jin Lee; sangjin@gnah.co.kr

Academic Editor: Wen-xie Xu

Gastroparesis following radiofrequency catheter ablation (RFCA) is a very rare complication, as only two cases have been reported in the English literature. A 42-year-old man underwent RFCA due to recurrent drug-resistant symptomatic atrial fibrillation. The patient complained of indigestion and early satiety 2 days after the procedure. Contrast-enhanced computed tomography and an upper gastrointestinal series of the abdomen showed a large amount of material remaining in the stomach area. All food material was removed by endoscopy, and the patient received medical treatment. We suggest a flow chart for diagnosis and treatment of AFGS based on the present case and previous cases. Endoscopic medical patent was designed on the basis of this case.

1. Introduction

The definition of gastroparesis is a delay in emptying of food from the stomach. The causes of gastroparesis are postvagotomy syndrome of a peptic ulcer, pancreatic adenocarcinoma, mesenteric vascular insufficiency, and systemic disease such as amyloidosis. Most patients with gastroparesis complain of abdominal distension and epigastric discomfort after eating. No ulcers or gastric outlet obstructions are found on an upper endoscopy exam. A gastrointestinal motility study is widely conducted to diagnose gastroparesis.

The radiofrequency catheter ablation (RFCA) procedure is widely performed to treat atrial fibrillation (AF). However, various complications have been reported. Thromboembolic events, tamponade, severe pulmonary vein stenosis, femoral pseudoaneurysm, and atrioesophageal fistula have been reported as complications of the RFCA procedure [1–3]. A few cases of vagus nerve injury due to RF ablation energy have been reported and retrospective studies have been conducted [4–6].

2. Case Report

A 59-year-old man presented with a history of paroxysmal palpitation for more than a few years. Symptom duration and frequency had been prolonged recently with a documented ECG. He was treated with digoxin, quinidine, propafenone, metoprolol, and amiodarone sequentially. However, his symptoms persisted. He was diagnosed with drug-refractory, symptomatic, chronic AF and underwent RFCA. The patient was transferred to the EP laboratory. After an esophagram, we positioned the catheters and performed a dual septal puncture. The baseline ECG indicated normal sinus rhythm. Ablation at the left superior pulmonary vein (LSPV) was started and electrical isolation of the LSPV, left inferior pulmonary

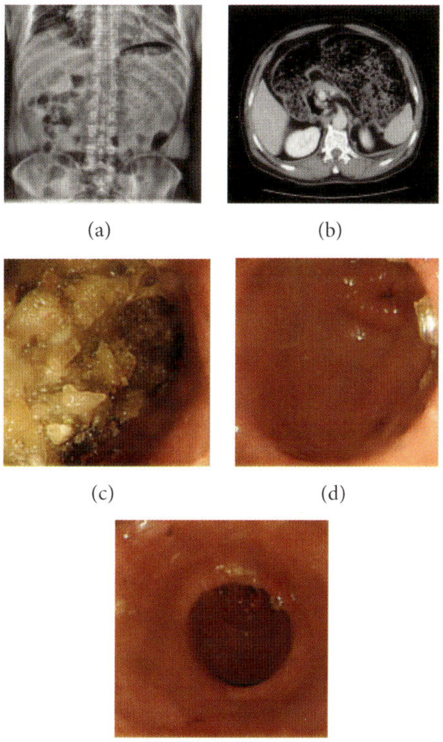

(a) (b) (c) (d) (e)

Figure 1: (a) Simple abdominal X-ray reveals a large amount of material in the stomach, suggesting severe gastric hypomotility. (b) Abdominopelvic computed tomography reveals a large amount of food material in the stomach, suggesting partial stricture in the postbulbar portion of the duodenum. (c) Endoscopic findings reveal large amounts of food stored in the gastric body and antrum. (d) The food was removed using a cap-fitted endoscope and a net over a period of days. (e) Peristaltic motion of the gastric antrum was normal and the pylorus opened and closed normally.

vein, right superior pulmonary vein, and right inferior pulmonary vein as well as a cavotricuspid isthmus block was completed. There was atrial flutter (AFL) on the left atrial side. An activation map was prepared. The AFL went through the roof and the perimitral area. We induced AF with ISO 5. After RFCA, he was admitted to the intensive care unit due to the long procedure time, 7 hours. No immediate complications were detected during the procedure. Sinus rhythm was maintained after the procedure. Patient has no underlying disease except for arrhythmia and did not complain of anxiety every day, before and after RFCA. But he complained of abdominal distension and epigastric discomfort after eating on hospital day 2. Bowel sounds were normal, and gas out was normal, but gastric distension was noted. He complained of epigastric pain, indigestion, and early satiety for 1 week.

To prove gastroparesis related with RFCA, we used simple abdomen X-ray, abdominal pelvic CT, and gastroscopy as a diagnostic method. A simple abdominal X-ray revealed a large amount of material in the stomach, suggesting severe gastric hypomotility. Abdominal pelvic CT revealed large amount of food in the stomach (Figures 1(a) and 1(b)).

Endoscopic findings revealed large amounts of food stored in the gastric body. Normal peristaltic motion of the gastric antrum and pylorus was observed (Figures 1(c), 1(d), and 1(e)). The food was removed using a cap-fitted endoscope and a net over a period of days. At the time of paralysis, specific lesions have not been found inside the gastrointestinal tract and biopsy was not performed. With suspected gastroparesis, he underwent a gastric emptying scan. The gastric emptying scan revealed delayed gastric emptying time with an almost flat time-activity curve. There still remained a large amount of contrast material in the 2-hour delayed image, suggesting severe gastric hypomotility (Figure 2(a)). He was treated with prokinetics (50 mg itopride three times daily) and antiulcer medication (100 mg rebamipide three times daily). After the start of treatment, digestive function and excretion function were improved by 20 percent in one week. Digestive function has been completely recovered in two months later. After normalization of gastrointestinal motility, there were no abnormal findings in the duodenum in follow-up gastroscopy examination (Figure 2(b)).

3. Discussion

The vagus nerve begins in the brain and extends into the abdomen. The vagus nerve is responsible for such varied tasks as heart rate, gastrointestinal peristalsis, sweating, and quite a few muscle movements in the mouth, including speech and

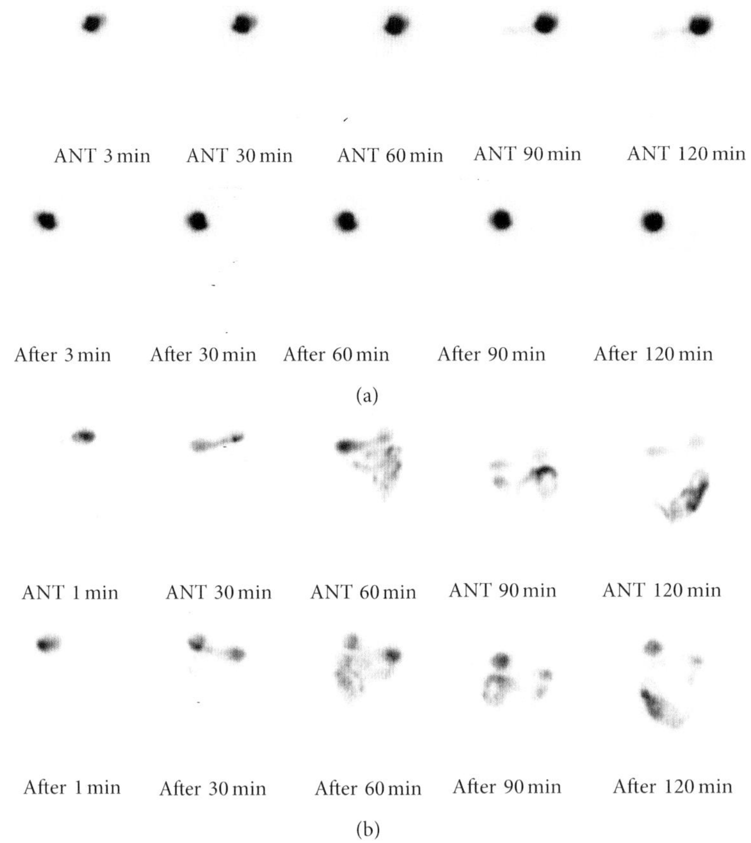

Figure 2: (a) Gastric emptying scan reveals delayed gastric emptying time with an almost flat time-activity curve. A large amount of contrast material remains in the 2-hour delayed image, suggesting severe gastric hypomotility. (b) Gastric emptying scan reveals delayed gastric emptying time, suggesting normal gastric motion.

keeping the larynx open for breathing. Digestive problems can sometimes occur as a result of vagus nerve damage. Persistent gastroparesis is often a symptom of nerve damage in this area. This is most commonly due to abnormalities or damage in the way the stomach and intestines contract. Decreased production of stomach acid is also a common symptom of this type of nerve damage [7].

Because the position of the vagus nerve is adjacent to the heart, gastroparesis due to the vagus nerve can occur due to various mechanical procedures such as postvagotomy syndrome for peptic ulcer or pancreatectomy due to pancreatic cancer. However, a vagus nerve injury due to electrical energy is very rare. Shah et al. reported four cases of acute delayed gastric emptying caused by vagus nerve injury after RF ablation for AF [2]. A case report of severe gastroparesis has been published recently [5]. Gastroparesis is observed as food retention via endoscopy and is supposedly caused by damage to the vagal nerve fibers surrounding the distal esophagus, as suggested in previous studies [5, 8]. Thus, delayed gastric emptying is considered a direct noncardiac complication of the ablation procedure.

We defined atrial fibrillation gut syndrome (AFGS) as symptoms of decreased gastrointestinal motility that occur after RFCA treatment. Our patient had no underlying disease other than AF, and digestive function was good. Because there was no underlying disease, we eliminated other causes for the gastroparesis. After treatment, severe abdominal distension findings revealed the gastroparesis findings, and AFGS was diagnosed. Although AFGS can occur based on treatment time, the vagus nerve tract, intensity of the electric force, treatment time, and RFCA site, it is reversible. RFCA treatment time is different according to the patient and center. In our center it took about 6 hours and it took up about 7 hours in this case. According to the existing literature, AFGS has been estimated by the treatment site and the amount of energy. Procedure time is also important, because a large amount of energy is transmitted in proportion to the time. In order to reduce the thermal injury to a minimum, we wrapped cooling pack to the portion of the neck in the procedure. We will prepare a prospective study on the effectiveness of the cooling pack to minimize the gastrointestinal paralysis on the above variables.

It took 6 months for the previous gastroparesis cases to recover to normal [5]. Our case was more serious, as the patient complained of terrible distension. However, gastric function completely recovered in 2 months with a rapid diagnosis, treatment, and exercise.

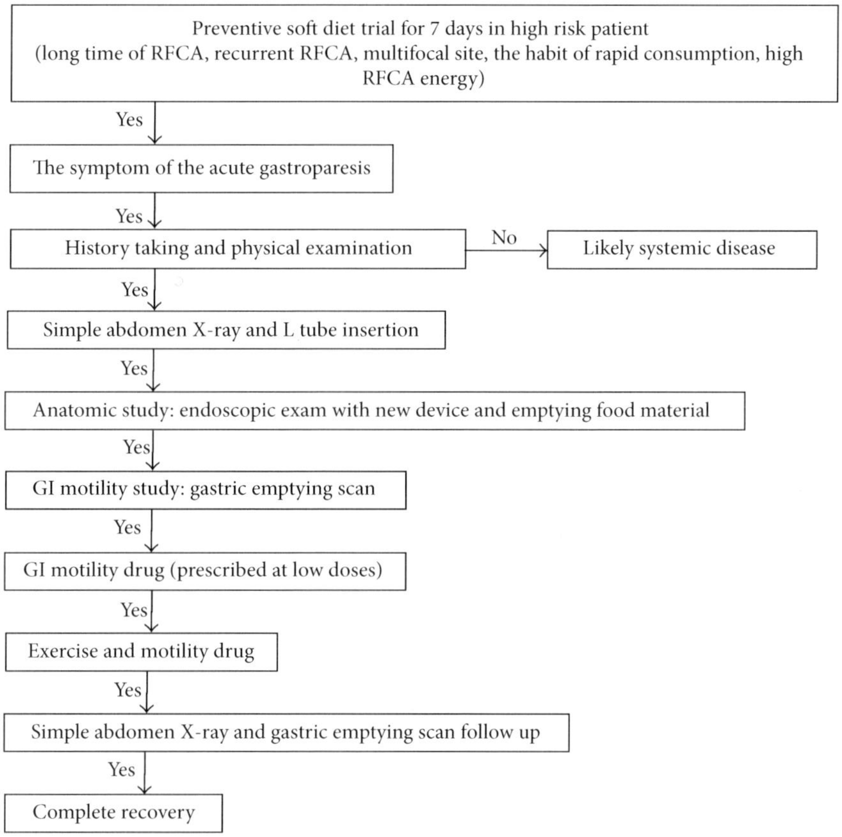

FIGURE 3: Flow chart of the diagnosis and treatment in our case and previous other cases.

It is believed that the recovery period can be reduced by rapid diagnosis and proper treatment and rehabilitation. We suggest a flow chart for diagnosis and treatment of AFGS based on the present case and previous cases. This flow chart can minimize the complications that occur after the operation in the AFGS high risk group. We recommend a soft diet in the high risk patient, as indicated in Figure 3, because it is easy to remove residual food material in cases of severe gastroparesis.

4. Conclusion

Although many complications can occur during RFCA, it is an absolutely necessary treatment for AF. AFGS is very unfamiliar complications to the cardiologists and gastroenterologists. It is difficult to predict AFGS on the basis of the patient symptoms. Our patient was the most serious case of AFGS that has been reported to date but shows that AFGS is fully reversible. In addition, this case presents the summary for diagnosing and treating AFGS to the RFCA practitioner. Considering these reversible and frequent AFGS complications, we think AFGS should be added to the common causative category of mechanical gastroparesis.

A feature of digestive tract paralysis due to vagus nerve damage is that movement of the wall of the digestive tract is paralyzed but movement of the pylorus is normal. Thus, the bowel is normal on a physical exam but retention of food material interferes with the pylorus. Removal of food is essential to resolve the abdominal distension and problem with the pylorus. According to our experience, endoscopic removal by colonoscopy is recommended for hardened food material.

Medical patent has been invented on the basis of the present case (patent number 10-2014-0102131, Republic of Korea) (Figure 4). Patent device is devised to eliminate gastric contents through the esophagus without surgery. By using the patent endoscope tube, sufficient internal space of the esophagus is ensured. Via a secure space, grinding endoscopic instrument is inserted and all of the gastric contents can be removed easily such as hematoma, foreign body, and food material. In future, fast diagnosis and treatment of AFGS will be possible. Various gastrointestinal foreign matter removals can be possible without surgery.

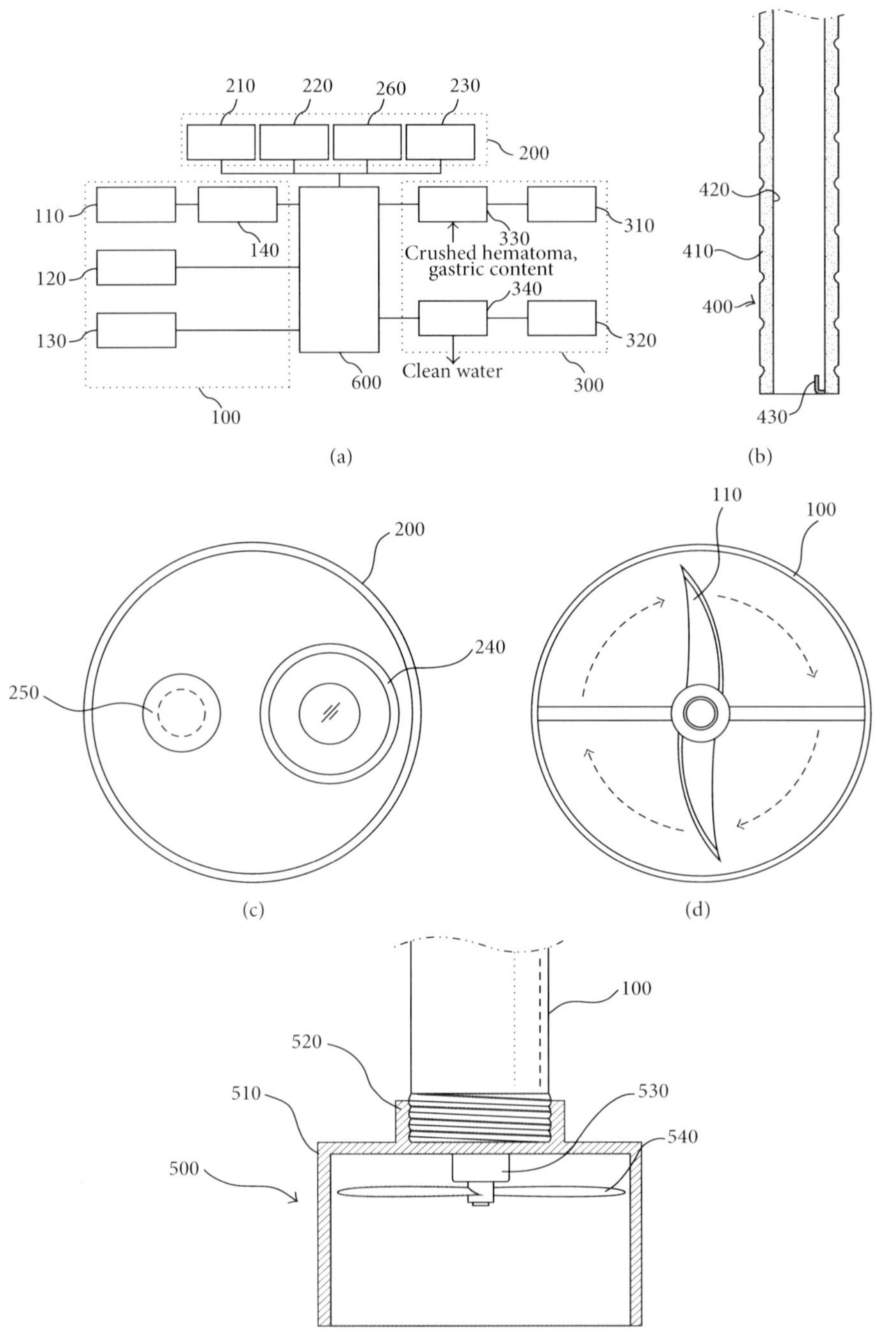

(100) Insertion tube
(110) Crushing unit
(120) Recording unit
(130) Illumination unit
(200) Irrigating and suction unit
(210) Operation buttons of crushing
(220) First irrigation button
(230) Suction button
(240) Suction tube
(250) Irrigation tube
(260) Second irrigation button
(300) Storage chamber
(310) Collection containers
(320) Storage container
(330) Pump
(340) Valve
(400) Guide tube
(410) Outer tube
(420) Inner tube
(500) Crushing device
(510) Mixer case
(520) Fastening parts
(530) Blade moving parts
(540) Blade
(600) Diagnosis parts

(e)

Figure 4: Continued.

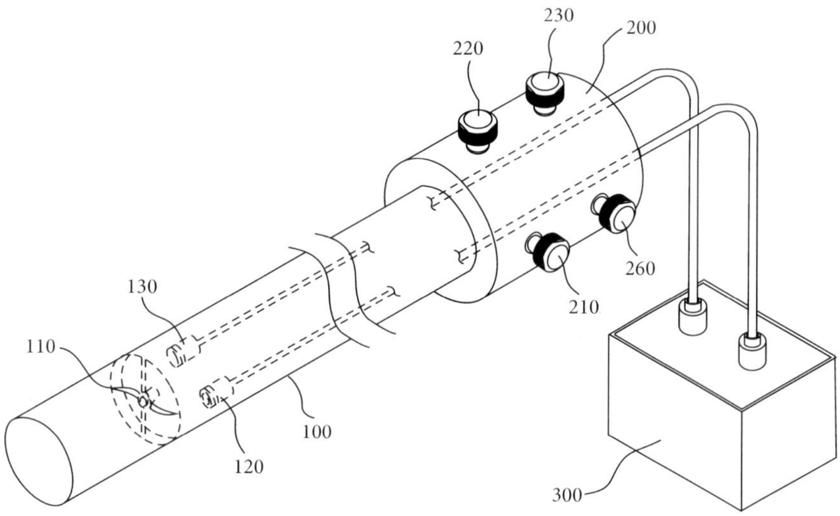

(100) Insertion tube
(110) Crushing unit
(120) Recording unit
(130) Illumination unit
(200) Irrigating and suction unit
(210) Operation buttons of crushing
(220) First irrigation button
(230) Suction button

(240) Suction tube
(250) Irrigation tube
(260) Second irrigation button
(300) Storage chamber
(310) Collection containers
(320) Storage container
(330) Pump
(340) Valve

(400) Guide tube
(410) Outer tube
(420) Inner tube
(500) Crushing device
(510) Mixer case
(520) Fastening parts
(530) Blade moving parts
(540) Blade
(600) Diagnosis parts

(f)

FIGURE 4: (a) Schematic control flow of the gastric content removing device; (b) endoscopic guide tube for evacuating gastric content; (c) irrigation and suction unit of the gastric contents; (d) mixer parts of crushing unit; (e) fastening parts of crushing unit; (f) appearance of the gastric content removing device.

Acknowledgment

The authors acknowledge the financial support for patent by Foundation for Industry Cooperation, University of Ulsan.

References

[1] C. Pappone, H. Oral, V. Santinelli et al., "Atrio-esophageal fistula as a complication of percutaneous transcatheter ablation of atrial fibrillation," *Circulation*, vol. 109, no. 22, pp. 2724–2726, 2004.

[2] D. Shah, J.-M. Dumonceau, H. Burri et al., "Acute pyloric spasm and gastric hypomotility: an extracardiac adverse effect of percutaneous radiofrequency ablation for atrial fibrillation," *Journal of the American College of Cardiology*, vol. 46, no. 2, pp. 327–330, 2005.

[3] N. Dagres, G. Hindricks, H. Kottkamp et al., "Complications of atrial fibrillation ablation in a high-volume center in 1,000 procedures: still cause for concern?" *Journal of Cardiovascular Electrophysiology*, vol. 20, no. 9, pp. 1014–1019, 2009.

[4] T. J. Bunch, K. A. Ellenbogen, D. L. Packer, and S. J. Asirvatham, "Vagus nerve injury after posterior atrial radiofrequency ablation," *Heart Rhythm*, vol. 5, no. 9, pp. 1327–1330, 2008.

[5] S. W. Choi, S. H. Kang, O. S. Kwon et al., "A case of severe gastroparesis: indigestion and weight loss after catheter ablation of atrial fibrillation," *Pacing and Clinical Electrophysiology*, vol. 35, no. 3, pp. e59–e61, 2012.

[6] H. Knopp, U. Halm, R. Lamberts et al., "Incidental and ablation-induced findings during upper gastrointestinal endoscopy in patients after ablation of atrial fibrillation: a retrospective study of 425 patients," *Heart Rhythm*, vol. 11, no. 4, pp. 574–578, 2014.

[7] K. L. D. Moore and F. Arthur, *Clinically Oriented Anatomy*, 7th edition, 2014.

[8] C. F. Pisani, D. Hachul, E. Sosa, and M. Scanavacca, "Gastric hypomotility following epicardial vagal denervation ablation to treat atrial fibrillation," *Journal of Cardiovascular Electrophysiology*, vol. 19, no. 2, pp. 211–213, 2008.

Self-Expandable Metal Stent Placement for Closure of a Leak after Total Gastrectomy for Gastric Cancer: Report on Three Cases and Review of the Literature

Dario Raimondo,[1] Emanuele Sinagra,[1,2,3] Tiziana Facella,[4] Francesca Rossi,[1] Marco Messina,[5] Massimiliano Spada,[5] Guido Martorana,[4] Pier Enrico Marchesa,[4] Rosario Squatrito,[6] Giovanni Tomasello,[3,7] Attilio Ignazio Lo Monte,[7] Giancarlo Pompei,[8] and Ennio La Rocca[6,9]

[1] *Gastroenterology and Endoscopy Unit, Fondazione Istituto San Raffaele-G. Giglio, Contrada Pietra Pollastra Pisciotto, 90015 Cefalù, Italy*
[2] *Ph.D. Course in Surgical Biotechnology and Regenerative Medicine, University of Palermo, Piazza delle Cliniche 2, 90100 Palermo, Italy*
[3] *Euro-Mediterranean Institute of Science and Technology (IEMEST), Via Emerico Amari 123, 90100 Palermo, Italy*
[4] *Surgery Unit, Fondazione Istituto San Raffaele-G. Giglio, Contrada Pietra Pollastra Pisciotto, 90015 Cefalù, Italy*
[5] *Oncology Unit, Fondazione Istituto San Raffaele-G. Giglio, Contrada Pietra Pollastra Pisciotto, 90015 Cefalù, Italy*
[6] *Internal Medicine Unit, Fondazione Istituto San Raffaele-G. Giglio, Contrada Pietra Pollastra Pisciotto, 90015 Cefalù, Italy*
[7] *Department of Surgical and Oncological Disciplines, University of Palermo, Piazza delle Cliniche 2, 90100 Palermo, Italy*
[8] *Pathology Unit, Fondazione Istituto San Raffaele-G. Giglio, Contrada Pietra Pollastra Pisciotto, 90015 Cefalù, Italy*
[9] *Unità Operativa di Medicina Interna e Trapiantologia, Ospedale San Raffaele, Via Olgettina 60, Milano, Italy*

Correspondence should be addressed to Emanuele Sinagra; emanuelesinagra83@googlemail.com

Academic Editor: Naohiko Koide

In the setting of the curative oncological surgery, the gastric surgery is exposed to complicated upper gastrointestinal leaks, and consequently the management of this problem has become more critically focused than was previously possible. We report here three cases of placement of a partially silicone-coated SEMS (Evolution Controlled Release Esophageal Stent System, Cook Medical, Winston-Salem, NC, USA) in patients who underwent total gastrectomy with Roux-en-Y end-to-side esophagojejunostomy for a gastric adenocarcinoma. The promising results of our report, despite the small number of patients, suggest that early stenting (through a partially silicone-coated SEMS) is a feasible alternative to surgical treatment in this subset of patients. In fact, in the treatment of leakage after total gastrectomy, plastic stents and totally covered metallic stents may not adhere sufficiently to the esophagojejunal walls and, as a result, migrate beyond the anastomosis. However, prospective studies with a larger number of patients might assess the real effectiveness and safety of this procedure.

1. Introduction

In the setting of the curative oncological surgery, the gastric surgery is exposed to complicated upper gastrointestinal leaks, and consequently the management of this problem has become more critically focused than was previously possible. The management of a patient with an upper gastrointestinal leak is complex and often involves treatment of sepsis, organ failure, and nutritional deficits in addition to treating the underlying leak [1]. The use of stents in the management of postoperative leaks has been reported with variable success [2–10].

We report here three cases of placement of a partially silicone-coated SEMS (Evolution Controlled Release

Esophageal Stent System, Cook Medical, Winston-Salem, NC, USA) in patients who underwent total gastrectomy with Roux-en-Y end-to-side esophagojejunostomy for a gastric adenocarcinoma.

2. Case Report 1

A 52-year-old woman was admitted to our hospital for abdominal pain and weight loss. Esophagogastroduodenoscopy (EGDS) showed a gastric lesion, which on histology was revealed to be a gastric adenocarcinoma. As a result, the patient underwent total gastrectomy with Roux-en-Y end-to-side esophagojejunostomy. A stapling esophagojejunostomy was performed: the anvil was secured in the esophagus with a purse-string suture; subsequently an end anastomosis stapler was inserted through the distal end of the Roux limb. The anastomosis was made on the antimesenteric side of the bowel. Once the anastomosis was complete, the end of the Roux limb was amputated with a single firing of a gastrointestinal anastomosis stapler. The enteric staple line was reinforced with interrupted Lembert sutures of 3–0 silk. Five days later, due to the onset of nausea and abdominal pain, EGDS was performed, showing a 2 cm fistula at the anastomosis, about 38 cm from the mouth (Figure 2). This was confirmed by gastrografin esophagography. The patient was started on total parenteral nutrition (TPN) (Figure 1) and empirical antibiotic therapy. The abdominal cavity drainage was performed maintaining a drainage tube for 15 days, which was removed; after that the disappearance of the abdominal effusion was demonstrated through abdominal ultrasound. Having deemed clipping treatment for this fistula unfeasible, we decided to insert a partially silicone-coated SEMS (Evolution Controlled Release Esophageal Stent System). The Evolution stent (Cook, Bloomington, IN, USA) is available as a partially or fully covered SEMS. The stent is encased (Figure 3) with silicone on its exterior and interior surfaces to prevent tumor ingrowth. A unique feature of Evolution delivery system is that it enables a controlled release and recapturability feature with a "point of no return" indicator. With each squeeze of the stent system's trigger-based introducer, a proportional length of the stent is deployed or recaptured. The diameter of the Evolution stent employed was 25 mm and 20 mm at the flare and at the shaft, respectively; the length was 10 cm. We chose this type of partially covered metallic stent in order to avoid the kind of stent migration described in some reports [9, 11, 12]. The stent was removed after six weeks. EGDS showed closure of the fistula. No clinical complications were observed, and the patient was able to start normal per os nutrition 7 days after the stent placement, once an upper X-ray series with gastrografin secured the disappearance of the contrast extravasation (Figure 4).

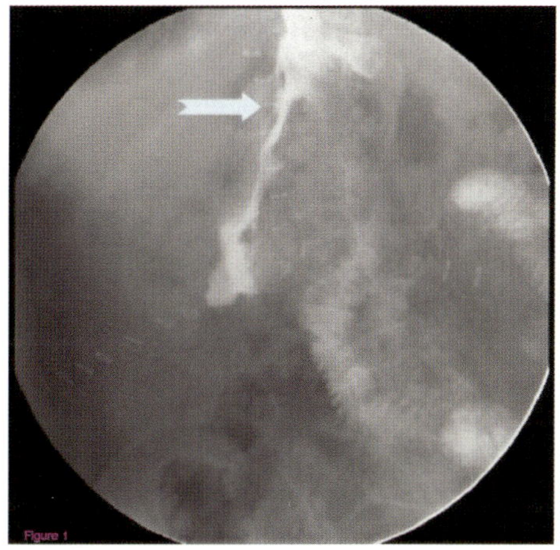

FIGURE 1: Gastrografin esophagography showing a 2 cm fistula at the anastomosis.

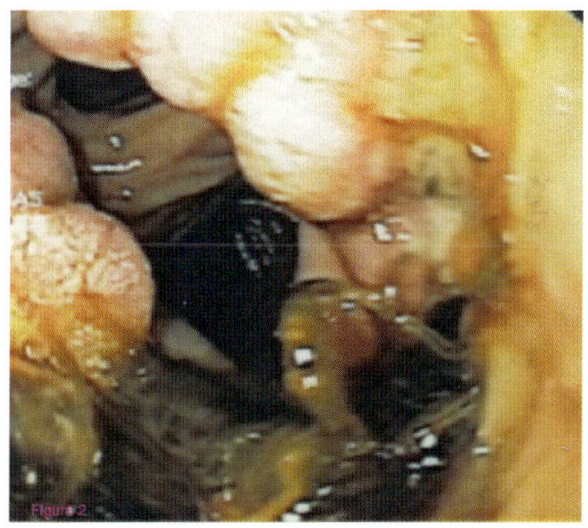

FIGURE 2: Endoscopic view of the fistula.

3. Case Report 2

Like the previous patient, a 71-year-old woman was admitted to our hospital for abdominal pain and weight loss. EGDS showed a gastric lesion, which on histology was revealed to be a gastric adenocarcinoma, and the patient underwent total gastrectomy with Roux-en-Y end-to-side esophagojejunostomy. A stapling esophagojejunostomy was performed, according to the aforementioned procedure. Eight days later, due to the onset of fever and abdominal pain, EGDS was performed, showing a 1.7 cm fistula at the anastomosis, about 40 cm from the mouth. This was confirmed by gastrografin esophagography. The patient was started on TPN and empirical antibiotic therapy. The abdominal cavity drainage was performed maintaining a drainage tube for 15 days, which was removed; after that the disappearance of the abdominal effusion was demonstrated through abdominal ultrasound. Having deemed clipping treatment for this fistula unfeasible, we decided, also in this patient, to insert a partially silicone-coated SEMS (Evolution Controlled Release Esophageal Stent System). The patient was able to start normal per os nutrition 7 days after the stent placement, once an upper X-ray series with gastrografin secured the disappearance of the contrast extravasation. The stent was removed after six weeks. EGDS showed closure of the fistula. Unfortunately, the patient died of a pulmonary embolism, ten days after stent removal.

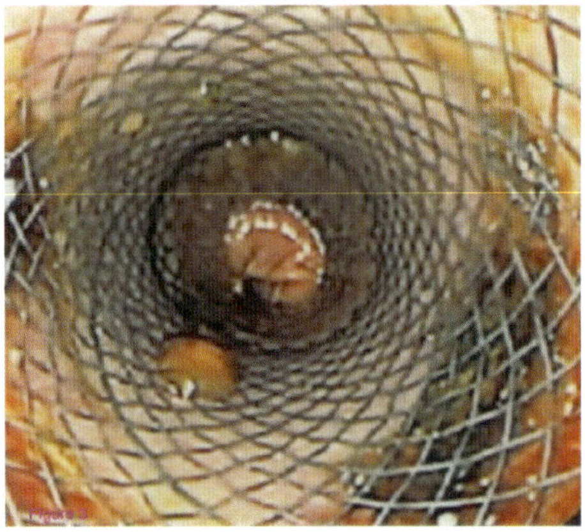

FIGURE 3: Endoscopic view of the placement of the stent.

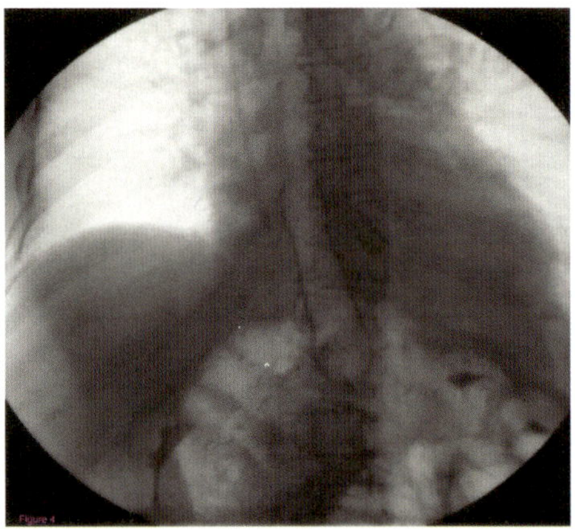

FIGURE 4: Gastrografin esophagography showing the absence of contrast extravasation, after the placement of the stent.

4. Case Report 3

Finally, a 66-year-old man was admitted to our hospital with severe anemia (6 g/dL), abdominal pain, and weight loss. Like in the cases reported above, EGDS showed a gastric lesion, which on histology was revealed to be a gastric adenocarcinoma, and the patient underwent total gastrectomy with Roux-en-Y end-to-side esophagojejunostomy. A stapling esophagojejunostomy was performed, according to the aforementioned procedure. Seven days later, EGDS was performed, due to the onset of severe nausea and fever, showing a 1.8 cm fistula at the anastomosis, about 38 cm from the mouth. This was confirmed by CT scan with gastrografin. The patient was started on TPN and empirical antibiotic (Figure 5) therapy. The abdominal cavity drainage was performed maintaining a drainage tube for 15 days, which was removed; after that the disappearance of the abdominal effusion was demonstrated through abdominal ultrasound. Having deemed clipping treatment for this fistula unfeasible, we decided, also in this patient, to insert a partially silicone-coated SEMS (Evolution Controlled Release Esophageal Stent System). The stent was removed after six weeks. Gastrografin esophagography showed no further contrast extravasation,

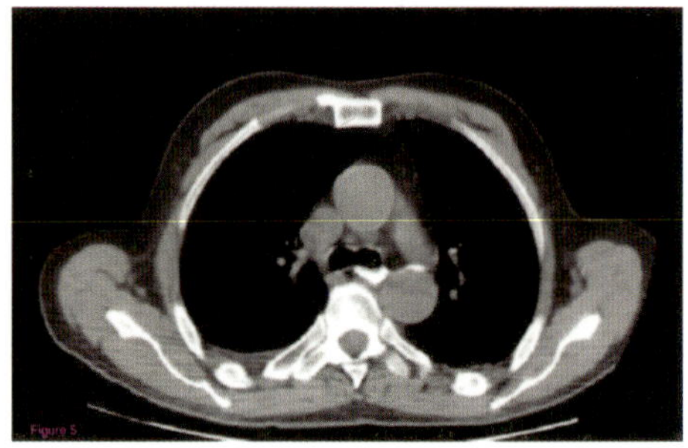

FIGURE 5: CT scan with gastrographin showing the contrast extravasation.

and EGD showed closure of the fistula. No clinical complications were observed, and the patient was able to start normal per os nutrition 7 days after the stent placement, once an upper X-ray series with gastrografin secured the disappearance of the contrast extravasation.

5. Discussion

The treatment of symptomatic leaks in patients who have undergone esophagojejunostomy is challenging, and leakage from the jejunal stump can be a potentially serious complication. Therapeutic options are surgical repair or resection or conservative management with cessation of oral intake and antibiotic therapy. Open surgical reintervention is associated with considerable risk, particularly in depleted patients [13].

This report provides further evidence that stenting for upper gastrointestinal leaks is a simple and robust technique and has the definite advantage of allowing early recommencement of enteral nutrition. In our small series, we report only three cases of anastomotic leaks after total gastrectomy for gastric cancer, which occurred in our center from January 2010 to December 2013, which were treated with SEMS placement, with a technical and clinical success rate of 100%. Stenting should be considered early in the management of patients with evolving sepsis from gastrointestinal leakage even where the defect is large. It is suitable for combination with laparoscopic, thoracoscopic, or open drainage when contamination is significant. Previous reports have suggested the effectiveness and the safety of this procedure [1, 14]. In the study performed by Babor and coworkers, in the setting of bariatric surgery, seven patients with staple line and anastomotic dehiscences and a single case of Boerhaave syndrome were treated by using a removable, polyester covered self-expanding metal stent (ELLA Boubella, Ella-CS, Hradec, Czech Republic). All patients had active severe sepsis and significant contamination in the abdomen or thorax at the time of stenting. In 4 cases, the stent was sutured in place with dissolvable synthetic sutures with suture bites incorporating the full thickness of the gut wall and the stent itself to prevent stent migration. All patients showed resolution of their intra-abdominal sepsis and were able to resume an oral diet after stenting; all stents were retrieved endoscopically after clinical resolution of the leak. Stent migration after leak resolution was observed in 3 patients. In patients with large defects or minimal anatomic barriers to stent migration, suture fixation stabilized the stent; there were no episodes of persistent leak or development of stricture in this series [1]. Eisendrath and coworkers also evaluated, in the setting of bariatric surgery, in a series of twenty-one patients which underwent endoscopic treatment for persisting large anastomotic leaks before considering redo surgery, whether endoscopic treatment may reduce reoperation rates [15]. In these patients, partially covered SEMS were used, followed by additional endoscopic procedures if the SEMS failed. SEMS insertion led to 62% (13/21) primary closures. Complementary endoscopic treatment led to 4 secondary closures. Total success rate was 81% (17/21). Interestingly, the success rates of endotherapy were 100% (8/8) in the gastric bypass group, 62.5% (5/8) in the SDS group, 75% (3/4) in the sleeve gastrectomy group, and 100% (1/1) for the Scopinaro procedure; furthermore, gastrocutaneous fistulas on a sleeve suture seemed to be the most difficult condition to treat (successfully treated in 60% of cases (6/10)) [15].

Recently, Shim and coworkers performed a prospective study to assess the clinical characteristics and therapeutic outcomes of SEMS and nonstent endoscopic therapy (NSET, which includes fibrin glue injection, endoclip, and other devices) for treatment of anastomotic leaks after total gastrectomy with the aim of assisting endoscopists in choosing a treatment method [16]. 13 patients treated with SEMS (with a total of 16 SEMS placement sessions) and 14 patients treated with NSET (with a total 21 NSET sessions) for anastomotic leaks after total gastrectomy were enrolled onto the study. At the end of the study, the successful sealing rate at the first attempt by SEMS was significantly better than that of NSET (80.0 versus 28.6%, $P = 0.036$), whereas the successful sealing rate after multiple endoscopic treatments was not statistically different (80.0 versus 64.3%, $P = 0.653$). The main reason for reintervention with SEMS was complications and with NSET was nonseal ($P = 0.004$). Interestingly, clinical outcomes including length of hospital stay, endoscopic treatment-related mortality, and all-cause mortality were not significantly different between the 2 groups [16].

An area of uncertainty regards the real knowledge of the migration rate of partially covered SEMS in this subset of patients, as well as how long the stent should be left in place to allow removability and avoid complications.

In our series the complete closures of the anastomotic leaks were achieved after 6 weeks of stent indwelling using partially covered metal stents in all 3 patients.

In an article of systematic review on temporary stent placement for benign rupture or anastomotic leaks of the esophagus, twenty-five studies made up of 267 patients who were treated with endoscopic placement of fully covered or partially covered SEMS or plastic stents were analyzed; the mean indwelling time of partially covered SEMS was 6 weeks. It was concluded that covered stent placement for a period of 6–8 weeks was safe and effective for benign esophageal ruptures and anastomotic leaks to heal [17]. An article from Lee and coworkers reported that healing of leaks after endoscopic placement of covered stents in patients with anastomotic leaks occurred in 4 out of 6 patients after 2 weeks of stent indwelling [18], while an article from Schubert and coworkers reported that a complete closure of the leakage after silicone-covered, self-expanding polyester stents in patients with thoracic esophageal anastomotic leaks was achieved in 11 of 12 patients after stent removal with a median stent retrieval time of 4 weeks (range 2–8 weeks) [9]. On the other hand, Eubanks and coworkers reported that healing of leaks after endoscopic placement of covered stents in patients with anastomotic leaks after bariatric surgery was achieved at a mean of 33 days [19], while Edwards and coworkers reported that acute anastomotic leaks after Roux-en-Y bypass had completely healed at a median of 44 days when self-expanding polyester stents were used [20]. Finally, Fischer and coworkers recently reported that the median stent indwelling time after using a specially designed partially covered self-expandable metal stent in 11 patients with upper GI anastomotic leaks was 24 (range 18–41) days [21].

Although stent migration remains a common problem when using fully covered metal stents in patients with postoperative anastomotic leaks, several novel fixation procedures were reported to eliminate migration of the fully covered metal stents, such as a stent fixation technique with a bridle which was created by delivering umbilical tape through each nostril [22] or through a novel stent insertion technique with a newly designed proximal-releasing, self-expanding metallic stent (PR-SEMS) and transnasal endoscope that can enable stent insertion without fluoroscopy as a new method to prevent stent migration [18].

It is worth mentioning, in the fields of leaks and perforation of the upper gastrointestinal tract, the use of endoscopic placed vacuum sponge therapy. In the study performed by Schorsch and coworkers, 17 cases of anastomotic leakage and 7 cases of iatrogenic perforation due to interventional endoscopy or rigid panendoscopy with either intraluminal or intracavitary endoscopic vacuum therapy were treated [23]. In 23 of 24 cases, the endoscopic treatment was successful. The median duration of therapy was 11 days (range 4–46 days). All 7 cases of iatrogenic perforation and 16 of 17 anastomotic leakage cases were cured after a median therapy duration of 5 and 12 days, respectively. According to the authors' experience, it has seemed to be the best choice for iatrogenic perforations and has been a potent supplement in the management of anastomotic leakages [23].

It is remarkable that in all patients of our series the length of the fistula did not exceed 2 cm and that no further complications, like abscesses of sepsis, were present; as a consequence, the shortness of the fistulae and the lack of abscesses, together with the prompt antibiotic therapy, are probably further reasons for the rapid healing of the leaks.

The promising results of our report suggest that early stenting (through a partially silicone-coated SEMS) is a feasible alternative to surgical treatment in this subset of patients. In fact, in the treatment of leakage after total gastrectomy, plastic stents and totally covered metallic stents may not adhere sufficiently to the esophagojejunal walls and, as a result, migrate beyond the anastomosis. However, prospective studies with a larger number of patients might assess the real effectiveness and safety of this procedure.

Authors' Contribution

Emanuele Sinagra and Dario Raimondo wrote the paper; Tiziana Facella and Francesca Rossi performed the endoscopies; Marco Messina, Rosario Squatrito, Giancarlo Pompei, and Massimiliano Spada followed clinically the patients; Guido Martorana and Pier Enrico Marchesa performed the surgical interventions; and Ennio La Rocca, Attilio Ignazio Lo Monte, and Giovanni Tomasello revised critically the paper.

References

[1] R. Babor, M. Talbot, and A. Tyndal, "Treatment of upper gastrointestinal leaks with a removable, covered, self-expanding metallic stent," *Surgical Laparoscopy, Endoscopy and Percutaneous Techniques*, vol. 19, no. 1, pp. e1–e4, 2009.

[2] S. H. Roy-Choudhury, A. A. Nicholson, K. R. Wedgwood et al., "Symptomatic malignant gastroesophageal anastomotic leak: management with covered metallic esophageal stents," *American Journal of Roentgenology*, vol. 176, no. 1, pp. 161–165, 2001.

[3] C. J. Brinster, S. Singhal, L. Lee, M. B. Marshall, L. R. Kaiser, and J. C. Kucharczuk, "Evolving options in the management of esophageal perforation," *Annals of Thoracic Surgery*, vol. 77, no. 4, pp. 1475–1483, 2004.

[4] C. Ott, N. Ratiu, E. Endlicher et al., "Self-expanding polyflex plastic stents in esophageal disease: various indications, complications, and outcomes," *Surgical Endoscopy and Other Interventional Techniques*, vol. 21, no. 6, pp. 889–896, 2007.

[5] F. B. Langer, E. Wenzl, G. Prager et al., "Management of postoperative esophageal leaks with the polyflex self-expanding covered plastic stent," *Annals of Thoracic Surgery*, vol. 79, no. 2, pp. 398–403, 2005.

[6] R. K. Freeman, A. J. Ascioti, and T. C. Wozniak, "Postoperative esophageal leak management with the Polyflex esophageal stent," *Journal of Thoracic and Cardiovascular Surgery*, vol. 133, no. 2, pp. 333–338, 2007.

[7] M. Hünerbein, C. Stroszczynski, K. T. Moesta, and P. M. Schlag, "Treatment of thoracic anastomotic leaks after esophagectomy with self-expanding plastic stents," *Annals of Surgery*, vol. 240, no. 5, pp. 801–807, 2004.

[8] J. M. Doniec, B. Schniewind, V. Kahlke, B. Kremer, and H. Grimm, "Therapy of anastomotic leaks by means of covered self-expanding metallic stents after esophagogastrectomy," *Endoscopy*, vol. 35, no. 8, pp. 652–658, 2003.

[9] D. Schubert, H. Scheidbach, R. Kuhn et al., "Endoscopic treatment of thoracic esophageal anastomotic leaks by using silicone-covered, self-expanding polyester stents," *Gastrointestinal Endoscopy*, vol. 61, no. 7, pp. 891–896, 2005.

[10] P. D. Siersema, "Treatment of esophageal perforations and anastomotic leaks: the endoscopist is stepping into the arena," *Gastrointestinal Endoscopy*, vol. 61, no. 7, pp. 897–900, 2005.

[11] P. Salminen, R. Gullichsen, and S. Laine, "Use of self-expandable metal stents for the treatment of esophageal perforations and anastomotic leaks," *Surgical Endoscopy and Other Interventional Techniques*, vol. 23, no. 7, pp. 1526–1530, 2009.

[12] D. Tuebergen, E. Rijcken, R. Mennigen, A. M. Hopkins, N. Senninger, and M. Bruewer, "Treatment of thoracic esophageal anastomotic leaks and esophageal perforations with endoluminal stents: efficacy and current limitations," *Journal of Gastrointestinal Surgery*, vol. 12, no. 7, pp. 1168–1176, 2008.

[13] C. M. Gelbmann, N. L. Ratiu, H. C. Rath et al., "Use of self-expandable plastic stents for the treatment of esophageal perforations and symptomatic anastomotic leaks," *Endoscopy*, vol. 36, no. 8, pp. 695–699, 2004.

[14] G. Curcio, F. Mocciaro, I. Tarantino et al., "Self-expandable metal stent for closure of a large leak after total gastrectomy," *Case Reports in Gastroenterology*, vol. 4, no. 2, pp. 293–297, 2010.

[15] P. Eisendrath, M. Cremer, J. Himpens, G. B. Cadière, O. le Moine, and J. Devière, "Endotherapy including temporary stenting of fistulas of the upper gastrointestinal tract after laparoscopic bariatric surgery," *Endoscopy*, vol. 39, no. 7, pp. 625–630, 2007.

[16] C. N. Shim, H. I. Kim, and W. J. Hyung, "Self-expanding metal stents or nonstent endoscopic therapy: which is better for anastomotic leaks after total gastrectomy ?" *Surgical Endoscopy*, vol. 28, no. 3, pp. 833–840, 2014.

[17] P. G. A. Van Boeckel, A. Sijbring, F. P. Vleggaar, and P. D. Siersema, "Systematic review: temporary stent placement for benign rupture or anastomotic leak of the oesophagus," *Alimentary Pharmacology and Therapeutics*, vol. 33, no. 12, pp. 1292–1301, 2011.

[18] K. M. Lee, S. J. Shin, J. C. Hwang et al., "Proximal-releasing stent insertion under transnasal endoscopic guidance in patients with postoperative esophageal leakage," *Gastrointestinal Endoscopy*, vol. 72, no. 1, pp. 180–185, 2010.

[19] S. Eubanks, C. A. Edwards, N. M. Fearing et al., "Use of endoscopic stents to treat anastomotic complications after bariatric surgery," *Journal of the American College of Surgeons*, vol. 206, no. 5, pp. 935–938, 2008.

[20] C. A. Edwards, P. T. Bui, J. A. Astudillo et al., "Management of anastomotic leaks after Roux-en-Y bypass using self-expanding polyester stents," *Surgery for Obesity and Related Diseases*, vol. 4, no. 5, pp. 594–599, 2008.

[21] A. Fischer, D. Bausch, and H.-J. Richter-Schrag, "Use of a specially designed partially covered self-expandable metal stent (PSEMS) with a 40-mm diameter for the treatment of upper gastrointestinal suture or staple line leaks in 11 cases," *Surgical Endoscopy and Other Interventional Techniques*, vol. 27, no. 2, pp. 642–647, 2013.

[22] C. D. Lyons, M. P. Kim, and S. H. Blackmon, "A novel fixation procedure to eliminate covered self-expanding metal stent migration," *Annals of Thoracic Surgery*, vol. 94, no. 5, pp. 1748–1750, 2012.

[23] T. Schorsch, C. Müller, and G. Loske, "Endoscopic vacuum therapy of anastomotic leakage and iatrogenic perforation in the esophagus," *Surgical Endoscopy and Other Interventional Techniques*, vol. 27, no. 6, pp. 2040–2045, 2013.

7

Psoas Muscle Infiltration Masquerading Distant Adenocarcinoma

Kamel A. Gharaibeh,[1] Arnaldo Lopez-Ruiz,[1] and Tauqeer Yousuf[1,2]

[1] *Department of Internal Medicine, University of Mississippi Medical Center, 2500 North State Street, Jackson, MS 39216, USA*
[2] *Division of Hospital Medicine, Department of Medicine, University of Mississippi Medical Center, 2500 North State Street, Jackson, MS 39216, USA*

Correspondence should be addressed to Arnaldo Lopez-Ruiz; alopezruiz@umc.edu

Academic Editor: Shiro Kikuchi

Malignant metastasis to the psoas muscle is rare. We report a case that clinically mimicked psoas abscess that was subsequently proven to be from metastatic disease secondary to adenocarcinoma of the duodenum. A 62-year-old male presented with a seven-month history of right lower quadrant abdominal pain and progressive dysphagia. CT scan of abdomen-pelvis revealed a right psoas infiltration not amenable to surgical drainage. Patient was treated with two courses of oral antibiotics without improvement. Repeated CT scan showed ill-defined low-density area with inflammatory changes involving the right psoas muscle. Using CT guidance, a fine needle aspiration biopsy of the right psoas was performed that reported metastatic undifferentiated adenocarcinoma. Patient underwent upper endoscopy, which showed a duodenal mass that was biopsied which also reported poorly differentiated adenocarcinoma. In this case, unresponsiveness to medical therapy or lack of improvement in imaging studies warrants consideration of differential diagnosis such as malignancy. Iliopsoas metastases have shown to mimic psoas abscess on their clinical presentation and in imaging studies. To facilitate early diagnosis and improve prognosis, patients who embody strong risk factors and symptoms compatible with underlying malignancies who present with psoas imaging concerning for abscess should have further investigations.

1. Introduction

The most frequent tumor of the duodenum is adenocarcinoma [1, 2]. Adenocarcinoma of the duodenum may arise from duodenal polyps observed in familial polyposis or Gardener's syndrome or be associated with celiac disease [3, 4]. The tumor can be located in any part of the duodenum but is most frequently found in the descending part. The most common metastatic sites of duodenal carcinoma are liver, lungs, lymph nodes, and peritoneum. To our knowledge, metastasis to skeletal muscle from duodenal carcinoma has never been described. Furthermore, skeletal muscle is a rare site for metastases which manifest clinically, but has a slightly higher reported autopsy incidence of 16–25% [5, 6]. Leukemia, high grade lymphomas, and carcinoma (originating from cervix, ovary, colon, stomach, lung, breast, and kidney) are the most frequent primary sources [5–7]. Skeletal metastatic lesions usually mimic the clinical presentation of abscess or hematomas [5, 8]. This fact constitutes the most frequent reason for delaying appropriate therapy of the underlying malignant process [5]. The purpose of this report is to describe perhaps the first case in the literature of iliopsoas metastasis from duodenal adenocarcinoma.

2. Case Report

A 62-year-old Caucasian male with history of chronic obstructive pulmonary disease, gastroesophageal reflux disease, and knee osteoarthritis presented with seven months history of gradual, dull, and constant abdominal pain affecting the right lower quadrant (RLQ). The pain radiated to his right groin and down his anterior right thigh. Patient also reported 10 months history of mild but persistent epigastric discomfort, dysphagia, and odynophagia with solids and liquids. The patient denied history of fever or chills but did report significant weight loss (>10 lb) and night sweats over the last six weeks. The patient had an extensive tobacco

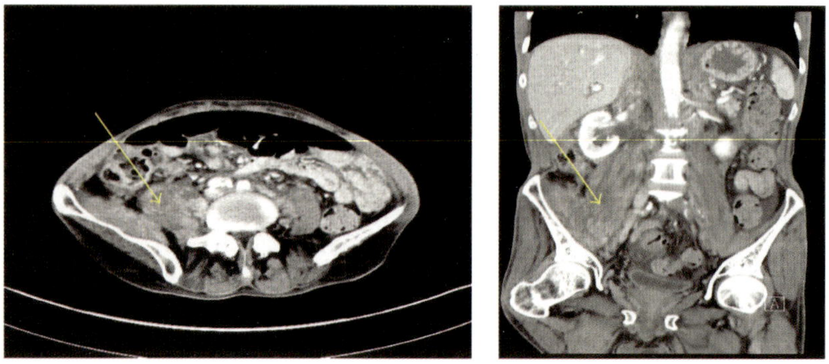

(a) (b)

Figure 1: (a) Contrast-enhanced axial CT image through upper pelvis demonstrate enlarged, heterogeneously enhancing right psoas and iliacus muscles with the muscles demonstrating increased and prominent striations (as pointed by arrow). Left psoas is normal. (b) Contrast-enhanced coronal CT image through the abdomen and the pelvis demonstrate enlarged, heterogeneously enhancing right psoas and iliacus muscles (as pointed by arrow) with lateral and anterior displacement of right kidney. No fluid collection is seen.

history of two packs-per-day for fifty years, as well as an extensive alcohol history despite abstinence the preceding months. Three months prior to admission to our service, patient underwent laparoscopic cholecystectomy due to the abdominal pain that was described above. However, his abdominal pain persisted postoperatively. Patient presented to our emergency department and was sent home on oral antibiotics for iliopsoas phlegmon as per CT findings thought to be secondary to infection. He presented for the second time two weeks later complaining of severe abdominal pain; repeat CT scan of abdomen and pelvis did not show any significant change in the iliopsoas phlegmon. Vital signs were within normal. Physical exam showed a cachectic man that appeared older than stated age. Abdomen was soft, nondistended and with moderate tenderness to palpation in RLQ and suprapubic area with no evidence of peritoneal inflammation. There were normal bowel sounds and no hepatosplenomegaly. The rest of the physical exam was normal. Initial laboratory results on admission revealed hemoglobin to be 12.6 g/L and otherwise normal CBC. Renal function was within normal. Total protein was 5.8 g/L, albumin was 2.9 g/L, alkaline phosphatase was 1619 mg/dL, ALT was 51 UI, AST was 43 UI, GGT was >1200 u/L, C-reactive protein was 3.7 mg/dL (normal range <5 mg/dL), and ESR was 52. Blood cultures were negative. An abdominal ultrasound reported normal liver measuring 15 cm, no definitive intrahepatic biliary dilatation and mild extrahepatic biliary dilation (CBD measuring 10 mm) that was likely related to cholecystectomy, suggested as not significant. Ultrasound was not done to evaluate psoas muscle. A repeated CT scan of abdomen-pelvis reported ill-defined areas of low density involving the right psoas muscle from origin to insertion and inflammatory changes along the right psoas muscle and right iliacus muscle (Figures 1(a) and 1(b)). Soft tissue lumbar MRI showed persistent thickening and heterogeneity of the entirety of the right iliopsoas musculature. Axial T1 post contrast MRI (images of the lumbar spine) showed normal appearing muscle segments on the left side. Significantly enlarged and enhancing right psoas and paraspinal musculature on the right side (Figure 2).

The differential diagnoses suggested by the radiologist were infectious process versus neoplastic infiltration. Given the malignant suspicious of the lesion, using CT guidance, a fine needle aspiration biopsy of the right psoas mass was performed. The core biopsy sections revealed atypical cells with high nuclear cytoplasmic ratio and hyperchromasia in an infiltrative pattern and were positive for cytokeratin immunostain confirming the diagnosis of metastatic poorly differentiated carcinoma (Figure 3). CT of head, neck, and chest was done because of significant smoking history, however, it was negative for any abnormality suggestive of malignancy. Given progressive dysphagia, patient underwent upper endoscopy, which revealed esophageal stricture that was dilated. Stomach showed no endoscopic evidence of ulcers or masses. Upon reaching the duodenum, ERCP was attempted for elevated alkaline phosphatase and GGT using regular scope but cannulation was not achieved; near the ampulla, a protruding luminal mass was seen in the second portion of the duodenum (Figure 4). Duodenal biopsy was taken which showed similar tumor cells in an infiltrative pattern consistent with poorly differentiated adenocarcinoma (Figure 5). Upon discussing the results with the patient, he refused any type of therapy and requested palliative care. He was discharged to hospice care facility.

3. Discussion

The clinical presentation of this patient was compatible with a "malignant psoas syndrome" that is usually secondary to infiltrating and metastatic processes [9]. Two very common differential diagnoses that must be considered in this condition are psoas abscess or psoas hematoma. However, in situations when psoas abscess is considered, the poor response to antibiotics and lack of improvement in the imaging studies after 3-4 weeks of therapy should encourage further investigation to rule out a malignant process [10]. It has been reported that 40% of the lesions initially considered as psoas abscess were found later to be lymphomas, sarcomas, or metastasis [8]. Our patient did not present any risk

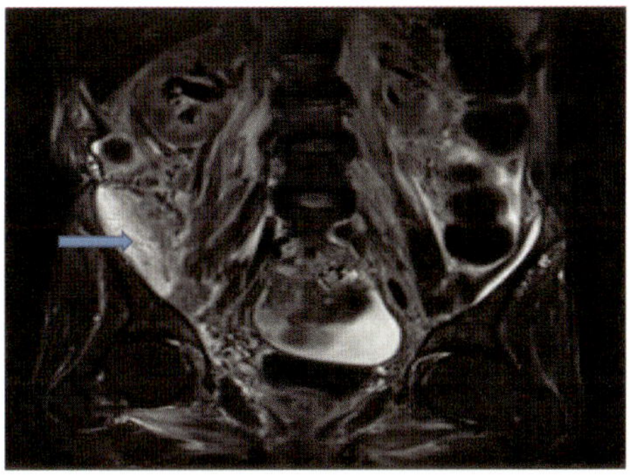

Figure 2: T2 coronal MR imaging showed enlarged predominantly hyperintense right psoas and iliopsoas (as pointed by arrow) without any discrete fluid collection. Right kidney displaced anteriorly and laterally.

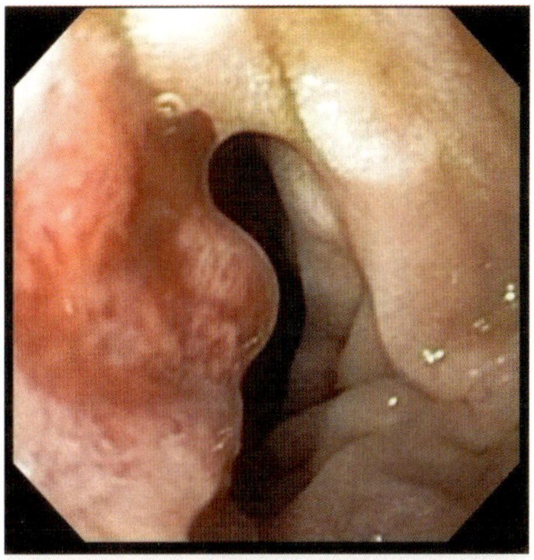

Figure 4: Duodenal mass.

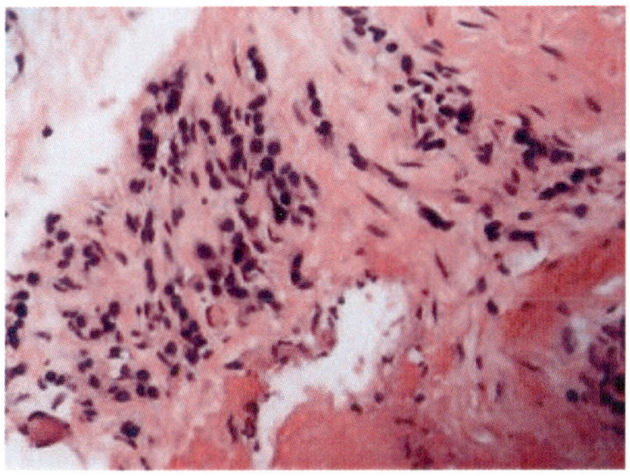

Figure 3: (H&E, 20x) CT-guided psoas muscle biopsy showing tumor cells in the dense fibroconnective tissue with background lymphocytes. The individual tumor cells are atypical, pleomorphic, and hyperchromatic in an infiltrative pattern and were cytokeratin positive, confirming the diagnosis of metastatic poorly differentiated carcinoma.

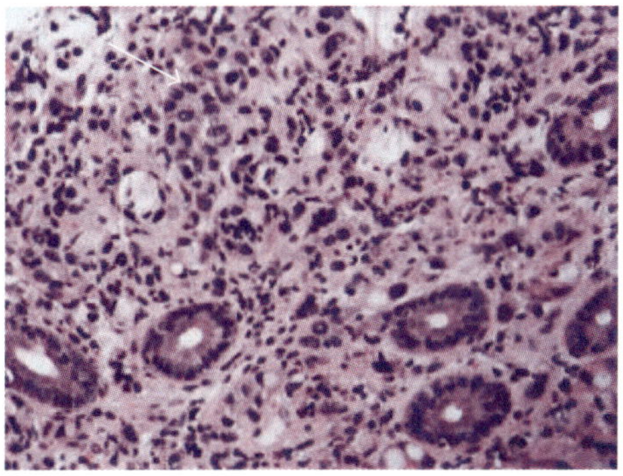

Figure 5: (H&E, 20x) Duodenal mass biopsy showing tumor cells in an infiltrative pattern interspersed within intestinal mucosa. The cells are hyperchromatic and pleomorphic and show abortive gland formation (arrow) consistent with poorly differentiated adenocarcinoma.

factor usually associated with psoas abscess [10, 11]. The clinical presentation with no fever, absence of leukocytosis, reduced C-reactive protein, negative blood cultures, and null improvement with antibiotics supported a noninfectious process. Given the strong history of smoking and chronic gastrointestinal symptoms (dysphagia and odynophagia) associated with significant weight loss, we ordered a CT scan abdomen-pelvis which showed an extensive enhancing lesion in the lower area of the right psoas. This study was not confirmatory for an abscess and was unable to show any endoluminal lesion in the small bowel or a direct extension from a tumoral process. It has been reported that muscle metastases appear as focal or diffuse areas of muscle enlargement, occasionally isodense, in noncontrast CT [12]. Contrast enhancement may provide further information on disease extent, but is nonspecific for the diagnosis of malignancy, as more than 50% of inflammatory diseases show rim enhancement postcontrast administration [13]. Some reports have shown that CT imaging give poor accuracy and sensitivity in the differentiation of iliopsoas neoplasm from abscess or hemorrhage [14]. We then evaluated this lesion by MRI, which highly suggested a malignant infiltration. Use of MRI for the diagnosis of psoas muscle disorders has been previously reported to present more than 90% sensitivity and to present higher specificity than CT for detection of sarcomas and metastatic lesions [15, 16]. In order to confirm our suspicions, we performed a CT guided biopsy which showed a metastatic poorly differentiated adenocarcinoma. Metastasis of carcinoma to the skeletal muscle is uncommon and generally found in patients with advanced-stage neoplasm. The prevalence of skeletal metastasis in the population with cancer is extremely low (0.03%) [17]. In addition, 90% of patients with skeletal muscle metastasis were found to have widespread metastatic lesions, brain, bone, and lungs being the most commons sites [18]. It is thought that constant muscle movement and the muscle's capability to remove lactic acid and free oxygen radicals produced by tumor contribute to the resistance of skeletal muscles for the metastatic process [19, 20]. Given the clinical presentation of gastrointestinal symptoms (dysphagia) and negative CT chest for lung malignancy, GI workup was started with an upper endoscopy, which was performed to locate the primary lesion. This study showed a large endoluminal mass in the second portion of the duodenum that was biopsied and later reported as poorly differentiated adenocarcinoma. To our surprise, this duodenal mass was not seen in the upper endoscopy performed in outside facility. This type of tumor is an extremely uncommon malignant lesion. The peak of frequency is the sixth decade. Signs and symptoms are unspecific and include abdominal pain (60%), weight loss (70%), nausea and vomiting (30%), jaundice (30%), and hemorrhage (40%) [21]. A palpable abdominal mass is found in less than 5% of the patients [22]. Five to 40% of the patients have distant metastases or peritoneal seeding at the time of diagnosis [23]. Complete surgical resection is the only hope for cure. Pancreatoduodenectomy and various types of lymphadenectomies have been advocated as the surgical procedure of choice because they offer the possibility of regional lymph node resection [24, 25]. Radiotherapy and chemotherapy have been used in few cases most often as an adjuvant postoperative treatment with no improvement in outcome. The 5-year survival rate varies widely according to the series published, but is generally reported to be >40% in case of curative resection and to less than 5% in cases of metastatic disease [23–25].

In summary, iliopsoas metastases may mimic psoas abscess or hematomas, both clinically (lower abdominal pain, decreased hip excursion) as well as at imaging (asymmetric swelling of psoas muscles with or without low attenuation regions showing heterogeneous enhancement that can be either unilateral or bilateral). In a patient who presents clinically with hip pain, flexion deformity, and limited extension, the characteristic imaging findings and relevant history will usually lead to the correct diagnosis. However, in a patient with unknown primary tumor but with risk factors (smoking) and chronic symptoms compatible with underlying malignancy who shows abnormalities on psoas muscle imaging, the possibility of metastases, although uncommon, should be considered.

References

[1] K. Lillemoe and A. L. Imbembo, "Malignant neoplasms of the duodenum," *Surgery Gynecology and Obstetrics*, vol. 150, no. 6, pp. 822–826, 1980.

[2] J. D. Cunningham, R. Aleali, M. Aleali, S. T. Brower, and A. H. Aufses, "Malignant small bowel neoplasms: histopathologic determinants of recurrence and survival," *Annals of Surgery*, vol. 225, no. 3, pp. 300–306, 1997.

[3] R. W. Burt, M. M. Berenson, R. G. Lee, K. G. Tolman, J. W. Freston, and E. J. Gardner, "Upper gastrointestinal polyps in Gardner's syndrome," *Gastroenterology*, vol. 86, no. 2, pp. 295–301, 1984.

[4] G. K. T. Holmes, G. I. Dunn, R. Cockel, and V. S. Brookes, "Adenocarcinoma of the upper small bowel complicating coeliac disease," *Gut*, vol. 21, no. 11, pp. 1010–1015, 1980.

[5] A. Sudo, Y. Ogihara, Y. Shiokawa, S. Fujinami, and S. Sekiguchi, "Intramuscular metastasis of carcinoma," *Clinical Orthopaedics and Related Research*, no. 296, pp. 213–217, 1993.

[6] M. E. Lampenfeld, M. A. Reiley, M. A. Fein, and C. J. Zaloudek, "Metastasis to skeletal muscle from colorectal carcinoma: a case report," *Clinical Orthopaedics and Related Research*, no. 256, pp. 193–196, 1990.

[7] P. P. McKeown, P. Conant, and L. E. Auerbach, "Squamous cell carcinoma of the lung: an unusual metastasis to pectoralis muscle," *Annals of Thoracic Surgery*, vol. 61, no. 5, pp. 1525–1526, 1996.

[8] J. B. Kenny, D. J. Widdowson, A. T. Carty, and C. E. Williams, "Malignent involvement of the iliopsoas muscle: CT appearances," *European Journal of Radiology*, vol. 10, no. 3, pp. 183–187, 1990.

[9] M. J. Stevens, C. Atkinson, and A. M. Broadbent, "The malignant psoas syndrome revisited: case report, mechanisms, and current therapeutic options," *Journal of Palliative Medicine*, vol. 13, no. 2, pp. 211–216, 2010.

[10] I. H. Mallick, M. H. Thoufeeq, and T. P. Rajendran, "Iliopsoas abscesses," *Postgraduate Medical Journal*, vol. 80, no. 946, pp. 459–462, 2004.

[11] T. Mückley, T. Schütz, M. Kirschner, M. Potulski, G. Hofmann, and V. Bühren, "Psoas abscess: the spine as a primary source of infection," *Spine*, vol. 28, no. 6, pp. E106–E113, 2003.

[12] J. B. Williams, R. A. Youngberg, L. T. Bui-Mansfield, and J. David Pitcher, "MR imaging of skeletal muscle metastases," *American Journal of Roentgenology*, vol. 168, no. 2, pp. 555–557, 1997.

[13] G. R. Avery, "Metastatic adenocarcinoma masquerading as a psoas abscess," *Clinical Radiology*, vol. 39, no. 3, pp. 319–320, 1988.

[14] L. Lenchik, D. J. Dovgan, and R. Kier, "CT of the iliopsoas compartment: value in differentiating tumor, abscess, and hematoma," *American Journal of Roentgenology*, vol. 162, no. 1, pp. 83–86, 1994.

[15] J. C. Weinreb, J. M. Cohen, and K. R. Maravilla, "Iliopsoas muscles: MR study of normal anatomy and disease," *Radiology*, vol. 156, no. 2, pp. 435–440, 1985.

[16] J. K. T. Lee and H. S. Glazer, "Psoas muscle disorders: MR imaging," *Radiology*, vol. 160, no. 3, pp. 683–687, 1986.

[17] C. L. Herring Jr., J. M. Harrelson, and S. P. Scully, "Metastatic carcinoma to skeletal muscle. A report of 15 patients," *Clinical Orthopaedics & Related Research*, no. 355, pp. 272–281, 1998.

[18] T. Arpaci, G. Ugurluer, T. Akbas, R. B. Arpaci, and M. Serin, "Imaging of the skeletal muscle metastases," *European Review for Medical and Pharmacological Sciences*, vol. 16, no. 15, pp. 2057–2063, 2012.

[19] S. Seely, "Possible reasons for the high resistance of muscle to cancer," *Medical Hypotheses*, vol. 6, no. 2, pp. 133–137, 1980.

[20] G. L. Nicolson and G. Poste, "Tumor implantation and invasion at metastatic sites.," *International Review of Experimental Pathology*, vol. 25, pp. 77–181, 1983.

[21] P.-L. Fagniez and N. Rotman, "Malignant tumors of the duodenum," in *Surgical Treatment: Evidence-Based and Problem-Oriented*, Zuckschwerdt, Munich, Germany, 2001.

[22] I. A. Spira, A. Ghazi, and W. I. Wolff, "Primary adenocarcinoma of the duodenum," *Cancer*, vol. 39, no. 4, pp. 1721–1726, 1977.

[23] D. M. Rose, S. N. Hochwald, D. S. Klimstra, and M. F. Brennan, "Primary duodenal adenocarcinoma: a ten-year experience with 79 patients," *Journal of the American College of Surgeons*, vol. 183, no. 2, pp. 89–96, 1996.

[24] N. Rotman, D. Pezet, P.-L. Fagniez, D. Cherqui, B. Celicout, and P. Lointier, "Adenocarcinoma of the duodenum: factors influencing survival," *British Journal of Surgery*, vol. 81, no. 1, pp. 83–85, 1994.

[25] H. Ohigashi, O. Ishikawa, S. Tamura et al., "Pancreatic invasion as the prognostic indicator of duodenal adenocarcinoma treated by pancreatoduodenectomy plus extended lymphadenectomy," *Surgery*, vol. 124, no. 3, pp. 510–515, 1998.

8

Portal Vein Thrombosis due to Prothrombin Gene Mutation following Sleeve Gastrectomy

Murad Baba,[1] Jordan Fakhoury,[2] and Amer Syed[1]

[1]*Department of Internal Medicine, Jersey City Medical Center, 355 Grand Street, Jersey City, NJ 07302, USA*
[2]*New York Institute of Technology College of Osteopathic Medicine, Old Westbury Northern Boulevard, Old Westbury, NY 11568, USA*

Correspondence should be addressed to Murad Baba; muurad@hotmail.com

Academic Editor: Olga I. Giouleme

Introduction. Portomesenteric thrombosis is increasingly recognized as a complication of laparoscopic sleeve gastrectomy (LSG). It often presents with abdominal pain. We present a mother and her son who both developed portal vein thrombosis (PVT) after LSG. *Case Description.* A 43-year-old woman presented complaining of sudden severe abdominal pain, two weeks after she had uncomplicated laparoscopic sleeve gastrectomy. CT scan of the abdomen and pelvis with IV contrast showed portal vein thrombosis and SMV thrombosis. Two weeks later her son had the same LSG for morbid obesity and presented with the same clinical picture. Thrombophilia workup showed heterozygous prothrombin gene mutation. *Conclusions.* A high index of suspicion is necessary to diagnose PVT; although rare, it can be potentially lethal. Anticoagulation therapy should be initiated immediately to limit the morbidities and improve the outcome. Patients with family history of thrombophilia should be investigated prior to any bariatric surgery and nonsurgical alternative treatments for morbid obesity should be strongly encouraged.

1. Introduction

The portal vein is formed by the splenic and superior mesenteric veins; it accounts for 75% of the blood supply to the liver (25% is accounted by the hepatic artery). Posterior to the neck of the pancreas, the portal vein originates from the union of the superior mesenteric and splenic veins. In the porta hepatis, the portal vein divides into the right and left branches that continue to their respective hepatic lobes, eventually emptying into hepatic sinusoids. Blood returning from the liver enters the inferior vena cava via the hepatic veins.

Portal vein thrombosis is a condition resulting from the formation of a blood clot in the extrahepatic portion of the portal vein. Local and systemic prothrombotic factors are both implicated in the development of PVTs. Infectious, inflammatory, and malignant conditions of the abdomen are the most commonly implicated local risk factors. Examples of systemic etiological factors include both congenital and acquired thrombophilic states. Recently, genetic polymorphisms such as Factor V Leiden and prothrombin 20210 gene mutation are being acknowledged as thrombogenic conditions resulting in splanchnic venous system clots [1].

According to the Centers for Disease Control and Prevention (CDC) more than 78 million Americans [2] (nearly one-third of all US adults) suffer from obesity. The American Society for Metabolic and Bariatric Surgery estimates that about 24 million have severe or morbid obesity [3]. Bariatric surgery has been shown to be the most effective and stable option of management for morbid obesity [4]. Surgery leads to significant weight loss and helps decrease the risks and improves or resolves more than 40 obesity-related diseases or conditions including certain cancers, type 2 diabetes, obstructive sleep apnea, and heart disease [5–7].

One common surgical procedure is the laparoscopic sleeve gastrectomy (LSG). LSG is a restrictive bariatric surgery procedure for high risk morbid obese patients, with lower incidence of complications and lower mortality rates in relation to the other bariatric operations. Beginning in the late 1990s, LSG was performed as the primary approach in bariatric surgeries before biliopancreatic diversion or Roux-en-Y gastric bypass [8]. This restrictive technique consisted of performing a longitudinal greater curvature gastrectomy

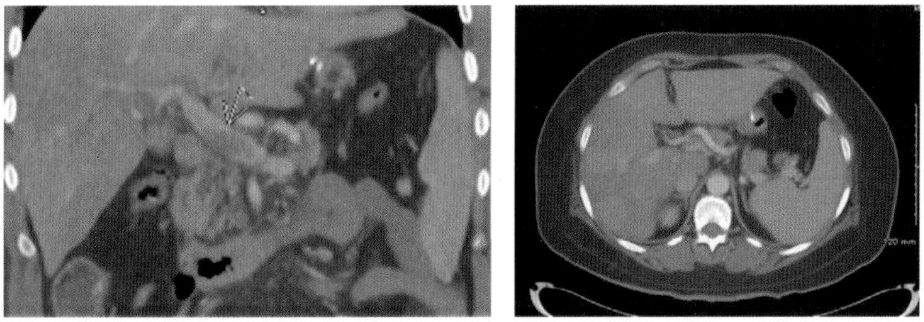

FIGURE 1: Contrast enhanced axial and coronal computed tomographic images of the abdomen. There is a lack of enhancement in the main portal vein (arrow) due to thrombosis.

starting proximal to the pylorus up to the gastroesophageal junction. The goal is to produce a restricted space with reduction in the size of the stomach to a 100 cc tube via greater curvature resection [9]. Although LSG is considered to be a safe procedure with fewer complications than other bariatric surgeries, there are still several complications to be considered [10]. An increasingly recognized yet rare complication of LSG is portomesenteric thrombosis. We report cases of postoperative PVT in a mother and her son who underwent LSG to treat morbid obesity.

2. Case Report

A 43-year-old female patient, with PMH significant for morbid obesity, diabetes mellitus, GERD, and psoriasis, presented to the emergency room complaining of sharp severe abdominal pain that started two days ago in the epigastric area, got worse gradually, and spreads to the upper abdomen with radiation to the back. It was associated with nausea, without any other symptoms. Two weeks ago she had a laparoscopic sleeve gastrectomy and was sent home with noncomplicated postoperative recovery. On physical examination, her vital signs showed tachycardia of 111 bpm; abdomen examination revealed tenderness on palpation of the upper abdomen more in the epigastric area. Labs showed she is anemic with Hb 10.5 with normal kidney function, liver function, lactic acid, and coagulation profile. Further workup was done including a CT scan of the abdomen and pelvis with IV contrast that showed partial thrombosis of the main portal vein with complete thrombosis of the left portal vein and anterior branch of right portal vein as shown in Figure 1, in addition to superior mesenteric vein thrombosis.

She was admitted and started on therapeutic anticoagulation and her diet resumed gradually as tolerated. Her hospital course was smooth, and she was discharged on Rivaroxaban/Xarelto PO. Thrombophilia workup showed that she is negative for Factor 5 Leiden mutation but positive for one copy of the G20210A mutation (heterozygous) in the prothrombin/factor 2 gene.

Two weeks later her son, a 23-year-old male with PMH of DM and morbid obesity, had a laparoscopic sleeve gastrectomy two weeks ago and presented with sharp abdominal pain in the epigastric area with radiation to whole abdomen, physical exam showed abdominal tenderness on palpation and voluntary guarding, labs revealed AST of 115, ALT of 185, and CT scan of the abdomen with IV contrast showed evidence of portal vein thrombosis and SMV thrombosis, with hepatic artery collaterals draining the liver. His thrombophilia workup showed the same gene mutation as his mother.

3. Discussion

Portal vein thrombosis (PVT) is rare; usually it is associated with liver cirrhosis or prothrombotic disorders. It can be complete or partial. Patients with acute PVT may present clinically without symptoms or can have abdominal pain.

Symptoms and signs of PVT in the postoperative period are often nonspecific especially in obese patients. Abdominal pain, nausea, and vomiting are the usual chief complaints. Patients may also present with fever and elevated white blood cell count. To establish diagnosis, ultrasonography with Doppler imaging, computed tomography (CT), and magnetic resonance (MR) of the abdomen have replaced the customary invasive test of portal venography and superior mesenteric arteriography [1]. Acute PVT appears as a filling defect in the lumen of the portal vein upon imaging with CT scan with contrast [11]. CT scan can also be helpful in determining if any bowel ischemia or infarction has occurred.

Laparoscopic sleeve gastrectomy has significantly increased in utilization through the United States medical centers surpassing gastric bypass since 2013. Becoming the most commonly performed bariatric surgery, it makes up over 60% of all weight loss surgeries performed [12]. Given that its popularity has dramatically increased, physicians must be aware of the possible complications that may be associated with this procedure.

More common acute complications of LSG include hemorrhage, staple line leak, and abscess formation while more common chronic complications include stricture formation, nutritional deficiencies, and GERD [13]. Portal and mesenteric vein thrombosis are considered rare complications; however, they may be difficult to diagnose and indeed lead to dire consequences. Portomesenteric venous thrombosis accounts for 5% to 15% of all mesenteric ischemic events [14]. Clinical presentations range from incidental findings in completely asymptomatic patients to emergency bowel infarctions and ischemia [15].

Treatment for patients diagnosed with acute PVT (as with our patient) must be started immediately: underlying conditions should be recognized and interventional therapy and/or surgery must be considered. Physicians must then investigate any hypercoagulable states and patients are subjected to 3–6 months of anticoagulation. If it is determined that patients are indeed hypercoagulable, long-term anticoagulation must be considered with the goal of recanalization of the portal vein [16]; if a hypercoagulable state is ruled out, anticoagulation should be stopped in 3–6 months.

Portomesenteric vein thrombosis has been reported with several other laparoscopic surgical procedures including splenectomy, right hemicolectomy, and cholecystectomy [17, 18]. It is still uncertain what during laparoscopic procedures leads to the increased risk of thrombosis. It has been hypothesized that hemodynamic changes in pneumoperitoneum due to increased intra-abdominal pressure may play a role in thrombosis [19]. Furthermore, visceral vasoconstriction due to an increase of vasopressin intraoperatively, the retention of CO_2 causing increased portal pressure, and patient positioning during surgery may all also affect portal blood flow. Several case reports [20–23] and studies [11, 24] have shown PVT occurring after laparoscopic sleeve gastrectomy. Most recently, a patient who underwent uncomplicated LSG presented two weeks after the surgery with epigastric pain was diagnosed with PVT, a case very similar to the one presented. However, the thrombophilia workup for that patient was unremarkable [20].

The risk of thromboembolism following bariatric surgery extends long after discharge from the hospital; this should raise the question of continuing thromboprophylaxis for several weeks postoperatively and it was suggested by some studies in the literature [25].

4. Conclusion

Portal vein thrombosis represents an important clinical problem encountered by physicians. A high index of suspicion is necessary to diagnose this rare, but potentially lethal, complication. LSG is a safe procedure with low morbidity. Patients with family history of thrombophilia should be investigated prior to any bariatric surgery and nonsurgical alternative treatments for morbid obesity should be strongly encouraged.

References

[1] S. Parikh, R. Shah, and P. Kapoor, "Portal vein thrombosis," *American Journal of Medicine*, vol. 123, no. 2, pp. 111–119, 2010.

[2] C. L. Ogden, M. D. Carroll, B. K. Kit, and K. M. Flegal, "Prevalence of childhood and adult obesity in the United States, 2011-2012," *Journal of the American Medical Association*, vol. 311, no. 8, pp. 806–814, 2014.

[3] American Society for Metabolic and Bariatric Surgery, *Fact Sheet*, American Society for Metabolic and Bariatric Surgery, Gainesville, Fla, USA, 2013.

[4] R. A. Weiner, "Indications and principles of metabolic surgery," *U.S. National Library of Medicine*, vol. 81, no. 4, pp. 379–396, 2010.

[5] S. Chikunguwo, P. W. Dodson, J. G. Meador et al., "Durable resolution of diabetes after roux-en-y gastric bypass associated with maintenance of weight loss," *Surgery for Obesity and Related Diseases*, vol. 5, no. 3, p. S1, 2009.

[6] L. M. Kaplan, "Body weight regulation and obesity," *Journal of Gastrointestinal Surgery*, vol. 7, no. 4, pp. 443–451, 2003.

[7] A. Kokkinos, K. Alexiadou, C. Liaskos et al., "Improvement in cardiovascular indices after Roux-en-Y gastric bypass or sleeve gastrectomy for morbid obesity," *Obesity Surgery*, vol. 23, no. 1, pp. 31–38, 2013.

[8] D. Cottam, F. G. Qureshi, S. G. Mattar et al., "Laparoscopic sleeve gastrectomy as an initial weight-loss procedure for high-risk patients with morbid obesity," *Surgical Endoscopy and Other Interventional Techniques*, vol. 20, no. 6, pp. 859–863, 2006.

[9] P. E. Roa, O. Kaidar-Person, D. Pinto, M. Cho, S. Szomstein, and R. J. Rosenthal, "Laparoscopic sleeve gastrectomy as treatment for morbid obesity: technique and short-term outcome," *Obesity Surgery*, vol. 16, no. 10, pp. 1323–1326, 2006.

[10] E. E. Frezza, S. Reddy, L. L. Gee, and M. S. Wachtel, "Complications after sleeve gastrectomy for morbid obesity," *Obesity Surgery*, vol. 19, no. 6, pp. 684–687, 2009.

[11] M. C. Haddad, D. C. Clark, H. S. Sharif, M. Al Shahed, O. Aideyan, and B. M. Sammak, "MR, CT, and ultrasonography of splanchnic venous thrombosis," *Gastrointestinal Radiology*, vol. 17, no. 1, pp. 34–40, 1992.

[12] J. V. Varela and N. T. Nguyen, "Laparoscopic sleeve gastrectomy leads the U.S. utilization of bariatric surgery at academic medical centers," *Surgery for Obesity and Related Diseases*, 2015.

[13] K. Sarkhosh, D. W. Birch, A. Sharma, and S. Karmali, "Complications associated with laparoscopic sleeve gastrectomy for morbid obesity: a surgeon's guide," *Canadian Journal of Surgery*, vol. 56, no. 5, pp. 347–352, 2013.

[14] J. H. Grendell and R. K. Ockner, "Mesenteric venous thrombosis," *Gastroenterology*, vol. 82, no. 2, pp. 358–372, 1982.

[15] A. W. James, C. Rabl, A. C. Westphalen, P. F. Fogarty, A. M. Posselt, and G. M. Campos, "Portomesenteric venous thrombosis after laparoscopic surgery: a systematic literature review," *Archives of Surgery*, vol. 144, no. 6, pp. 520–526, 2009.

[16] B. Condat, F. Pessione, S. Hillaire et al., "Current outcome of portal vein thrombosis in adults: risk and benefit of anticoagulant therapy," *Gastroenterology*, vol. 120, no. 2, pp. 490–497, 2001.

[17] K. W. Millikan, S. M. Szczerba, J. M. Dominguez, R. McKenna, and J. C. Rorig, "Superior mesenteric and portal vein thrombosis following laparoscopic-assisted right hemicolectomy. Report of a case," *Diseases of the Colon and Rectum*, vol. 39, no. 10, pp. 1171–1175, 1996.

[18] U. Haglund, K. Norlen, I. Rasmussen et al., "Complications related to pneumoperitoneum," in *Complications of Laparoscopic Surgery*, R. W. Bailey and J. L. Flowers, Eds., pp. 45–48, Quality Medical, St. Louis, Mo, USA, 1995.

[19] N. Abu-Jkeim, A. Al-Hazmi, A. A. M. Alawad et al., "Portal vein thrombosis following laparoscopic sleeve gastrectomy: a rare case report," *International Journal of Case Reports and Images*, vol. 6, no. 9, pp. 556–559, 2015.

[20] B. Berthet, E. Bollon, R. Valero, M. Ouaissi, I. Sielezneff, and B. Sastre, "Portal vein thrombosis due to factor 2 leiden in the post-operative course of a laparoscopic sleeve gastrectomy for morbid obesity," *Obesity Surgery*, vol. 19, no. 10, pp. 1464–1467, 2009.

[21] J. M. Rosenberg, M. Tedesco, D. C. Yao, and D. Eisenberg, "Portal vein thrombosis following laparoscopic sleeve gastrectomy for morbid obesity," *Journal of the Society of Laparoendoscopic Surgeons*, vol. 16, no. 4, pp. 639–643, 2012.

[22] R. Lopez and R. Flint, "Portal vein thrombosis as a complication of laparoscopic sleeve gastrectomy," *The New Zealand Medical Journal*, vol. 126, no. 1386, pp. 103–105, 2013.

[23] J. Salinas, D. Barros, N. Salgado et al., "Portomesenteric vein thrombosis after laparoscopic sleeve gastrectomy," *Surgical Endoscopy*, vol. 28, no. 4, pp. 1083–1089, 2014.

[24] D. Goitein, I. Matter, A. Raziel et al., "Portomesenteric thrombosis following laparoscopic bariatric surgery: incidence, patterns of clinical presentation, and etiology in a bariatric patient population," *The JAMA Surgery*, vol. 148, no. 4, pp. 340–346, 2013.

[25] K. E. Steele, M. A. Schweitzer, G. Prokopowicz et al., "The long-term risk of venous thromboembolism following bariatric surgery," *Obesity Surgery*, vol. 21, no. 9, pp. 1371–1376, 2011.

9

Diagnosis and Treatment of Esophageal Granular Cell Tumor: A Case Report and Review of the Literature

Ramin Niknam,[1] Kamran Bagheri Lankarani,[2] and Bita Geramizadeh[3]

[1] *Gastroenterohepatology Research Center, Shiraz University of Medical Sciences, Shiraz, Iran*
[2] *Health Policy Research Center, Shiraz University of Medical Sciences, Shiraz, Iran*
[3] *Department of Pathology, Transplant Research Center, Shiraz University of Medical Sciences, Shiraz, Iran*

Correspondence should be addressed to Ramin Niknam; niknamramin@yahoo.com

Academic Editor: Naohiko Koide

Gastrointestinal granular cell tumors are uncommon. The most common site of gastrointestinal granular cell tumor (GCT) is esophagus. We report a case of esophageal GCT incidentally diagnosed by endoscopy. The lesion was evaluated by endoscopic ultrasonography and resected using the endoscopic technique without complication.

1. Introduction

Granular cell tumor (GCT) was described in 1926 by Abrikossoff [1]. These tumors may arise in different organs [2]. The origin of GCTs is the Schwann cell. These tumors consist of fusiform and polygonal cells in compact nests with dark nuclei and abundant eosinophilic granular cytoplasm [3, 4].

The most common site of gastrointestinal GCTs is esophagus that only a few cases have been reported in the literature [4–6]. In this report, we described a case of esophageal GCT treated by the endoscopic technique. We also review some literature on diagnosis and management of GCTs.

2. Case Report

A 50-year-old woman presented to our center with dyspepsia from three months prior to evaluation. Past medical history was unremarkable. The physical examination was normal. Upper gastrointestinal endoscopy was performed for evaluation of cause of dyspepsia. Endoscopy identified a firm submucosal yellow lesion, measuring approximately 10 mm and located 30 cm distal from the incisor teeth (Figure 1). The stomach and duodenum were normal. Biopsies by forceps were taken from the esophageal lesion. The histologic assessment was in favor of GCT.

Endoscopic ultrasonography (EUS) was performed by linear echo with frequency of 10 MHZ. EUS identified a submucosal lesion with a diameter of 12 mm. It was a nonhomogeneous hyperechoic solid lesion with clear border with no extension to muscularis layer and without mediastinal adenopathies (Figure 1).

The patient was considered for endoscopic resection of lesion. After deep sedation with intravenous Propofol (Lipuro-1%), submucosal injection of 5 ml diluted epinephrine solution (0.01 mg/ml) with 0.5 ml methylene blue was done using a sclerotherapy needle (ENDO-FLEX-Germany). After creation of the submucosal fluid bulging, the resection of lesion was performed using a monofilament rotatable polypectomy snare (Boston; 20 mm; output setting: cut 40 watts; coagulation 40 watts) without any complication (Figure 2). The resected specimen was removed by basket. The size of specimen was 12×5 mm with yellow color (Figure 2). The specimen was fixed in 10% formalin and transferred to the lab for histologic assessment.

In histologic examination, the diagnosis of GCT was confirmed. Histological analysis of specimen revealed nests of medium-sized cells with abundant eosinophilic granular cytoplasm with bland looking nuclei without any atypia or pleomorphism (Figure 3).

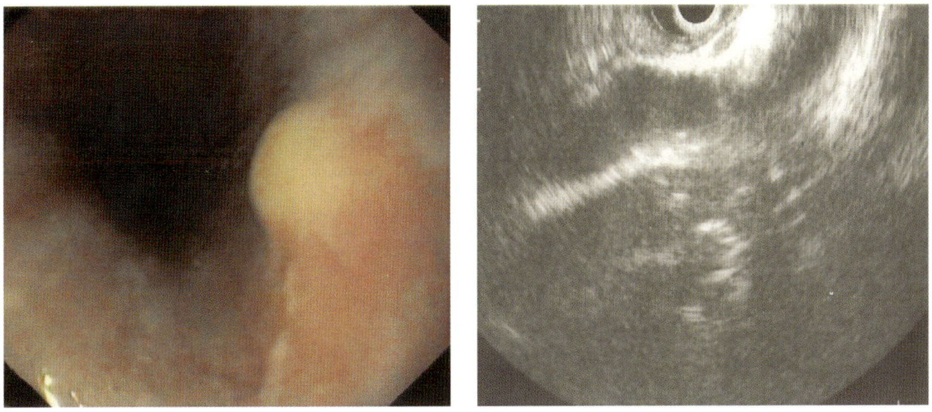

(a) (b)

FIGURE 1: Endoscopic view of an elevated yellow submucosal lesion in esophagus (a). Endosonographic image showed a nonhomogeneous hyperechoic submucosal lesion with a diameter of 12 mm and without extension to muscularis layer (b).

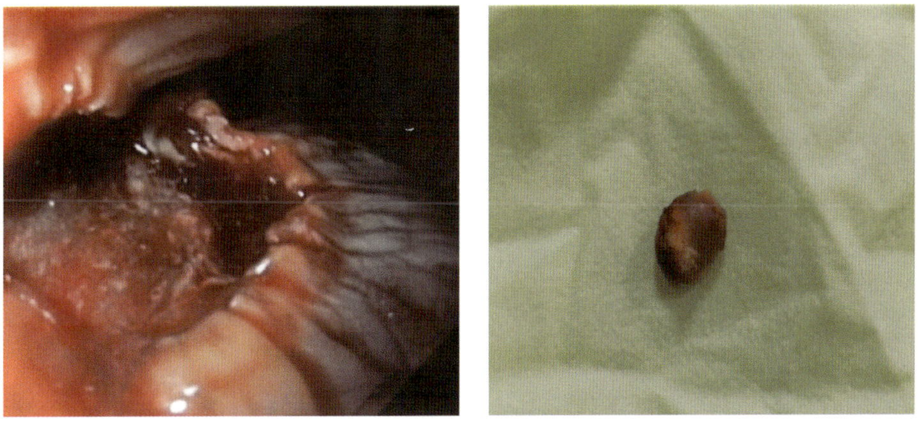

(a) (b)

FIGURE 2: Endoscopic view of the esophagus after endoscopic treatment of tumor (a). Gross appearance of the tumor after endoscopic treatment (b).

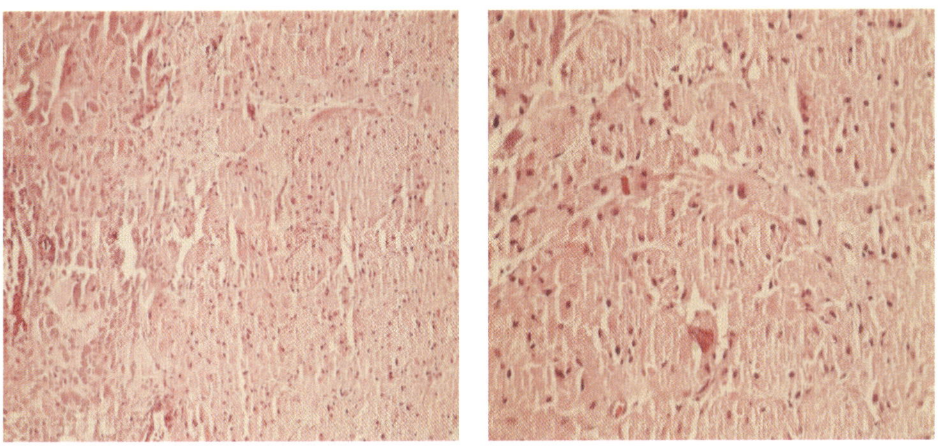

(a) (b)

FIGURE 3: Section of the esophageal wall (a) showed nests of medium-sized cells with abundant eosinophilic granular cytoplasm (H&E ×100). High power view of the tumor in the esophageal wall (b) showed the above-mentioned cells with bland looking nuclei without any atypia or pleomorphism (H&E ×400).

Follow-up endoscopy 9 months after removal of tumor showed complete healing of the site of resection in esophagus.

3. Discussion

The most common site of GCTs is tongue although these tumors may arise in other organs [2]. Gastrointestinal GCTs are uncommon. The most common site of gastrointestinal GCTs is esophagus that approximately 270 cases have been reported in the literature [4–6]. Esophageal GCTs usually appear as a white-gray to yellow submucosal mass that may be mistaken for other lesions such as lipoma, leiomyoma, and cyst [2, 4].

Esophageal GCTs are usually asymptomatic and found incidentally during endoscopy. The tumor may present with dysphagia when it is larger than 1 cm [2, 4, 7–9].

Although most esophageal GCTs have a benign clinical course, malignant tumors were reported in the literature. Malignant GCTs are usually larger than 4 cm [4, 10] with rapid growth and invasion of the adjacent tissues and high recurrence rate after excision [2, 11]. Tumor cell spindling and necrosis, increased mitotic activity with pleomorphism, and large nucleoli with high nuclear to cytoplasmic ratio are histologic evidence in favor of malignant GCTs [12].

EUS is useful technique for deciding the type of management of GCTs [4, 13]. EUS pattern of esophageal GCTs appears as a solid hypoechoic lesion with a smooth borders and mildly inhomogeneous echo pattern [2, 14]. They usually originate in the muscularis mucosa or submucosal layer of the esophagus. For evaluation of the role of EUS in the diagnosis of GCTs, a study in 15 patients with esophageal GCTs was performed by Palazzo et al. They concluded that EUS can contribute to planning the management of GCTs [14].

In order to compare EUS findings and histopathological analysis of resected submucosal lesions, Yazumi et al. studied 18 consecutive patients with esophageal submucosal tumors (5 GCTs and 13 leiomyomas). They concluded that EUS is useful for differentiating esophageal GCTs from leiomyomas [15].

The optimum management of GCTs is controversial [12]. Endoscopic follow-up for asymptomatic tumors less than 10 mm, endoscopic resection for tumors 10–20 mm [4, 12, 16, 17], and surgical excision for tumors more than 20 mm or symptomatic patient [12, 18] are generally recommended.

Similar to our case, Nakajima et al. reported a case of esophageal GCT diagnosed by endoscopic biopsy and EUS that treated by endoscopic submucosal dissection. They concluded that ESD is a safe and accurate procedure for GCTs [4]. De Ceglie et al. also reported a case of esophageal GCT diagnosed by endoscopic biopsy and EUS that was treated by EMR without any complication [2].

Similar to some reports, GCT in our patient was incidentally diagnosed by endoscopy [7, 9]. Because of the size of tumor 10–20 mm, similar to some reports, we treated the tumor by endoscopic resection [4, 16, 17].

Based on our experience and other published reports [2, 4, 14] we recommend that the submucosal lesion of esophagus can be evaluated by biopsy and EUS. If biopsy and/or EUS finding shows high possibility for diagnosis of GCT, endoscopic treatment can be safely scheduled for the tumors with size 10–20 mm.

Authors' Contributions

Ramin Niknam was the physician in charge and assisted in study supervision, endoscopic resection, and manuscript writing. Kamran Bagheri Lankarani conducted the endoscopic ultrasonography evaluation. Bita Geramizadeh helped in histology evaluation.

Acknowledgments

The authors would like to acknowledge the Center for Development of Clinical Research of Nemazee Hospital, Shiraz University of Medical Sciences, Shiraz, Iran, for editorial assistance.

References

[1] A. Abrikossoff, "Über Myome ausgehend von der quergestreiften willkürlichen Muskulatur," *Virchows Archiv für pathologische Anatomie und Physiologie und für klinische Medizin*, vol. 260, no. 1, pp. 215–233, 1926.

[2] A. De Ceglie, B. Gatteschi, S. Blanchi, F. Scotto, A. Pellecchia, and M. Conio, "Esophageal granular cell tumor treated by endoscopic mucosal resection. A case report and review of the literature," *Digestive Diseases and Sciences*, vol. 50, no. 10, pp. 1875–1879, 2005.

[3] A. Giacobbe, D. Facciorusso, P. Conoscitore, F. Spirito, M. M. Squillante, and M. Bisceglia, "Granular cell tumor of the esophagus," *American Journal of Gastroenterology*, vol. 83, no. 12, pp. 1398–1400, 1988.

[4] M. Nakajima, H. Kato, H. Muroi et al., "Esophageal granular cell tumor successfully resected by endoscopic submucosal dissection," *Esophagus*, vol. 8, no. 3, pp. 203–207, 2011.

[5] E. E. Lack, G. F. Worsham, M. D. Callihan et al., "Granular cell tumor: a clinicopathologic study of 110 patients," *Journal of Surgical Oncology*, vol. 13, no. 4, pp. 301–316, 1980.

[6] S. Perçinel, B. Savaş, G. Yilmaz et al., "Granular cell tumor of the esophagus: three case reports and review of the literature," *The Turkish Journal of Gastroenterology*, vol. 19, no. 3, pp. 184–188, 2008.

[7] J. R. Goldblum, T. W. Rice, G. Zuccaro, and J. E. Richter, "Granular cell tumors of the esophagus: a clinical and pathologic study of 13 cases," *The Annals of Thoracic Surgery*, vol. 62, no. 3, pp. 860–865, 1996.

[8] B. Geramizadeh and P. Ali Nowshadi, "Photoclinic," *Archives of Iranian Medicine*, vol. 16, no. 1, Article ID 013161, pp. 59-60, 2013.

[9] T. Toyanaga, M. Man-I, D. Ivanov et al., "The results and limitations of endoscopic submucosal dissection for colorectal tumors," *Acta Chirurgica Iugoslavica*, vol. 55, no. 3, pp. 17–23, 2008.

[10] J. C. Fanburg-Smith, J. M. Meis-Kindblom, R. Fante, and L.-G. Kindblom, "Malignant granular cell tumor of soft tissue: diagnostic criteria and clinicopathologic correlation," *The American Journal of Surgical Pathology*, vol. 22, no. 7, pp. 779–794, 1998.

[11] J. Orlowska, J. Pachlewski, A. Gugulski, and E. Butruk, "A conservative approach to granular cell tumors of the esophagus: four case reports and literature review," *American Journal of Gastroenterology*, vol. 88, no. 2, pp. 311–315, 1993.

[12] L. De Rezende, A. J. Lucendo, and H. Álvarez-Argüelles, "Granular cell tumors of the esophagus: report of five cases and review of diagnostic and therapeutic techniques," *Diseases of the Esophagus*, vol. 20, no. 5, pp. 436–443, 2007.

[13] D. U. Kim, G. H. Kim, D. Y. Ryu et al., "Endosonographic features of esophageal granular cell tumors using a high-frequency catheter probe," *Scandinavian Journal of Gastroenterology*, vol. 46, no. 2, pp. 142–147, 2011.

[14] L. Palazzo, B. Landi, C. Cellier et al., "Endosonographic features of esophageal granular cell tumors," *Endoscopy*, vol. 29, no. 9, pp. 850–853, 1997.

[15] S. Yazumi, R. Takahashi, T. Kajiyama et al., "Comparison of histological analysis and endosonographic features in esophageal granular cell tumors," *Digestive Endoscopy*, vol. 15, no. 4, pp. 284–288, 2003.

[16] S. Okahara, S. Tanaka, and K. Haruma, "A case of granular cell tumor of the esophagus resected endoscopically," *The Hiroshima Medical Association*, vol. 48, pp. 810–814, 1995.

[17] I. Yasuda, E. Tomita, K. Nagura, Y. Nishigaki, O. Yamada, and H. Kachi, "Endoscopic removal of granular cell tumors," *Gastrointestinal Endoscopy*, vol. 41, no. 2, pp. 163–167, 1995.

[18] D. S. Coutinho, J. Soga, T. Yoshikawa, K. Miyashita, O. Tanaka, K. Sasaki et al., "Granular cell tumors of the esophagus: a report of two cases and review of the literature," *The American Journal of Gastroenterology*, vol. 80, pp. 758–762, 1985.

10

Amyand's Hernia: Rare Presentation of a Common Ailment

Sanjeev Singhal,[1] Anu Singhal,[2] Sanjay Singh Negi,[3] Rahul Tugnait,[1] Pankaj Kumar Arora,[1] Bishwanath Tiwari,[1] Pawan Malik,[1] Lav Gupta,[1] Amit Bimal,[1] Abhishek Gupta,[1] Rahul Gupta,[1] Pushkar Chouhan,[1] and ChandraKant Singh[1]

[1] *Department of Surgery, Northern Railway Central Hospital, Basant Lane, New Delhi 110055, India*
[2] *Department of Radiology, ESI PGIMSR, Basaidarapur, Ring Road, New Delhi 110015, India*
[3] *GI and HPB Surgery, Dr. BL Kapoor Memorial Hospital, Pusa Road, New Delhi 110005, India*

Correspondence should be addressed to Anu Singhal; drsinghal_anu@yahoo.co.in

Academic Editor: I. Michael Leitman

Inguinal hernia with vermiform appendix as content is known as Amyand's hernia. It is a rare entity but we encountered four cases within six months. A 52-year-old female had high grade fever and evidence of inflammatory pathology involving the ileocaecal region. She was initially managed conservatively and subsequently underwent exploratory laparatomy. The appendix was perforated and herniating in the inguinal canal. Appendectomy was done with herniorrhaphy without mesh placement. A 74-year-old male with bilateral inguinal hernia, of which, the right side was more symptomatic, underwent open exploration. Operative findings revealed a lipoma of the sac and a normal appearing appendix as content. Contents were reduced without appendectomy and mesh hernioplasty was performed. A 63-year-old male with an obstructed right sided hernia underwent emergency inguinal exploration which revealed edematous caecum and appendix as content without any inflammation. Contents were reduced without any resection. Herniorrhaphy was performed without mesh placement. A 66-year-old male with an uncomplicated right inguinal hernia underwent elective surgery. The sac revealed an appendix with adhesions at the neck. Contents were reduced after adhesiolysis and hernioplasty was performed with mesh placement. Emphasis is made to the rarity of disease, variation in presentation, and difference in treatment modalities depending upon the state of appendix.

1. Introduction

Various organs have been described as contents of inguinal hernia. Of these, one of the rarest is the vermiform appendix. The incidence of having a normal appendix within the inguinal hernial sac varies from 0.5% to 1%. Appendicitis in the inguinal canal occurs even less frequently, with the reported incidence being between 0.07% and 0.13%. However, incidence as high as 1% has also been reported. Perforated appendix and periappendicular abscess formation within an inguinal hernia sac is even rarer. The incidence of appendicitis in general population is about 8% but only around 0.1% of all cases of appendicitis present in an inguinal hernia [1–4]. The term Amyand's hernia has been used to describe varying clinical scenarios like (a) the occurrence of an inflamed appendix within an inguinal hernia (b), finding a perforated appendix within an inguinal hernia (c), or the presence of a noninflamed appendix within an irreducible inguinal hernia [5]. This anomaly was first described by Amyand in 1735. The eponym Amyand's hernia was first coined by Creese in 1953 and then by Hiatt and Hiatt in 1988, followed by Hutchinson in 1993 [1].

We encountered 4 cases of this rare disease over a relatively short period of about 6 months. This prompted us to present our series of cases along with a detailed review of literature.

2. Case 1

A 52-year-old lady presented with discomfort in right inguinal region. Ultrasound (USG) revealed a small collection in the inguinal canal which was aspirated. She was treated conservatively with antibiotics. After 2 weeks, she again presented with high grade fever, pain in the right iliac fossa and

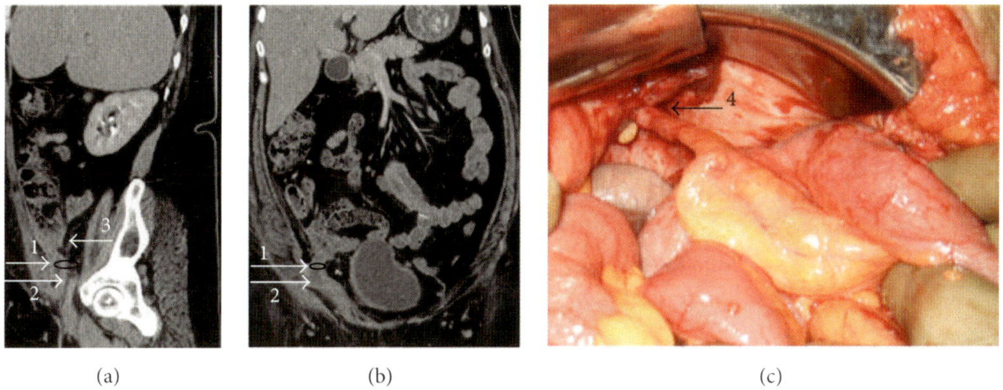

FIGURE 1: (a) and (b) display the sagittal and coronal views, respectively, of CECT of the first case: 1, black ring depicts the region of right deep ring defect; 2 depicts the herniating appendix; and 3 denotes the caecum. (c) is an operative photograph of the first case showing 4, the inflamed appendix from caecum to its entry in the inguinal canal.

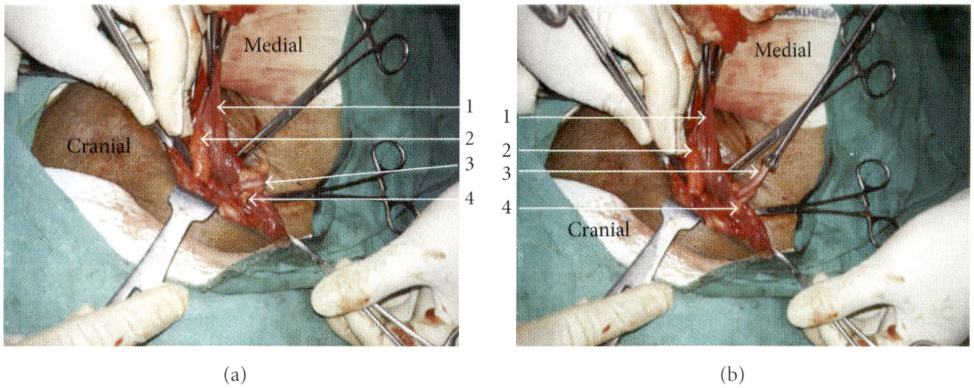

FIGURE 2: (a) and (b) are operative photographs of the second case showing 1, the opened right indirect hernial sac; 2, lipoma of the sac wall; 3, normal healthy appendix as a content of the sac; and 4, a normal healthy mesoappendix.

inguinal area, and a lump in the right iliac fossa. Computed tomography (CT) revealed a mass in right iliac fossa where appendix could not be delineated (Figures 1(a) and 1(b)). She was worked up for possible appendicitis or abdominal Koch's with infection tracking along ilioinguinal nerve, but all investigations were noncontributory. Her symptoms did not subside even after 6 weeks of antibiotic therapy and a repeat CT was again indicative of inflammatory pathology in the ileocaecal area. She underwent exploratory laparotomy with lower midline incision. The operative findings included perforated appendix herniating into the right inguinal canal (Figure 1(c)) with periappendicular abscess formation and an umbilical hernia. Appendectomy with drainage of pus, lavage of peritoneal cavity, and primary closure of the hernial defects in the inguinal and umbilical region were done. Postoperatively she developed a small collection in the surgical site which was aspirated under USG guidance. She has recurrence of the umbilical hernia but has otherwise remained comfortable over last 8 months of follow-up.

3. Case 2

A 74-year-old gentleman presented with swellings in both inguinal areas, right more than left, which were gradually progressive over the previous 6 months. The swellings increased on standing and walking but the right sided swelling was not completely reducible. He was a known case of hypertension and coronary artery disease and had undergone bypass surgery 13 years back. A diagnosis of bilateral indirect inguinal hernia, right more than left, was made. He underwent unilateral open inguinal hernia surgery under local anaesthetic block, because of poor cardiac status. Right side was operated as it was partially irreducible and more symptomatic. Operative findings included a lipoma of the sac wall and a normal looking appendix as content of the indirect hernial sac (Figures 2(a) and 2(b)). The adhesions at the neck of the sac were separated and the contents reduced. Mesh hernioplasty was performed using a composite mesh of polypropylene and poliglecaprone. Patient had an uneventful postoperative recovery and is maintaining good health on 6-month follow-up.

4. Case 3

A 63-year-old gentleman presented with a longstanding right sided inguinal hernia which had become irreducible for 1 day. The patient had associated history of nonpassage of stools and flatus along with multiple episodes of bilious projectile vomiting over the same duration. He had tachycardia, and on examination there was an irreducible right sided inguinal

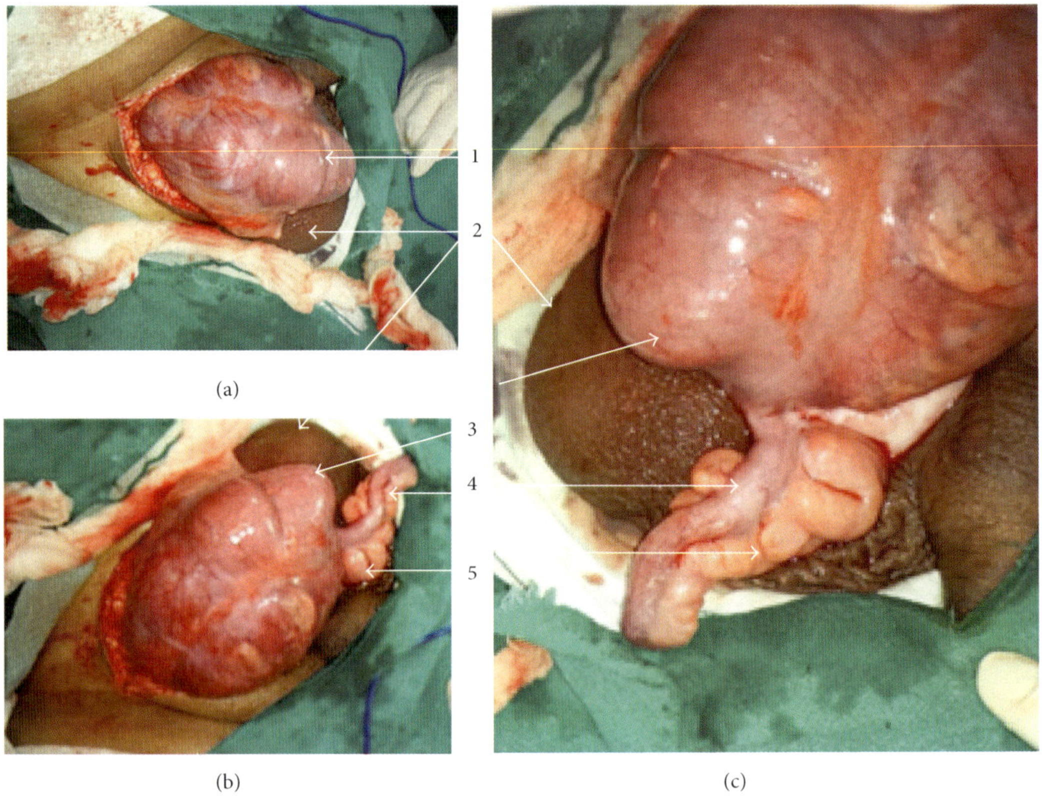

FIGURE 3: (a), (b), and (c) are operative photographs of the third case showing 1, the obstructed right sided hernial sac; 2, scrotum; 3, caecum; 4, appendix; and 5, mesoappendix. The caecum, appendix, and mesoappendix are edematous but otherwise healthy and show no signs of inflammation.

hernia with tenderness and erythema of the overlying skin. A provisional diagnosis of obstructed right sided inguinal hernia with impending strangulation was made. Patient was taken up for emergency surgery.

Intraoperatively, an obstructed indirect sac was found with the level of obstruction at deep ring. It had caecum and appendix as contents. The bowel, though oedematous, was viable and healthy (Figures 3(a), 3(b), and 3(c)). The obstruction was relieved, contents were reduced, and herniorrhaphy (Bassini's repair) was performed. The patient had an uneventful recovery and is in good health on a 5-month follow-up.

5. Case 4

A 66-year-old male patient presented with history of left inguinal swelling for 6 months which was reducible and used to increase in size on straining. After thorough examination it was diagnosed as left indirect uncomplicated inguinal hernia. Patient had no significant comorbidities. He was taken up for surgery after all necessary investigations and preanaesthetic fitness.

He underwent hernioplasty under inguinal block. Intraoperatively an indirect sac was found and dissected free of cord structures. On opening, it revealed appendix as content. There were flimsy adhesions of mesoappendix with the neck of the sac (Figures 4(a) and 4(b)). The adhesions were gently broken and appendix was reduced. Hernioplasty was completed using a composite mesh of polypropylene and poliglecaprone. Patient had an uneventful postoperative recovery and has remained comfortable over last 3 months of follow-up.

6. Discussion

Amyand's hernia, which means the presence of a normal or pathological appendix as a content of inguinal hernia, is a rare clinical entity. D'Alia et al. reported an incidence of just 0.08%, in 1341 patients of inguinal hernias over a 13-year period in Messina University Hospital in 2003 [7]. Presence of appendicitis in inguinal hernia is even more uncommon. Solecki et al. observed that acute appendicitis was found in 0.62% of all groin hernia sacs [8] whereas Ryan reported that only 11 of 8,692 cases of acute appendicitis occurred in external hernia of all forms [9]. The incidence of acute appendicitis occurring in a hernial sac varies between the 0.13% reported by Ryan in 1937 and the 1% reported by Carey in 1967 [10]. Thomas et al. reported only 7 cases of acute appendicitis occurring in an external hernia sac during 8 years [11]. In a review of 18 cases, the median age was 42 years, with the oldest age noted in literature being 89 years. However, age of these cases ranges from 3 weeks to 88 years [12]. It is more common in men and almost always on the right side probably because of the normal anatomical position of the appendix and also because right sided inguinal herniae are more common. Left sided Amyand's herniae are even rarer. They may be associated with situs inversus, malrotation,

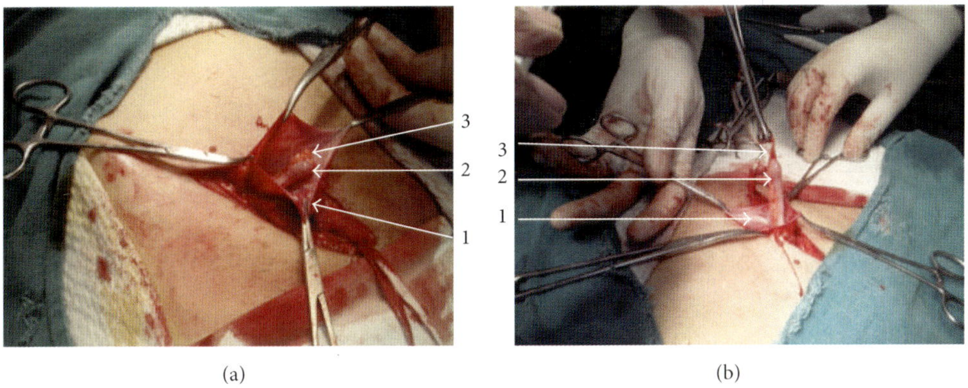

FIGURE 4: (a) and (b) are operative photographs of the fourth case showing 1, the opened right indirect hernial sac; 2, normal healthy appendix as a content of the sac; and 3, a normal healthy mesoappendix.

or a very mobile caecum [2]. Though all our cases were right sided, one was in a female. All our male patients were over 60 years and the female patient was 52 years old. The average age of our patients was 63.75 years.

Appendix in a hernial sac was first reported in a femoral hernia, in 1731 by De Garengeot [13]. Appendix in an inguinal hernia was first reported by Amyand, sergeant surgeon to King George II of England, on December 6, 1735. His patient was Hanvil Anderson, an 11-year-old boy, with an appendiceal abscess, presenting with "a fistula between the scrotum and thigh." He treated the child by a transhernial appendectomy and pathology revealed a chronically inflamed appendix included within the inguinal hernia sac and perforated by a previously swallowed pin. He not only described the first case of appendicitis in the inguinal canal (later named as Amyand's hernia), but also performed the world's first recorded successful appendectomy. The patient eventually recovered and was "discharged with a truss, which he was ordered to wear for some time." The case was published in the Philosophical Transactions of the Royal Society of London. Though the appendectomy was successful, the hernia later recurred [4, 13–15]. Therefore, in his honour, an inguinal hernia containing the vermiform appendix, whether it is inflamed or not, is called "Amyand's hernia." Interestingly the first appendicectomy performed in USA by Robert J Hall a century and a half later, in 1886, was also performed in a case of perforated appendix within an inguinal hernia, another example of Amyand's hernia [16].

The pathophysiology of appendicitis in Amyand's hernia is unknown. Majority of the cases have appendicitis incarcerated in a hernia. Weber et al. proposed that, due to herniation, the appendix becomes more vulnerable to microtrauma causing inflammation and adherence of appendix to the hernial sac due to fibrosis. This hypothesis that inflammatory swelling may lead to incarceration and subsequent impaired blood supply and bacterial overgrowth was supported by several other authors. Muscle contraction and changes in abdominal pressure cause compression of appendix resulting in decreased blood supply and secondary inflammation [1, 2]. It is difficult to determine whether appendicitis is the main pathology or if the primary event is strangulation of the herniated appendix, leading to ischemic necrosis and secondary inflammation.

Preoperative diagnosis requires high index of clinical suspicion as there are no typical or pathognomonic symptoms. Clinical picture may vary depending on the extent of periappendicular inflammation and the presence or absence of peritoneal contamination. It is a differential diagnosis of an irreducible inguinal hernia and inguinal lymphadenitis as well as an acute scrotum. It may present as a strangulated hernia, testicular torsion or tumors, epididymitis, a fistula or an abscess of the scrotum, thigh, or abdominal wall, or an incidental finding. Tenderness over McBurney's point is usually absent [5, 17]. Due to these facts, it is difficult to reach a clinical diagnosis of Amyand's hernia. Diagnosis is usually made intraoperatively when the patient undergoes surgical exploration. In one review of 60 cases over a 12-year period, only one case was diagnosed preoperatively [18]. Laermans et al. in 2003 reported only two cases where diagnosis was established prior to surgery. Ultrasound often demonstrates a potentially inflammatory mass within the hernial sac. An abdominal CT scan could diagnose the condition but is usually not performed [5, 17]. Diagnosis is made by demonstration of an inguinal herniation containing a blind-ending tubular structure with thickened walls, in connection with the caecum. Multiplanar reconstructions are most useful in order to better visualize the appendix and demonstrate its relationship with surrounding structures [17]. The CT scan done in our first case could only pick up the abnormality retrospectively.

There are two issues in treatment of Amyand's hernia, whether to perform an appendectomy or not and whether or not to use mesh in hernia repair. The presence or absence of inflammation of appendix is an important determinant of appropriate treatment. If appendicitis is present, a transherniotomy appendectomy is advocated. Associated intra-abdominal abscess should be drained either percutaneously or by open drainage. In presence of pus or perforation of the organ, mesh repair is contraindicated due to increased risk of complications. A normal looking appendix in the hernial sac does not always require appendectomy. Appendectomy adds the risk of infection to an otherwise clean

Table 1: Classification of Amyand's hernias and their plan of management [6].

Classification	Description	Surgical management
Type I	Normal appendix in inguinal hernia	Hernia reduction; mesh repair; appendectomy in young patients
Type II	Acute appendicitis within an inguinal hernia and no abdominal sepsis	Appendectomy through hernia; primary repair of hernia; no mesh
Type III	Acute appendicitis within an inguinal hernia or the abdominal wall or peritoneal sepsis	Laparotomy; appendectomy; primary repair of hernia; no mesh
Type IV	Acute appendicitis within an inguinal hernia with related or unrelated abdominal pathology	Management as detailed above for hernia type I–III and treat the second pathology as appropriate

procedure. Superficial wound infection increases morbidity; and deep infection may contribute to hernia recurrence [14]. However, Ofili reported two patients who developed acute appendicitis after repair of inguinal herniae which contained the appendix, along with 11 patients who had appendicectomies at the time of herniorrhaphy, without developing any wound infections or hernia recurrences. He, therefore, advocated "incidental" appendicectomies [19]. Whether to remove or leave behind a normal appendix is a clinical dilemma because no evidence-based information exists. The decision should be based on common sense, taking into account the patient's age, life expectancy, life-long risk of developing acute appendicitis, and the size and overall anatomy of the appendix. Also, in cases where there is no inflammation, and appendix has merely been reduced, there is no contraindication to using a mesh [14], though some authorities recommend that the use of synthetic mesh should be avoided even if the appendix appears normal, as subclinical contamination is bound to occur [2].

A scheme of classification and management has been given by Losanoff and Basson [6] (Table 1).

We conclude that the presence of the appendix in an inguinal hernial sac, referred to as "Amyand's hernia," is a rare entity and appendicitis within the hernial sac is even less frequently encountered. Preoperative diagnosis is difficult and the condition is usually diagnosed intraoperatively. Surgeons should be aware of the condition and the recommended line of management, so that they are able to offer appropriate treatment.

Consent

Authors have taken a fully informed consent from all patients for identity blinded publication of their case. They have also taken approval of the scientific and ethical committee of the institute for the same case.

Authors' Contribution

All authors have contributed significantly to the paper in terms of clinical material, radiological diagnosis, surgical craft, and final preparation of the paper.

References

[1] S. M. Ali, K. A. Malik, and H. Al-Qadhi, "Amyand's Hernia: study of four cases and literature review," *Sultan Qaboos University Medical Journal*, vol. 12, no. 2, pp. 232–236, 2012.

[2] K. A. Malik, "Left sided Amyand's hernia," *Journal of the College of Physicians and Surgeons Pakistan*, vol. 20, no. 7, pp. 480–481, 2010.

[3] C.-M. Kwok, C.-H. Su, W.-K. Kwang, and Y.-C. Chiu, "Amyand's Hernia—case report and review of the literature," *Case Reports in Gastroenterology*, vol. 1, no. 1, pp. 65–70, 2007.

[4] I. Sengul, D. Sengul, and D. Aribas, "An elective detection of an Amyand's hernia with an adhesive caecum to the sac: report of a rare case," *North American Journal of Medical Sciences*, vol. 3, no. 8, pp. 391–393, 2011.

[5] J. Fernando and S. Leelaratna, "Amyand's hernia," *Ceylon Medical Journal*, vol. 47, no. 2, article 71, 2002.

[6] J. E. Losanoff and M. D. Basson, "Amyand hernia: a classification to improve management," *Hernia*, vol. 12, no. 3, pp. 325–326, 2008.

[7] C. D'Alia, M. G. Lo Schiavo, A. Tonante et al., "Amyand's hernia: case report and review of the literature," *Hernia*, vol. 7, no. 2, pp. 89–91, 2003.

[8] R. Solecki, A. Matyja, and W. Milanowski, "Amyand's hernia: a report of two cases," *Hernia*, vol. 7, no. 1, pp. 50–51, 2003.

[9] W. J. Ryan, "Hernia of the vermiform appendix," *Annals of Surgery*, vol. 106, no. 1, pp. 135–139, 1937.

[10] L. C. Carey, "Acute appendicitis occurring in hernias: a report of 10 cases," *Surgery*, vol. 61, no. 2, pp. 236–238, 1967.

[11] W. F. G. Thomas, K. D. J. Vowles, and R. C. N. Williamson, "Appendicitis in external herniae," *Annals of the Royal College of Surgeons of England*, vol. 64, no. 2, pp. 121–122, 1982.

[12] H. A. D. V. Cunha, R. D. Sugahara, and M. V. Castilho, "Amyand's hernia," *Revista do Colegio Brasileiro de Cirurgioes*, vol. 36, no. 3, pp. 279–280, 2009.

[13] K. Ballas, Th. Kontoulis, Ch. Skouras et al., "Unusual findings in inguinal hernia surgery: report of 6 rare cases," *Hippokratia*, vol. 13, no. 3, pp. 169–171, 2009.

[14] K. Psarras, M. Lalountas, M. Baltatzis et al., "Amyand's hernia-a vermiform appendix presenting in an inguinal hernia: a case series," *Journal of Medical Case Reports*, vol. 5, article 463, 2011.

[15] C. Amyand, "Of an inguinal rupture, with a pin in the appendix caeci, incrusted with stone; and some observations on wounds in the guts," *Philosophical Transactions of the Royal Society of London*, vol. 39, no. 436–444, pp. 329–342, 1736.

[16] L. Flood, K. H. Chang, and O. J. McAnena, "A rare case of Amyand's hernia presenting as an enterocutaneous fistula," *Journal of Surgical Case Reports*, vol. 7, article 6, 2010.

[17] S. Laermans, P. Aerts, and R. De Man, "Amyand's hernia: inguinal hernia with acute appendicitis," *Journal Belge de Radiologie*, vol. 90, no. 6, pp. 524–525, 2007.

[18] R. V. Weber, Z. C. Hunt, and J. G. Kral, "Amyand's hernia: etiologic and therapeutic implications of two complications," *Surgical Rounds*, vol. 22, pp. 552–556, 1999.

[19] O. P. Ofili, "Simultaneous appendectomy and inguinal herniorrhaphy could be beneficial," *Ethiopian Medical Journal*, vol. 29, no. 1, pp. 37–38, 1991.

11

Epigenetic Alterations in a Gastric Leiomyoma

M. T. Branham,[1] M. Pellicer,[2] E. Campoy,[1] M. Palma,[3] A. Correa,[4] and M. Roqué[1]

[1] *Institute of Histology and Embryology (IHEM-CCT-CONICET) and School of Medical Sciences, National University of Cuyo, M5502JMA Mendoza, Argentina*
[2] *Pathology Laboratory, J5402EQC San Juan, Argentina*
[3] *Surgery Unit, San Martin Hospital, E3100 Entre Ríos, Argentina*
[4] *Surgery Unit, Español Hospital, M5501 Mendoza, Argentina*

Correspondence should be addressed to M. T. Branham; mbranham@fcm.uncu.edu.ar

Academic Editor: Haruhiko Sugimura

Leiomyomas constitute 2.5% of all resected neoplasms of the stomach. They are usually asymptomatic, but may present mucosal ulceration. Aberrant DNA methylation is a well-defined epigenetic change in human neoplasms; however, gene-acquired methylation may not necessarily be related with a malignant phenotype. In this report we analyzed in a gastric leiomyoma, the methylation status of 84 CpGI in tumor suppressor and DNA repair genes. We analyzed the tumor center (TC) and tumor periphery (TP) separately. We found aberrant methylation in 2/84 CpGI in the TC portion, that is, *MLH1* and *MSH3*, and 5/84 CpGI in the TP, that is, *MLH1*, *MSH3*, *APC*, *MSH6*, and *MGMT*. The gene with the highest methylation percentage in the TC and TP was *MLH1*. Given that *MLH1* methylation has been associated with microsatellite instability, we analyzed the status of the microsatellite Bat-26. We found that neither the TC nor the TP presented instability. The methylation of *MLH1*, *MGMT*, and *APC* has been described in GISTs, but to the best of our knowledge this is the first time that the methylation of these genes has been associated with gastric leiomyoma. Further research should be conducted to identify reliable molecular markers that could differentiate between GISTs and gastric leiomyomas.

1. Introduction

Gastric leiomyomas account for 2.5% of gastric neoplasms. Although most of them are asymptomatic, patients may present upper gastrointestinal hemorrhage [1, 2]. Endoscopically, gastric leiomyomas appear as a large submucosal lesion, and generally endoscopic biopsies are not deep enough to be of any diagnostic value [3]. Pathologically, most of these tumors are composed of spindle cells and display smooth muscle differentiation. Leiomyomas are defined as being desmin and actin positive and c-Kit (or CD117) negative tumors [4].

Tumorigenesis is the result of a multistep process characterized by the accumulation of genetic and epigenetic alterations leading to uncontrolled growth. Among epigenetic modifications, the most studied event in human neoplasms is the deregulation of methylation of DNA, giving rise to widespread changes in the methylome patterns during tumor progression [5]. The epigenome of tumors is characterized by global DNA hypomethylation and by gene-specific hypermethylation. Gene silencing by CpG islands (CpGI) hypermethylation in gene promoters can modulate pathways that control the basic function of the cell by acting directly on tumor suppressor genes and caretaker genes and indirectly on oncogenes through their regulators [5].

Gene expression profile studies have demonstrated that some genes are hypermethylated in gastric GISTs (gastro intestinal stromal tumors) [6–8], but, to our knowledge, there is no information of the methylation profile of gastric leiomyomas.

The objective of this study was to analyze by methyl specific-multiplex ligation probe amplification (MS-MLPA) the methylation status of tumor suppressor and DNA repair genes in a gastric leiomyoma.

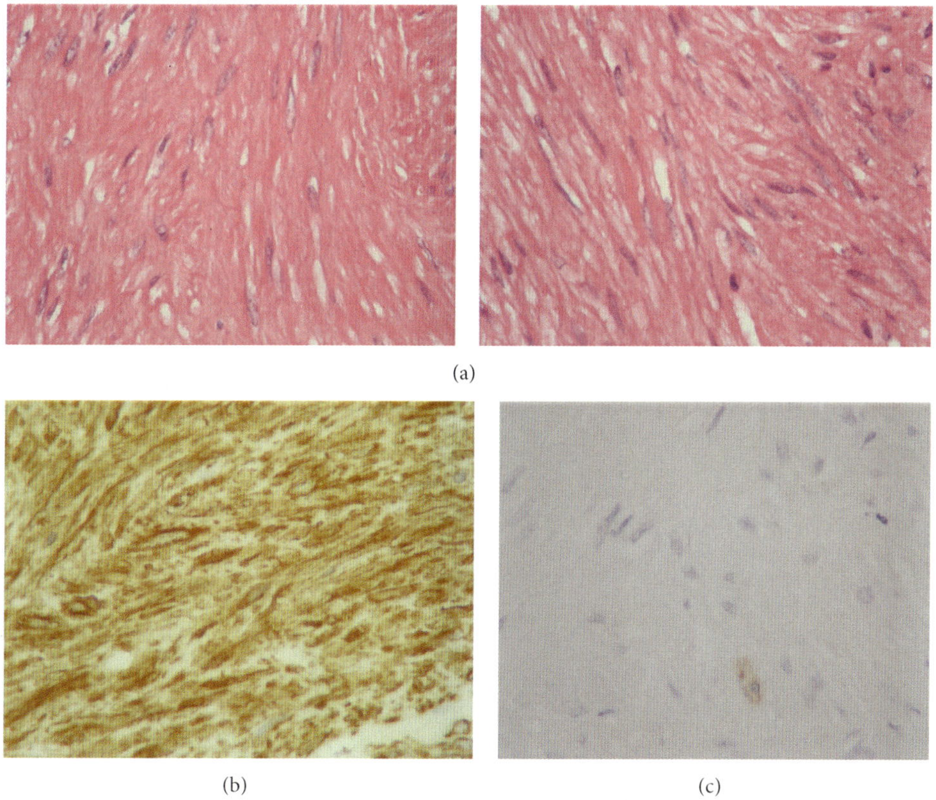

FIGURE 1: Histopathological images of the gastric leiomyoma analyzed. (a) Intersecting bundles of bland spindle cells in TC (left) and in TP (right). (b) Strong smooth muscle actin immunoreactivity. (c) Negative immunostain with CD117 (a positive mastocyte is shown as positive internal control).

2. Case Report

A 63-year-old Hispanic female presented with history of melena for two days. Upon clinical examination the patient mentioned that she was treated for *H. pylori* infection 15 years before. No other constitutional symptoms were present. Upper gastrointestinal endoscopy was performed, showing an ulcerated submucosal tumor localized on the cardial region. Upper endoscopic ultrasonography (EUS) evidenced a submucosal lesion, of about 50 mm with decreased echogenicity and homogeneous structure, and no necrotic areas. The lesion belonged to the muscular layer, and EUS suggested GIST (gastrointestinal stromal tumor). Multisided tomography revealed that the lesion was 5 cm and showed no evidence of other lesions in the abdominal area. The patient was scheduled for laparoscopic surgery and was discharged from the hospital eleven days after the operation.

2.1. Histopathology. The histopathological diagnosis for the submucosal lesion was gastric leiomyoma, characterized by a proliferation of bland, spindle-shaped cells with elongated nuclei and eosinophilic fibrillary cytoplasm without necrosis and atypia (Figure 1). The mitotic index (number of mitoses per 50 high-power fields, HPF) was <2/50 HPF. The immunohistochemistry assay indicated diffuse positivity for vimentin, smooth muscle actin, and desmin and negative staining for c-Kit/CD117, CD34, cytokeratins AE1/AE2, and S-100. The morphology of the lesion along with the immunohistochemical features supported the diagnosis of leiomyoma.

2.2. Methylation Analysis. MS-MLPA assay was performed by kits ME001, ME002, ME003, ME0024, and ME011 according to manufacturer's, MRC-Holland, Amsterdam, The Netherlands, instructions (http://www.mlpa.com/) on DNA obtained from the formalin fixed embedded tumor. The methylation status of 84 CpGIs in 41 cancer related genes was assessed (Table 1). We have established a cut-off threshold by considering a region to show methylation if the dosage ratio was >8% [9]. Due to tumor heterogeneity and in order to analyze if there were epigenetic differences between different regions of the tumor, we analyzed separately the tumor center (TC) and the tumor periphery (TP). We found aberrant methylation in 2/84 CpGI in the TC portion, that is, one site localized at 485 nt before the transcription start site (TSS) of *MSH3* and one site at 382 nt before TSS of *MLH1*. Even though both genes presented methylation percentages above the established cut-off level, it is interesting to mention that they differed significantly: 11.6% and 52.9%, respectively (Figure 2, green bars). The peripheric portion of the tumor presented a different profile: 5/84 CpG sites were aberrantly methylated, from which 2 sites were shared with the center portion, that is, *MSH3* and *MLH1*, and 3 sites were exclusively methylated

Table 1: List of genes analyzed in the gastric leiomyoma. Gene names and gene symbols are according to the HGNC database.

Gene symbol	Gene name
APC	Adenomatous polyposis coli
ATM	Ataxia telangiectasia mutated
BCL2	B-cell CLL/lymphoma 2
BNIP3	BCL2/adenovirus E1B 19 kDa interacting protein 3
BRCA1	Breast cancer 1
BRCA2	Breast cancer 2
CACNA1A	Calcium channel, voltage-dependent, P/Q type, alpha 1A subunit
CACNA1G	Calcium channel, voltage-dependent, P/Q type, alpha 1B subunit
CADM1	Cell adhesion molecule 1
CCND2	Cyclin D2
CD44	CD44 molecule
CDH13	Cadherin 13
CDKN1B	Cyclin-dependent kinase inhibitor 1B
CDKN2A	Cyclin-dependent kinase inhibitor 2A
CHFR	Checkpoint with forkhead ring finger domains
CREM	cAMP responsive element modulator
DAPK1	Death-associated protein kinase 1
DLC1	DLC1 Rho GTPase activating protein
ESR1	Estrogen receptor 1
FHIT	Fragile histidine triad
GATA5	GATA binding protein 5
GSTP1	Glutathione S-transferase pi 1
H2AFX	H2A histone family, member X
HIC1	Hypermethylated in cancer 1
HLTF	Helicase-like transcription factor
ID4	Inhibitor of DNA binding 4, dominant negative helix-loop-helix protein
MGMT	O-6-Methylguanine-DNA methyltransferase
MLH1	MutL homolog 1
MLH3	MutL homolog 3
MSH2	MutS homolog 2
MSH3	MutS homolog 3
MSH6	MutS homolog 6
PAH	Phenylalanine hydroxylase
PAX5	Paired box 5
PAX6	Paired box 6
PMS2	PMS2 postmeiotic segregation increased 2
PRDM2	PR domain containing 2, with ZNF domain
PTCH1	Patched 1
PTEN	Phosphatase and tensin homolog
PYCARD	PYD and CARD domain containing
RARB	Retinoic acid receptor beta
RASSF1	Ras association domain family member 1A
RB1	Retinoblastoma 1
RUNX3	Runt-related transcription factor 3
SCGB3A1	Secretoglobin, family 3A, member 1
SFRP4	Secreted frizzled-related protein 4
SFRP5	Secreted frizzled-related protein 5
STK11	Serine/threonine kinase 11
TGIF1	TGFB-induced factor homeobox 1
THBS1	Thrombospondin 1
TIMP3	TIMP metallopeptidase inhibitor 3
TP53	Tumor protein p53
TP73	Tumor protein p73
TWIST1	Twist family bHLH transcription factor 1
VHL	Von Hippel-Lindau tumor suppressor
WT1	Wilms tumor 1

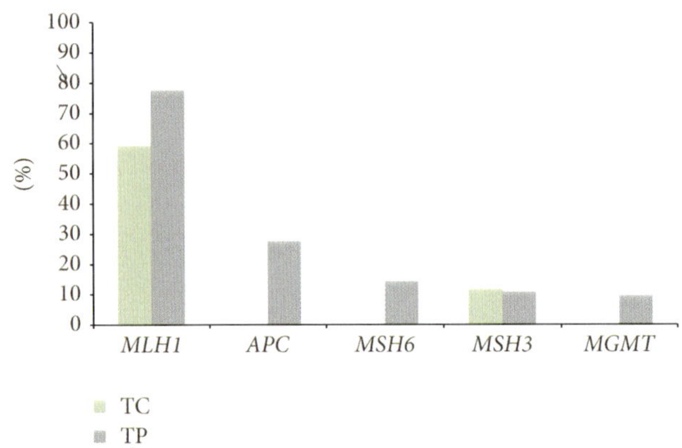

Figure 2: Genes methylated in a gastric leiomyoma. Grey bars represent the genes methylated in the tumor periphery and green bars represent the genes methylated in the tumor center.

in the tumor periphery, that is, *MSH6*, *MGMT*, and *APC* (Table 2). As a control, MS-MLPA assay was performed in normal tissue (i.e., leucocytes of healthy patients); we determined that there was no aberrant methylation in the regions analyzed. The percentages of methylation in the TP were 10.8%, 77%, 14.3%, 9.5%, and 27.7%, respectively (Figure 2, grey bars). Even though the methylated genes differed between the TC and the TP, it is interesting to mention that *MLH1* was shared by both and presented the highest percentage of methylation (52.9% and 77%, resp.). To analyze whether methylation affected gene expression, we performed qRT-PCR assays on 2 cell lines (MDA-MB231 and MCF-7) which presented different percentages of APC promoter methylation (0% and 52%, resp.); we confirmed that the methylation of APC on the CpG site −21 nt before TSS reduces gene expression (data not shown). The methylation of *MLH1* at 382 nt before TSS has been previously shown to provoke downregulation of gene expression [10].

Given that *MLH1* methylation is associated with microsatellite instability (MSI) in sporadic endometrial and

TABLE 2: List of methylated genes in the gastric leiomyoma studied. Gene names and gene symbols are according to the HGNC database; CpG site locations are mentioned based on the MRC-Holland data sheets. TP indicates tumor periphery and TC tumor center.

Gene symbol	Name	CpG location	Sample	Mehtylation %
APC	Adenomatous polyposis coli	21 nt before TSS	TP	27.7
			TC	0
MGMT	O-6-Methylguanine-DNA Methyltransferase	233 nt after TSS	TP	9.5
			TC	0
MSH6	mutS homolog 6	317 nt before TSS	TP	14.3
			TC	0
MLH1	MutL Homolog 1	382 nt before TSS	TP	77.6
			TC	59.2
MSH3	mutS homolog 3	485 nt before TSS	TP	10.8
			TC	11.6

TSS: transcription start site. nt: nucleotide.

colorectal cancers [11, 12], we decided to analyze MSI in the gastric leiomyoma. To evaluate MSI, we analyzed by PCR the status of the mononucleotide microsatellite Bat-26 in the tumor center and periphery. This microsatellite has been shown to be highly efficient and sensitive to determine MSI-H when used as a single marker [13, 14]. Interestingly, Bat-26 was stable in the TC as well as in the TP portion of the gastric leiomyoma analyzed. When we tested Bat-26 status in 5 nontumoral tissues and in peripheral blood of healthy patients, none of these tissues presented Bat-26 instability.

3. Discussion

The onset and progression of tumorigenesis involves a cascade of genetic and/or epigenetic events. Results from recent investigations have shown that DNA methylation profiles contain tumor type-specific signatures which, in the future, could serve as biomarkers for clinical outcome [15]. Hypermethylation at the promoter region of several genes has been shown to be an important mechanism in gene silencing. However, gene-acquired methylation may not necessarily be related with malignant phenotype [16, 17]. In this report, we show that a gastric leiomyoma, considered a benign disease, presents methylation in 2–5 of 84 analyzed CpGI, varying in different tumor parts.

The methylation percentage in the overall sample varied widely (from 9.5% to 77%) for the different genes (Figure 1). This wide-ranging methylation levels could be indicating that the aberrant hypermethylation occurs at different sites and times, and, therefore, probably the genes with higher methylation levels (such as *MLH1* or *APC*) were the first ones to be epigenetically altered during tumoral progression. Considering that *MLH1* presents a high methylation percentage, we hypothesize that its methylation could be an initial epigenetic event during gastric leiomyoma formation.

Given that *MLH1* methylation is associated with MSI in several tumors [11, 12], we analyzed the status of the mononucleotide microsatellite Bat-26. As we mentioned before, neither the TC nor the TP portion presented Bat-26 instability. We speculate that the gastric leiomyoma analyzed is not MSI-H due to Bat-26 stability, but we cannot discard MSI-L or MSI-S. It is interesting to mention that the fact that MLH1 is methylated and MSI is stable has been also described by other authors and several hypotheses have been proposed. For example, studies performed by Esteller and colleagues on endometrial atypical hyperplasia concluded that MLH1 promoter methylation is an early event and in some cases may precede a detectable MSI phenotype [18]. Therefore, a possible explanation could be that the leiomyoma presents MLH1 methylation as an early event, lacking yet MSI signs. In another work performed by Kanaya et al. the authors studied the region 700 bp upstream of MLH1 promoter region covering 48 CpG sites; they classified the methylation status as full (over 80% of CpGs were methylated), partial (10–80%), or nonmethylation (less than 10%). The authors concluded that the degree, rather than region-specific methylation of CpG islands, is critical for MSI phenotype [19].

The genes found methylated in the gastric leiomyoma play different functions in the cell: *MLH1*, *MSH3*, *MGMT*, and *MSH6* participate in DNA repair functions whereas *APC* gene participates in cell proliferation. The methylation of *MLH1*, *MGMT*, and *APC* has been previously described in GISTs, but to the best of our knowledge this is the first time that the methylation of these genes has been associated with gastric leiomyoma, which is considered a benign disease. Interestingly, we also found that there were differentially methylated genes between GISTs and the gastric leiomyoma. For example, in a study performed by House et al., the authors determined that the most frequently methylated genes in GISTs (in decreasing frequency) are *MGMT*, *p16*, *RASSF1A*, *E-cadherin*, and *MLH1* [6]. In another report performed by Saito et al., the authors determined that, besides *MLH1* and *MGMT*, GISTs also presented methylation in *MINT2*, *p73*, *p16*, *E-cadherin*, *MINT1*, *p15*, and *MINT3*. Moreover, the methylation of *RASSF1A* progressively increased from small to malignant GISTs and *p16* was specifically methylated in malignant-prone and malignant GIST [8]. Note that neither *RASSF1*, *p16*, nor *p73* is methylated in the studied gastric leiomyoma. These epigenetic differences between malignant GISTs and gastric leiomyoma have not been described before.

To the best of our knowledge this is the first report showing the methylation profile of a gastric leiomyoma. Further research should be conducted to identify reliable and accurate molecular markers that could help in the differentiation between GISTs and gastric leiomyomas.

Acknowledgments

This work lacked specific grant and was partially supported by National Cancer Institute of Argentina and by the National University of Cuyo, Argentina.

References

[1] A. K. Madan, C. T. Frantzides, A. Keshavarzian, and C. Smith, "Laparoscopic wedge resection of gastric leiomyoma," *JSLS*, vol. 8, no. 1, pp. 77–80, 2004.

[2] B. K. Morgan, C. Compton, M. Talbert, W. J. Gallagher, and W. C. Wood, "Benign smooth muscle tumors of the gastrointestinal tract: a 24-year experience," *Annals of Surgery*, vol. 211, no. 1, pp. 63–66, 1990.

[3] A.-W. N. Meshikhes, E. A. Al-Khalaf, and S. H. Al-Bahar, "Gastric leiomyoma. Is there an association with *Helicobacter pylori*?" *Saudi Medical Journal*, vol. 25, no. 11, pp. 1758–1759, 2004.

[4] M. Miettinen, L. H. Sobin, and M. Sarlomo-Rikala, "Immunohistochemical spectrum of GISTs at different sites and their differential diagnosis with a reference to CD117 (KIT)," *Modern Pathology*, vol. 13, no. 10, pp. 1134–1142, 2000.

[5] M. Esteller, "Molecular origins of cancer: epigenetics in cancer," *The New England Journal of Medicine*, vol. 358, no. 11, pp. 1148–1159, 2008.

[6] M. G. House, M. Guo, D. T. Efron et al., "Tumor suppressor gene hypermethylation as a predictor of gastric stromal tumor behavior," *Journal of Gastrointestinal Surgery*, vol. 7, no. 8, pp. 1004–1014, 2003.

[7] Y. Okamoto, A. Sawaki, S. Ito et al., "Aberrant DNA methylation associated with aggressiveness of gastrointestinal stromal tumour," *Gut*, vol. 61, no. 3, pp. 392–401, 2012.

[8] K. Saito, S. Sakurai, T. Sano et al., "Aberrant methylation status of known methylation-sensitive CpG islands in gastrointestinal stromal tumors without any correlation to the state of *c-kit* and *PDGFRA* gene mutations and their malignancy," *Cancer Science*, vol. 99, no. 2, pp. 253–259, 2008.

[9] M. T. Branham, D. M. Marzese, S. R. Laurito et al., "Methylation profile of triple-negative breast carcinomas," *Oncogenesis*, vol. 1, no. 7, article e17, 2012.

[10] L. H. Jensen, A. A. Rasmussen, L. Byriel et al., "Regulation of MLH1 mRNA and protein expression by promoter methylation in primary colorectal cancer: a descriptive and prognostic cancer marker study," *Cellular Oncology*, vol. 36, no. 5, pp. 411–419, 2013.

[11] X. Li, X. Yao, Y. Wang et al., "*MLH1* promoter methylation frequency in colorectal cancer patients and related clinicopathological and molecular features," *PLoS ONE*, vol. 8, no. 3, Article ID e59064, 2013.

[12] I. Zighelboim, P. J. Goodfellow, F. Gao et al., "Microsatellite instability and epigenetic inactivation of *MLH1* and outcome of patients with endometrial carcinomas of the endometrioid type," *Journal of Clinical Oncology*, vol. 25, no. 15, pp. 2042–2048, 2007.

[13] M. S. Cicek, N. M. Lindor, S. Gallinger et al., "Quality assessment and correlation of microsatellite instability and immunohistochemical markers among population—and clinic-based colorectal tumors: results from the colon cancer family registry," *Journal of Molecular Diagnostics*, vol. 13, no. 3, pp. 271–283, 2011.

[14] K. Imai and H. Yamamoto, "Carcinogenesis and microsatellite instability: the interrelationship between genetics and epigenetics," *Carcinogenesis*, vol. 29, no. 4, pp. 673–680, 2008.

[15] A. Al-Kaabi, L. W. van Bockel, A. J. Pothen, and S. M. Willems, "$P16^{INK4A}$ and $p14^{ARF}$ gene promoter hypermethylation as prognostic biomarker in oral and oropharyngeal squamous cell carcinoma: a review," *Disease Markers*, vol. 2014, Article ID 260549, 8 pages, 2014.

[16] A. O. O. Chan, S. K. Lam, B. C.-Y. Wong, Y.-L. Kwong, A. Rashid, and G. Tamura, "Gene methylation in non-neoplastic mucosa of gastric cancer: age or *Helicobacter pylori* related?" *The American Journal of Pathology*, vol. 163, no. 1, pp. 370–373, 2003.

[17] D. M. Marzese, F. E. Gago, J. I. Orozco, O. M. Tello, M. Roqué, and L. M. Vargas-Roig, "Aberrant DNA methylation of cancer-related genes in giant breast fibroadenoma: a case report," *Journal of Medical Case Reports*, vol. 5, article 516, 2011.

[18] M. Esteller, R. Levine, S. B. Baylin, L. H. Ellenson, and J. G. Herman, "*MLH1* promoter hypermethylation is associated with the microsatellite instability phenotype in sporadic endometrial carcinomas," *Oncogene*, vol. 17, no. 18, pp. 2413–2417, 1998.

[19] T. Kanaya, S. Kyo, Y. Maida et al., "Frequent hypermethylation of *MLH1* promoter in normal endometrium of patients with endometrial cancers," *Oncogene*, vol. 22, no. 15, pp. 2352–2360, 2003.

12

Acute Pancreatitis Secondary to Hemobilia after Percutaneous Liver Biopsy: A Rare Complication of a Common Procedure, Presenting in an Atypical Fashion

Ramy Mansour and Justin Miller

Genesys Regional Medical Center Gastroenterology, 1 Genesys Parkway, ATTN: Medical Education, Grand Blanc, MI 48439, USA

Correspondence should be addressed to Ramy Mansour; ramyjm@gmail.com

Academic Editor: Engin Altintas

Percutaneous Liver Biopsy is an often-required procedure for the evaluation of multiple liver diseases. The complications are rare but well reported. Here we present a case of a 60-year-old overweight female who underwent liver biopsy for elevated alkaline phosphatase. She developed acute pancreatitis secondary to hemobilia, with atypical signs and symptoms, following the biopsy. She never had the classic triad of RUQ pain, jaundice, and upper GI hemorrhage. There were also multiple negative imaging studies, thus complicating the presentation. She was successfully treated with ERCP, sphincterotomy, balloon sweep, and stent placement. Angiography and transcatheter embolization were not required.

1. Introduction

Histological assessment of the liver is the gold standard for many liver and biliary disorders. Percutaneous liver biopsy (PLB) is the most commonly utilized method of obtaining tissue for analysis. Image guidance is preferred, though not mandatory, by current guidelines [1]. The complications are rare but well reported and include pain, hematoma, pneumothorax, hemobilia, peritonitis, sepsis, abscess, and death [2]. Here we present a case of one rare complication, with atypical signs and symptoms, following an image guided PLB.

2. Case Report

We present a case of a 60-year-old overweight female with a past medical history of type 2 diabetes, hypothyroidism, hyperlipidemia, hypertension, and internal hemorrhoids presented to her primary care physician for a health maintenance exam. She does not drink alcohol, is a lifelong nonsmoker, and denies illicit drug use. Past surgeries included cholecystectomy and total abdominal hysterectomy. She does not take antiplatelet and anticoagulant medications. She complained of hematuria during the review of systems. A CT scan was performed without contrast for the hematuria and revealed diffuse hepatic steatosis. A follow-up MRI Liver with Gadavist revealed hepatosplenomegaly with hepatic steatosis with no evidence of liver masses. Upon further discussion, she revealed complaints of pruritus. Labs were drawn after the imaging and revealed the following: AST 48 U/L (10-35 U/L), ALT 46 U/L (6-29 U/L), alkaline phosphatase 333 U/L (33-130 U/L), total bilirubin 0.4 mg/dl (0.2-1.2 mg/dl), and GGT 861 U/L (3-70 U/L) (Table 1).

She was ultimately referred to a gastroenterologist and further serologic testing was performed. She had a negative viral hepatitis panel, smooth muscle antibody, immunoglobulin-G, anti-Mitochondrial Antibody (AMA), iron saturation, ferritin, alpha-one antitrypsin genotype, and ceruloplasmin. She was a nondrinker. She had metabolic risk factors for nonalcoholic fatty liver disease but the elevated alkaline phosphatase prompted further work-up. She underwent subcostal CT guided core liver biopsy with a 17-gauge guide needle and an 18-gauge core biopsy needle inserted coaxially. Four total passes were made and ranged in size from 0.6 to 1.5 cm. The patient tolerated the procedure well. The liver biopsy revealed abundant central zone macrovesicular

Table 1: Laboratory values before and after biopsy and ERCP.

Lab	Pre-Biopsy	7 Days Post-Biopsy	12 Days Post-Biopsy	17 Days Post-Biopsy	18 Days Post-Biopsy (Day of ERCP)	2 Months Post-ERCP
Alk Phos (U/L)	262	687	1186	889	850	280
Bilirubin (g/dL)	0.5	1.2	4.8	3.1	3.2	0.7
Lipase (U/L)			1002	2235		
AST (U/L)	32	173	273	87	152	26
ALT (U/L)	24	87	220	75	103	18
Hgb (g/dL)	11.3	12.0	11.2	10.1	7.5	10.7

steatosis and a large amount of ballooning hepatocytes with Mallory-Denk bodies, consistent with steatohepatitis with fibrosis. Elevations in alkaline phosphatase can be seen in up to 1/3 of patients with nonalcoholic steatohepatitis [3], as was the case in this patient.

Two days after the biopsy, she began experiencing intermittent bouts of acute chest and epigastric abdominal pain with nausea, nonbloody emesis, and increasing stool frequency. She had several visits to the emergency department and was found to have worsening alkaline phosphatase and bilirubin levels. On postbiopsy day twelve, she had an elevated lipase of 1002 U/L (normal 20-50 U/L), but MRI/MRCP failed to reveal any abnormalities, though she was pain-free at the time of the study. The pain continued intermittently but would resolve spontaneously, with work-ups and imaging modalities (US and CT imaging) revealing no defining etiology. Seventeen days status after liver biopsy, she presented again with acute onset of epigastric pain, sharp, severe, nonradiating, and associated with nonbloody emesis, and no melena. She was found to have an elevated alkaline phosphatase and bilirubin once again but also a lipase of 2235 U/L (normal 25-50 U/L). Contrasted CT scan, ordered urgently and performed while the pain was present, finally showed pancreatitis with hyperdense material within the common bile duct.

She was referred to a tertiary center for further management. She initially underwent EGD that failed to reveal any abnormalities, including any signs of bleeding. She subsequently underwent ERCP with sphincterotomy and 9-12 mm balloon sweep of small blood clot from the left intrahepatic duct (Figures 1, 2, and 3). A 10 French by 7 cm stent was placed in the common bile duct and there was adequate bile flow. There was no evidence of further bleeding and no need for embolization. She had no further bouts of abdominal complaints.

A follow-up ERCP was performed 8 weeks later and a 9-12 mm balloon sweep with contrast was performed that did not reveal any biliary dilation or obstruction. The stent was removed successfully. Biliary drainage was noted to be adequate after procedure. Her alkaline phosphatase and bilirubin returned to their baseline prior to the liver biopsy (Table 1). She did not have any recurrence or relapse of her symptoms. There were no further signs of bleeding and her hemoglobin returned to baseline.

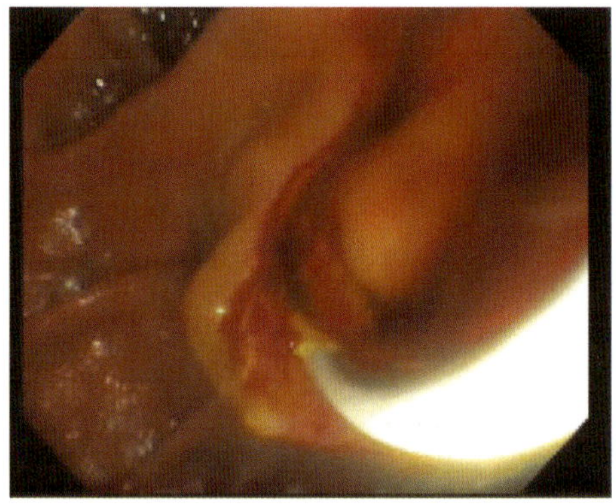

Figure 1: Blood coming from CBD on ERCP.

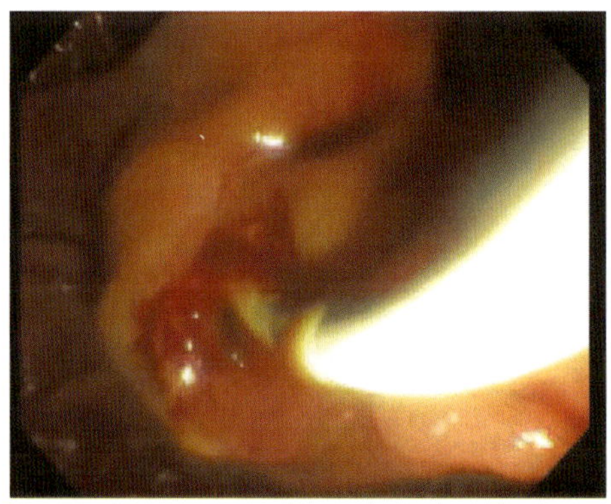

Figure 2: Blood clot being removed from ampulla during ERCP.

3. Discussion

Hemobilia was first theorized in 1654 by Frances Glisson on postmortem examination of a man who was stabbed by a sword in the liver and died from a GI hemorrhage [4]. It was seen throughout the years and eventually recognized antimortem. The classic triad of right upper quadrant (RUQ) pain, jaundice, and upper GI hemorrhage was first described in 1871 by Quincke [5]. Hemobilia had a grave prognosis, as there were limited treatment options. Several surgical approaches were attempted, but most were unsuccessful. In 1976, Walter was the first at successfully treating hemobilia

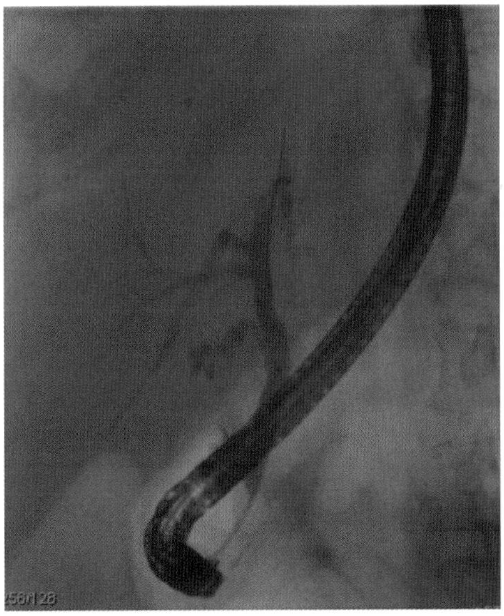

Figure 3: ERCP Fluoroscopy showing biliary tree with no abnormalities. However when the left intrahepatic duct was swept with a 9-12 balloon, a small amount of blood and a blood clot was evacuated.

with transcather embolization, and this has become the standard of therapy for treatment ever since [3]. However, its utility is limited to the amount of bleeding, requiring a bleeding rate of at least 0.5 to 1.0 ml/min.

Hemobilia as a complication of PLB was first reported in 1967 [6]. In a large case series of reported complications of liver biopsy, only 4 out of 68,276 patients had hemobilia [2]. The average time between liver biopsy and hemobilia onset is 5 days [7]. Several studies have described acute pancreatitis secondary to biliary obstruction from hemobilia and clot formation [8–19], the first of which was in 1975 [20]. The first cases of ERCP with sphincterotomy for treatment of acute pancreatitis secondary to hemobilia after PLB were in 1999 [11, 12]. Only three other cases since then have utilized ERCP for diagnosis and therapy of this rare adverse event [8, 9, 18].

The number of passes required during liver biopsy has been associated with a higher complication rate [1, 21, 22]. In one study by Perrault et al., the rate of complication was statistically significant when a biopsy was completed with more than 4 passes in a transthoracic approach, but not with the subcostal approach [22]. The subcostal approach was used in this patient.

4. Conclusion

A high index of suspicion is required to make this diagnosis. The classic triad of RUQ pain, jaundice, and upper GI hemorrhage was not observed in this case, thus delaying the diagnosis. Also, the timing of the MRI, ultrasounds, and CT scans played a role in the eventual diagnosis. The patient had intermittent symptoms and there was no evidence of acute pathology when the patient had imaging when the pain was not present. We theorize that this was likely due to spontaneous passage of the clot through the ampulla. The dilation and debris seen in the bile ducts and inflammatory changes seen in the pancreas were only noted when the patient was having severe pain at the time of imaging. There was also minimal evidence of bleeding (melena, hematochezia, decrease in hemoglobin, or elevation in BUN) until the diagnosis was already established by imaging and the patient was already scheduled for ERCP. During the ERCP, there were no abnormalities noted on fluoroscopy (Figure 3). However, since the suspected diagnosis was hemobilia with clot, the ducts were swept and ultimately revealed blood clot within the left intrahepatic biliary system (Figure 2).

Patients who suffer this rare complication of PLB historically underwent transcatheter embolization for treatment. In the case of this patient, embolization would likely not have been successful, as the patient had limited signs of bleeding and may have not been brisk enough to be picked up on standard angiography. ERCP with sphincterotomy and stent placement should be considered as an adequate adjunct treatment option, as this is the fourth case report that suggests success with ERCP treatment alone. It could also be suggested that a balloon sweep with sphincterotomy and stent placement should be performed when the diagnosis is suspected, even if this is not confirmed with cross sectional imaging or fluoroscopy at the time of ERCP.

Consent

Consent was obtained from the patient to publish information relating to case details.

Disclosure

Ramy Mansour is the primary author. Justin Miller is a contributing author and the guarantor.

References

[1] D. C. Rockey, S. H. Caldwell, Z. D. Goodman, R. C. Nelson, and A. D. Smith, "Liver biopsy," *Hepatology*, vol. 49, no. 3, pp. 1017–1044, 2009.

[2] F. Piccinino, E. Sagnelli, G. Pasquale, and G. Giusti, "Complications following percutaneous liver biopsy. a multicentre retrospective study on 68,276 biopsies," *J Hepatol*, vol. 2, pp. 165–173, 1986.

[3] M. H. Sleisenger, M. Feldman, L. S. Friedman, and L. J. Brandt, *Sleisenger & Fordtran's gastrointestinal and liver disease: Pathophysiology, diagnosis, management*, MD Consult, St. Louis, Mo, USA, 2010.

[4] F. Glisson, *Anatomia Hepatis*, Janssonium and Weyerstraten, Amsterdam, Netherlands, 1st edition, 1654.

[5] H. Quincke, "Ein Fall von Aneurysma der Leberarterie," *Klin Wochenschr*, vol. 8, pp. 349–351, 1871.

[6] E. F. Cox, "Hemobilia Following Percutaneous Needle Biopsy of the Liver," *JAMA Surgery*, vol. 95, no. 2, pp. 198–201, 1967.

[7] S. W. Merrell and P. D. Schneider, "Hemobilia–evolution of current diagnosis and treatment," *Western Journal of Medicine*, vol. 155, pp. 621–625, 1991.

[8] W. Albuquerque, V. Arantes, K. de Paula Farah, and J. R. Lambertucci, "Acute pancreatitis and acute cholecystitis caused by hemobilia after percutaneous ultrasound-guided liver biopsy," *Endoscopy*, vol. 37, no. 11, pp. 1159-1160, 2005.

[9] A. Nowak, M. Hartleb, M. Kohut, E. Nowakowska-Duława, and J. Pilch-Kowalczyk, "Haemobilia causing acute pancreatitis after percutaneous liver biopsy," *Journal of Hepatology*, vol. 43, no. 2, p. 366, 2005.

[10] V. I. Machicao, F. J. Lukens, S. M. Lange, and J. S. Scolapio, "Arterioportal fistula causing acute pancreatitis and hemobilia after liver biopsy," *Journal of Clinical Gastroenterology*, vol. 34, no. 4, pp. 481–484, 2002.

[11] A. Sood, V. Midha, A. Kumar, and N. Sood, "Acute pancreatitis with hemobilia following percutaneous liver biopsy.," *Indian Journal of Gastroenterology*, vol. 21, no. 2, pp. 81-82, 2002.

[12] T. Asselah, B. Condat, A. Sibert et al., "Haemobilia causing acute pancreatitis after percutaneous liver biopsy: Diagnosis by magnetic resonance cholangiopancreatography," *European Journal of Gastroenterology & Hepatology*, vol. 13, no. 7, pp. 877–879, 2001.

[13] J. A. Gómez-Valero, J. Sardi, J. Vilaseca, M. P. Lafuente, and J. R. Malagelada, "Pancreatitis and haemobilia due to arterioportal fistula after percutaneous liver biopsy resolved by selective arterial embolization," *European Journal of Gastroenterology & Hepatology*, vol. 13, no. 6, pp. 727–730, 2001.

[14] P. Jornod, P. H. Wiesel, P. Pescatore, and J.-J. Gonvers, "Hemobilia, a rare cause of acute pancreatitis after percutaneous liver biopsy: Diagnosis and treatment by endoscopic retrograde cholangiopancreatography," *American Journal of Gastroenterology*, vol. 94, no. 10, pp. 3051–3054, 1999.

[15] H. J. Kim, J. H. Shin, Y. Y. Lee et al., "Hemobilia causing acute biliary pancreatitis after percutaneous liver biopsy," *Endoscopy*, vol. 31, no. 3, pp. S18–S19, 1999.

[16] E. C. Van Os and B. T. Petersen, "Pancreatitis secondary to percutaneous liver biopsy-associated hemobilia," *American Journal of Gastroenterology*, vol. 91, no. 3, pp. 577–580, 1996.

[17] X. de Ribot, F. Casellas, M. Papo, J. Vilaseca, M. Moreiras, and J. R. Malagelada, "Hemobilia causing acute pancreatitis after percutaneous liver biopsy," *Journal of Clinical Gastroenterology*, vol. 21, no. 2, pp. 171-172, 1995.

[18] L. R. Peña, T. L. Horn, and C. B. Cross, "Acute pancreatitis secondary to hemobilia after percutaneous liver biopsy," *Therapeutic Advances in Gastroenterology*, vol. 2, no. 3, pp. 165–168, 2009.

[19] D. S. Zhang, Z. Metwalli, and K. B. Hussain, "Arterial-Portal Fistula After Percutaneous Liver Biopsy in Hepatic Allograft Causing Hemobilia and Pancreatitis," *Clinical Gastroenterology and Hepatology*, vol. 15, no. 1, pp. e3–e4, 2017.

[20] H. C. Redman and R. R. Joseph, "Hemobilia and pancreatitis as complications of a percutaneous transhepatic cholangiogram," *American Journal of Digestive Diseases*, vol. 20, no. 7, pp. 691–698, 1975.

[21] A. Grant and J. Neuberger, "Guidelines on the use of liver biopsy in clinical practice," *Gut*, vol. 45, no. 4, pp. IV1–IV11, 1999.

[22] J. Perrault, D. B. McGill, B. J. Ott et al., "Liver biopsy: complications in 1000 inpatients and outpatients," *Gastroenterology*, vol. 74, pp. 103–106, 1978.

13

Ulcerating Ileocolitis in Severe Amatoxin Poisoning

Matthias Peter Hilty,[1] Marcel Halama,[2] Anne-Katrin Zimmermann,[3] Marco Maggiorini,[1] and Andreas Geier[2]

[1] *Medical Intensive Care Unit, University Hospital of Zurich, Rämistrasse 100, 8091 Zurich, Switzerland*
[2] *Department of Gastroenterology and Hepatology, University Hospital of Zurich, Rämistrasse 100, 8091 Zurich, Switzerland*
[3] *Department of Pathology, University Hospital of Zurich, Rämistrasse 100, 8091 Zurich, Switzerland*

Correspondence should be addressed to Matthias Peter Hilty; matthias.hilty@usz.ch

Academic Editor: Christoph Vogt

Amatoxin poisoning is still associated with a great potential for complications and a high mortality. While the occurrence of acute gastroenteritis within the first 24 hours after amatoxin ingestion is well described, only very few descriptions of late gastrointestinal complications of amatoxin poisoning exist worldwide. We present the case of a 57-year-old female patient with severe amatoxin poisoning causing fulminant but reversible hepatic failure that on day 8 after mushroom ingestion developed severe abdominal pain and watery diarrhea. Ulcerating ileocolitis was identified by computed tomography identifying a thickening of the bowel wall of the entire ileum and biopsies taken from the ileum and large bowel revealing distinct ileitis and proximally accentuated colitis. The absence of discernible alternative etiologies such as infectious agents makes a causal relationship between the ulcerating ileocolitis and the amatoxin poisoning likely. Diarrhea and varying abdominal pain persisted over several weeks and clinical follow-up after six months showed a completely symptom-free patient. The case presented highlights the importance to consider the possibility of rare complications of *Amanita* intoxication in order to be able to respond to them early and adequately.

1. Introduction

Amanita is a genus of fungi in the phylum of basidiomycota consisting of around 600 known species [1]. Many of them are toxic and are easily misrecognized macroscopically by untrained individuals such as amateur mushroom hunters, leading to 205 cases of reported poisonings in Europe between 1971 and 1980, with an overall mortality of 22.4%, in the subpopulation of children less than 10 years even of 51.3% [2]. Incidence may have increased to date to around 50 per year in Europe [3] and somewhat less in the USA [4]. In Europe, mainly *Amanita phalloides* poisoning is described. Toxicity is attributable to amatoxins, a group of several polypeptides composed of around 35 amino acids that act as inhibitors of eukaryotic RNA polymerase II [2, 5] and therefore inhibit mRNA synthesis, leading to cell death. Through first-pass effect and a high level of metabolism, hepatocytes as a cell population are mainly affected, but there are also reports of kidney toxicity [6] and rarely late gastrointestinal toxicity [7]. Clinically, amatoxin poisoning initially manifests with gastroenteritis and an apparent recovery after 24 to 36 hours, coinciding with the onset of dose-dependent fulminant hepatic and multisystem organ failure [8].

2. Case Report

A 57-year-old female patient presented on day 3 after ingestion of approximately 200 g of self-collected mushrooms with a history of severe gastroenteritis beginning on day 1 and lasting through admission. On the day of admission, she became increasingly weak, providing her with the reason to seek medical attention. Otherwise, the patient had no medical record of any significance. The patient presented with stable cardiovascular and pulmonary function, afebrile, with diffuse abdominal tenderness and lively bowel sounds. There were no mushroom residues available for examination by an expert, but *Amanita phalloides* intoxication, which was highly compatible with the description of the patient and the clinical course, was proven via detection of α-amanitin

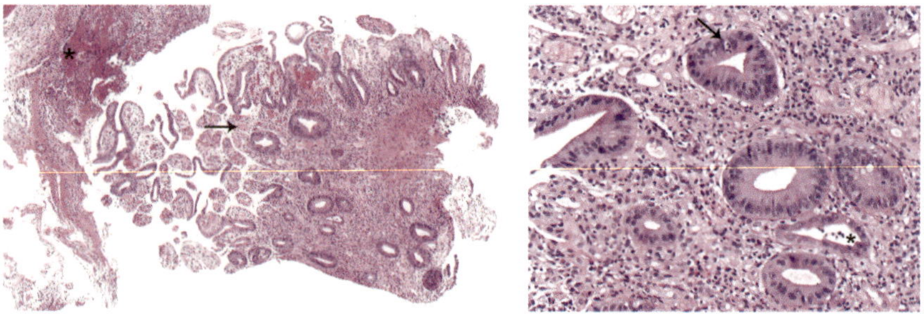

(a) (b)

FIGURE 1: Biopsy of the ileum. (a) Biopsy of the ileum with acute ulcerating inflammation and fibrinoleukocytic exudate (∗). Enteric architecture is changed with only fragmented residual villi and loss of Paneth cells. Mucosal vessels are heavily dilated (→) (40x magnification). (b) The lamina propria is filled by a dense mixed inflammatory infiltrate. Some neutrophilic granulocytes invade the epithelium of the crypts (→). In the lower right corner of the picture a residual crypt with atrophic epithelium and intraluminal cell detritus can be seen (∗). The epithelial cells show regeneratory and reactive changes with enlargement of the nuclei and prominent nucleoli (200x magnification).

TABLE 1: Toxin quantification and inflammatory and organ function parameters at admission with treatment initiation with silibinin and fluimucil and during the initial three days (I + 3 through I + 5), the onset of abdominal symptoms (I + 8), and dismissal from hospital (I + 17). Note the peak of liver injury and dysfunction at I + 4 with rapid recovery and the marked increase in inflammatory parameters at onset of abdominal symptoms.

Days after ingestion	I + 3 hospital admission, treatment initiation	I + 4	I + 5	I + 8 abdominal symptoms	I + 17 dismissal from hospital
Alpha-amanitin (urine) [μg/L]	42.4	2.9	Below threshold (<1.5)	—	—
C-reactive protein [mg/L]	15	24	36	85	5
Lactate [mmol/L]	2.3	2.4	1.1	—	—
Creatinine [μmol/L]	274	94	64	67	83
Blood urea nitrogen [mmol/L]	17.6	14.8	9.6	3.2	1.7
Aspartate-aminotransferase [U/L]	1249	5235	2998	727	30
Alanine-aminotransferase [U/L]	1380	6894	5430	120	19
Factor V [%]	35	Below threshold (<10)	49	121	138
INR [1]	1.6	2.7	1.7	1.2	1.1

in the urine using ELISA (Buehlmann Laboratories, Schonenbuch, Switzerland) with a maximal concentration of 42.2 μg/L on admission on day 3. Directly on admission, intravenous silibinin (Legalon SIL, Rottapharm, Monza, Italy) and acetylcysteine (Fluimucil 10%, Zambon Pharma, Milan, Italy) and multiple dose oral activated charcoal therapy were initiated at the intensive care unit according to current guidelines [9]. Silibinin was administered intravenously at 20 mg/kg per day for three days after a loading dose of 5 mg/kg; acetylcysteine was administered intravenously at 150 mg/kg over 1 hour, followed by 12.5 mg/kg over 4 hours and 6.25 mg/kg over 16 hours. At admission on day 3, liver enzymes were already elevated, reaching maximum on day 4 with alanine aminotransferase levels of 6894 U/L, aspartate aminotransferase of 5232 U/L, and lactate dehydrogenase of 10596 U/L. Alkaline phosphatase and γ-glutamyl transferase levels remained normal. As a measure of liver function, factor V activity was nondetectable on day 4, with factor II activity at 29% (60–150) and factor VII activity at 25% (60–150); the international normalized ratio (INR) was 2.7. Fortunately, liver function improved without further interventions on day 7 (Table 1). The patient initially also presented with renal failure. Renal ultrasonography studies were normal; however a calculated fractional excretion of urea of 65% hinted at an intrarenal pathology. Renal failure was completely reversible by day 4 without need for renal replacement therapy. On day 8, however, the patient developed severe abdominal pain, tenderness on examination with signs of peritonitis especially in the lower right quadrant, accompanied by watery diarrhea and an elevation of inflammatory parameters. Cardiovascular and pulmonary function remained stable. Abdominal computed tomography showed a thickening of the bowel wall of the entire ileum and no other pathologies. On day 12 after mushroom ingestion gastrointestinal biopsies were taken from the ileum and the large bowel; see Figures 1 and 2. Diagnostic findings were most prominent in the mucosa of the ileum and the cecum and decreased towards the rectum. The mucosa of the ileum showed, in addition to acute cryptitis

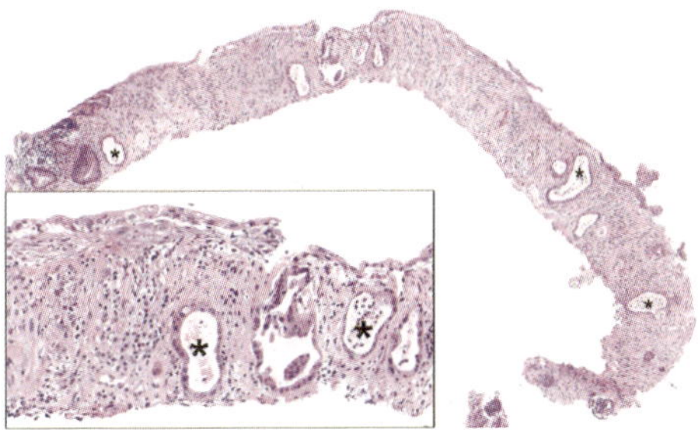

FIGURE 2: Biopsy of the cecum, showing rarefication and atrophy of the crypts, dilation of the lumina with intraluminal cell detritus (∗), and fibrosis of the lamina propria. Epithelial cells present reactive, respectively, regeneratory nuclear atypia in the context of inflammation (40x magnification); for details see the inset (200x magnification).

and ulcerating inflammation with fibrinoleukocytic exudate (pseudomembranes), regenerating changes of the epithelium. Acute erosive and ulcerating inflammatory changes together with a rarefication and atrophy of crypts, fibrosis of the lamina propria, and regenerating epithelial changes were most prominent in the cecum. These findings of a distinct ileitis and proximally accentuated colitis are not specific. Architectural and regenerating epithelial changes and fibrosis indicate a sustained or previous damage of the mucosa. Screening for Clostridium difficile toxin using ELISA as well as cultures for Clostridium difficile and *Salmonella*, *Shigella*, and *Campylobacter* species remained negative. With supportive therapy, gastrointestinal symptoms as well as inflammatory markers showed a tendency to regression so that the patient could be dismissed in good shape on day 17 after ingestion of *Amanita*. Diarrhea and varying abdominal pain persisted over several weeks thereafter. Clinical follow-up after six months showed a completely symptom-free patient.

3. Discussion and Conclusions

Worldwide, only a few cases of late gastrointestinal complications of *Amanita* intoxication have been reported [7]. Supported by the absence of other possible etiologies such as the detection of infectious agents, in our reported case, the impressive manifestation of ulcerating ileocolitis may be directly due to amatoxins, which could be detected in high concentrations in the patient's urine. Even though urine toxin concentration does not correlate as well with the clinical manifestations of the intoxication as the amount of toxin ingested per body weight [2], patient history also indicates a fairly high amount of ingested fungus, as 50 g of *Amanita phalloides* may already contain a lethal dose of toxin for an adult. Still, other possible causes of ulcerating ileocolitis cannot entirely be excluded even in the absence of known triggers such as nonsteroidal anti-inflammatory drugs or known ischemia. Renal failure can be the result of direct kidney damage due to amatoxins [6] as is at least in part suggested by the increased fractional excretion of urea; however, a combined prerenal etiology is likely in light of the rapid and complete amelioration following adequate volume management. Specific treatment to *Amanita* intoxication is available and was administered early in our case. Silibinin, an extract of the Mediterranean milk thistle (*Silybum marianum*), acts as specific inhibitor of amatoxin uptake into hepatocytes and may improve survival [10]. N-Acetyl cysteine, presumably acting through its antioxidant effects, has also recently been shown to significantly improve survival [11]. Finally, multiple dose activated charcoal administered until at least day 4 after ingestion removes the amatoxins from the enterohepatobiliary recirculation and thereby improves total toxin clearance [12]. Plasma exchange has also been discussed [13, 14], but there is little data about the risk-benefit-ratio. The effect of all of these treatment modalities on late gastrointestinal complications however is, to our knowledge, unknown. Clinical knowledge about the possibility of late gastrointestinal manifestations of *Amanita* intoxication was probably more common in the seventh and eighth decade of the twentieth century [15, 16], even though it remains important to generate and distribute knowledge about it, especially since *Amanita* intoxication is a permanent threat to the population and still remains difficult to treat. Also, further research is needed to possibly draw a connection between amatoxins and direct action on the bowel and to understand the specific mechanisms that may be involved. The case presented highlights the importance to consider the possibility of rare complications of *Amanita* intoxication in order to be able to respond to them early and adequately.

References

[1] J. McNeill, *International Code of Botanical Nomenclature*, International Association for Plant Taxonomy, Bratislava, Slovakia, 2006.

[2] C. Karlson-Stiber and H. Persson, "Cytotoxic fungi—an overview," *Toxicon*, vol. 42, no. 4, pp. 339–349, 2003.

[3] Y. Iliev, S. Andonova, and V. Akabaliev, "Our experience in the treatment of acute *Amanita phalloides* poisoning," *Folia Medica*, vol. 41, no. 4, pp. 30–37, 1999.

[4] K. J. Berger and D. A. Guss, "Mycotoxins revisited: part I," *Journal of Emergency Medicine*, vol. 28, no. 1, pp. 53–62, 2005.

[5] P. A. Horgen, A. C. Vaisius, and J. F. Ammirati, "The insensitivity of mushroom nuclear RNA polymerase activity to inhibiton by amatoxins," *Archives of Microbiology*, vol. 118, no. 3, pp. 317–319, 1978.

[6] P. L. West, J. Lindgren, and B. Z. Horowitz, "Amanita smithiana mushroom ingestion: a case of delayed renal failure and literature review," *Journal of Medical Toxicology*, vol. 5, no. 1, pp. 32–38, 2009.

[7] F. Eyer, N. Felgenhauer, and T. Zilker, "The development of a toxic megacolon due to *Amanita phalloides* poisoning. A rare complication," *Deutsche Medizinische Wochenschrift*, vol. 129, pp. 137–140, 2004.

[8] L. Giannini, A. Vannacci, A. Missanelli et al., "Amatoxin poisoning: a 15-year retrospective analysis and follow-up evaluation of 105 patients," *Clinical Toxicology*, vol. 45, no. 5, pp. 539–542, 2007.

[9] F. Enjalbert, S. Rapior, J. Nouguier-Soulé, S. Guillon, N. Amouroux, and C. Cabot, "Treatment of amatoxin poisoning: 20-Year retrospective analysis," *Journal of Toxicology—Clinical Toxicology*, vol. 40, no. 6, pp. 715–757, 2002.

[10] K. Letschert, H. Faulstich, D. Keller, and D. Keppler, "Molecular characterization and inhibition of amanitin uptake into human hepatocytes," *Toxicological Sciences*, vol. 91, no. 1, pp. 140–149, 2006.

[11] P. Poucheret, F. Fons, J. C. Doré, D. Michelot, and S. Rapior, "Amatoxin poisoning treatment decision-making: Pharmaco-therapeutic clinical strategy assessment using multidimensional multivariate statistic analysis," *Toxicon*, vol. 55, no. 7, pp. 1338–1345, 2010.

[12] A. Jaeger, F. Jehl, F. Flesch, P. Sauder, and J. Kopferschmitt, "Kinetics of amatoxins in human poisoning: therapeutic implications," *Journal of Toxicology: Clinical Toxicology*, vol. 31, no. 1, pp. 63–80, 1993.

[13] S. Jander, J. Bischoff, and B. G. Woodcock, "Plasmapheresis in the treatment of Amanita phalloides poisoning. II. A review and recommendations," *Therapeutic Apheresis*, vol. 4, no. 4, pp. 308–312, 2000.

[14] Y. Hiroshima, H. Nakae, and K. Gommori, "Amanita ibotengutake intoxication treated with plasma exchange," *Therapeutic Apheresis and Dialysis*, vol. 14, no. 5, pp. 483–484, 2010.

[15] C. Busi, L. Fiume, D. Costantino, M. Langer, and F. Vesconi, "Amanita toxins in gastroduodenal fluid of patients poisoned by the mushroom, *Amanita phalloides*," *The New England Journal of Medicine*, vol. 300, no. 14, p. 800, 1979.

[16] L. Fiume, M. Derenzini, V. Marinozzi, F. Petazzi, and A. Testoni, "Pathogenesis of gastro-intestinal symptomatology during poisoning by *Amanita phalloides*," *Experientia*, vol. 29, no. 12, pp. 1520–1521, 1973.

Left Colon Diverticulitis Presenting as Perforated Lumbar Abscess: A Case Report and Review of the Current Literature

Daniel Paramythiotis, Konstantinia Kofina, Vassileios N. Papadopoulos, and Antonios Michalopoulos

1st Propedeutic Surgical Clinic, Aristotle's University of Thessaloniki, AHEPA University Hospital, Stilponos Kyriakidi 1, 54636 Thessaloniki, Greece

Correspondence should be addressed to Daniel Paramythiotis; danosprx@med.auth.gr

Academic Editor: Antonio Macrì

Diverticular perforation is a common complication of diverticulitis and can lead to the creation of abscesses. The presence of such abscesses on the abdominal wall is rare and can lead to misdiagnosis. We present the case of a patient with abdominal pain and the formation of a large left lumbar abscess due to perforation of a diverticulum of the left colon and our surgical treatment of choice with favorable results.

1. Introduction

Diverticular disease affects mainly patients over forty years of age especially in the western countries, with left colon representing the most common site of presentation [1]. Most patients remain asymptomatic, while 20% of cases present symptoms [2]. Risk factors include obesity, smoking, and low-fiber diet, but the pathophysiology may also include a connection between diverticulitis, inflammatory disease, and irritable bowel syndrome [3]. Possible complications include abscesses, perforation, strictures, or the formation of fistula, altogether of a rate of 25% [2].

Actually, diverticulum perforation may, usually, lead to abscess formation because of the inflammation of the nearby structures through tissue continuity. However, the presence of an abscess on the abdominal wall due to such perforation is rare. We present the rare case of a patient with a large perforated left lumbar abscess and vague abdominal pain that was diagnosed as diverticular perforation and was treated surgically, following the existing guidelines [4].

2. Case Report

A 50-year-old male patient was admitted at the Emergency Department of our clinic complaining about mild diffuse abdominal pain, with no specific location of tenderness. This pain presented the previous day, along with fever up to 38.3°C. He did not mention any other symptoms, such as nausea, appetite loss, or bowel dysfunction. Prior to our examination, the patient was referred to the Internal Medicine Emergency Department, where he was scheduled to have a blood test and an X-ray examination of the abdomen (Figure 2). His laboratory values included WBC 8.43 K/μL with 74.5% neutrophils, Hb 11.2 gr/dL, and Ht 34.3%. His vital signs were between normal ranges. From his medical history he revealed two episodes of acute diverticulitis during the past five years (five and three years before this admission, each), for which he followed conservative treatment. At the time of admission, he was not on immunosuppressant or any other medication.

During the clinical examination, a mild diffuse sensitivity during palpation of the left abdominal area was observed, without any specific signs of abdominal pain. However, the patient's inspection revealed an abscess in the left lumbar area, which, according to the patient, was present for about three months and tended to reduce in size after defecation. The abscess seemed uncomplicated, not too large, and manageable through drainage under local anesthesia on bedside. Therefore, it was incised, but almost two liters of pus-like fluid was drained (Figure 1). Even though there was no clinical suspicion for the performance of an abdominal CT prior to the drainage, the quantity and quality of the drained fluids made it necessary to carry out this examination for further

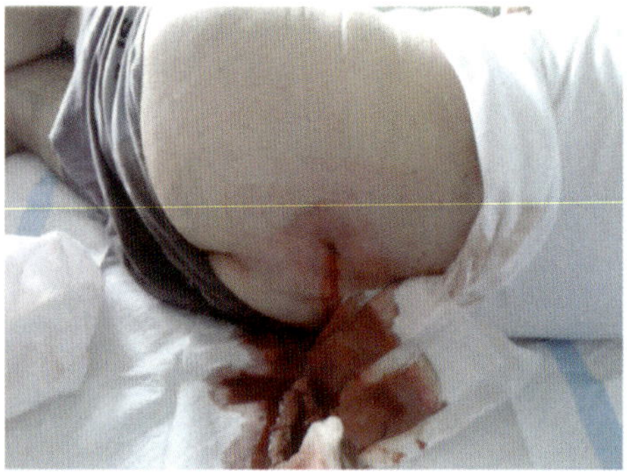

Figure 1: Image of left lumbar abscess drainage due to perforated diverticulitis.

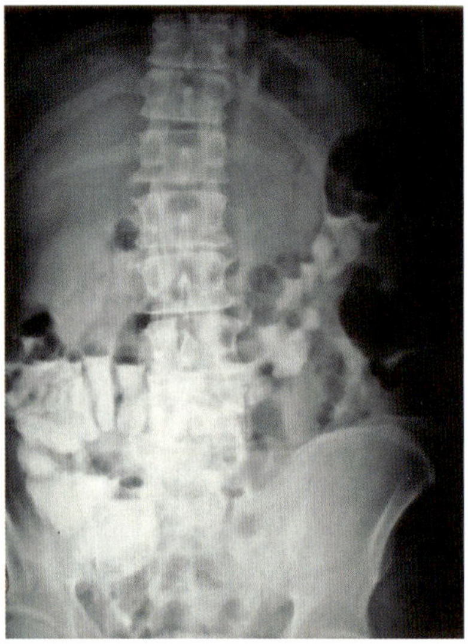

Figure 2: Abdominal X-ray showing inflammation at the left lumbar area.

control. The CT revealed the presence of free air in the lumbar wall, in the abscess area (but not in the abdomen), as well as signs of inflammation (Figures 3(a) and 3(b)).

Due to these imaging findings in combination with the patient's condition, we decided to perform an exploratory laparotomy, during which a perforated diverticulum of the left colon was revealed. This perforation led to the inflammation of the posterior abdominal wall through tissue continuity and resulted in the formation of the lumbar abscess. However, there were no signs of generalized peritonitis, as the fascia was not infected. The inflamed segment of the colon was excised at healthy margins and an end-to-end anastomosis was performed (Figures 4, 5(a), and 5(b)). The postoperative period was uneventful and the patient was discharged on the seventh day after surgery with the wall trauma on a good condition and with a recommendation of antibiotic uptake for the following two weeks.

3. Discussion

Diverticulitis is staged according to the classic Hinchey classification as pericolic abscess or phlegmon (Hinchey I), pelvic, abdominal, or retroperitoneal abscess (Hinchey II), generalized purulent peritonitis (Hinchey III), and generalized fecal peritonitis (Hinchey IV). Many other classifications have been reported also (Hughes, modified Hinchey, Köhler, Hansen/Stock, and Siewert) [5]. The usual presentation of a diverticulum perforation is acute abdominal pain and peritonitis. However, it can also appear with nontypical signs, through complications such as chronic abscesses, the creation of fistulae, and bowel obstruction. Therefore, cases have been reported that presented with colovesical and colovaginal fistulae [6], perianal fistulae [7], abscess formation on the abdominal wall [1], the thigh [6], or the renal fossa during end-stage renal disease [8], subcutaneous emphysema [9], and a perforation in a lumbar hernia [10].

In our case, the perforation appeared as a left lumbar area abscess of three-month duration, for which the patient did not seek treatment before, as he did not present any other symptoms. Apart from our case, only two other cases have been described clearly as an abscess in the lumbar area following diverticulum perforation in the literature (Table 1) [11, 12]. It is believed that recurrent attacks of diverticulitis provoke scarring and adhesion formation, so localized perforations and abscesses may appear instead of generalized peritonitis [4].

The management of acute diverticulitis includes fluid and antibiotic support, percutaneous drain abscess drainage or resection, and 1- or 2-stage anastomosis, depending on each individual case [13]. The first colon resection for the treatment of a diverticular perforation was reported by Mayo in 1907. New strategies in the management of perforated diverticular disease suggest that, in patients with Hinchey I and Hinchey II perforated diverticulitis, we should first perform laparoscopic lavage and secondly colonic resection and anastomosis at the same time. In Hinchey III and Hinchey IV perforated diverticulitis, the colorectal surgical specialists recommend either emergent definitive sigmoid resection with primary anastomosis with or without protective ileostomy formation or Hartmann's procedure [14].

Many studies have shown improved results through primary anastomosis, depending on the surgeon's experience [15], while others consider it as a frequent surgery with no higher morbidity or mortality in comparison to Hartmann's procedure [16]. In our case, resection of the damaged colon

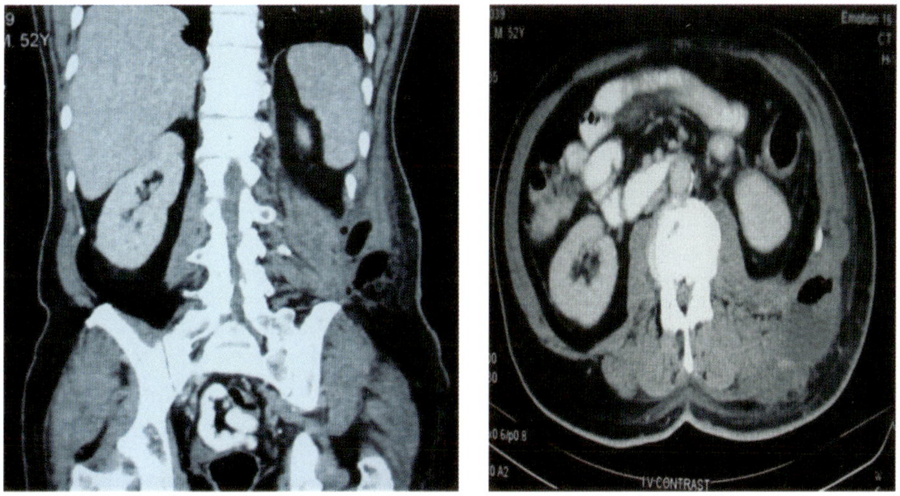

(a) (b)

Figure 3: Abdominal CT scans revealed a perforated diverticulitis of the sigmoid colon causing subcutaneous inflammation and free gas in the tissue of the posterior abdominal wall and lumbar area.

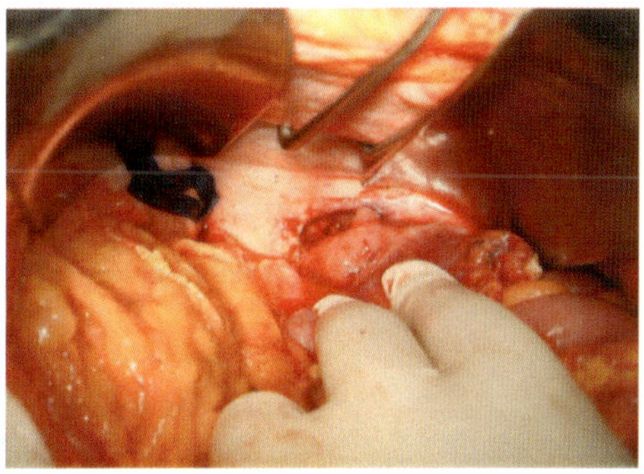

Figure 4: Intraoperative image of the loft colon perforation.

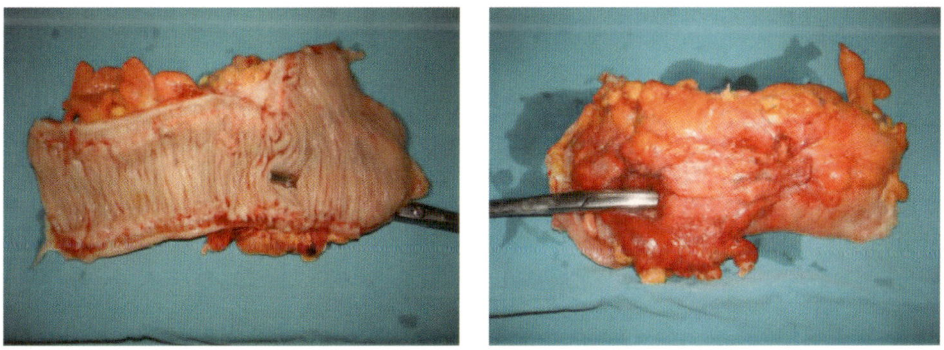

(a) (b)

Figure 5: Postoperative excised left colon specimen.

Table 1: Lumbar abscesses due to diverticular perforation: three reported cases and treatment of choice.

Authors	Year	Patients	Treatment
Green and Joypaul [11]	2009	1	Sigmoid colectomy and primary anastomosis
Coulier et al. [12]	2012	1	2-step surgical approach
Paramythiotis et al.	2015	1	Elective sigmoid dissection and primary anastomosis

and primary end-to-end anastomosis were considered viable and the recovery of the patient was uneventful.

Abdominal CT is the imaging examination of choice, as it sets the definite diagnosis, shows the extent of abdominal inflammation, and excludes any other causes of acute abdominal pain [9]. In our case, a CT was immediately performed after the lumbar abscess drainage because, in combination with the abdominal pain, the X-ray findings, and the medical history, a clinical suspicion of diverticular perforation was set. The early diagnosis is crucial, as a delayed diagnosis of such perforation is associated with high mortality. As this presentation of diverticular perforation is not typical, a surgeon should be always aware of this possibility and prevent any misdiagnosis.

4. Conclusion

The diagnosis of a diverticular perforation, especially when it appears with nonspecific symptoms as a lumbar area abscess, may be difficult to establish and is often misinterpreted. A detailed clinical history must be taken and the patient should be examined thoroughly. Imaging findings such as CT can help in the differential diagnosis and lead to the precise diagnosis and to early surgical treatment.

References

[1] R. Vasileios, G. Anna, L. Christos, T. Asimina, P. Sofia, and K. Vasiliki, "Abdominal wall abscess due to acute perforated sigmoid diverticulitis: a case report with MDCT and US findings," *Case Reports in Radiology*, vol. 2013, Article ID 565928, 5 pages, 2013.

[2] R. C. Spiller, "Changing views on diverticular disease: impact of aging, obesity, diet, and microbiota," *Neurogastroenterology and Motility*, vol. 27, no. 3, pp. 305–312, 2015.

[3] K. Moubax and D. Urbain, "Diverticulitis: new insights on the traditional point of view," *Acta Gastro-Enterologica Belgica*, vol. 78, no. 1, pp. 38–48, 2015.

[4] V. Naraynsingh, R. Maharaj, D. Hassranah, S. Hariharan, D. Dan, and A. P. Zbar, "Perforated left-sided diverticulitis with faecal peritonitis: is the Hinchey classification the best guide for surgical decision making?" *Techniques in Coloproctology*, vol. 15, no. 2, pp. 199–203, 2011.

[5] B. R. Klarenbeek, N. de Korte, D. L. van der Peet, and M. A. Cuesta, "Review of current classifications for diverticular disease and a translation into clinical practice," *International Journal of Colorectal Disease*, vol. 27, no. 2, pp. 207–214, 2012.

[6] P. B. Murphy and P. Belliveau, "Left-sided sigmoid diverticulitis presenting as right-sided thigh abscess," *International Surgery*, vol. 97, no. 4, pp. 285–287, 2012.

[7] I. B. Amor, R. Kassir, E. Bachir, H. Katharina, T. Debs, and J. Gugenheim, "Perforated diverticulitis of the sigmoid colon revealed by a perianal fistula," *International Journal of Surgery Case Reports*, vol. 8, pp. 73–75, 2015.

[8] S.-Y. Li, J.-K. Jiang, Y.-H. Chang, T.-C. Wu, W.-C. Yang, and Y.-Y. Ng, "Recurrent retroperitoneal abscess due to perforated colonic diverticulitis in a patient with polycystic kidney disease," *Journal of the Chinese Medical Association*, vol. 72, no. 3, pp. 153–155, 2009.

[9] R. Kassir, K. Abboud, J. Dubois et al., "Perforated diverticulitis of the sigmoid colon causing a subcutaneous emphysema," *International Journal of Surgery Case Reports*, vol. 5, no. 12, pp. 1190–1192, 2014.

[10] F. S. Frueh, R. N. Vuille-Dit-Bille, D. A. Raptis, H. Notter, and B. S. Muff, "Perforated sigmoid diverticulitis in a lumbar hernia after iliac crest bone graft—a case report," *BMC Surgery*, vol. 14, article 46, 2014.

[11] B. R. Green and V. Joypaul, "Left sided diverticulitis presenting as a right lumbar fistula: a case report," *Cases Journal*, vol. 2, no. 8, article 7146, 2009.

[12] B. Coulier, M. Gogoase, A. Ramboux, and F. Pierard, "Extra-abdominal lumbar abscesses caused by retroperitoneal gastrointestinal perforations through the lumbar triangle of Petit: report of two cases diagnosed by CT," *Abdominal Imaging*, vol. 37, no. 6, pp. 1122–1128, 2012.

[13] A. V. Weizman and G. C. Nguyen, "Diverticular disease: epidemiology and management," *Canadian Journal of Gastroenterology*, vol. 25, no. 7, pp. 385–389, 2011.

[14] F. A. Moore, F. Catena, E. E. Moore, A. Leppaniemi, and A. B. Peitzmann, "Position paper: management of perforated sigmoid diverticulitis," *World Journal of Emergency Surgery*, vol. 8, no. 1, pp. 55–65, 2013.

[15] M. S. Jafferji and N. Hyman, "Surgeon, not disease severity, often determines the operation for acute complicated diverticulitis," *Journal of the American College of Surgeons*, vol. 218, no. 6, pp. 1156–1161, 2014.

[16] L. Reyes-Espejel, M. Ruiz-Campos, J. Correa-Rovelo, and S. García-Osogobio, "Sigmoidectomy with primary anastomosis for complicated diverticulitis," *Revista de Gastroenterología de México*, vol. 80, no. 4, pp. 255–259, 2015.

15

Clinical Outcome of a Portosplenomesenteric Venous Thrombosis in Necrotizing Acute Pancreatitis with Protein C and S Deficiency Treated by Anticoagulation Therapy Alone

Firmin Ankouane,[1] Mathurin Kowo,[1] Bernadette Ngo Nonga,[2] Eric Magny,[3] Edith Hell Medjo,[3] and Elie Claude Ndjitoyap Ndam[4]

[1] *Department of Internal Medicine and Specialties, Faculty of Medicine and Biomedical Sciences, University of Yaounde 1, Yaounde University Teaching Hospital, Yaoundé, Cameroon*
[2] *Department of Surgery and Specialties, Faculty of Medicine and Biomedical Sciences, University of Yaounde 1, Yaounde University Teaching Hospital, Yaoundé, Cameroon*
[3] *Department of Radiology and Imaging, Faculty of Medicine and Biomedical Sciences, University of Yaounde 1, Yaoundé, Cameroon*
[4] *Department of Internal Medicine and Specialties, Faculty of Medicine and Biomedical Sciences, University of Yaounde 1, Yaounde General Hospital, Yaoundé, Cameroon*

Correspondence should be addressed to Firmin Ankouane; ankouaneandoulo@yahoo.com

Academic Editor: Hideto Kawaratani

Cases of splanchnic venous thrombosis have not been described in Cameroon. Their prevalence in acute pancreatitis is variable. With the emergence of acute intra-abdominal infections including typhoid fever and peritoneal tuberculosis in situations of acquired immunodeficiency syndrome, these cases will become frequent. We report the case of a portosplenomesenteric venous thrombosis related to necrotizing acute pancreatitis associated with proteins C and S deficiency, in a 46-year-old Cameroonian man, without particular past medical history. He was admitted for abdominal pain which had been evolving for 3 weeks and accompanied by vomiting. In the absence of hemorrhagic risk factor, the patient received low molecular weight heparin followed by oral warfarin. The abdominal ultrasound check on the 12th day showed a partial recanalization of venous thrombosis. The abdominal contrast-enhanced CT scanner at day 30 on oral anticoagulation therapy showed collateral vessels and small bowel edema. At the same time the upper gastrointestinal endoscopy showed grade II esophageal varices. We have maintained oral anticoagulation therapy. This case highlights that an early effective anticoagulation heparin therapy is needed for a clear benefit in case of suspected PSMVT. It is certain that the sooner the treatment is given, the better outcome will be.

1. Introduction

Venous thrombosis is a multifactorial disease resulting from the dynamic interaction between genetic and acquired risk factors. The common inflammatory causes of splanchnic venous thrombosis (SVT) are acute abdominal pathologies [1]. The portosplenomesenteric venous thrombosis (PSMVT) is rare [2]. In acute pancreatitis (AP) it has been found to be related to the severity of the pancreatitis. Necrotizing AP is accompanied by perivascular inflammation, pancreatic necrosis, and compression by peripancreatic collections or pseudocysts as well as protein C and S deficiency [2–4].

The use of unfractionated heparin or low molecular weight heparin followed by oral vitamin K antagonists is the common approach to anticoagulation [2]. The complications directly related to SVT are rare but PSMVT is associated with a more dismal prognosis [5]. We are reporting here the first case of PSMVT complicating a necrotizing pancreatitis which was associated with protein C and S deficiency.

2. Case Presentation

A 46-year-old Cameroonian man, living in North Cameroon, was admitted to the Yaoundé University Teaching Hospital

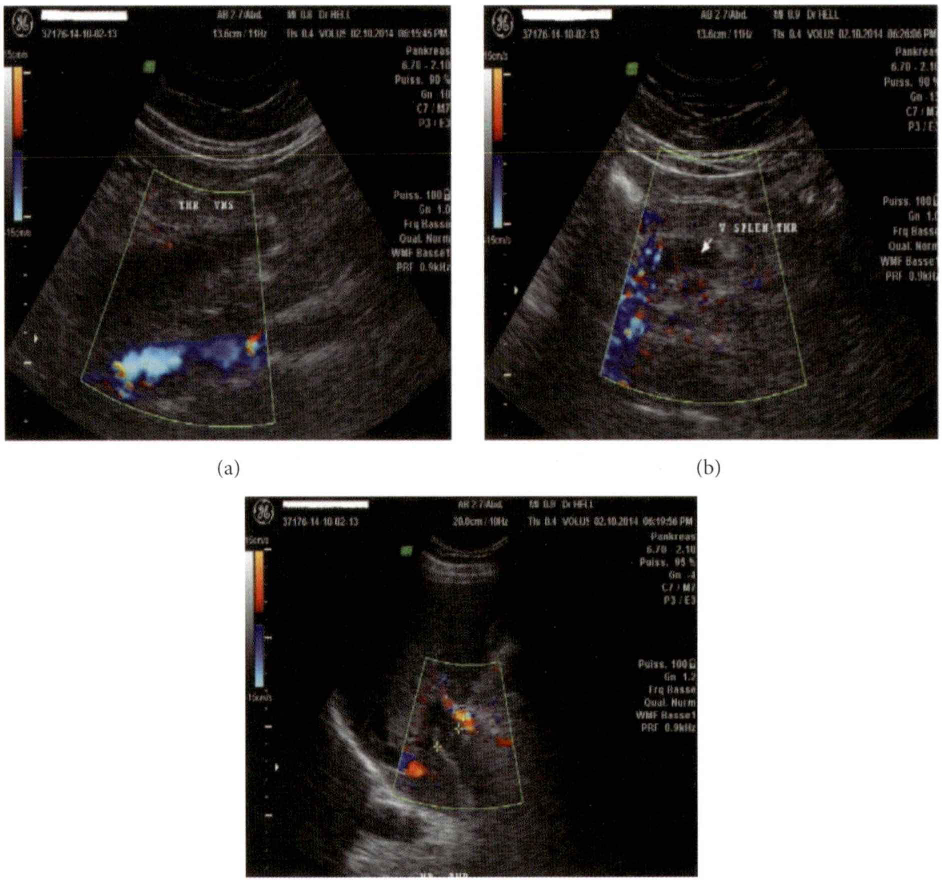

(a) (b) (c)

Figure 1: Doppler ultrasonography: showing in (a) the superior mesenteric vein thrombosis, in (b) the splenic vein thrombosis, and in (c) the portal vein thrombosis. With the permission of Medical Imaging Centre (MIC) in Yaoundé.

for diffuse abdominal pain accompanied by abdominal distension and vomiting for three-week duration. This was treated as a gastroduodenal ulcer without accurate diagnosis on endoscopy. His past medical history was unremarkable. The physical exam revealed a distended and tympanic abdomen, diffusely tender with no guarding. There was no palpable mass and bowel sounds were present. The digital rectal exam elicited pains on both sides. On admission, he has a low grade fever with a temperature of 38.2°C; the blood pressure was 113/82 mm Hg, and the heart rate 102 beats/minute. The laboratory tests (hemogram and biochemistry) were normal except for a C-reactive protein of 160 mg/L (standards: less than 6 mg/L), the lipase of 6xULN (upper limit of normal), and mild hepatic cytolysis (ALT greater than 3xULN). The tests of the hepatitis B surface antigen, the anti-hepatitis C virus antibodies, and the human immunodeficiency virus (HIV) were negative. Abdominal Doppler ultrasonography revealed an extensive venous thrombosis of the portal, splenic, and mesenteric veins (Figure 1). The abdominal contrast-enhanced CT scanner confirmed the extended thrombosis and highlighted an infiltration of the proximal pancreas associated with inflammatory flows in the peritoneum (Figure 2).

The diagnosis of necrotizing AP complicated by PSMVT was done. In the absence of significant contraindications factor, the patient received low molecular weight heparin (enoxaparin 1 mg/kg subcutaneously twice daily), followed by oral warfarin on the 10th day, dose adjusted according to the International Normalized Ratio (INR). The repeated abdominal Doppler ultrasound on the 12th day from admission showed a partial recanalization of the extensive venous thrombosis, confirmed by the abdominal contrast-enhanced CT scanner on 30th day which showed collateral vessels and small bowel edema (Figure 3). For accurate diagnosis, specific tests have shown normal serum lipids, and the tests for anti-nuclear antibodies, anti-native DNA antibodies, and antiphospholipids were negative; the hemoglobin electrophoresis was AA type. On the contrary, the functional test of protein C (STA Stachrom) showed a serum rate of 25% (normal range: 80–130%, Cerba Laboratories, France) and that of the protein S (STA Staclot) was 50% (normal range: 70–130%, Cerba Laboratories, France). Upper gastrointestinal endoscopy performed three months after follow-up showed grade II esophageal varices (Figure 4). There were no adverse effects on anticoagulation after three months of follow-up.

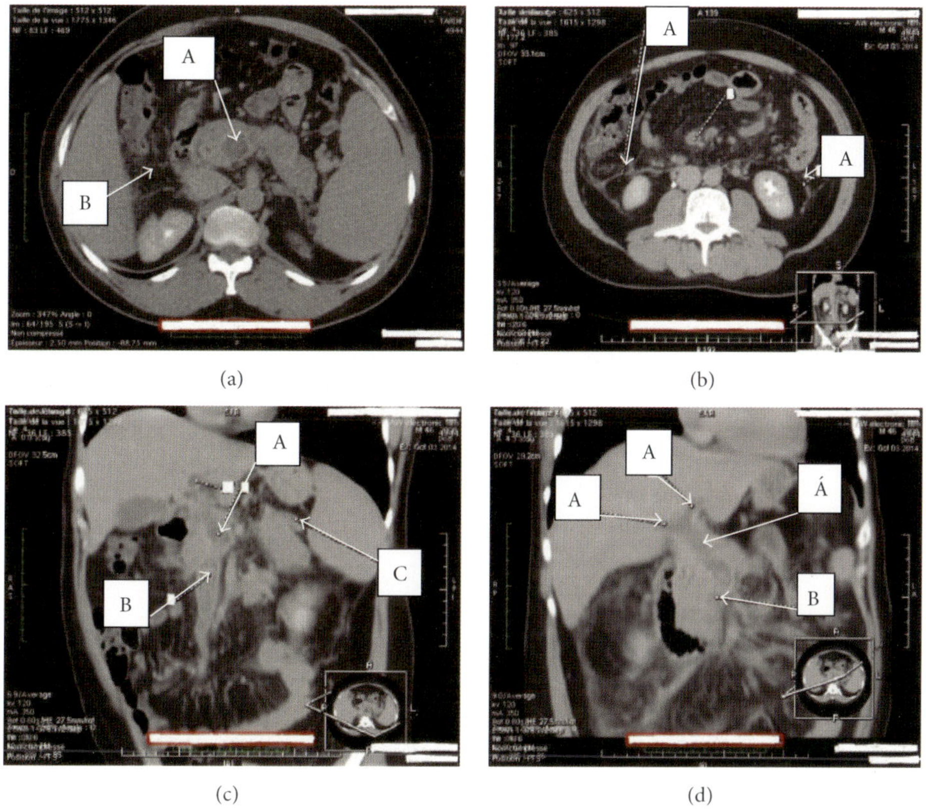

Figure 2: Abdominal contrast-enhanced CT scanner (hospital admission): (a) an edematous pancreas in (A) the superior mesenteric vein thrombosis and (B) the infiltration of the peripancreatic fat. (b) (A) Inflammatory flows. (c) (A) The portal venous thrombosis, (B) the superior mesenteric venous thrombosis, and (C) the splenic venous thrombosis. (d) (A) The thrombosis of the left and right branches of the portal vein and (B) the superior mesenteric venous thrombosis and distal branches. Light Speed CT-16 (GE Medical Systems, USA). Contrast: iobitridol 300 mg/mL (Xenetix, Guerbet, Roissy CDG Cedex, France). With the permission of the Cathedral Medical Center (CMC), Yaoundé.

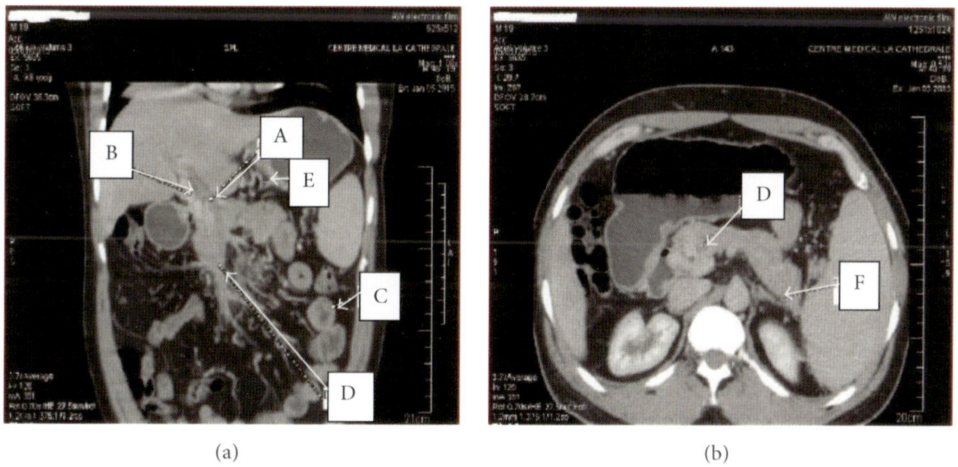

Figure 3: Abdominal contrast-enhanced CT scanner: control after three months on oral anticoagulation. (a) Partial recanalization of the portal venous thrombosis (A) and the superior mesenteric venous thrombosis (D), the portal cavernoma (B) and gastric collateral vessels (E), and thickening of the small intestinal bowel (C). (b) Superior mesenteric venous partial recanalization (D) and residual inflammatory flows (F). Light Speed CT-16 (GE Medical Systems, USA), contrast: iobitridol 300 mg/mL (Xenetix, Guerbet, Roissy CDG Cedex, France). With the permission of the Cathedral Medical Center (CMC), Yaoundé.

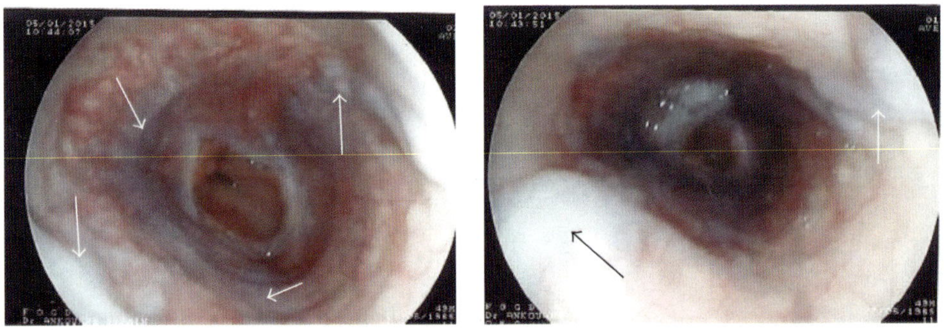

FIGURE 4: Upper gastrointestinal endoscopy performed after three months on oral anticoagulation. Arrows show medium varices occupying the circumference of the esophageal lumen. Fujinon EG250PE5, Japan. With the permission of the Cathedral Medical Center (CMC) in Yaoundé.

3. Discussion

Vascular complications have been associated with AP and these include SVT (1-2%) [5]. The different causes for splanchnic vein thrombosis are well established in the following list.

Known Causes of Splanchnic Vein Thrombosis

(1) Abdominal disorders and postoperative state are as follows:

(a) acute:

(i) pancreatitis*,
(ii) peritonitis and intra-abdominal sepsis*,
(iii) inflammatory bowel disease,
(iv) diverticulitis,
(v) splenectomy,
(vi) abdominal operations*,
(vii) sclerotherapy for esophageal varices,
(viii) blunt abdominal trauma;

(b) chronic:

(i) cirrhosis and portal hypertension,
(ii) neoplasm*.

(2) Prothrombotic states are as follows:

(i) Antithrombin III deficiency.
(ii) Protein C deficiency.
(iii) Protein S deficiency.
(iv) Factor V Leiden.
(v) G20210A mutation in prothrombin gene.
(vi) Antiphospholipid antibodies.
(vii) Hyperhomocysteinemia.

(3) Hematologic disorders are as follows:

(i) Polycythemia vera*.
(ii) Essential thrombocythemia*.
(iii) Idiopathic myelofibrosis.
(iv) Paroxysmal nocturnal hemoglobinuria* (PNH).

(4) Hormones are as follows:

(i) Oral contraceptives*.
(ii) Hormonal replacement therapy.
(iii) Pregnancy.
(iv) Puerperium.

(5) Autoimmune disorders are as follows:

(i) Behçet's disease.
(ii) Hypereosinophilic syndrome.

(6) Miscellaneous causes are as follows:

(i) Decompression sickness.
(ii) Cytomegalovirus.

(7) New biological markers of subclinical disorders are as follows:

(i) JAK2 mutation.
(ii) CD55 and CD59 (PNH clone).

*This factor is among the more common causes of splanchnic vein thrombosis.

Among these, the splenic venous thrombosis is the most common due to its proximity with the pancreas, far ahead of portal venous thrombosis and the superior mesenteric venous thrombosis [3, 5, 11–13]. Portosplenomesenteric venous thrombosis is very rare and it is extremely variable; this is the first case of PSMVT associated with AP reported from Cameroon; both diseases are very rare in our environment and have not been reported in the literature. For example, in a two-year prospective study, Gonzelez et al. [2] reported one case out of 127 patients admitted for AP.

In the context of the AP, inflammatory phenomena largely explain the occurrence of thrombosis. They include local prothrombotic intraendothelial phenomena [2, 6]. In the majority of cases, the development of PSMVT is associated with the presence, location, and extension of the pancreatic necrosis [2, 3].

Systemic activation of the coagulation system commonly occurs in over half of the critically ill patients with severe AP, and coagulation disorders are related to the severity of the disease [4]. Thus, they frequently include a deficit in proteins C and S [4]. The protein C and S deficiency, which are natural anticoagulants in blood and have an essential role in the regulation of the coagulation, are a known cause of SVT [7]. The AP of our observation was associated with deficiency in proteins C (25%) and S (50%) and inflammatory phenomena. Previous human studies have shown low activity of protein C in severe AP [4, 8]. Evaluation of the coagulation and the endogenous protein C/Antithrombin III system shows that nonsurvivors in severe AP have significantly lower levels of protein C and Antithrombin III than survivors [4, 9, 10]. Also, in severe AP, protein C pathway defects have been shown to be associated with development of organ failure [10]. In our case, a repeat assay on day 90 after presentation shows that protein C and S values were within their normal ranges, which suggests that this deficiency was acquired, due to AP. In our milieu, the prevalence of protein C and S deficiency in a healthy population is unknown. We believe that AP preceded the onset of PSMVT and protein C and S deficiency is a result of the pancreatic necrosis. Diverticulitis is another possible cause of SVT in this patient. However, abdominal CT scanner showed diverticula of the colon without inflammatory signs on them.

It has been reported that SVT can lead to bleeding, bowel ischemia, and liver failure, but the signs and symptoms may overlap with those of AP [2, 11, 12]. Thus, in this case, it was difficult to distinguish between symptoms related to the AP and those related to venous thrombosis.

The combination of Doppler ultrasonography and CT scanner increases the diagnostic sensitivity. Doppler ultrasonography and CT scanner have a negative predictive value of 98% and 100%, respectively. Both tests enable showing pseudoaneurysm, intrapseudocystic bleeding, intra-abdominal collections, venous thrombosis, and varices [11, 12]. We performed both exams for diagnosis in this case.

There is no randomized study related to the use of anticoagulants in acute SVT. The use of unfractionated heparin or low molecular weight heparin during hospital stay followed by oral vitamin K antagonists is the common approach to anticoagulation [13]. The doses of anticoagulation treatment and its duration are not well defined [13]. Whatever the type of treatment used, full recanalization is rare. It has been found only in 1/3 of cases, especially in the recently formed thrombosis [2, 3, 13, 14]. The percentage of that recanalization depends on how early the anticoagulant therapy is given [2, 13, 15]. We started the anticoagulation treatment 3 weeks after the onset of symptoms and we observed a partial recanalization on the 12th day of treatment. The delay of treatment in relation with the installation of thrombosis is difficult to specify in this case. This partial recanalization is probably related to a delay in starting the treatment.

Other invasive approaches such as thrombolysis and transjugular intrahepatic portosystemic stent-shunt (TIPS) exist [16]. Surgical thrombectomy has been reported, especially in patients with high risk of complications to anticoagulation and thrombolytic treatment [17].

Apart from visceral ischemia, PSMVT may be accompanied by hemorrhage. The incidence of this complication is not well defined. In a previous retrospective study concerning 53 patients with AP, Heider et al. [18] reported that gastric variceal bleeding from AP-induced SVT occurs in only 4% of the cases. The majority of patients with PSMVT develop collateral vessels and more than a quarter presented varices on endoscopy [3, 19]. This case developed collateral vessels, esophageal varices, and small bowel edema on anticoagulation three months following abdominal complaints onset.

In conclusion, we report a clinical outcome of PSMVT in necrotizing AP with combined deficiency of proteins C and S in 46-year-old Cameroonian man treated with anticoagulation alone. This case highlights that an early effective anticoagulation heparin therapy is needed for a clear benefit in case of suspected PSMVT. It is certain that the sooner the treatment is given, the better the outcome will be.

Authors' Contribution

Firmin Ankouane is major contributor in drafting and writing the paper. Mathurin Kowo contributed to medical case management during admission and writing. Edith Hell Medjo performed the abdominal ultrasound color Doppler, Eric Magny performed computed tomography examination, and Bernadette Ngo Nonga analyzed and interpreted the patient data. Elie Claude Ndjitoyap Ndam approved the final version of the paper. All authors read and approved the final paper.

Acknowledgments

The authors sincerely appreciate the patient for his availability and endurance, Professor Ngu Blackett K. Head of the Internal Medicine and Specialties, and all the paramedical staff of the Internal Medicine and Specialties of the Yaoundé University Teaching Hospital who took care of the patient.

References

[1] E. W. Mohamed, "A case of portal vein thrombosis associated with acute cholecystitis/pancreatitis or coincidence," *Hepatobiliary and Pancreatic Diseases International*, vol. 5, no. 2, pp. 308–310, 2006.

[2] H. J. Gonzelez, S. J. Sahay, B. Samadi, B. R. Davidson, and S. H. Rahman, "Splanchnic vein thrombosis in severe acute pancreatitis: a 2-year, single-institution experience," *HPB*, vol. 13, no. 12, pp. 860–864, 2011.

[3] J. Easler, V. Muddana, A. Furlan et al., "Portosplenomesenteric venous thrombosis in patients with acute pancreatitis is associated with pancreatic necrosis and usually has a benign course," *Clinical Gastroenterology and Hepatology*, vol. 12, no. 5, pp. 854–862, 2014.

[4] S. S. Badhal, S. Sharma, A. Saraya, and A. K. Mukhopadhyay, "Prognostic significance of D-dimer, natural anticoagulants and routine coagulation parameters in acute pancreatitis," *Tropical Gastroenterology*, vol. 33, no. 3, pp. 193–199, 2012.

[5] S. Harris, N. A. Nadkarni, H. V. Naina, and S. S. Vege, "Splanchnic vein thrombosis in acute pancreatitis: a single-center experience," *Pancreas*, vol. 42, no. 8, pp. 1251–1254, 2013.

[6] N. A. Nadkarni, S. Khanna, and S. S. Vege, "Splanchnic venous thrombosis and pancreatitis," *Pancreas*, vol. 42, no. 6, pp. 924–931, 2013.

[7] A. J. Lucendo Villarín, G. Carrión Alonso, S. Martín Chávarri, M. Allona Krauel, and J. R. Prado Rodríguez, "Acute pancreatitis and protein C deficiency caused by mesenteric venous thrombosis," *Revista Espanola de Enfermedades Digestivas*, vol. 98, no. 7, pp. 553–554, 2006.

[8] V. Pettilä, L. Kyhälä, M.-L. Kylänpää et al., "APCAP-activated protein C in acute pancreatitis: a double-blind randomized human pilot trial," *Critical Care*, vol. 14, no. 4, article R139, 2010.

[9] D. Radenković, D. Bajec, A. Karamarkovic et al., "Disorders of hemostasis during the surgical management of severe necrotizing pancreatitis," *Pancreas*, vol. 29, no. 2, pp. 152–156, 2004.

[10] O. Lindstrom, L. Kylänpää, P. Mentula et al., "Upregulated but insufficient generation of activated protein C is associated with development of multiorgan failure in severe acute pancreatitis," *Critical Care*, vol. 10, no. 1, article R16, 2006.

[11] S. Parikh, R. Shah, and P. Kapoor, "Portal vein thrombosis," *The American Journal of Medicine*, vol. 123, no. 2, pp. 111–119, 2010.

[12] W. Jiang, J. Zhou, L. Ke et al., "Splanchnic vein thrombosis in necrotizing acute pancreatitis: detection by computed tomographic venography," *World Journal of Gastroenterology*, vol. 20, no. 44, pp. 16698–16701, 2014.

[13] W.-S. Park, H.-I. Kim, B.-J. Jeon, S.-H. Kim, and S.-O. Lee, "Should anticoagulants be administered for portal vein thrombosis associated with acute pancreatitis?" *World Journal of Gastroenterology*, vol. 18, no. 42, pp. 6168–6171, 2012.

[14] A. Plessier, S. Darwish-Murad, M. Hernandez-Guerra et al., "Acute portal vein thrombosis unrelated to cirrhosis: a prospective multicenter follow-up study," *Hepatology*, vol. 51, no. 1, pp. 210–218, 2010.

[15] A. R. Alvi, S. Khan, S. K. Niazi, M. Ghulam, and S. Bibi, "Acute mesenteric venous thrombosis: improved outcome with early diagnosis and prompt anticoagulation therapy," *International Journal of Surgery*, vol. 7, no. 3, pp. 210–213, 2009.

[16] T. Opitz, A. B. Buchwald, T. Lorf, D. Awuah, G. Ramadori, and W. Nolte, "The transjugular intrahepatic portosystemic stent-shunt (TIPS) as rescue therapy for complete Budd-Chiari syndrome and portal vein thrombosis," *Zeitschrift fur Gastroenterologie*, vol. 41, no. 5, pp. 413–418, 2003.

[17] S. Vedantham, "Interventional approaches to deep vein thrombosis," *American Journal of Hematology*, vol. 87, supplement 1, pp. S113–S118, 2012.

[18] T. R. Heider, S. Azeem, J. A. Galanko et al., "The natural history of pancreatitis-induced splenic vein thrombosis," *Annals of Surgery*, vol. 239, no. 6, pp. 876–882, 2004.

[19] E. Andersson, D. Ansari, and R. Andersson, "Major haemorrhagic complications of acute pancreatitis," *British Journal of Surgery*, vol. 97, no. 9, pp. 1379–1384, 2010.

16

Resolution of Fundic Gland Polyposis following Laparoscopic Magnetic Sphincter Augmentation and Subsequent Cessation of Proton Pump Inhibitors

Joel R. Brockmeyer,[1] Erin E. Connolly,[2] Richard J. Wittchow,[3] and Shanu N. Kothari[2]

[1] *Minimally Invasive Bariatric Surgery and Advanced Laparoscopy Fellowship, Gundersen Medical Foundation, 1900 South Avenue, La Crosse, WI 54601, USA*
[2] *Department of General and Vascular Surgery, Gundersen Health System, 1900 South Avenue, La Crosse, WI 54601, USA*
[3] *Department of Pathology, Gundersen Health System, 1900 South Avenue, La Crosse, WI 54601, USA*

Correspondence should be addressed to Shanu N. Kothari; snkothar@gundersenhealth.org

Academic Editor: Haruhiko Sugimura

Gastric polyps occur from a variety of sources and are found commonly on upper endoscopy. We present the case of a 49-year-old female who presented for evaluation for antireflux surgery with a history of fundic gland polyposis who required twice-daily proton pump inhibitors (PPIs) for control of her gastric reflux. After verifying that she met criteria for surgery, she underwent an uncomplicated laparoscopic magnetic sphincter augmentation placement. With the cessation of PPIs following surgery, the fundic gland polyposis resolved. Fundic gland polyps may occur sporadically or within certain syndromes, such as familial adenomatous polyposis. Multiple possible inciting factors exist, including the use of PPIs. This is the first reported case of the resolution of numerous fundic gland polyps following the completion of laparoscopic magnetic sphincter augmentation.

1. Introduction

Gastric polyps occur from a variety of sources and are found commonly on upper endoscopy. Due to the high prevalence of gastroesophageal reflux disease in the United States, many patients receive proton pump inhibitors (PPIs). A possible side effect of PPIs is the development of fundic gland polyps [1]. We describe a patient with multiple fundic gland polyps who had resolution of the polyps with the use of magnetic sphincter augmentation leading to cessation of PPIs.

2. Case Presentation

A 49-year-old female presented for evaluation for antireflux surgery. She had a 20-year history of heartburn and frequent acid brash. Until recently, her symptoms were well controlled with twice-daily PPI use with occasional additional over-the-counter antacids used. She had undergone upper endoscopy multiple times over the past 20 years that revealed short segment Barrett esophagus and numerous polyps ranging in size from ten to twenty millimeters (Figure 1).

Previous endoscopic biopsies of the innumerable stomach polyps showed fundic gland polyps. She was followed up by gastrointestinal medicine, with upper endoscopy and biopsies yearly. The most recent upper endoscopy one month before surgical evaluation revealed a normal appearing esophagus and innumerable polyps between 10 and 20 mm in size within the body of the stomach. Five of the largest gastric polyps were resected. Pathologic evaluation showed benign fundic gland polyps (Figure 2).

She underwent an esophageal impedance study after stopping her PPI for three weeks. Her DeMeester score was calculated as 20.6 (normal less than 14.7). Acid exposure time was increased in the upright position, 11.7% (normal less than 6.3%). Her total acid exposure time was elevated to 6.8% (normal less than 4.2%). The patient had a positive reflux symptom index for stomach burning of 100% and a positive reflux symptom association probability for heartburn

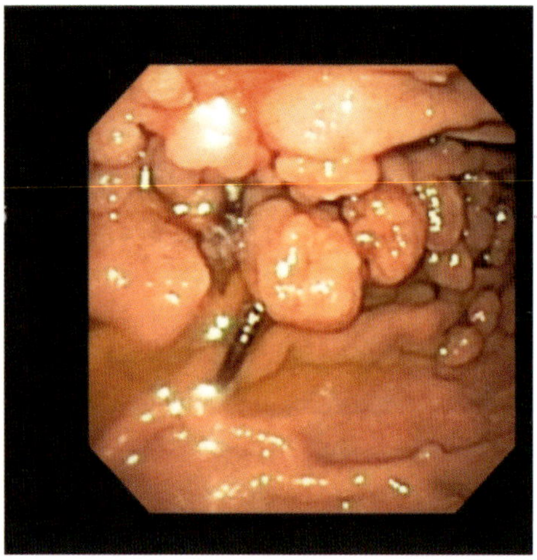

Figure 1: Upper endoscopy image taken prior to magnetic sphincter augmentation that shows multiple large polyps. Biopsy showed fundic gland polyps.

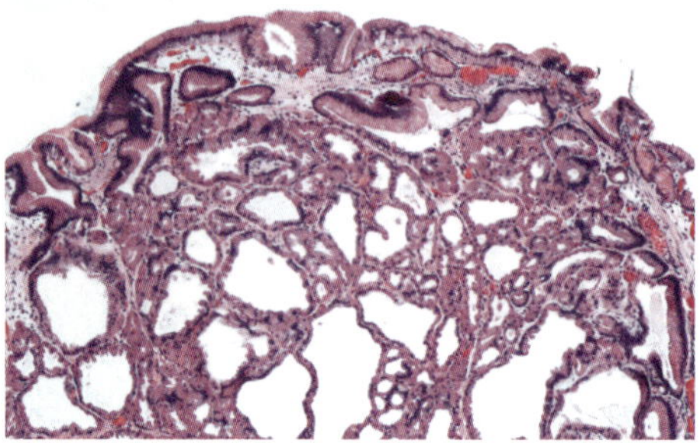

Figure 2: Fundic gland polyp, Hematoxylin and Eosin stain, 40x magnification.

of 100%. Esophageal manometry showed normal esophageal motility. Fluoroscopic upper gastrointestinal swallow study showed reflux without any hiatal hernia or other anatomic defects.

After discussion with the patient regarding laparoscopic fundoplication versus laparoscopic magnetic sphincter augmentation (MSA) (LINX, Torax Inc., Minneapolis, Minnesota, USA), the patient underwent laparoscopic MSA. The operation was completed without incident, and a 15-bead MSA device was placed around the lower esophageal sphincter. She was instructed to eat frequently to actuate the device at least every 4 hours. All antacid therapy was discontinued. She was seen in follow-up three weeks after surgery where she reported being free of reflux symptoms with only occasional dysphagia about three times per week.

The patient was seen nine months after MSA in the gastroenterology clinic for surveillance of her gastric polyps. She remained off all of her antacid medications and had no recurrent symptoms during that time. Surveillance upper endoscopy revealed a grossly normal esophagus. Biopsies of the gastroesophageal junction were obtained, revealing only benign mucosa with no further Barrett epithelium identified.

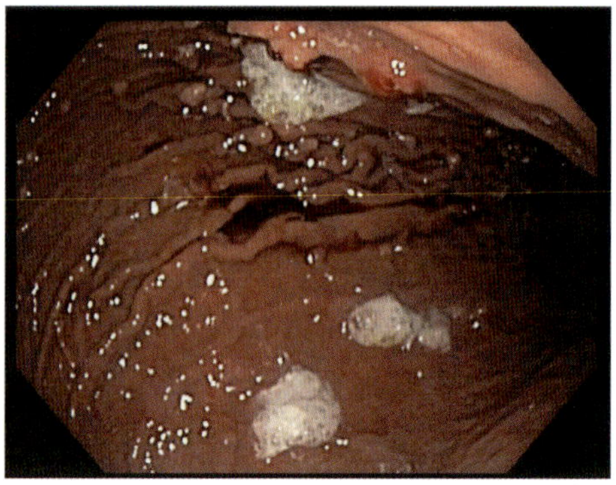

Figure 3: Upper endoscopy image following magnetic sphincter augmentation and cessation of all antacid medications showing minimal polyps that were biopsied and showed hyperplastic polyps.

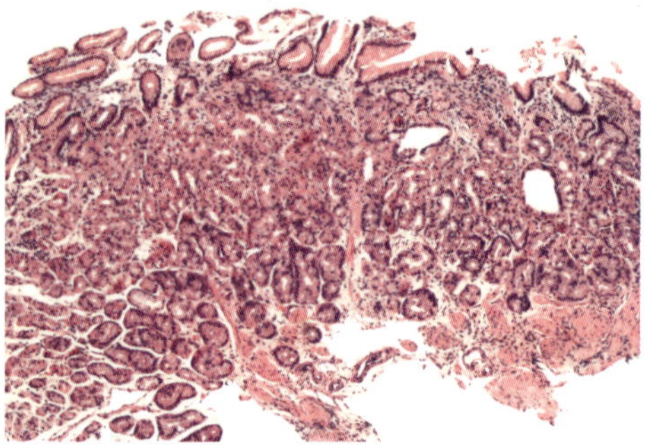

Figure 4: Mild chronic gastritis and reduction of fundic gland polyps, Hematoxylin and Eosin stain, 40x magnification.

Multiple polyps less than 5 mm in size were found in the body of the stomach with a drastic reduction in the number of polyps found prior to her MSA (Figure 3). Biopsies of these polyps revealed only mild chronic gastritis and a reduction of fundic gland polyps (Figure 4). The remainder of the endoscopy was normal. She has continued to do well since surgery without return of her reflux symptoms.

3. Discussion

Fundic gland polyps are the most common gastric polyps and account for about half of all benign gastric polyps [2]. First described in 1977, they are usually located in the body or fundus of the stomach and appear as sessile, shiny, translucent, pale to pinkish in color polyps with tiny surface blood vessels [3]. The polyps can be single or multiple and are characterized by cystically dilated fundic glands lined by flattened parietal cells, chief cells, and mucous neck cells [2]. No dysplastic morphology is seen in the overlying surface and foveolar gastric epithelium. Inflammatory changes in the polyps are minimal or absent and the surrounding gastric tissue is usually normal [3].

Fundic gland polyps may be sporadic or syndromic and are associated with familial adenomatous polyposis (FAP) and attenuated familial adenomatous polyposis (AFAP) [4].

Sporadic polyps are found on about 2% of all upper endoscopies and in 12.5 to 84% of patients with FAP [2]. In FAP-associated fundic gland polyps, inactivating mutations in the APC tumor suppressor gene on chromosome 5q have been found. In sporadic fundic gland polyps, activating mutations of the β-catenin gene are sometimes found. The difference in the genetic etiology of fundic gland polyps likely causes the difference in the dysplasia risk between the two, as FAP- and AFAP-associated fundic gland polyps have been found to have 41% rate of dysplasia. Sporadic fundic gland polyps have minimal risk of malignant transformation and rarely any dysplasia [4].

Few factors have been found to correlate with the development of sporadic fundic gland polyps. A negative relationship between *H. pylori* infection and fundic gland polyps has been found [4]. No definite predilection has been found based on sex or race [3]. The association with PPIs has been postulated, first by Dr. Graham in 1992 [5]. This has been substantiated by further studies. Jalving and colleagues performed a prospective study on 599 consecutive patients undergoing upper endoscopy [6]. They found that long-term PPI use was associated with an increased risk of fundic gland polyps. Patients on PPIs for 1–5 years had an odds ratio (OR) of 2.2 (95% CI: 1.3–3.8) of having fundic gland polyps on upper endoscopy, while patients on PPIs for longer than 5 years had an OR of 3.8 (95% CI: 2.2–6.7). Short-term therapy was not associated with development of fundic gland polyps. A similar conclusion was made by Ally et al., in a retrospective study of elective upper endoscopy results. They found a risk of developing fundic gland polyps when patients had been on PPIs for two years or longer [1]. Zelter and colleagues performed a large prospective study on 1780 patients who underwent upper endoscopy over a one-year period [7]. They found gastric polyps in 129 patients (7.2%) with 77 of those polyps identified as fundic gland polyps. Proton pump inhibitor use was detected in 49 patients with fundic gland polyps (63.6%) and 264 patients without fundic gland polyps (15.5%). In their study, women and older patients (58 years versus 50 years) were more likely to develop fundic gland polyps. Proton pump inhibitor use was the most significant predictor for development of fundic gland polyps. A possible mechanism for the development of fundic gland polyps in patients on PPIs was proposed by Cats et al., who suggested that fundic gland polyps develop as a consequence of mechanical obstruction of gastric glands by hyperplastic parietal cells [8]. Long-term administration of PPIs has been shown to cause parietal cell hyperplasia secondary to PPI-induced hypergastrinemia [9]. Protrusion of hyperplastic parietal cells into the glandular lumina of gastric fundic glands causes narrowing and obstruction of the glandular lumina and cystic dilatation of fundic glands, characteristic of fundic gland polyps [8].

Despite the proposed mechanism, some debate still exists about the causation of fundic gland polyps by long-term PPI use. Vieth and Stolte completed a retrospective study over a one-year period [10]. The frequency of fundic gland polyps in 2,251 patients on PPI therapy without *H. pylori* infection was compared to a control group of 28,096 patients not on PPI therapy without *H. pylori* infection. The rate of fundic gland polyps was the same in the two groups, 5.2% in PPI group and 5.0% in control group. No other significant differences were found between the two groups in relation to gastritis, age, or sex. Bearing this study in mind, more studies seem to show a correlation between long-term PPI use and fundic gland polyp development than not.

In fundic gland polyps associated with FAP, predilection for dysplasia and development of gastric adenocarcinoma is known to exist [1]. While the vast majority of sporadic fundic gland polyps are benign and pose no risk of malignant degeneration, several cases of malignant degeneration have been reported in the literature. Low-grade and high-grade dysplasia have been found within fundic gland polyps in large series [11, 12]. Those cancers that do develop in fundic gland polyps may be a different subtype of gastric adenocarcinoma [13]. Jeong and colleagues also describe a case of a fundic gland polyp containing signet-ring cell carcinoma. While these rare cases have been reported of cancer arising within a fundic gland polyp, these polyps are still considered benign.

By comparison, hyperplastic polyps (HPPs) are a very common gastric polyp and the most common epithelial polyp of the stomach [14]. They are found throughout the stomach and are sometimes mistaken endoscopically for cancer [15]. Hyperplastic polyps have a slight preference for the antrum [14]. Hyperplastic polyps arise in mucosa affected by chronic inflammation, such as autoimmune gastritis, *H. pylori* gastritis, or postantrectomy stomach [15]. Microscopically, HPPs contain hyperplastic, elongated, or dilated foveolae that are mixed with variable amounts of inflamed stroma. The foveolae lining is composed of mature gastric mucus cells with abundant cytoplasm, except in areas of surface erosions, where nuclear enlargement and depletion of cytoplasmic mucin may cause a regenerative appearance [16]. The genetic pathogenesis of HPPs remains largely unknown with the K-*ras* protooncogene a potential source. The suggested pathogenesis is that HPPs are the result of prominent, reparative, or regenerative phenomena [14]. The rate of dysplasia or adenocarcinoma within HPPs is relatively rare but has been reported in the literature at 1.9%–19% [15]. Most studies seem to suggest that larger HPPs are more likely to harbor adenocarcinoma [14].

Magnetic sphincter augmentation is a newer technology for the surgical treatment of reflux disease in patients with normal anatomy and absence of large hiatal hernia. It has been shown to be a safe procedure with minimal complications, the most common being dysphagia [17]. Patients are candidates for the surgery if they have typical gastroesophageal reflux disease symptoms that are documented on esophageal pH studies and normal esophageal manometry studies and a hiatal hernia less than 3 cm in size and use a daily PPI with some relief. Pertinent to this case, patients have had great success at stopping all antacid therapy. Ganz et al. showed a PPI use rate of only 13% at 3 years in the initial MSA study [18].

In this patient, implantation of MSA allowed for cessation of her PPI therapy. With the likely correlation between PPI use and the development of fundic gland polyps, the innumerable fundic gland polyps resolved leaving only a few FGPs and mild gastritis that can be more easily followed up.

This is the first reported case of the resolution of numerous fundic gland polyps following the completion of laparoscopic MSA. Due to the successful cessation of proton pump inhibitors in patients following MSA, it should be considered in all eligible patients with multiple fundic gland polyps to allow patients to stop PPIs and have resolution of their reflux symptoms.

References

[1] M. R. Ally, G. R. Veerappan, C. L. Maydonovitch et al., "Chronic proton pump inhibitor therapy associated with increased development of fundic gland polyps," *Digestive Diseases and Sciences*, vol. 54, no. 12, pp. 2617–2622, 2009.

[2] S. C. Abraham, B. Nobukawa, F. M. Giardiello, S. R. Hamilton, and T. T. Wu, "Sporadic fundic gland polyps: common gastric polyps arising through activating mutations in the β-catenin gene," *American Journal of Pathology*, vol. 158, no. 3, pp. 1005–1010, 2001.

[3] H. J. Freeman, "Proton pump inhibitors and an emerging epidemic of gastric fundic gland polyposis," *World Journal of Gastroenterology*, vol. 14, no. 9, pp. 1318–1320, 2008.

[4] A. Spiegel, P. Stein, M. Patel, R. Patel, and E. Lebovics, "A report of gastric fundic gland polyps," *Gastroenterology and Hepatology*, vol. 6, no. 1, pp. 45–48, 2010.

[5] J. R. Graham, "Gastric polyposis: onset during long-term therapy with omeprazole," *Medical Journal of Australia*, vol. 157, no. 4, pp. 287–288, 1992.

[6] M. Jalving, J. J. Koornstra, J. Wesseling, H. M. Boezen, S. De Jong, and J. H. Kleibeuker, "Increased risk of fundic gland polyps during long-term proton pump inhibitor therapy," *Alimentary Pharmacology and Therapeutics*, vol. 24, no. 9, pp. 1341–1348, 2006.

[7] A. Zelter, J. L. Fernández, C. Bilder et al., "Fundic gland polyps and association with proton pump inhibitor intake: a prospective study in 1,780 endoscopies," *Digestive Diseases and Sciences*, vol. 56, no. 6, pp. 1743–1748, 2011.

[8] A. Cats, B. Ed Schenk, E. Bloemena et al., "Parietal cell protrusions and fundic gland cysts during omeprazole maintenance treatment," *Human Pathology*, vol. 31, no. 6, pp. 684–690, 2000.

[9] T. Nishi, H. Makuuchi, and W. M. Weinstein, "Changes in gastric ECL cells and parietal cells after long-term administration of high-dose omeprazole to patients with Barrett's esophagus," *Tokai Journal of Experimental and Clinical Medicine*, vol. 30, no. 2, pp. 117–121, 2005.

[10] M. Vieth and M. Stolte, "Fundic gland polyps are not induced by proton pump inhibitor therapy," *American Journal of Clinical Pathology*, vol. 116, no. 5, pp. 716–720, 2001.

[11] T. T. Wu, S. Kornacki, A. Rashid, J. H. Yardley, and S. R. Hamilton, "Dysplasia and dysregulation of proliferation in foveoral and surface epithelia of fundic gland polyps from patients with familial adenomatous polyposis," *American Journal of Surgical Pathology*, vol. 22, no. 3, pp. 293–298, 1998.

[12] S. W. Carmack, R. M. Genta, C. M. Schuler, and M. H. Saboorian, "The current spectrum of gastric polyps: a 1-year national study of over 120,000 patients," *The American Journal of Gastroenterology*, vol. 104, no. 6, pp. 1524–1532, 2009.

[13] H. Ueyama, T. Yao, Y. Nakashima et al., "Gastric adenocarcinoma of fundic gland type (chief cell predominant type): proposal for a new entity of gastric adenocarcinoma," *The American Journal of Surgical Pathology*, vol. 34, no. 5, pp. 609–619, 2010.

[14] R. Jain and R. Chetty, "Gastric hyperplastic polyps: a review," *Digestive Diseases and Sciences*, vol. 54, no. 9, pp. 1839–1846, 2009.

[15] S. C. Abraham, V. K. Singh, J. H. Yardley, and T. T. Wu, "Hyperplastic polyps of the stomach: associations with histologic patterns of gastritis and gastric atrophy," *American Journal of Surgical Pathology*, vol. 25, no. 4, pp. 500–507, 2001.

[16] S. C. Ming, "Malignant potential of gastric polyps," *Gastrointestinal Radiology*, vol. 1, no. 1, pp. 121–125, 1976.

[17] J. C. Lipham, P. A. Taiganides, B. E. Louie, R. A. Ganz, and T. R. Demeester, "Safety analysis of first 1000 patients treated with magnetic sphincter augmentation for gastroesophageal reflux disease," *Diseases of the Esophagus*, vol. 28, no. 4, pp. 305–311, 2015.

[18] R. A. Ganz, J. H. Peters, S. Horgan et al., "Esophageal sphincter device for gastroesophageal reflux disease," *The New England Journal of Medicine*, vol. 368, no. 8, pp. 719–727, 2013.

Infected Renal Cyst as a Complication of Dropped Gallstones during Laparoscopic Cholecystectomy

Chelsea Kennedy-Snodgrass,[1] Vivian Keenan,[2] and Douglas S. Katz[3]

[1]*NYU Winthrop Hospital, Department of Internal Medicine, 259 1st Ave, Mineola, NY 11501, USA*
[2]*NYU Winthrop Hospital, Department of Pulmonary and Critical Care, 259 1st Ave, Mineola, NY 11501, USA*
[3]*NYU Winthrop Hospital, Department of Radiology, 259 1st Ave, Mineola, NY 11501, USA*

Correspondence should be addressed to Chelsea Kennedy-Snodgrass; chelsea.kennedy-snodgrass@nyulangone.org

Academic Editor: I. Michael Leitman

Dropped gallstones are a relatively common complication, occurring in 3% to 32% of laparoscopic cholecystectomies performed, depending on various intraoperative risk factors. However, complications arising from dropped gallstones are relatively rare, occurring in fewer than 1% of such patients, and can include abscesses and inflammatory masses confined to the subhepatic space, presenting days to years later. We report a patient who developed an infected renal cyst as a result of dropped gallstones, which created a fistula from the duodenum to a previously simple right renal cyst, which was initially identified on an abdominal CT scan. Dropped gallstones can result in substantial morbidity in a minority of patients following cholecystectomy performed for cholecystitis, and a high clinical as well as radiological index of suspicion may be required for accurate early recognition and treatment.

1. Introduction

One of the most common major abdominal surgical procedures performed is laparoscopic cholecystectomy (LC), which is the standard of care for routine gallbladder removal [1, 2]. Overall, complication rates for LC are lower than for open cholecystectomy, likely reflecting that open procedures are reserved for complex elective cases or for complicated laparoscopic procedures which require conversion to an open cholecystectomy [3, 4]. LC, however, more frequently results in injury to the common bile duct and complications from dropped gallstones [3]. Complications which can arise from dropped gallstones in the setting of cholecystitis include abscesses and inflammatory masses which are generally confined to the subhepatic space or the retroperitoneum below the subhepatic space; however, uncommon and unusual complications have also occurred including broncholithiasis, hernia sac stones, and calculi migrating near or into the ovaries or fallopian tubes [3, 5, 6]. We describe an unusual case of a patient who developed an infected renal cyst as a result of dropped gallstones, which created a fistula from the duodenum to a previously simple right renal cyst, which was identified on an abdominal computed tomography (CT) performed 59 days following laparoscopic cholecystectomy.

2. Case Presentation

A 45-year-old male presented to our hospital with diaphoresis, chills, and worsening right flank pain. He had a past medical history of cirrhosis due to alcoholism and portal hypertension with esophageal varices managed with prior transjugular intrahepatic portosystemic shunt (TIPS) procedure. He had a history of hepatic encephalopathy, hypertension, and type II diabetes. He had a recent admission to another institution for septic shock secondary to recurrent cholecystitis and had recently had an LC fifty-eight days prior. The patient was admitted to the outside hospital fifty-nine days prior to admission to our institution for subacute cholecystitis, which had initially required a cholecystostomy drain on prior admissions, and then ultimately an LC at that hospital. The gallbladder was not noted to be perforated, but the procedure was complicated by dropped gallstones, some

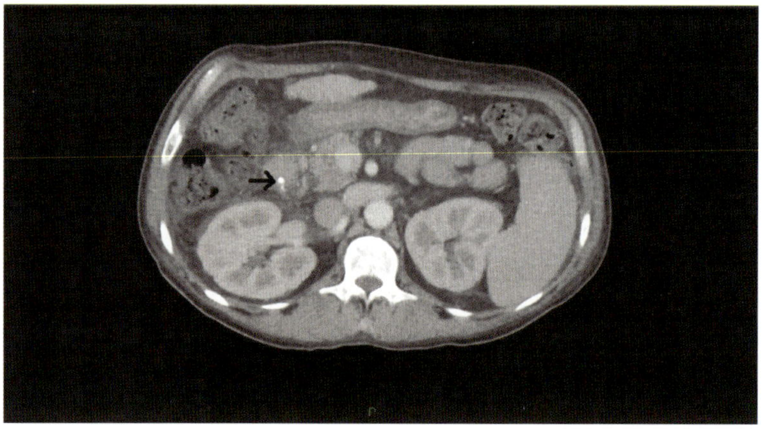

(a) Axial CT image of the abdomen obtained with IV contrast on patient's admission to our institution, demonstrates two retained, dropped gallstones (black arrow) from the previous cholecystectomy, forming a fistulous tract from the posterior aspect of the second portion of the duodenum and an adjacent right renal cyst

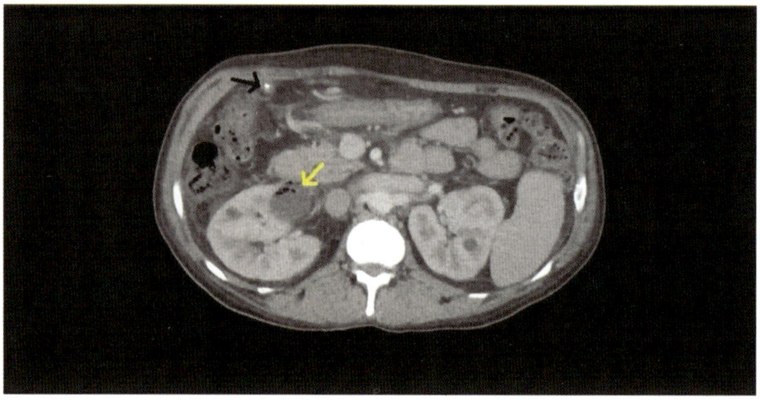

(b) Axial CT image at a slightly lower level than in Figure 1(a) shows an infected right renal cyst with pockets of gas (yellow arrow). There is an additional retained gallstone in a laparoscopic cholecystectomy port (black arrow)

FIGURE 1

of which were retrieved as stated in the operative report. On the current admission, the patient was hypotensive requiring vasopressors and was anemic and thrombocytopenic, requiring blood and platelet transfusions.

A CT scan of the abdomen and pelvis with IV contrast was performed on admission demonstrating residual gallstones in the gallbladder fossa and/or cystic duct remnant and multiple small fluid collections and/or forming granulomatous masses surrounding additional retained/dropped gallstones in the surgical tracts and vicinity. A fistula with gallstones was also seen extending through the posterior and inferior wall of the second portion of the duodenum, to the anterior and superior aspect of a right renal cyst, which measured 3.4 cm x 3.0 cm and which contained gas in its superior aspect (Figures 1(a) and 1(b)). A previous CT of the abdomen and pelvis performed with IV contrast sixty-five days prior to admission and seven days prior to the LC demonstrated a simple right renal cyst in the location of the now complex and infected cyst, measuring 2.8 cm x 2.5 cm (Figure 2).

Drainage of the infected renal cyst seen on the initial CT was considered; however, the cyst was relatively small and inaccessible. A repeat CT of the abdomen and pelvis with oral and IV contrast was performed four days after admission due to concern for abscess formation as the patient continued to have right flank pain. The CT demonstrated an unchanged superinfected cyst in the right kidney, with the fistula tract still visible, and heterogeneous retention of IV contrast in the right kidney, which was consistent with associated pyelonephritis (Figures 3(a) and 3(b)).

On initial presentation, the patient was noted to have a history of *Klebsiella pneumoniae* and vancomycin-resistant enterococcus (VRE) in the cholecystectomy drain and was treated for the gallstone abscess and fistula accordingly with meropenem as there was no other source of infection. Blood cultures were later positive for *K. pneumoniae* and VRE. The patient was ultimately treated with linezolid and meropenem was deescalated to ceftriaxone.

Discussion between the patient's outside hepatologist, the abdominal radiologist, the interventional radiologist, and the gastroenterologists determined that the most likely etiology of the initial sepsis was an infected renal cyst secondary to an infected dropped gallstone. The patient was ultimately

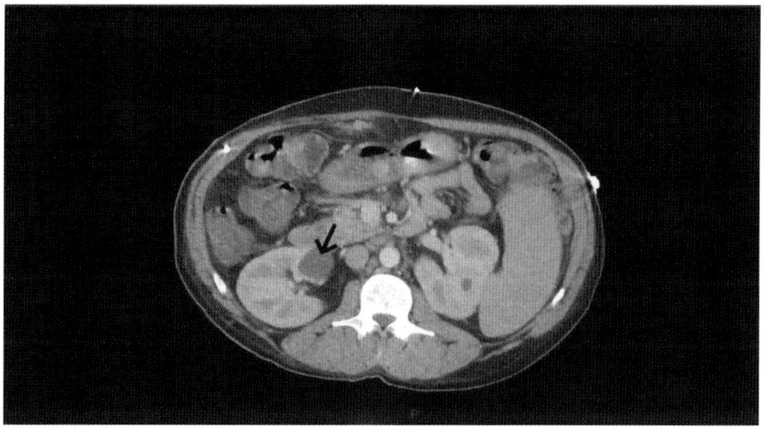

FIGURE 2: Axial image from CT of the abdomen with IV contrast obtained 65 days prior to admission revealed a simple right renal cyst (black arrow) in the location of the now infected cyst.

transferred to the outside hospital where he previously had his cholecystectomy for surgical follow-up.

3. Discussion

Laparoscopic cholecystectomy is the current accepted standard of treatment for symptomatic gallbladder disease [7]. Although morbidity rates for laparoscopic cholecystectomy are lower than for open cholecystectomy, complications can include bile duct injury, biliary leakage, and infection due to dropped gallstones in the setting of acute or chronic cholecystitis [7–9]. It is thought that gallbladder perforation and subsequent dropped gallstones may occur more often during LC than during open cholecystectomy due to excessive traction on the gallbladder during dissection from the liver, accidental entrance into the gallbladder during the dissection itself, or the elevated pressures on the gallbladder as it is extracted from the abdomen through a small incision [2, 10]. The incidence of gallbladder perforation reported varies widely, from 3% to 32%; however, the incidence of clinically significant events due to dropped gallstones is rare, occurring in fewer than 1% of such patients [1, 2, 8, 10–12].

Dropped gallstones are often located near the liver, in Morison's pouch, in the gallbladder fossa, and in the pelvis, but occasionally can be found elsewhere, including the left abdomen and even the thorax, due to concurrent fistulization [1]. Such dropped gallbladder calculi in the setting of cholecystitis can be retrieved intraoperatively by irrigating and suctioning the abdominal/pelvic cavity, by collection with a sponge, or recovered postoperatively by percutaneous interventional radiologic, laparoscopic, or open surgical techniques [7]. Recovery can be difficult as was demonstrated in our patient, as the operative report noted that all dropped gallstones were thought to have been retrieved. Dropped gallstones have a low incidence of complications, especially in the setting of a routine cholecystectomy not performed for acute or subacute infection, but can potentially cause a range of postoperative complications [3]. In the setting of acute cholecystitis, dropped gallstones are more likely to have infectious complications [13]. The most common complication of dropped gallstones is intraperitoneal abscess formation with or without transabdominal fistula [11]. These abscesses or inflammatory masses containing the gallstones or gallstone fragments are generally limited to the subhepatic space or to the retroperitoneum below the subhepatic space [5]. Uncommon presentations of spilled gallstones have included urinary tract involvement, obstructive cholangitis, secondary acute appendicitis, and even intestinal volvulus or intestinal obstruction [11]. These complications from dropped calculi may not present until many years following the initial surgery in some patients [3]. Several cases have been reported of abscesses occurring a decade after LC with gallstone spillage due to Actinomyces infection [14–16]. Due to the wide range of possible complications and the potentially extended time-interval between cholecystectomy and clinical presentation, dropped gallstones may not be considered in the differential diagnosis, leading to inaccurate diagnosis and inappropriate treatment.

In patients with suspected spilled gallstones, ultrasound and especially CT are recommended for evaluation of possible abscesses and associated complications [5]. Ultrasound may be a more sensitive modality for detection of dropped gallstones; however, imaging depth is limited due to beam penetration [17]. Gallstones with high calcium content will appear as high attenuation foci on CT; however, pure cholesterol stones may go undetected [1]. Unenhanced CTs should be used for stone identification as adjacent inflammation may enhance with contrast and obscure the stone [17]. When diagnosing complications resulting from dropped gallstones, it is important that their characteristic CT appearance be recognized, because such calculi with associated collections or granuloma formation can mimic other diseases, including tumors or bowel obstruction [8].

Our patient is the first reported case, to our knowledge, of an infected renal cyst resulting from dropped gallstones in the setting of cholecystitis, with a fistula between the duodenum and a previously simple renal cyst. This case highlights the diverse range of complications and therefore the wide variety of presenting signs and symptoms which can occur from spilled gallstones in this setting. Though rare as a

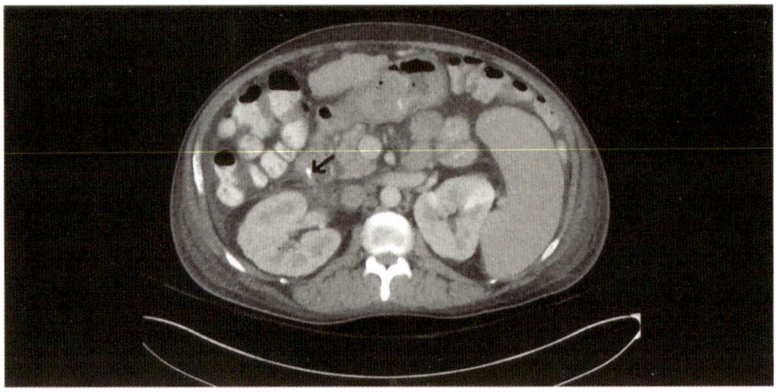

(a) Axial image of CT abdomen with IV contrast obtained 4 days after admission to our institution shows the fistula tract at the posterior aspect of the second portion of the duodenum with two adjacent calculi (black arrow). Also note retained contrast in the left kidney from the previous CT, indicating associated pyelonephritis

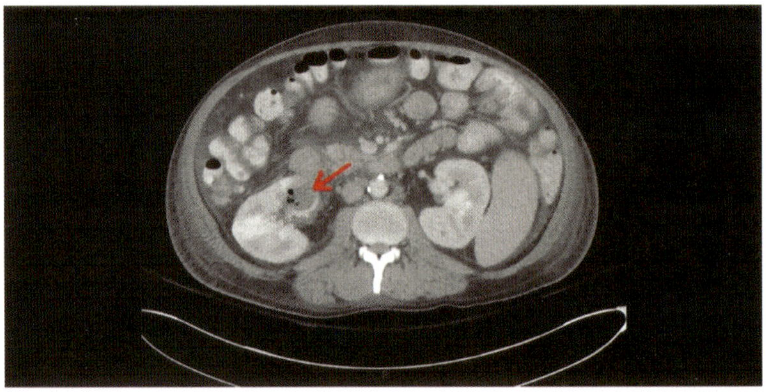

(b) Axial CT image at a slightly lower level than in Figure 3(a) shows right perinephric inflammation associated with the infected renal cyst with gas (red arrow). Also note bilateral retained contrast in the kidneys from the previous CT, indicating pyelonephritis

FIGURE 3

major complication, dropped gallstones during laparoscopic cholecystectomy can result in significant morbidity, and a high clinical as well as radiological index of suspicion may be required for early recognition and treatment.

Consent

Patient has been sufficiently anonymized according to the International Committee of Medical Journal Editors' recommendations.

References

[1] L. Nayak, C. O. Menias, and G. Gayer, "Dropped gallstones: spectrum of imaging findings, complications and diagnostic pitfalls," *British Journal of Radiology*, vol. 86, no. 1028, 2013.

[2] M. T. Brueggemeyer, A. K. Salba, and L. C. Thibodeaux, "Abscess formation following spilled gallstones during laparoscopic cholecystectomy," *JSLS*, vol. 1, pp. 145–152, 1997.

[3] J. Zehetner, A. Shamiyeh, and W. Wayand, "Lost gallstones in laparoscopic cholecystectomy: all possible complications," *The American Journal of Surgery*, vol. 193, no. 1, pp. 73–78, 2007.

[4] F. Coccolini, F. Catena, M. Pisano et al., "Corrigendum to "Open versus laparoscopic cholecystectomy in acute cholecystitis. Systematic review and meta-analysis"," *International Journal of Surgery*, vol. 18, pp. 196–204, 2015.

[5] M. M. Morrin, J. B. Kruskal, M. G. Hochman, P. F. Saldinger, and R. A. Kane, "Radiologic features of complications arising from dropped gallstones in laparoscopic cholecystectomy patients," *American Journal of Roentgenology*, vol. 174, no. 5, pp. 1441–1445, 2000.

[6] P. K. Papasavas, P. F. Caushaj, and D. J. Gagné, "Spilled gallstones after laparoscopic cholecystectomy," *Journal of Laparoendoscopic & Advanced Surgical Techniques*, vol. 12, no. 5, pp. 383–386, 2002.

[7] K. Singh, M. L. Wang, E. Ofori, W. Widmann, A. Alemi, and M. Nakaska, "Gallstone abscess as a result of dropped gallstones during laparoscopic cholecystectomy," *International Journal of Surgery Case Reports*, vol. 3, no. 12, pp. 611–613, 2012.

[8] A. R. Tumer, Y. N. Yüksek, A. C. Yasti, U. Gözalan, and N. A. Kama, "Dropped gallstones during laparoscopic cholesystectomy: the consequences," *World Journal of Surgery*, vol. 29, no. 4, pp. 437–440, 2005.

[9] I. Triantafyllidis, N. Nikoloudis, N. Sapidis, M. Chrissidou, I. Kalaitsidou, and T. Chrissidis, "Complications of laparoscopic cholecystectomy: Our experience in a district general hospital," *Surgical Laparoscopy Endoscopy & Percutaneous Techniques*, vol. 19, no. 6, pp. 449–458, 2009.

[10] T. Sathesh-Kumar, A. P. Saklani, R. Vinayagam, and R. L. Blackett, "Spilled gall stones during laparoscopic cholecystectomy: a review of the literature," *Postgraduate Medical Journal*, vol. 80, no. 940, pp. 77–79, 2004.

[11] A. J. Nooghabi, M. Hassanpour, and A. Jangjoo, "Consequences of lost gallstones during laparoscopic cholecystectomy: a review article," *Surgical Laparoscopy Endoscopy & Percutaneous Techniques*, vol. 26, no. 3, pp. 183–192, 2016.

[12] J. G. Brockmann, T. Kocher, N. J. Senninger, and G. M. Schürmann, "Complications due to gallstones lost during laparoscopic cholecystectomy: an analysis of incidence, clinical course, and management," *Surgical Endoscopy*, vol. 16, no. 8, pp. 1226–1232, 2002.

[13] J. C. Woodfield, M. Rodgers, and J. A. Windsor, "Peritoneal gallstones following laparoscopic cholecystectomy: incidence, complications, and management," *Surgical Endoscopy*, vol. 18, no. 8, pp. 1200–1207, 2004.

[14] D. Stupak, S. Cohen, F. Kasmin, Y. Lee, and J. H. Siegel, "Intra-abdominal actinomycosis 11 years after spilled gallstones at the time of laparoscopic cholecystectomy," *Surgical Laparoscopy Endoscopy & Percutaneous Techniques*, vol. 17, no. 6, pp. 542–544, 2007.

[15] A. Ladic, I. Petrovic, G. Augustin et al., "Hemoptysis as an early symptom of abdominal actinomycosis with thoracic extension ten years after cholecystectomy with retained gallstone," *Surgical Infections*, vol. 14, no. 4, pp. 408–411, 2013.

[16] J. M. Vyas, A. Kasmar, H. R. Chang, J. Holden, and E. Hohmann, "Abdominal abscesses due to actinomycosis after laparoscopic cholecystectomy: case reports and review.," *Clinical infectious diseases : an official publication of the Infectious Diseases Society of America*, vol. 44, no. 2, p. -4, 2007.

[17] N. K. Ramamurthy, V. Rudralingam, D. F. Martin, S. W. Galloway, and S. A. Sukumar, "Out of sight but kept in mind: complications and imitations of dropped gallstones," *American Journal of Roentgenology*, vol. 200, no. 6, pp. 1244–1253, 2013.

The Traumatic Tube: Bleeding Rectal Ulcer Caused by Flexi-Seal Device

Abhinav Tiwari,[1] Himani Sharma,[1] Khola Qamar,[2] Yaseen Alastal,[2] Thomas Sodeman,[2] and Ali Nawras[2]

[1]*Department of Internal Medicine, University of Toledo Medical Center, Toledo, OH, USA*
[2]*Department of Gastroenterology, University of Toledo Medical Center, Toledo, OH, USA*

Correspondence should be addressed to Abhinav Tiwari; Abhinav.tiwari@utoledo.edu

Academic Editor: Hideto Kawaratani

Diarrhea and fecal incontinence are common in critically ill patients and present a challenging problem in patient management. The Flexi-Seal® Fecal Management System is a device to divert the stools away from the patient, thus improving the care to patients with fecal incontinence. There have been only few case reports describing the complications with the use of this device. Here, we present a case of a 77-year-old woman who was admitted due to massive hematochezia while on anticoagulation. She was found to have a large rectal ulcer caused by the Flexi-Seal device, used during the last hospital stay for fecal incontinence. Flexi-Seal device can be effective for the management of incontinence; however, caution should be exercised during handling and pressure from the retention balloon should be relieved periodically.

1. Introduction

Fecal incontinence is not uncommon in acutely ill hospitalized patients, occurring in up to 33% of critically ill patients often in association with diarrhea [1]. The etiology of diarrhea or fecal incontinence, in critically ill patients, is often unknown and can be multifactorial. Managing diarrhea in such patients presents a challenging problem in patient management as it can lead to breakdown of skin, ulceration, and infection [2]. Flexi-Seal Fecal Management system (FSFMS) (ConvaTec Professional Services) was designed to provide a safe and effective diversion of liquid stool away from the skin and has been adopted by many intensive care units (ICUs). These devices reduce the need for labor-intensive nursing care, decrease the risk of perianal skin breakdown, and decrease transmission of fecal microbiota. These devices consist of a soft silicon catheter and a retention balloon that is inflated with 45 ml of saline or water. This balloon is inflated in the rectum to form a seal that prevents seepage of fecal contents around it. These devices are often believed to be safe and effective, and some studies have demonstrated their successful use in patients with diarrhea [3]. However, there have been few cases in the literature describing the adverse effects from the pressure necrosis or traumatic removal of such devices. Such complications include rectal ampullary ulcers, rectal fissures, and fatal bleeding due to rectal trauma. Although limited, such reports suggest that these devices may have a higher morbidity risk than previously believed. Here, we present a case of a 77-year-old woman who developed hematochezia while on anticoagulation. Further investigation revealed bleeding rectal ulcer secondary to the recent use of the Flexi-Seal system.

2. Case Report

A 77-year-old female with a history of interstitial lung disease was admitted to ICU due to multiple episodes of lower gastrointestinal bleeding. Vital signs revealed a blood pressure of 98/68 mm Hg, heart rate of 102 beats per minute, respiratory rate of 18/min, and temperature of 97.5 degrees Fahrenheit. Rectal examination was unremarkable except for bright red blood on the examining finger. Laboratory workup revealed a WBC count of 8.6 × 109/L, hemoglobin level of 8.9 g/dL, and platelet count of 250,000/μL. Seven days before the current admission, she was discharged after an extended stay in ICU for respiratory failure requiring

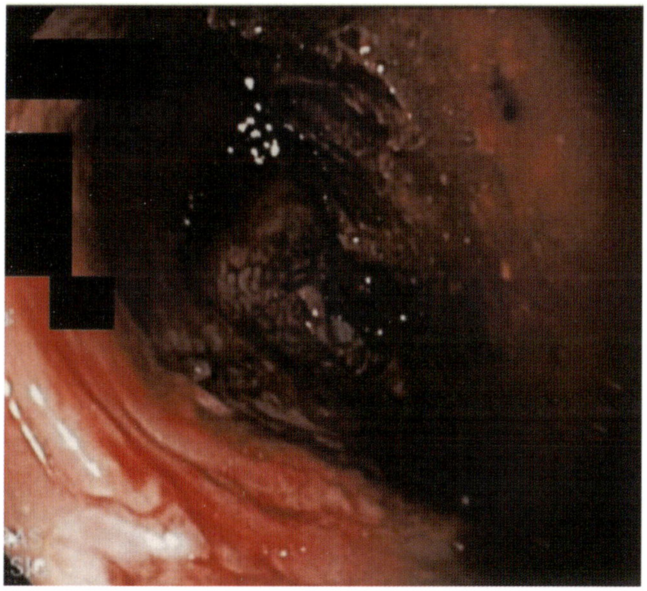

Figure 1: Flexible sigmoidoscopy showing a circumferential rectal ulcer with erythematous mucosa.

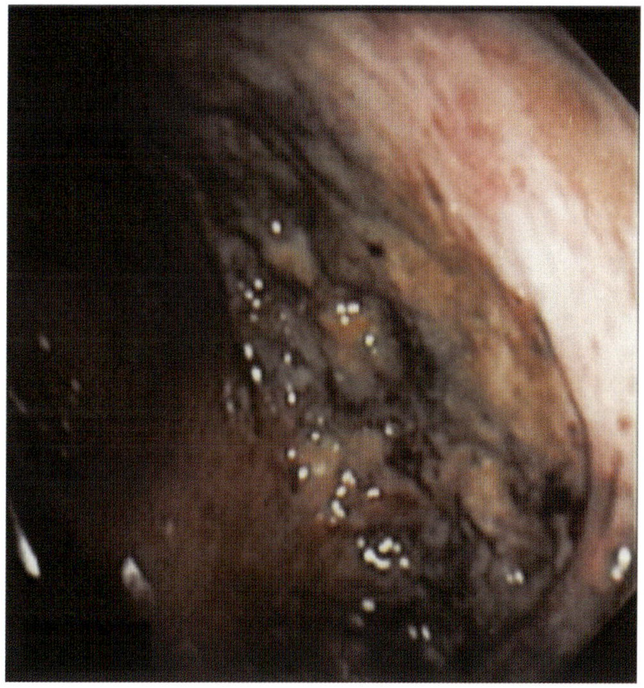

Figure 2: Flexible sigmoidoscopy showing a part of circumferential ulcer in the rectum.

intubation and mechanical ventilation. She was diagnosed with bilateral lower extremity deep vein thrombosis and was discharged on apixaban. Hemoglobin level was 10.3 g/dL at the time of discharge. During the current hospitalization, apixaban was held, and the patient was given intravenous fluids. Gastroenterology consultation was obtained, and an esophagogastroduodenoscopy (EGD) was performed to rule out rapid upper gastrointestinal (GI) bleeding. EGD was unremarkable with no evidence of fresh or old blood until the second part of the duodenum. Flexible sigmoidoscopy showed some retained stool in the rectum. However, there was a large area of ulceration and erythema involving most of the circumference of the rectal wall (Figures 1 and 2). This ulcerated area extended up to 15 cm from the anal verge. The scope was advanced up to 35 cm from the anal verge and rest of the colonic mucosa was normal. Multiple biopsies taken from the ulcer edge revealed necrotic epithelium with no evidence of dysplasia or malignancy. Chart review revealed that the patient had Flexi-Seal system placed for low-volume diarrhea during the last hospital stay. Flexi-Seal was placed for a total of 9 days and removed after stool output slowed down. Otherwise, there was no history of rectal trauma or rectal surgery in the past.

Bleeding ceased after anticoagulation was discontinued and an inferior vena cava (IVC) filter was placed to prevent pulmonary embolism. The patient was discharged without anticoagulation. There was no subsequent episode of GI bleeding.

3. Discussion

Diarrhea and fecal incontinence are a widespread problem in critically ill patients [4–6]. Critical illness is by itself a risk factor for diarrhea, while other factors include physiological stress, medications (magnesium, laxatives), lack of fibers in enteral feed, and alteration in intestinal flora due to antibiotic use [4, 7]. Diarrhea can compromise the management of the patient and cause considerable morbidity due to skin breakdown and infection. Recently, the use of indwelling intrarectal fecal collection systems has gained popularity because of their effectiveness in diverting fecal material away from the patient. The Flexi-Seal device (FMS; ConvaTec, Division of E.R. Squibb & Sons, LLC, Princeton, NJ) is the most widely used device designed to be used continuously for up to 30 days.

The first report describing the potential adverse effects of the Flexi-Seal system was a prospective, multicenter, clinical study involving 42 patients [3]. This study reported 2 cases of generalized skin breakdown and one case of rectal bleeding resulting from pressure ulceration. Subsequently, there have been a handful of reports of adverse effects arising from the use of such device. There are 9 case reports in the literature reporting 13 patients who had lower GI bleeding secondary to either an ulcer or laceration secondary to use of Flexi-Seal device.

Page et al. (2008) reported the case of a 65-year-old man who developed severe bleeding from the rectal mucosa due to a laceration, 6 cm from the anal verge, which was sutured. This laceration was attributed to the use of the Flexi-Seal system for six days [8]. Bright et al. [9] reported lower GI bleeding in a 79-year-old man 11 days after insertion of a Flexi-Seal device. Colonoscopy findings at the time were suggestive of pressure necrosis in the rectal area. Mesenteric angiography showed extravasation of contrast material from a branch of the superior rectal artery, and coil embolization was successfully performed. Sparks et al. (2010) reported 3 cases of massive GI bleeding associated with the use of the Flexi-Seal device [10]. The first patient, a 72-year-old woman, presented with two episodes of lower GI bleeding due to a rectal laceration 4 cm proximal to the dentate line. The laceration was sutured after the second episode of bleeding. The second patient was a 54-year-old woman on warfarin who also presented with lower GI bleeding secondary to a tear of the anterior rectal wall 3 cm from the anal verge. The tear was treated with direct pressure, application of thrombin, and suture ligation. The third patient was a 59-year-old man on warfarin who was admitted due to a single episode of GI bleeding secondary to a mucosal ulcer in the proximal part of the anal canal. No treatment other than reversal of anticoagulation was required. Monge et al. (2011) reported two patients with rectal hemorrhage associated with the Flexi-Seal device [11]. The first patient was a 71-year-old man on prophylactic dose enoxaparin who presented with rectal hemorrhage 25 days after insertion of the device. Endoscopy revealed a mucosal ulcer in the distal part of the rectum. The second patient was a 67-year-old woman who had two episodes of rectal bleeding secondary to a mucosal ulcer in the posterior distal part of the rectum. Walsh and Sanders (2010) reported a case of fatal hemorrhage arising from a rectal ulcer caused by rectal tube [12]. The patient died despite clipping, banding, and injecting the lesion with epinephrine.

Reynolds and van Haren (2012) reported a case in which a 50-year-old man on heparin developed lower GI bleeding five days after insertion of a Flexi-Seal device [13]. Endoscopy revealed a mucosal ulcer in the distal part of the rectum 10 cm from the anal verge. The lesion was cauterized, injected with epinephrine, and suture-ligated. Mulhall and Jindal (2013) reported a case of a 58-year-old man with lower GI bleeding 13 days after insertion of the Flexi-Seal device [14]. Angiography revealed bleeding from a medial branch of the superior rectal artery which was then embolized. Eleven days later, the patient developed another episode of massive rectal bleeding and colonoscopy showed a posterior rectal laceration that was not actively bleeding and an anterior rectal ulcer with active hemorrhage. Hemostasis of the ulcer was achieved by suture ligation and application of topical thrombin. Popek and Senagore (2013) reported two cases of Flexi-Seal device-related complication [15]. The first case involved a 60-year-old woman who developed bright red blood per rectum from a bleeding rectal ulcer for which a clip was placed. Two weeks later, the patient again developed rectal bleeding, and an angiogram identified a bleeding vessel in the rectum, which was suture-ligated. The second patient was a 39-year-old patient admitted for sepsis and multiple organ failure. Three weeks after placement of the Flexi-Seal device, he began having bright red blood per rectum. Flexible sigmoidoscopy demonstrated a pulsatile vessel in the rectum, and the patient was taken to the operating room for suture ligation of the vessel. Shaker et al. (2014) reported a case of a 75-year-old female with atrial fibrillation on warfarin [16]. She developed lower GI bleeding 12 days after insertion of the Flexi-Seal device. CT angiogram showed that the bleeding was originating from the distal rectum. Flexible sigmoidoscopy showed severe ulceration involving the whole circumference of the rectum and evidence of active bleeding from a small artery. Hemostasis was achieved via argon-beam photocoagulation, a hemostatic stitch to the bleeding point, and packing of the rectum with alginate ribbon.

Whiteley et al. published a retrospective study analyzing the complications of Flexi-Seal in acute care setting [17]. The records of 50 patients who had a total of 69 study FMS inserted (mean: 1.4 FMS) were included in the study. Most patients (37, 74%) experienced no complications; 7 (14%) had their retention balloon overinflated but suffered no injury to the rectal mucosa; 4 (8%) experienced temporary anal atony; and 2 (4%) suffered excessive leak of stool around the device.

The pathophysiology of rectal ulceration or laceration due to the Flexi-Seal device is due to the pressure exerted by the retention balloon that, when inflated with saline, allows the catheter to remain anchored in the rectal ampulla. Build-up of semisolid fecal material above the level of the balloon may also contribute towards pressure necrosis, a mechanism similar to stercoral perforation caused by fecal impaction in severely constipated patients [18]. Therefore, the retention balloon should be periodically deflated to allow the fecal build-up to flow around the tubing and to release pressure on the mucosal wall.

This is the second case report in the literature of circumferential rectal ulceration secondary to a Flexi-Seal device. Our patient was on anticoagulation, which might have triggered bleeding from the rectal ulcer. However, as described above, there have been cases where the patient had substantial lower GI bleeding without anticoagulation.

In conclusion, Flexi-Seal is a useful device for controlling fecal incontinence. However, it is important to exercise caution with prolonged use of this device. Patients on anticoagulation should be closely monitored for any signs of lower gastrointestinal hemorrhage. The continued need for the utilization of this device should be assessed daily, and a low threshold for removal should be employed.

References

[1] D. Z. Bliss, S. Johnson, K. Savik, C. R. Clabots, and D. N. Gerding, "Fecal incontinence in hospitalized patients who are acutely ill," *Nursing Research*, vol. 49, no. 2, pp. 101–108, 2000.

[2] M. Gray, C. Ratliff, and A. Donovan, "Perineal skin care for the incontinent patient," *Advances in Skin & Wound Care*, vol. 15, no. 4, pp. 170–178, 2002.

[3] A. Padmanabhan, M. Stern, J. Wishin, M. Mangino, K. Richey, and M. DeSane, "Clinical evaluation of a flexible fecal incontinence management system," *American Journal of Critical Care*, vol. 16, no. 4, pp. 384–393, 2007.

[4] P. Wiesen, A. Van Gossum, and J.-C. Preiser, "Diarrhoea in the critically ill," *Current Opinion in Critical Care*, vol. 12, no. 2, pp. 149–154, 2006.

[5] T. W. J. Kelly, K. M. Hillman, and M. R. Patrick, "Study of diarrhea in critically ill patients," *Critical Care Medicine*, vol. 11, no. 1, pp. 7–9, 1983.

[6] J. M. Beitz, "Faecal incontinence in acutely and critically ill patients: options in management," *Ostomy Wound Manage*, vol. 52, pp. 56–58, 2006.

[7] V. K. Sabol and K. K. Carlson, "Diarrhea: applying research to bedside practice," *AACN Advanced Critical Care*, vol. 18, no. 1, pp. 32–44, 2007.

[8] B. P. Page, S. A. Boyce, C. Deans, and J. Camilleri-Brennan, "Significant rectal bleeding as a complication of a fecal collecting device: report of a case," *Diseases of the Colon and Rectum*, vol. 51, no. 9, pp. 1427–1429, 2008.

[9] E. Bright, G. Fishwick, D. Berry, and M. Thomas, "Indwelling bowel management system as a cause of life-threatening rectal bleeding," *Case Reports in Gastroenterology*, vol. 2, no. 3, pp. 351–355, 2008.

[10] D. Sparks, D. Chase, B. Heaton, L. Coughlin, and J. Metha, "Rectal trauma and associated hemorrhage with the use of the ConvaTec flexi-seal fecal management system: report of 3 cases," *Diseases of the Colon and Rectum*, vol. 53, no. 3, pp. 346–349, 2010.

[11] F. J. Monge, I. Á. Angorrilla, E. S. Aguado, and F. R. Ruiz, "Ulceración rectal como una complicación del uso de sistema de control fecal fexi-seal: relato de casos," *Revista da Escola de Enfermagem da USP*, vol. 45, no. 5, pp. 1256–1259, 2011.

[12] W. J. Walsh and K. Sanders, "Fatal hemorrhage from a rectal ulcer due to a rectal tube: a rare complication," *American Journal Of Respiratory And Critical Care Medicine*, vol. 181, 2010.

[13] M. G. Reynolds and F. van Haren, "A case of pressure ulceration and associated haemorrhage in a patient using a faecal management system," *Australian Critical Care*, vol. 25, no. 3, pp. 188–194, 2012.

[14] A. M. Mulhall and S. K. Jindal, "Massive gastrointestinal hemorrhage as a complication of the flexi-seal fecal management system," *American Journal of Critical Care*, vol. 22, no. 6, pp. 537–543, 2013.

[15] S. Popek and A. Senagore, "Indwelling rectal tubes: An unusual cause of significant rectal bleeding in two critically ill patients," *American Surgeon*, vol. 79, no. 2, pp. 219-220, 2013.

[16] H. Shaker, E. J. Maile, and K. J. Telford, "Complete circumferential rectal ulceration and haemorrhage secondary to the use of a faecal management system," *Therapeutic Advances in Gastroenterology*, vol. 7, no. 1, pp. 51–55, 2014.

[17] I. Whiteley, G. Sinclair, A. M. A. Lyons, and R. Riccardi, "A retrospective review of outcomes using a fecal management system in acute care patients," *Ostomy/Wound Management*, vol. 60, no. 12, pp. 37–43, 2014.

[18] C. Oakenful and A. L. Lambrianides, "Stercoral perforation of the rectum," *EMA - Emergency Medicine Australasia*, vol. 23, no. 2, pp. 224–227, 2011.

19

A Case of Segmental Arterial Mediolysis Presenting as Mucosal Gastric Hematoma

Shunsuke Sakuraba,[1] Hajime Orita,[1] Shuhei Ueda,[1] Satoshi Tokuda,[1] Tomoaki Ito,[1] Tomoyuki Kushida,[1] Mutsumi Sakurada,[1] Hiroshi Maekawa,[1] Ryo Wada,[2] and Koichi Sato[1]

[1] *Department of Surgery, Juntendo Shizuoka Hospital, Shizuoka, Japan*
[2] *Department of Pathology, Juntendo Shizuoka Hospital, Shizuoka, Japan*

Correspondence should be addressed to Shunsuke Sakuraba; lunlun8shunsuke@gmail.com and Hajime Orita; oriori@juntendo.ac.jp

Academic Editor: Yoshihiro Moriwaki

Background. Although segmental arterial mediolysis (SAM) has been increasingly recognized as arteriopathy and there are some case reports about SAM, it is still very rare. It is characterized clinically by aneurysm, dissection, stenosis, and occlusion within splanchnic arterial branches, causing intra-abdominal hemorrhage or bowel ischemia. Mortality is as high as 50% in acute events. *Case Presentation.* A 51-year-old man was referred to our hospital with hematemesis. Gastroscopy revealed a submucosal-like tumor on the posterior wall of gastric angle with ulceration. Computed tomography indicated a tumor measuring 65 × 50 mm in the stomach, which was suspected to have invaded into the pancreas. Significant hematemesis recurred; the patient developed shock and underwent emergency distal gastrectomy, distal pancreatectomy, and splenectomy. The pathology and the clinical course were compatible with SAM splenic artery rupture causing retroperitoneal hemorrhage that penetrated into the stomach. After that surgery, aneurysm of common hepatic artery ruptured and coil embolization was performed. *Conclusion.* SAM is an important cause of intra-abdominal or retroperitoneal hemorrhage in patients without underlying disease. SAM typically presents as intra-abdominal hemorrhage, but, in this case, the retroperitoneal hemorrhage penetrated into the stomach and it looked like a submucosal tumor.

1. Introduction

Segmental arterial mediolysis (SAM), previously called segmental mediolytic arteritis (SMA), is a rare nonarteriosclerotic, noninflammatory vascular disease first described in 1976 by Slavin and Gonzalez-Vitale [1–3]. Though reports about SAM have become much more frequent as knowledge about the disease and use of thin slice computed tomographic angiography have increased [4], the incidence is still only about 1 per 100,000 per year. The etiology is unknown but it is said that alpha-1 adrenergic receptors and beta-2 agonists such as ractopamine can cause similar condition. Ractopamine is used in many countries as a partitioning agent in pigs, but in Japan this agent is not permitted. A definite diagnosis is determined histologically and it is characterized by vacuolization and lysis of the outer media of arterial wall. Disease lesions typically occur in a skip pattern within splanchnic arterial branches, leading to aneurysm, dissection, stenosis, and occlusion. As an arteriopathy, SAM is similar to inflammatory vasculitis, collagen vascular disease, and fibromuscular dysplasia (FMD), so excluding these diseases is necessary. This disease is difficult to diagnose presymptomatically; therefore most cases present as spontaneous intra-abdominal hemorrhage, and a few cases appear as bowel ischemia, hematuria, or hemobilia. Particularly, bleeding sometimes causes a fatal result and may require urgent treatment. Coil embolization is currently well recognized as the first-line treatment whenever conservative therapy is not feasible, and the affected artery can be sacrificed. If embolization can cause distal ischemia or result in failure, surgical intervention is necessary.

In this case, we report a case of SAM with heterochronic vessel rupture of the splenic and common hepatic arteries, treated by surgical intervention and coil embolization.

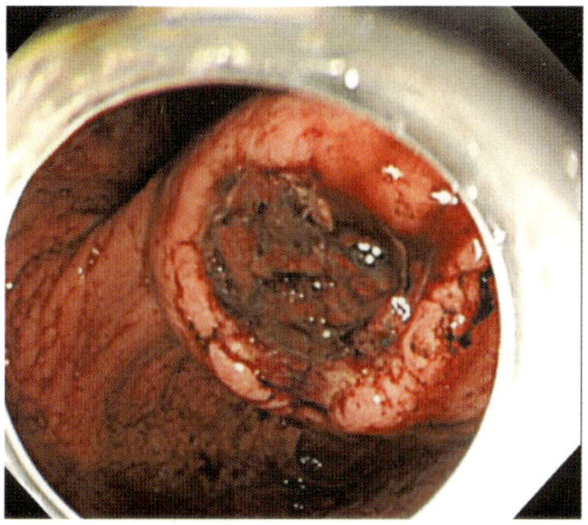

FIGURE 1: Gastroscopy revealed a submucosal-like tumor on the posterior wall of gastric angle with superficial ulceration.

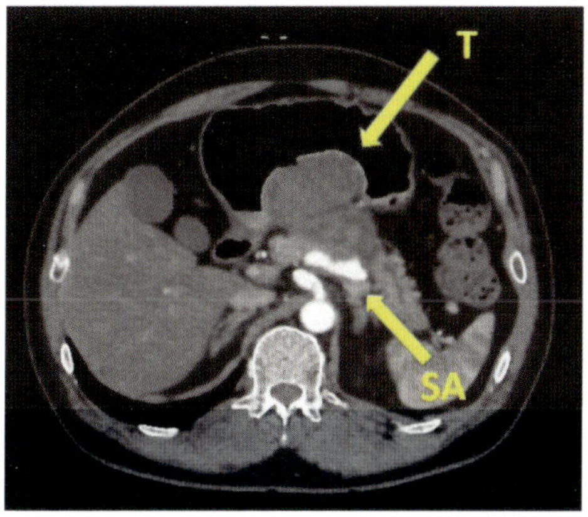

FIGURE 2: Computed tomography indicated a tumor measuring 65× 50 mm in the stomach, which was suspected to have invaded into the pancreas, but no metastatic lesions were detected. T: tumor; SA: splenic.

2. Case Presentation

The patient was a 51-year-old man who presented to the Emergency Department with hematemesis. His past medical history was unremarkable and he took no drugs. Physical examination revealed normal vital signs. On abdominal examination, the patient had no masses, muscle guarding, or rebound. Complete blood count revealed anemia with hemoglobin of 9.2. C-reactive protein (CRP) was normal, and the remainder of the serologic and immunologic workup was within normal limits. Gastroscopy revealed a submucosal-like tumor on the posterior wall of gastric angle with superficial ulceration (Figure 1). There were blood clots on top of the tumor, but no active bleeding existed; therefore we did not perform endoscopic hemostasis technique. Computed tomography indicated a tumor measuring 65 × 50 mm in the stomach, which was suspected to have invaded into the pancreas, but no metastatic lesions were detected (Figure 2). Magnetic resonance imaging also revealed a mass, having a high signal in the diffusion-weighted image (DWI) in the stomach, and the mass was also growing into the pancreas. At first, we considered the tumor as a malignant submucosal tumor such as GIST in the stomach or NET in the pancreas. General condition after hospital admission was stable, so we decided to perform an operation on suspicion of submucosal tumor, originating in the stomach or pancreas. During the preoperative period, massive hematemesis occurred with bright red blood with hemostatic shock. Emergency distal gastrectomy, distal pancreatectomy, and splenectomy were performed. The resected specimen consisted mostly of a hematoma and some vessel wall but did not have any malignant cells (Figure 3). We checked preoperative CT angiogram retrospectively and it indicated dissection of common hepatic artery as well as aneurysms of the common hepatic artery (maximum diameter, 8 mm) and bilateral renal artery (maximum diameter, 5 mm) (Figures 4(a), 4(b), and 4(c)). The tumor was close to splenic artery; therefore he was diagnosed with vessel rupture of splenic artery causing retroperitoneal hemorrhage and a hematoma that penetrated into the stomach.

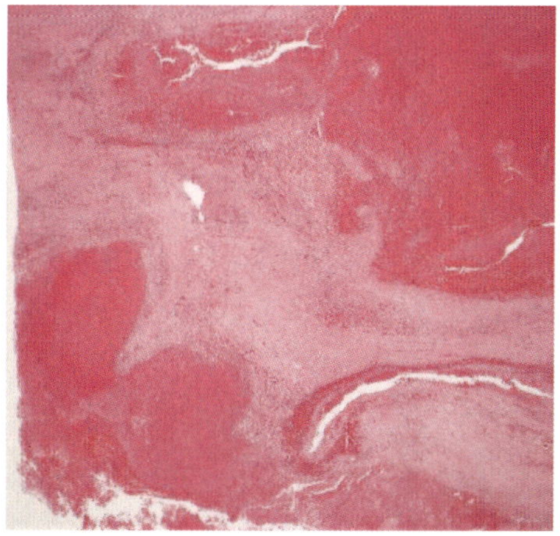

FIGURE 3: The resected specimen consisted mostly of a hematoma and some vessel wall.

On postoperative day 21, he exhibited peritoneal irritation in the form of a rigid board-like abdomen with shock vital signs. Emergency CTA showed a dissection and vessel rupture of aneurysm of common hepatic artery, causing intra-abdominal hemorrhage, so he underwent emergency coil embolization (Figures 5(a) and 5(b)).

Follow-up was done every 6 months, and CTA one year after the first operation indicated the aneurysms (maximum diameter, 5 mm) of the bilateral renal arteries remained.

3. Discussion

SAM is a nonarteriosclerotic, noninflammatory vascular disease that commonly presents as spontaneous intra-abdominal hemorrhage from middle-size splanchnic arterial branches. Abdominal pain, anemia, and shock are the main symptoms. Some cases present as bowel ischemia, hematuria, and hemobilia, but this is rare. Bleeding from the splanchnic artery sometimes causes a fatal results, so prompt diagnosis and treatment are required. To diagnose SAM, computed tomographic angiography (CTA), especially thin slice CTA, is very helpful. Digital subtraction angiography (DSA) is also

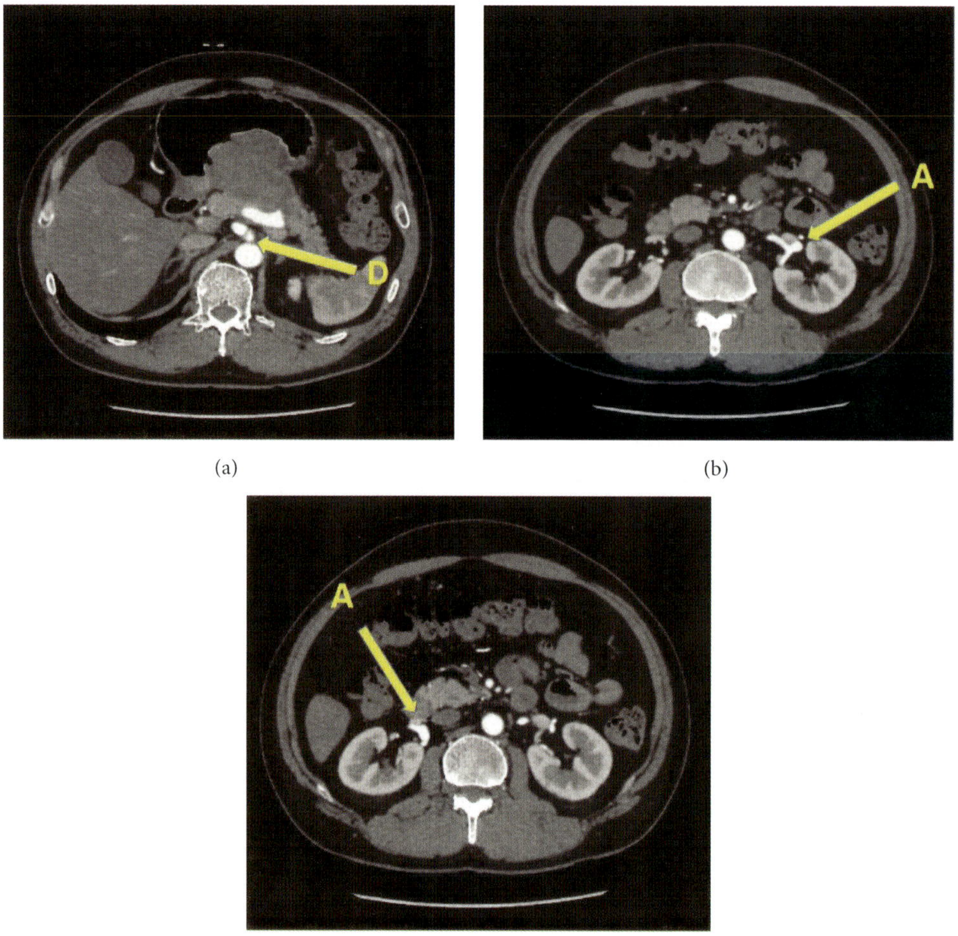

(a) (b) (c)

Figure 4: CT angiogram indicated dissection of common hepatic artery as well as aneurysms of the common hepatic artery (maximum diameter, 8 mm) and bilateral renal artery (maximum diameter, 5 mm). D: dissection; A: aneurysm.

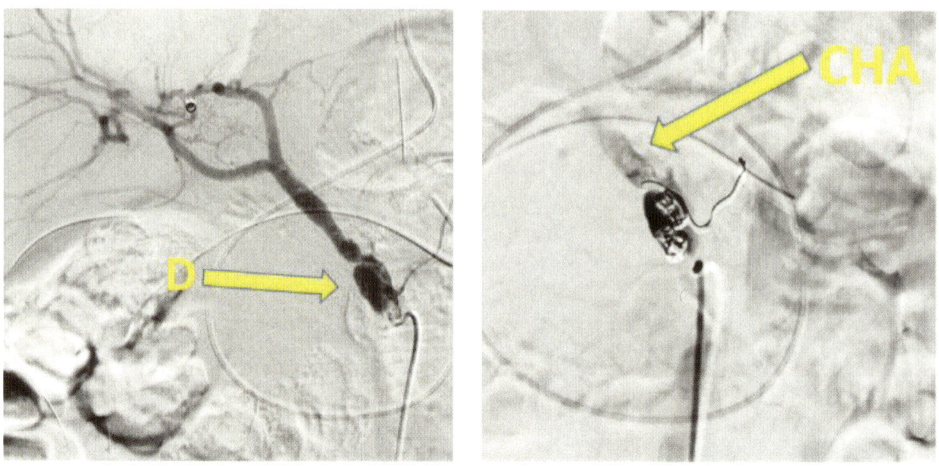

(a) (b)

Figure 5: Coil embolization was performed for the aneurysm of common hepatic artery. D: dissection; CHA: common hepatic artery.

useful because when the lesion is identified, we can treat it with embolization. For radiographic features, CT scans typically show mesenteric or intraperitoneal hemorrhage, and CTA and arteriography features include fusiform aneurysms, stenosis, dissections, and occlusions within the splanchnic arteries. A pattern of aneurysms and stenosis in series is characteristic, the "string-of-beads" appearance. Pathology is the diagnostic gold standard, and the underlying histological process is lysis of the smooth muscle of the outer media of the arterial wall. In cases in which collecting a specimen is not viable, CTA helps us to discover SAM lesions and it is thought to be sufficient to diagnose SAM [5]. It affects the visceral arteries of the abdomen in a skip pattern, most commonly affecting the medium size branches of the superior mesenteric artery. Included in the differential diagnosis are inflammatory arteritis, collagen vascular disease, mycotic aneurysms, cystic medial necrosis seen in type IV Ehlers Danlos and Marfan's syndrome, and fibromuscular dysplasia (FMD) which are also important to consider [6, 7]. Laboratory markers of inflammation, differences in distribution, age, gender, and stigma may help to distinguish these diseases.

Typically, SAM presents in middle-aged or elderly patients with no underlying disease, and laboratory markers of inflammation or collagen disease are absent. Because some angiographic findings are similar to fibromuscular dysplasia (FMD) findings, SAM is considered by some researchers to be an early lesion, a variant of FMD [2, 8–10]. However, FMD occurs mainly in young to middle-aged women, and the pattern of arterial involvement is different [5, 11]. Based on the standard treatment for intra-abdominal hemorrhage, the course of treatment is mainly divided into two ways, embolization and surgical intervention. Because the etiology is not inflammatory or autoimmune, immunosuppressive agents are counterproductive. Treatment with embolization is the first choice but if it results in failure, surgical intervention, such as resection of the injured arteries or artery bypass, is necessary [11]. Preventive embolization for a lesion discovered incidentally may be recommended depending on the size of aneurysm. The prognosis if the acute event is adequately treated is good. With time, the lesions may resolve or remain unchanged [5, 12].

This case differs in that the CT scan showed dissection of the common hepatic artery and aneurysms of the common hepatic artery, splenic artery, and bilateral renal arteries. At first, the splenic artery ruptured, resulting in a retroperitoneal hematoma which penetrated into the stomach and masked as a submucosal tumor. Because the chief complaint was not typical intra-abdominal hemorrhage but hematemesis, at first we considered tumors such as GIST or NET.

SAM typically presents as intra-abdominal hemorrhage, but there are a few cases in which bleeding occurs into the bowel lumen. If we diagnosed SAM based on the CTA findings, the first-line treatment for the hematemesis would be coil embolization. We should keep in mind the possibility of SAM alternatively presenting as digestive tract hemorrhage, for which surgery is preferred.

4. Conclusion

SAM is an important cause of intra-abdominal or retroperitoneal hemorrhage in patients without underlying disease. SAM typically presents as intra-abdominal hemorrhage, but in this case, the retroperitoneal hemorrhage penetrated into the stomach and it looked like a submucosal tumor.

References

[1] R. E. Slavin and J. C. Gonzalez-Vitale, "Segmental mediolytic arteritis: a clinical pathologic study," *Laboratory Investigation*, vol. 35, pp. 23–29, 1976.

[2] R. E. Slavin, K. Saeki, B. Bhagavan, and A. E. Maas, "Segmental arterial mediolysis: A precursor to fibromuscular dysplasia?" *Modern Pathology*, vol. 8, no. 3, pp. 287–294, 1995.

[3] R. E. Slavin, L. Cafferty, and J. Cartwright, "Segmental Mediolytic Arteritis," *The American Journal of Surgical Pathology*, vol. 13, no. 7, pp. 558–568, 1989.

[4] A. Ro, N. Kageyama, A. Takatsu, and T. Fukunaga, "Segmental arterial mediolysis of varying phases affecting both the intra-abdominal and intracranial vertebral arteries: An autopsy case report," *Cardiovascular Pathology*, vol. 19, no. 4, pp. 248–251, 2010.

[5] M. Michael, U. Widmer, S. Wildermuth, A. Barghorn, S. Duewell, and T. Pfammatter, "Segmental arterial mediolysis: CTA findings at presentation and follow-up," *American Journal of Roentgenology*, vol. 187, no. 6, pp. 1463–1469, 2006.

[6] R. E. Slavin, "Segmental arterial mediolysis: A clinical-pathologic review, its role in fibromuscular dysplasia and description and differential diagnosis of the masquerader-muscular artery cystic necrosis," *World Journal of Cardiovascular Diseases*, vol. 03, no. 01, pp. 64–81, 2013.

[7] N. Garg and F. S. Keller, "Segmental arterial mediolysis, a vasculitis mimic: Case report and review of literature," *International Journal of Diagnostic Imaging*, vol. 1, no. 2, p. 101, 2014.

[8] R. J. Chan, T. A. Goodman, T. H. Aretz, and J. T. Lie, "Segmental mediolytic arteriopathy of the splenic and hepatic arteries mimicking systemic necrotizing vasculitis," *Arthritis & Rheumatology*, vol. 41, no. 5, pp. 935–938, 1998.

[9] J. T. Lie, "Segmental mediolytic arteritis: not an arteritis but a variant of arterial fibromuscular dysplasia," *Archives of Pathology & Laboratory Medicine*, vol. 116, pp. 238–241, 1992.

[10] R. E. Slavin, "Segmental arterial mediolysis: course, sequelae, prognosis, and pathologic-radiologic correlation," *Cardiovascular Pathology*, vol. 18, no. 6, pp. 352–360, 2009.

[11] J. C. Baker-LePain, D. H. Stone, A. N. Mattis, M. C. Nakamura, and K. H. Fye, "Clinical diagnosis of segmental arterial mediolysis: Differentiation from vasculitis and other mimics," *Arthritis Care & Research*, vol. 62, no. 11, pp. 1655–1660, 2010.

[12] T. Juvonen, O. Niemelä, A. Reinilä, J. Nissinen, and M. I. Kairaluoma, "Spontaneous intraabdominal haemorrhage caused by segmental mediolytic arteritis in a patient with systemic lupus erythematosus-an underestimated entity of autoimmune origin?" *European Journal of Vascular and Endovascular Surgery*, vol. 8, no. 1, pp. 96–100, 1994.

Fenofibrate: A Nonlithogenic Means of Recurrent Drug-Induced Pancreatitis

Thamer Kassim,[1] **Joy-Marie Hermes**,[2] **Abdullah Abdussalam**,[3]
Ahmed Aly,[4] **and Subhash Chandra**[3]

[1] *Department of Medicine, Division of General Internal Medicine, Creighton University, Omaha, NE, USA*
[2] *Creighton University School of Medicine, Omaha, NE, USA*
[3] *Department of Medicine, Division of Gastroenterology, Creighton University, Omaha, NE, USA*
[4] *Department of Radiology, Creighton University, Omaha, NE, USA*

Correspondence should be addressed to Subhash Chandra; subhash.chandra@alegent.org

Academic Editor: R. J. L. F. Loffeld

Medications account for a small portion of the various etiologies of acute pancreatitis. Prompt identification of drugs as the inciting factor decreases disease recurrence and unnecessary invasive diagnostic intervention. This case is a report of fenofibrate-induced acute pancreatitis including a disease recurrence with continuation of fenofibrate which subsequently resolved after drug discontinuation. The patient underwent invasive diagnostic evaluation including endoscopic ultrasound with fine needle aspiration and endoscopic retrograde cholangiopancreatography (ERCP). Based on exclusion of other disease etiologies and a positive drug rechallenge, fenofibrate fits as a class 1A medication in the classification of drug-induced pancreatitis.

1. Introduction

The etiology of acute pancreatitis is identified in 70-90% of cases. Gallstones (up to 45%) and alcohol use (up to 35%) overwhelmingly produce most cases. Other precipitating factors include hypertriglyceridemia, ERCP, hypercalcemia, smoking, scorpion venom, malignancy, infection, and trauma (10% combined) [1]. The remaining 10-30% of cases are classified as idiopathic pancreatitis [1, 2]. This percentage continues to shrink with improvement of diagnostic modalities and increased literature regarding drug-induced pancreatitis, which accounts for approximately 2% of cases [2, 3].

Drug-induced pancreatitis is a diagnosis fraught with difficulty. It is made when symptoms resolve with drug cessation and recur in accordance with a rechallenge of the same drug [4]. In this report, we examine a case of fenofibrate-induced recurrent pancreatitis.

2. Case Presentation

A 79-year-old male with a medical history of cholelithiasis, for which he underwent cholecystectomy 11 years ago, hyperlipidemia, essential hypertension, and paroxysmal atrial fibrillation was admitted for mild acute pancreatitis. His presentation included severe epigastric pain radiating to the back, lipase of 1840 u/L, and no organ failure. He denied fever, chills, or body aches. The patient denied alcohol consumption and reported to have quit smoking 41 years ago. Liver chemistries, serum bilirubin, serum triglycerides, and immunoglobulin subclasses were within normal limits (Table 1). Abdominal CT scan demonstrated peripancreatic haziness consistent with noncomplicated acute pancreatitis (Figure 1). Home medications included atorvastatin for several years and the addition of 160 mg fenofibrate six months prior to admission. These medications were held upon admission but resumed at discharge. Full medication lists on admission and at discharge are shown in (Table 2). The patient was managed with fluid resuscitation and pain control. The patient recovered well and was able to tolerate regular diet without any pain or nausea. The patient was discharged in a stable condition after three hospital admission days, and lipase level at the day of discharge was 307 u/l.

Three days later, the patient returned with similar symptoms. Lipase levels were >30,000 u/l (Table 1), and

TABLE 1: Laboratory markers: initial admission; second admission after drug rechallenge.

Laboratory test	Initial Admission	Second admission - 72 hours after discharge	Reference range
Pancreatic enzymes			
Amylase (u/l)	158	671	20 - 90
Lipase (u/l)	1840 307 at discharge	>30,000	73-393
Basic metabolic panel			
Glucose (mg/dl)	101	75	70 - 100
Sodium (mmol/L)	136	138	135 - 145
Potassium (mmol/L)	4.2	3.6	3.7 - 5.1
Chloride (mmol/L)	104	102	96 - 110
Carbon dioxide (mmol/L)	24.0	28	22.0 - 32.0
Calcium (mg/dl)	9.0	8.8	8.5 - 10.5
Creatinine (mg/dl)	1.46	1.36	0.60 - 1.30
Blood urea nitrogen mg/dl	22	17	6 - 24
Glomerular filtration rate (mL/min/1.73 m2)	45	49	>=90
Anion Gap (mmol/L)	12	12	<=20
Hepatic function panel			
Alanine aminotransferase (u/l)	28	44	12 - 78
Aspartate aminotransferase (u/l)	33	37	10 - 40
Alkaline Phosphatase (u/l)	61	86	33 - 138
Total bilirubin (mg/dl)	1.1	0.5	0.0 - 1.5
Total protein (gm/dl)	7.5	7.4	6.0 - 8.4
Albumin (gm/dl)	3.4	3.3	3.5 - 5.0
Immunoglobulin subclasses			
IgG Subclass 1 (mg/dl)	626		405 - 1011
IgG Subclass 2 (mg/dl)	498		169 - 786
IgG Subclass 3 (mg/dl)	33		11 - 85
IgG Subclass 4 (mg/dl)	19		3 - 201
Other laboratory tests			
Triglycerides (mg/dl)	74		<149
White blood cell (k/ul)	14.7	10.8	4.0-12.0
Hemoglobin (gm/dl)	15.2	14.1	13.5-17.5
Platelets (k/ul)	237	298	140-440

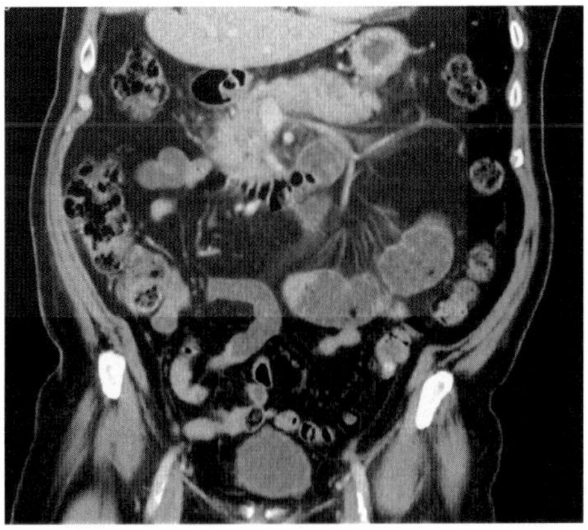

FIGURE 1: Coronal contrast enhanced CT image showing a homogenously enhancing bulky pancreas with peripancreatic haziness (arrows) with no evidence of collections consistent with noncomplicated acute interstitial pancreatitis.

TABLE 2: Complete medication list prior to each admission and on discharge.

On first admission	At first discharge	On second admission	At second discharge
Atorvastatin 20 mg ever night	Atorvastatin 20 mg ever night	Atorvastatin 20 mg ever night	Allopurinol 300 mg daily
Fenofibrate 160 mg every night	Fenofibrate 160 mg every night	Fenofibrate 160 mg every night	Acetaminophen 500 mg every 6 hours PRN
Allopurinol 300 mg daily	Allopurinol 300 mg daily	Allopurinol 300 mg daily	Lisinopril 10 mg daily
Acetaminophen 500 mg every 6 hours PRN	Acetaminophen 500 mg every 6 hours PRN	Acetaminophen 500 mg every 6 hours PRN	Warfarin 5 mg daily
Lisinopril 10 mg daily	Lisinopril 10 mg daily	Lisinopril 10 mg daily	Propafenone 225 mg daily
Warfarin 5 mg daily	Warfarin 5 mg daily	Warfarin 5 mg daily	Fluticasone 2 sprays in each nostril every night
Propafenone 225 mg daily	Propafenone 225 mg daily	Propafenone 225 mg daily	Multivitamin (centrum silver) every day
Fluticasone 2 sprays in each nostril every night	Fluticasone 2 sprays in each nostril every night	Fluticasone 2 sprays in each nostril every night	Vitamin C (ascorbic acid) 1000 mg every day
Multivitamin (centrum silver) every day	Multivitamin (centrum silver) every day	Multivitamin (centrum silver) every day	
Vitamin C (ascorbic acid) 1000 mg every day	Vitamin C (ascorbic acid) 1000 mg every day	Vitamin C (ascorbic acid) 1000 mg every day	
Co-Q 100 mg every day	Co-Q 100 mg every day	Co-Q 100 mg every day	

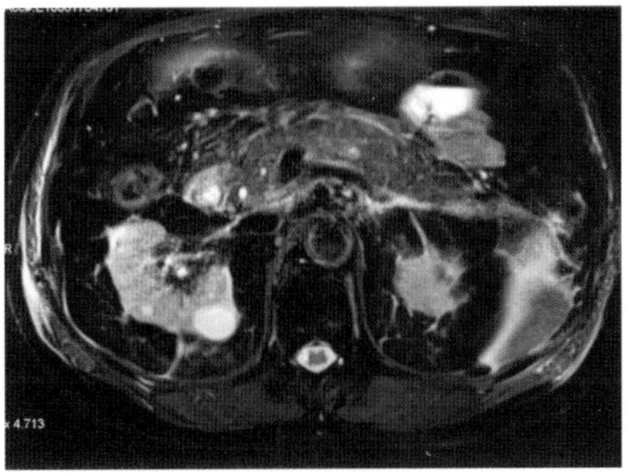

FIGURE 2: Fat suppressed T2W axial image showing both peripancreatic haziness and edema (arrows) consistent with acute interstitial pancreatitis.

magnetic resonance cholangiopancreatography showed acute interstitial edematous pancreatitis (Figure 2). The patient was treated conservatively with intravenous fluid resuscitation, pain control, and nothing per mouth until his symptoms resolved. Four days after his second admission, the patient recovered well and was discharged home in a stable condition. Fenofibrate and atorvastatin were discontinued (Table 2).

Two months later, the patient remained asymptomatic and returned for further workup to rule out an alternative cause to fenofibrate-induced pancreatitis. Endoscopic ultrasound (EUS) was done, which showed a 12 mm x 20 mm pancreatic head mass without pancreatic duct stenosis, strictures, or dilation. There were no common bile duct abnormalities. Fine needle aspiration was performed, and cytology was negative for malignant cells. Endoscopic retrograde cholangiopancreatography (ERCP) was performed to place a prophylactic pancreatic duct stent. Cholangiogram revealed a normal biliary system without dilation or strictures. The biliary tree was swept, and nothing was found. A prophylactic pancreatic duct stent was placed and a prophylactic sphincterotomy was performed. No recurrence of pancreatitis has occurred as of 6-month follow-up.

Given the course of the patient's illnesses in relation to fenofibrate usage, the timespan of drug initiation, and the fact that he had been taking atorvastatin for many years without previous signs or symptoms of acute pancreatitis, we hypothesize that his recurrent disease is probably due to the use of fenofibrate.

3. Discussion

Drug-induced pancreatitis accounts for 0.1%-2% of all cases of acute pancreatitis. Diagnosis of drug-induced pancreatitis is made when symptoms resolve with drug cessation and recur in accordance with a rechallenge of the same drug [4]. The disease is classified, from class I to IV, based on the number of cases reported, demonstration of a consistent latency, and reaction with rechallenge [5]. Three patterns of consistent latency are noted: a short latency of less than 24 hours, an intermediate latency of 24 hours to 30 days, and a long latency of greater than 30 days [5].

Typically, severity of drug-induced pancreatitis ranges from mild to moderate, but severe and even fatal cases may occur. The mechanism behind the condition remains controversial and varies between different offending medications [4]. Possible mechanisms include pancreatic duct constriction, cytotoxic effects, hypersensitivity reactions, and accumulation of toxic metabolites. Some drugs may cause pancreatitis indirectly by inducing hyperlipidemia or hypercalcemia [4, 6].

Lipid-modifying treatment with fibrates has been associated with the development of acute pancreatitis [7, 8]. According to the Coronary Drug Research Project, clofibrate was associated with a 50% increased risk of developing cholelithiasis or cholecystitis versus placebo, thus increasing the risk of acute pancreatitis [7]. Fenofibrate is believed to be less likely to induce gallstone formation while bezafibrate may raise biliary cholesterol concentration, thereby increasing the potential for gallstone formation and possibly resulting in acute pancreatitis [8]. However, there is limited data to support this theory.

Prior case reports have implicated clofibrate and bezafibrate as potential precipitating causes of acute pancreatitis [9, 10]. The only case involving fenofibrate-associated pancreatitis was reported by McDonald et al. [1] (2002) in which a patient on simvastatin, a class 1A medication, and fenofibrate developed acute pancreatitis. In their report, there was no rechallenge as the patient expired during a complicated hospital course.

Our patient was on atorvastatin, a class III medication, for many years without complications. He developed acute pancreatitis subsequent to the addition of fenofibrate six months prior to his initial presentation. The patient developed a recurrence of pancreatitis within 72 hours of fenofibrate rechallenge. In addition, the patient had a prior cholecystectomy and an EUS was negative for biliary stones, strictures, dilations, sludge, and chronic pancreatitis. A 12 mm x 20 mm pancreatic mass was found without pancreatic duct stenosis, strictures, or dilation and FNA revealed no malignant cells. Given that all other known causes of acute pancreatitis were ruled out, along with a positive rechallenge to the medication, we theorize that fenofibrate was a probable cause of recurrent drug-induced pancreatitis. Also, it is possible that the combination of fenofibrate and statin use can increase the risk for the disease. Furthermore, we believe that fenofibrate may produce pancreatitis by a different mechanism than previously theorized in literature, as there was no evidence of biliary stones or sludge in this case.

4. Conclusion

This case identifies fenofibrate as a probable cause of drug-induced pancreatitis, in addition to highlighting the importance of medication review in patients presenting with recurrent disease. We hypothesize that the mechanism of action regarding fenofibrate-induced pancreatitis is separate from the previously stated mechanism of lithogenic potential of other lipid lowering agents. It is also possible that the combination of fenofibrate with a statin can increase the risk of recurrent drug-induced pancreatitis.

References

[1] K. B. McDonald, B. G. Garber, and M. M. Perreault, "Pancreatitis associated with simvastatin plus fenofibrate," *Annals of Pharmacotherapy*, vol. 36, no. 2, pp. 275–279, 2002.

[2] P. Somani, T. Sunkara, and M. Sharma, "Role of endoscopic ultrasound in idiopathic pancreatitis," *World Journal of Gastroenterology*, vol. 23, no. 38, pp. 6952–6961, 2017.

[3] R. D. Bowers, S. M. Valanejad, and A. A. Holombo, "Mirtazapine-induced pancreatitis—a case report," *Journal of Pharmacy Practice*, 2018.

[4] M. R. Jones et al., "Drug-induced acute pancreatitis: a review," *The Ochsner Journal*, vol. 15, pp. 45–51, 2015.

[5] N. Badalov, R. Baradarian, K. Iswara, J. Li, W. Steinberg, and S. Tenner, "Drug-induced acute pancreatitis: an evidence-based review," *Clinical Gastroenterology and Hepatology*, vol. 5, no. 6, pp. 648.e3–661.e3, 2007.

[6] W. Y. Hung, "Contemporary review of drug-induced pancreatitis: A different perspective," *World Journal of Gastrointestinal Pathophysiology*, vol. 5, no. 4, p. 405, 2014.

[7] The Coronary Drug Project Research Group, "Gallbladder disease as a side effect of drugs influencing lipid metabolism experience in the coronary drug project," *The New England Journal of Medicine*, vol. 296, no. 21, pp. 1185–1190, 1977.

[8] D. Preiss, M. J. Tikkanen, P. Welsh et al., "Lipid-modifying therapies and risk of pancreatitis: A meta-analysis," *Journal of the American Medical Association*, vol. 308, no. 8, pp. 804–811, 2012.

[9] N. Gang, P. Langevitz, and A. Livneh, "Relapsing acute pancreatitis induced by re-exposure to the cholesterol lowering agent bezafibrate," *American Journal of Gastroenterology*, vol. 94, no. 12, pp. 3626–3628, 1999.

[10] M. Miettinen, O. Turpeinen, and M. J. Karvonen, "A co-operative trial in the primary prevention of ischaemic heart disease using clofibrate.," *British Heart Journal*, vol. 42, no. 3, pp. 370-371, 1979.

21

When the Benign Pneumatosis Intestinalis Becomes No Longer Benign: A Rare Case of Bowel Perforation in a Patient with Systemic Sclerosis

Jian Guan,[1] Alvina Munaf,[1] Alric V. Simmonds,[2] and Irteza Inayat[3]

[1]*Department of Internal Medicine, Graduate Medical Education, Florida Hospital, 2501 N. Orange Suite 235, Orlando, FL 32804, USA*
[2]*Department of General Surgery, Graduate Medical Education, Florida Hospital, 2415 N. Orange Ave., Suite 400, Orlando, FL 32804, USA*
[3]*Central Florida Hepatology & Gastroenterology, Florida Hospital, 2415 N. Orange Ave., Suite 200, Orlando, FL 32804, USA*

Correspondence should be addressed to Jian Guan; jianguan@bu.edu

Academic Editor: Chia-Tung Shun

Systemic sclerosis is a multisystem disease featured with autoimmunity and organ fibrosis. Although gastrointestinal (GI) tract involvement is common in patients with systemic sclerosis, colonic perforation is extremely rare. Benign pneumatosis intestinalis, a phenomenon more frequently seen in rheumatologic conditions, makes the diagnosis of colonic perforation even more challenging. We report a unique case of colonic perforation in a patient with chronic systemic sclerosis. This patient initially presented with mild abdominal pain and hematemesis. Urgent upper endoscopy was unremarkable and radiology showed stable pneumatosis intestinalis. Due to worsening abdominal pain, laparotomy exploration was performed and colonic perforation with transmural ischemic necrosis was found.

1. Introduction

Systemic scleroderma or systemic sclerosis is a chronic multisystem disease featured with generalized vasculopathy, activation of immune response, and progressive fibrosis of the skin and internal organs [1]. Gastrointestinal (GI) tract involvement is very common in patients with systemic sclerosis and dysmotility is the primary manifestation [2]. GI Symptoms are usually nonspecific, including dysphagia, heartburn, nausea, vomiting, abdominal pain, and distention [3]. It is not uncommon to see chronic bowel dilation, pseudo-obstruction, and benign pneumatosis intestinalis on imaging, but these conditions are typically managed conservatively [2]. The bowel perforation is a rare but serious complication of systemic sclerosis with GI involvement [4, 5]. Timely and accurate differentiation of true bowel perforation from benign pneumatosis intestinalis can be challenging.

2. Case Description

A 78-year-old woman with a long-standing history of anticentromere antibody positive systemic sclerosis with limited skin involvement (CREST syndrome) initially presented to emergency room (ER) for a one-day history of hematemesis and mild abdominal pain. Her medical history was remarkable for peripheral artery disease and duodenal arteriovenous malformation. At presentation, her vital signs were within normal limits and her physical examination revealed mild periumbilical tenderness and decreased bowel sounds without significant signs of peritonitis. Laboratory studies revealed a WBC count of $29X10^{\wedge 3}/\mu l$ and a hemoglobin of 4.7 g/L which acutely declined compared with her baseline hemoglobin of 9.5 g/L. Renal/liver function tests were within normal limits. Elevated venous lactate level was noted. Patient received intravenous fluid resuscitation and empirical piperacillin/tazobactam as well as 2 units of red blood cells

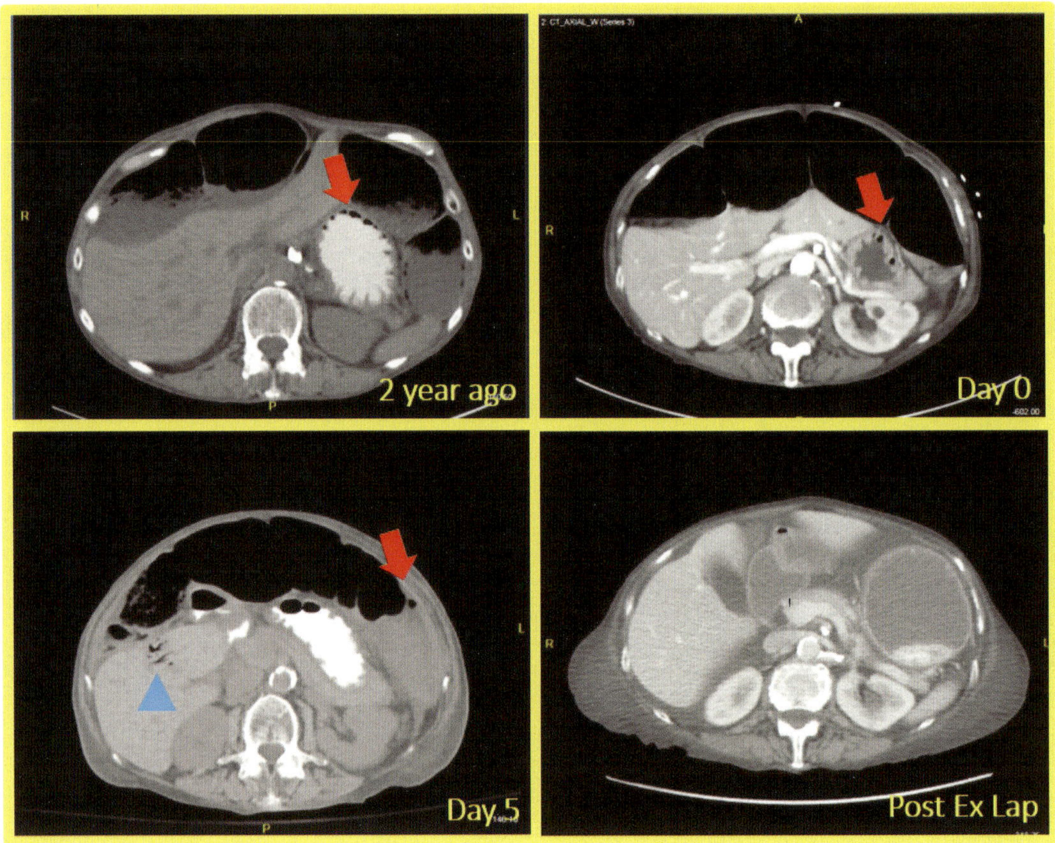

Figure 1: CT of abdomen revealed chronic bowel dilation and pneumatosis intestinalis ((a) and (b)); emergency of portal vein gas and worsening pneumatosis intestinalis (c); improvement after subtotal colectomy (d). Red arrow: pneumatosis intestinalis; blue arrow: portal vein gas.

transfusion in ER. A subsequent computed tomography (CT) scan of the abdomen that showed significantly dilated colon and pneumatosis intestinalis (Figure 1). No surgical intervention was deemed necessary per general surgery consultation, considering that the pneumatosis intestinalis was stable compared to the previous CT findings two years ago and the absence of acute peritonitis sign. Patient was then admitted to ICU for close monitoring and management of acute on chronic anemia from GI bleeding. Urgent esophagogastroduodenoscopy (EGD) only identified Barrett's-type esophageal mucosa, erosive gastritis without actively bleeding lesion. Patient was discharged home on the 4th day of hospitalization after tolerating liquid food. However, she was brought back to ER for severe lower abdominal pain just a few hours after discharge. The abdominal pain was sharp, constant, and nonradiating. No melena or hematochezia was reported. On examination, absent bowel sounds and abdominal distention without rebound tenderness or guarding were noted. Her laboratory evaluation was significant for leukocytosis and hypokalemia. Repeated CT scan of abdomen/pelvis showed distended small and large bowel loops, portal venous gas, and pneumatosis within the jejunum and colon (Figure 1). Clinical diagnosis of bowel perforation was made, for which patient underwent emergent exploratory laparotomy. Patchy necrosis throughout the large intestine and a perforated lesion in the ascending colon were identified during the operation. Subtotal colectomy, omentectomy, and end ileostomy were performed. Pathological findings were consistent with colonic perforation with transmural ischemic necrosis and fibrosis (Figure 2). CT angiography and conventional angiogram were performed to determine the culprit artery for bowel ischemia and identified a noncritical stenosis in superior mesenteric artery (Figure 3). Patient was then transferred to ICU for postoperative care. Patient's recovery was complicated with ventilation dependent respiratory failure and another episode of bowel perforation. Given her advanced age, comorbidities, and poor prognosis, end-of-life care was discussed with family members, and they decided to initiate comfort care after a prolonged hospital stay.

3. Discussion

Although systemic sclerosis is generally perceived as an orphan disease, its incidence was found to be comparable with the incidences of other well-known diseases such as esophageal cancer [6]. Although exact mechanism of systemic sclerosis remains unclear, [7] evidence suggests that autoimmunity mediated endothelial cell injury, ischemia-reperfusion injury, and generation of reactive oxygen species

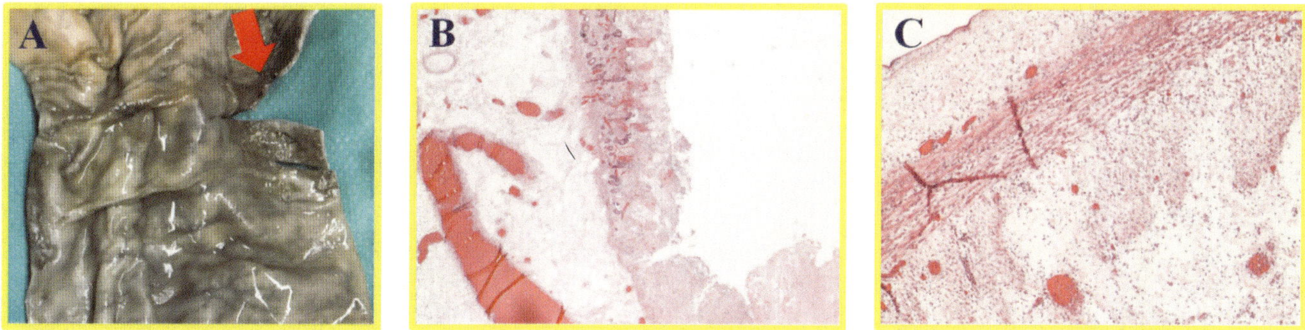

(a) (b) (c)

FIGURE 2: Perforation site in the ascending colon. (a) Gross image of perforation site in ascending colon. (b,c) H&E staining revealed the extensive mucosal necrosis or ulceration and overlying fibrinopurulent exudate.

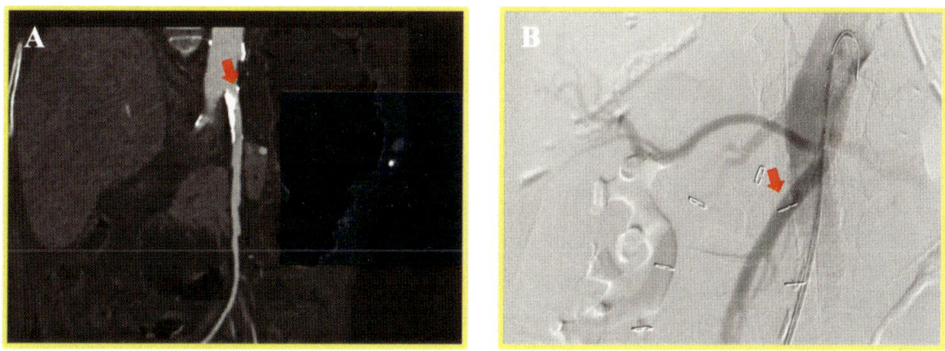

(a) (b)

FIGURE 3: CT angiography abdomen revealed stenosis of mesenteric artery (a). Arteriogram indicated patent mesenteric artery (b). Arrow: mesenteric artery.

and proinflammatory cytokines lead to vasculopathy and fibrosis in systemic sclerosis.[7]

GI tract involvement is seen in nearly 90% of patients with systemic sclerosis [3]. Dysmotility in systemic sclerosis is caused by abnormal compliance of bowel wall and reduced contractile function due to myopathy, neuropathy, and fibrosis [2]. Among all of GI complications of systemic sclerosis, pneumatosis intestinalis is probably the most challenging one to diagnose and manage, partially due to the unspecificity of its clinical presentation and potential detrimental consequence [8]. Pneumatosis intestinalis, defined as a cluster of intramural air in small or large intestinal wall, is a relatively infrequent finding and typically associated with secondary cause including autoimmune disease, trauma, and inflammatory diseases [9]. Close monitoring and conservative management such as gastric decompression, bowel rest, and antibiotics are typically recommended.

The bowel perforation is an extremely rare but detrimental complication of systemic sclerosis with GI tract involvement. The common risk factors of bowel perforation including atrophy of intestinal wall, stercoral ulceration from chronic dilation, and fecal impaction are frequently present in patients with systemic sclerosis. The first two cases of bowel perforation in patients with systemic sclerosis were reported in 1970s [4, 5]. More recently, a few reports have linked the use of octreotide or complication of gastrointestinal procedure with bowel perforation [10].

In our case, the cause for the bowel perforation was probably multifactorial (Figure 4). Atrophy of intestinal wall secondary to vasculopathy, inflammation, and fibrosis, as well as chronic dilation induced stercoral ulceration, might be the driving forces for the development of bowel perforation. Acute anemia from GI bleeding in the setting of preexisting atherosclerotic disease involving superior mesenteric artery led to acute bowel ischemia, which exaggerated the process of bowel perforation. There are several learning points in this unique case. Physicians should fully assess the overall clinical manifestation and risk factors, rather than being falsely reassured by radiologically "stable" pneumatosis intestinalis. Premature discharge in her first hospitalization could have been avoided if we had a high suspicion of a ruptured viscus rather than a benign pneumatosis intestinalis.

To sum up, benign pneumatosis intestinalis can be asymptomatic and managed medically in patients with systemic sclerosis; however, bowel perforation needs to be considered in the differential diagnosis in selected cases.

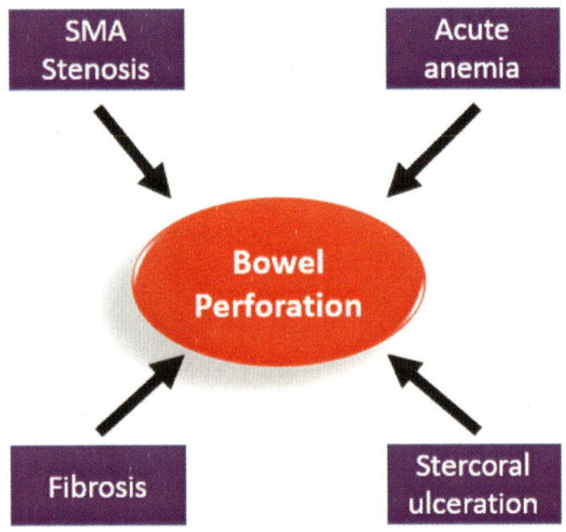

FIGURE 4: Scheme of the factors contributing to the bowel perforation in this case.

Disclosure

Abstract of this article was invited for poster presentation in the National American College of Physician (San Diego CA 2017).

References

[1] C. P. Denton and D. Khanna, "Systemic sclerosis," *The Lancet*, vol. 390, no. 10103, pp. 1685–1699, 2017.

[2] Y. Alastal, T. A. Hammad, A. Renno et al., "Gastrointestinal manifestations associated with systemic sclerosis: Results from the nationwide inpatient sample," *Annals of Gastroenterology*, vol. 30, no. 5, pp. 498–503, 2017.

[3] A. B. Shreiner, C. Murray, C. Denton, and D. Khanna, "Gastrointestinal manifestations of systemic sclerosis," *Journal of Scleroderma and Related Disorders*, vol. 1, no. 3, pp. 247–256, 2018.

[4] J. C. Robinson and S. L. Teitelbaum, "Stercoral ulceration and perforation of the sclerodermatous colon: Report of two cases and review of the literature," *Diseases of the Colon & Rectum*, vol. 17, no. 5, pp. 622–632, 1974.

[5] M. I. V. Jayson, J. Gough, P. R. Salmon, T. Poliness, and R. L. Bishton, "Spontaneous bowel perforation in intestinal scleroderma: first report of a non-fatal case," *Postgraduate Medical Journal*, vol. 48, no. 555, pp. 56–58, 1971.

[6] A. Fischer, E. Zimovetz, C. Ling, D. Esser, and N. Schoof, "Humanistic and cost burden of systemic sclerosis: A review of the literature," *Autoimmunity Reviews*, vol. 16, no. 11, pp. 1147–1154, 2017.

[7] M. Furue, C. Mitoma, H. Mitoma et al., "Pathogenesis of systemic sclerosis—current concept and emerging treatments," *Immunologic Research*, vol. 65, no. 4, pp. 790–797, 2017.

[8] A. Balbir-Gurman, O. R. Brook, I. Chermesh, and Y. Braun-Moscovici, "Pneumatosis cystoides intestinalis in scleroderma-related conditions," *Internal Medicine Journal*, vol. 42, no. 3, pp. 323–329, 2012.

[9] L.-L. Wu, Y.-S. Yang, Y. Dou, and Q.-S. Liu, "A systematic analysis of pneumatosis cystoids intestinalis," *World Journal of Gastroenterology*, vol. 19, no. 30, pp. 4973–4978, 2013.

[10] H. Oiwa, Y. Ikemoto, K. Mandai, K. Koide, T. Nishida, and Y. Tabe, "A case of systemic sclerosis sine scleroderma associated with perforation of an afferent loop after subtotal gastrectomy with Billroth 2 anastomosis for its severe gastrointestinal involvement," *Modern Rheumatology*, vol. 15, no. 5, pp. 371–373, 2005.

22

Cannabinoid Hyperemesis Syndrome: A Case Report of Cyclic Severe Hyperemesis and Abdominal Pain with Long-Term Cannabis Use

Julia Hermes-Laufer,[1] Lola Del Puppo,[1] Ihsan Inan,[2] François-Xavier Troillet,[3] and Omar Kherad[1,4]

[1] *Department of Internal Medicine, Hôpital de La Tour, Avenue J.-D.-Maillard 3, 1217 Geneva, Switzerland*
[2] *Department of Visceral Surgery, Clinique Générale Beaulieu, Chemin de Beau Soleil 20, 1206 Geneva, Switzerland*
[3] *Department of Gastroenterology, Hôpital de La Tour, Avenue J.-D.-Maillard 3, 1217 Geneva, Switzerland*
[4] *Faculty of Medicine, University of Geneva, Geneva, Switzerland*

Correspondence should be addressed to Julia Hermes-Laufer; julia.laufer@gmail.com

Academic Editor: Stephanie Van Biervliet

Introduction. Cannabinoid Hyperemesis Syndrome (CHS) is a rare condition that includes cyclic severe vomiting in subjects who have been consuming large doses of cannabis for several years. One of the major diagnostic criteria is the alleviation of symptoms by hot showers. The syndrome was first described in 2004 and is so far neither completely understood nor well known. The latter leads to continued morbidity in concerned subjects and unnecessary expenses for futile investigations. Standard treatments of vomiting as 5-HT3 or D2-receptor antagonists have been shown to be ineffective in alleviating the symptoms. The only long-term satisfying treatment option is the complete abstinence from cannabis consumption. *Case Summary.* In this case report we describe a 26-year-old male Caucasian long-term cannabis consumer who repeatedly presented in our emergency room with cyclic severe nausea and vomiting ceased by hot showers and resistant to all other treatments. The final diagnosis was not established until his third visit to the ER. *Conclusion.* CHS is an important differential diagnosis in patients who present with cyclic vomiting and abdominal pain with a history of long-term cannabis use. Recognition of this syndrome is important in order to avoid unnecessary clinical testing and to help the patients break the cycle of drug use.

1. Introduction

Cannabis is a commonly used recreational drug, which contains the principal psychoactive component delta 9-tetrahydrocannabinol (THC). Cannabis use is associated with several short- and long-term side effects such as changes in mood, impaired memory, impaired attention, depression, and anxiety and it is correlated with schizophrenia [1, 2]. However, cannabis use also has a therapeutic dimension due to its antiemetic and appetite-enhancing effects that is why it is sometimes used as a treatment for oncological patients suffering from nausea, vomiting, and loss of appetite during or after chemotherapy [3, 4]. The Cannabinoid Hyperemesis Syndrome is rare and was first described in the year 2004 by Allen et al. [5] and 2009 by Sontineni et al. [6] who first tried to establish diagnostic criteria. It has a delay in onset and is hence mostly observed in subjects who have been consuming large doses of cannabis over a period of several years. The syndrome can lead to complications like metabolic alkalosis, hypokalemia, acute kidney injury [7], or injuries of the oesophagus. Diagnostic criteria were renewed after a case series of 98 patients of Mayo Clinic in 2012 and include severe cyclic nausea and vomiting, resolution with cannabis cessation, relief of symptoms with hot showers or baths, abdominal pain, and weekly use of marijuana as major criteria [8] (see "Proposed Clinical Criteria by Simonetto et al. Mayo Clinic, 2012 [8]"). Faced with patients presenting the underdiagnosed CHS, physicians often perform ample and expensive investigations and workups that are futile in many cases. The only satisfying treatment is the complete abstinence from cannabis use.

Proposed Clinical Criteria by Simonetto et al. Mayo Clinic, 2012 [8]

Long-term cannabis use: essential for diagnosis

Major features:

(i) Severe cyclic nausea and vomiting
(ii) Resolution with cannabis cessation
(iii) Relief of symptoms with hot showers or baths
(iv) Abdominal pain: epigastric our periumbilical
(v) Weekly use of marijuana

Supportive features:

(i) Age less than 50 years
(ii) Weight loss of >5 kg
(iii) Morning predominance of symptoms
(iv) Normal bowel habits
(v) Negative laboratory and radiographic and endoscopic test results

2. Case Presentation

2.1. Personal History of the Patient. A 26-year-old male Caucasian patient presents three times to our emergency room with recurrent vomiting and colicky abdominal pain during the years 2014 and 2015. Every time he reports at least 20 episodes of vomiting a day and a strong abdominal pain (8/10) predominantly in the epigastric region. During the crises, he is unable to intake liquids or food out of fear of triggering vomiting. Episodes last about 24 to 48 hours and are refractory to all standard treatments for nausea and vomiting. His personal medical history reveals Gilbert's syndrome and a myringoplasty at the age of 5. The patient consumes cannabis twice a day since at least 10 years alongside an alcohol consumption which is reported to be irregular with 3 portions a week in average. He has been presenting these episodes in an irregular pattern for about 5 years with a duration of 1-2 days. The patient does not present fever and reports to have rather liquid stools, without meeting criteria for diarrhea. Before his hospitalization, several blood tests, enhanced abdominal CT-scan, and abdomen ultrasound have been performed ambulatory to investigate his symptoms. Blood tests, including complete blood count, glucose, basic metabolic panel, and pancreatic and hepatic enzymes, were normal. Radiological workup describes sludge and small gall stones within the gall bladder without evidence of acute cholecystitis. Considering the history with the atypical pain pattern and vomiting, the diagnosis of symptomatic gall stone disease was retained and a laparoscopic cholecystectomy was performed in August 2015. After an initial clinical improvement, the patient relapses and presents the same symptoms few weeks later, without any change in intensity.

2.2. Physical Examination and Other Tests. At our ER department, the patient had normal vital signs and no fever and physical examination was normal except for dehydration and light epigastric tenderness during abdominal examination. A neurological assessment was negative for any focal neurological deficit. Blood tests showed a slight leukocytosis (12 Giga/l) and slight hypokalemia (3.4 mmol/l). Hepatic profile showed typical signs of Gilbert's syndrome with an elevated total and unconjugated bilirubin without any other abnormalities. Stool cultures appeared to be negative. An esophagogastroduodenoscopy did not show any signs of ulceration or gastritis and the biopsies proved to be negative for a *Helicobacter pylori* infection. A cerebral MRI ruled out central causes of vomiting. A second abdominal CT-scan excluded any intra-abdominal pathology, especially no sign of superior mesenteric artery syndrome. Metabolic tests excluded diabetes mellitus, porphyria, and adrenal and thyroid diseases. The patient did not respond to standard treatments of nausea and vomiting as metoclopramide, ondansetron, or droperidol. The only effective measure to calm his abundant vomiting was hot showers or baths. The symptoms ceased right away after standing under hot water during his inpatient stay.

2.3. Treatment and Follow-Up. The patient was discharged from the hospital after two days with the recommendation to completely stop the consumption of cannabis. Follow-up nine months after discharge revealed that the patient had smoked cannabis again about two weeks after discharge in October 2015 with a relapse of symptoms and then never consumed cannabis again. He has been completely free of episodes of vomiting and abdominal pain since this time.

3. Discussion

Cannabis is of extraordinary cultural importance as it is the most commonly used illicit drug worldwide and ranks on the third place of recreational drugs behind alcohol and tobacco [9]. Every year about 130–230 million people use cannabis as a recreational drug [10] whereupon the percentage of legal and medical use is rising since a strong legalization movement has been established in people and governments of several countries over the last few years. It is therefore crucial to have solid evidence based information about all its possible health risks. There are many well explored short- and long-term side effects such as changes in mood, impaired memory, impaired attention, depression anxiety, and its correlation with schizophrenia [1, 2, 11].

The exact mechanisms of how and by which receptors the effects of THC are mediated in the human body are not yet completely understood. There are two main G-protein coupled receptors: the CB1 and CB2 receptor. The CB1 receptor is found in the central and peripheral nervous system, for example, in the hippocampus, the basal ganglia, and the cerebellum as well as in the enteric nervous system, and plays a neuromodulator role [12]. We know less about the CB2 receptor which is found primarily in immune cells and seems to have immunomodulatory effects [4, 13]. THC modulates the hypothalamus-pituitary axis by a diminution of secretion of anterior pituitary hormones like prolactin, growth hormone, thyroid hormone, or gonadotropin as well as an augmentation of corticotropin secretions [13]. These changes in the hypothalamus-pituitary-adrenal axis might also implicate changes in the thermoregulation. In a mouse model a decrease in body temperature has been described after the administration of THC [14] which might be an approach to a possible explanation of the compulsive bathing behavior in CHS patients.

The antiemetic effect of cannabis is mediated by an activation of CB-1 receptors in the brainstem and the enteric nervous system [15]. We still lack understanding of how a paradoxical hyperemetic effect can develop in long-term users, although several hypotheses were established during the last years. THC is lipophilic and accumulates in body fat, which serves as a long-term storage and probably liberates THC due to lipolysis in times of food deprivation and stress [13]. This might be one of the key aspects in the development of the CHS considering that mostly long-term users are concerned. However, since only a very small percentage of long-term cannabis consumers develop a CHS we need to identify risk factors for the development. Galli et al. proposed that the genetic polymorphisms in the cytochrome P450 enzymes and resulting in these possible excessive levels of emetogenic cannabinoid metabolites might be the cause [13].

Another important aspect is the quality of THC as a partial agonist on cannabinoid CB1 receptors. In case of chronic use and high tissue concentrations the antagonist nature of THC may emerge and induce a sudden withdrawal [16]. A sudden cessation from prolonged cannabis use might induce hyperemesis as already stated by Allen et al. in 2004 [5]. A downregulation of receptor density and desensitization of transduction mechanisms (tolerance) which can rapidly develop in case of chronic use [17] can also induce the transformation of THC from a partial agonist to an antagonist on CB1 receptors.

Eventually THC delays gastric emptying through the CB1 receptors found on the gastrointestinal system [18]. This effect has proven to be resistant to the development of tolerance [19].

Given the high prevalence of chronic cannabis abuse we presume that the syndrome is often underdiagnosed or misdiagnosed as cyclic vomiting or psychogenic vomiting. Further studies are warranted to better understand the pathophysiology and to identify risk factors as well as to validate the diagnostic criteria. Meanwhile, clinicians must evoke this diagnosis to avoid extensive workup and sometimes even futile surgery. Many of these patients relapse upon resuming cannabis because of their perception that it will have beneficial effects on nausea. Patient education should therefore be provided with emphasis on the paradoxical nature of the symptoms of CHS.

4. Conclusion

The Cannabinoid Hyperemesis Syndrome is a challenging differential diagnosis in patients who present with cyclic vomiting and abdominal pain with history of cannabis use. Recognition of this syndrome is important in order to avoid costly and unnecessary clinical testing and to help the patient understand and break the cycle of drug use. We emphasize the importance of a complete anamnestic inquiry concerning drug consumption and relief by hot showers or baths in those patients.

Abbreviations

CHS:	Cannabinoid Hyperemesis Syndrome
ER:	Emergency room
5-HT3 receptor:	5-hydroxytryptamine 3 (serotonin) receptor
US:	Ultrasound
THC:	Delta 9-tetrahydrocannabinol.

Additional Points

Availability of Data and Materials. The authors agree to make the raw data and materials described in our manuscript freely available.

Consent

Written informed consent was obtained from the patient for publication of this case report and any accompanying images.

Authors' Contributions

Julia Hermes-Laufer cowrote the manuscript. Omar Kherad cowrote and reviewed the manuscript. Lola Del Puppo, Ihsan Inan, and François-Xavier Troillet reviewed the manuscript. All authors read and approved the final manuscript.

Acknowledgments

This case report was supported by ward doctors with regard to the acquisition of data. The authors are thankful to the patient's mother for support given in providing data.

References

[1] National Institutes of Drug Abuse website: NIDA Info Facts: Marijuana, National Institute on Drug Abus, https://www.drugabuse.gov/publications/drugfacts/marijuana.

[2] J. D. Foley, "Adolescent use and misuse of marijuana," *Adolescent Medicine Clinics*, vol. 17, no. 2, pp. 319–334, 2006.

[3] D. Walsh, K. A. Nelson, and F. A. Mahmoud, "Established and potential therapeutic applications of cannabinoids in oncology," *Supportive Care in Cancer*, vol. 11, no. 3, pp. 137–143, 2003.

[4] M. Davis, V. Maida, P. Daeninck, and J. Pergolizzi, "The emerging role of cannabinoid neuromodulators in symptom management," *Supportive Care in Cancer*, vol. 15, no. 1, pp. 63–71, 2007.

[5] J. H. Allen, G. M. de Moore, R. Heddle, and J. C. Twartz, "Cannabinoid hyperemesis: cyclical hyperemesis in association with chronic cannabis abuse," *Gut*, vol. 53, no. 11, pp. 1566–1570, 2004.

[6] S. P. Sontineni, S. Chaudhary, V. Sontineni, and S. J. Lanspa, "Cannabinoid hyperemesis syndrome: clinical diagnosis of an underrecognised manifestation of chronic cannabis abuse," *World Journal of Gastroenterology*, vol. 15, no. 10, pp. 1264–1266, 2009.

[7] J. Habboushe and J. Sedor, "Cannabinoid hyperemesis acute renal failure: a common sequela of cannabinoid hyperemesis syndrome," *American Journal of Emergency Medicine*, vol. 32, no. 6, pp. 690.el–690.e2, 2014.

[8] D. A. Simonetto, A. S. Oxentenko, M. L. Herman, and J. H. Szostek, "Cannabinoid hyperemesis: a case series of 98 patients," *Mayo Clinic Proceedings*, vol. 87, no. 2, pp. 114–119, 2012.

[9] Global Drug Survey, 2014, https://www.globaldrugsurvey.com/past-findings/the-global-drug-survey-2014-findings/.

[10] United Nations Office of Drugs and Crime, World Drug Report 2015, https://www.unodc.org/documents/wdr2015/World_Drug_Report_2015.pdf.

[11] S. R. Childers and C. S. Breivogel, "Cannabis and endogenous cannabinoid systems," *Drug and Alcohol Dependence*, vol. 51, no. 1-2, pp. 173–187, 1998.

[12] M. R. Elphick and M. Egertová, "The neurobiology and evolution of cannabinoid signalling," *Philosophical Transactions of the Royal Society of London B: Biological Sciences*, vol. 356, no. 1407, pp. 381–408, 2001.

[13] J. A. Galli, R. A. Sawaya, and F. K. Friedenberg, "Cannabinoid hyperemesis syndrome," *Current Drug Abuse Reviews*, vol. 4, no. 4, pp. 241–249, 2011.

[14] K. Hayakawa, K. Mishima, M. Nozako et al., "Δ^9-Tetrahydrocannabinol (Δ^9-THC) prevents cerebral infarction via hypothalamic-independent hypothermia," *Life Sciences*, vol. 80, no. 16, pp. 1466–1471, 2007.

[15] N. A. Darmani, "Mechanisms of broad-spectrum antiemetic efficacy of cannabinoids against chemotherapy-induced acute and delayed vomiting," *Pharmaceuticals*, vol. 3, no. 9, pp. 2930–2955, 2010.

[16] N. A. Darmani, "Cannabinoid-induced hyperemesis: a conundrum—from clinical recognition to basic science mechanisms," *Pharmaceuticals (Basel)*, vol. 3, no. 7, pp. 2163–2177, 2010.

[17] B. R. Martin, L. J. Sim-Selley, and D. E. Selley, "Signaling pathways involved in the development of cannabinoid tolerance," *Trends in Pharmacological Sciences*, vol. 25, no. 6, pp. 325–330, 2004.

[18] R. W. McCallum, I. Soykan, K. R. Sridhar, D. A. Ricci, R. C. Lange, and M. W. Plankey, "Delta-9-tetrahydrocannabinol delays the gastric emptying of solid food in humans: A Double-blind, Randomized Study," *Alimentary Pharmacology and Therapeutics*, vol. 13, no. 1, pp. 77–80, 1999.

[19] R. Abalo, P. A. Cabezos, V. López-Miranda et al., "Selective lack of tolerance to delayed gastric emptying after daily administration of WIN 55,212-2 in the rat," *Neurogastroenterology and Motility*, vol. 21, no. 9, p. 1002–e80, 2009.

23

Esophageal Lichen Planus: Understanding a Potentially Severe Stricturing Disease

Bharat Rao,[1,2] Abhishek Gulati,[1,2] Blair Jobe,[3,4] and Shyam Thakkar[1,2]

[1]*Department of Gastroenterology, Allegheny Health Network, Pittsburgh, PA, USA*
[2]*Allegheny Center for Digestive Health, 1307 Federal Street, Suite 301, Pittsburgh, PA 15212, USA*
[3]*Department of Surgery, Allegheny Health Network, Pittsburgh, PA, USA*
[4]*Esophageal and Lung Institute, 4815 Liberty Avenue, Mellon Pavilion, Suite 158, Pittsburgh, PA 15224, USA*

Correspondence should be addressed to Bharat Rao; bharatkrao@gmail.com

Academic Editor: Tetsuo Hirata

A 67-year-old woman with a long-standing history of recurrent dysphagia and esophageal strictures failed to respond to aggressive antireflux management. She required multiple dilations for symptomatic strictures that were discovered throughout the esophagus. Intralesional, topical, and systemic glucocorticoid therapies were utilized without resolution in symptoms. Several years after initial presentation, histopathology ultimately demonstrated lichenoid features and a diagnosis of esophageal lichen planus (ELP) was confirmed. However, as her symptoms had already become significantly disabling with severe strictures that carried an increased risk of endoscopic complications with dilation, she ultimately decided to undergo an esophagectomy for definitive treatment. Moreover, ELP may often go unrecognized for several years. Clinicians should consider ELP in the differential for dysphagia in middle- to elderly-aged women with or without a known history of lichen planus (LP) especially for those with findings of multiple or proximal strictures.

1. Introduction

Lichen planus (LP), an inflammatory disorder with an unknown etiology, commonly manifests in the oral mucosa and skin [1]. LP though may involve much less common sites including the esophagus [2]. It is not uncommon to take few to several years to correctly diagnose esophageal lichen planus (ELP) due to unfamiliarity with the disease, often nonspecific endoscopic and histopathology findings, and the possibility of ELP being the first manifestation of LP [3, 4]. We present our own experience of a patient with a severe case of ELP in order to further the understanding of this potentially chronic and debilitating stricturing disease. Important concepts to diagnosis ELP early in its course along with management strategies are reviewed.

2. Case Presentation

A 67-year-old woman presented with a long-standing history of dysphagia and recurrent strictures. She did not have typical heartburn or regurgitation symptoms consistent with reflux disease. Her medical history included psoriasis and hypothyroidism. Exam findings of oral lesions or skin findings consistent with LP were not identified.

Laboratory investigations were remarkable for a positive antinuclear antibody with titres of 1 : 320 in a homogenous pattern with other autoimmune markers being nonreactive. Hepatitis C antibody was also nonreactive. Histopathology specimens predominantly showed nonspecific findings of acute and chronic inflammation suggestive of reflux disease.

She underwent multiple esophagogastroduodenoscopies (EGD) with findings of mucosal friability, webs, and strictures (Figures 1–3). Initial examinations revealed strictures in the lower third of the esophagus. Later, strictures were discovered in both the proximal and mid-esophagus. Strictures ranged in diameter within 9–14 mm.

Initial treatment consisted of twice daily proton pump inhibitor (PPI) for initially suspected reflux esophagitis, which offered no improvement in symptoms. A trial of

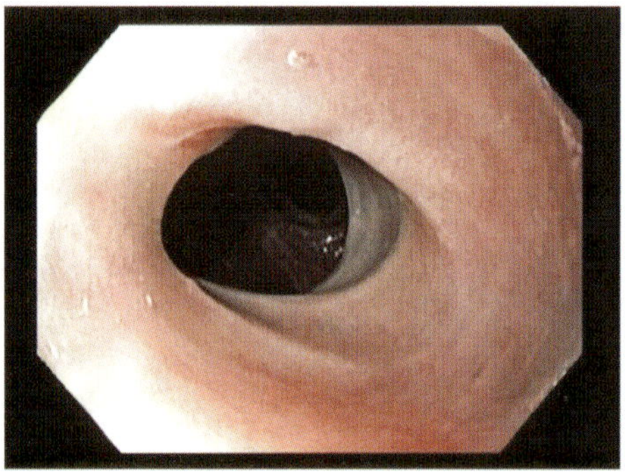

Figure 1: Stricture in the lower third of esophagus.

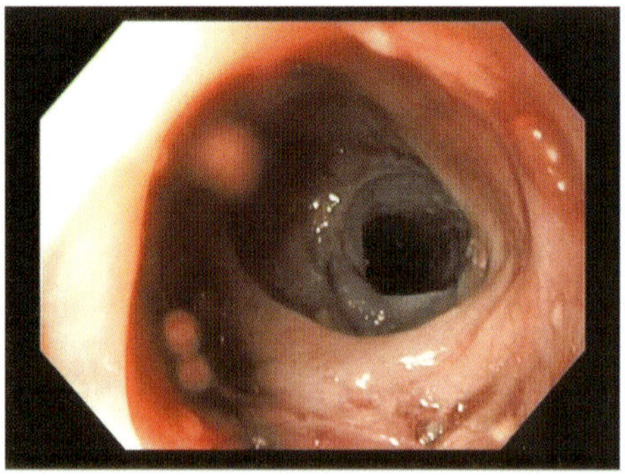

Figure 2: Stricture in the middle third of esophagus.

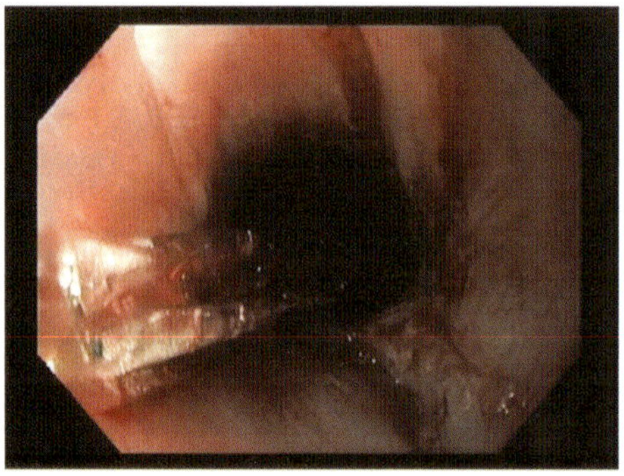

Figure 3: Proximal stricture treated with dilatation.

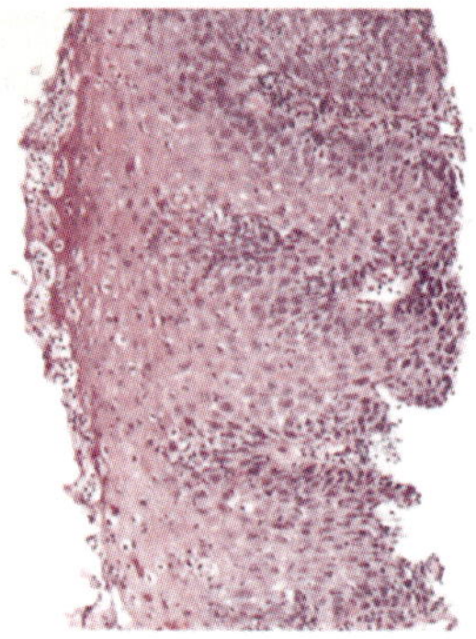

Figure 4: Esophageal squamous epithelium with H&E staining at 100x magnification. Findings showing lymphocytic infiltrate in the basal layer and scattered apoptotic keratinocytes (Civatte bodies).

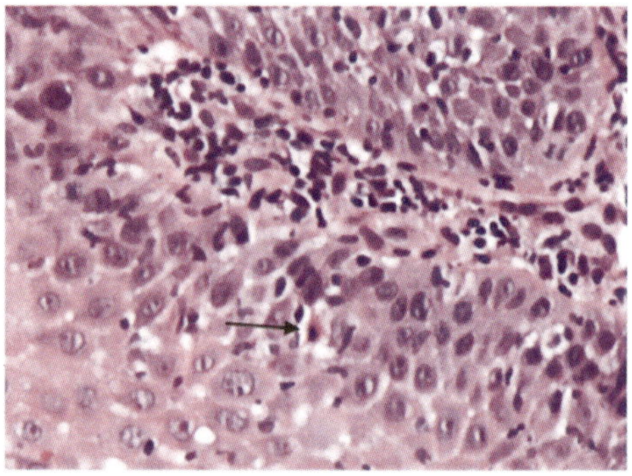

Figure 5: Esophageal squamous epithelium with H&E staining at 200x magnification with black arrow showing a Civatte body.

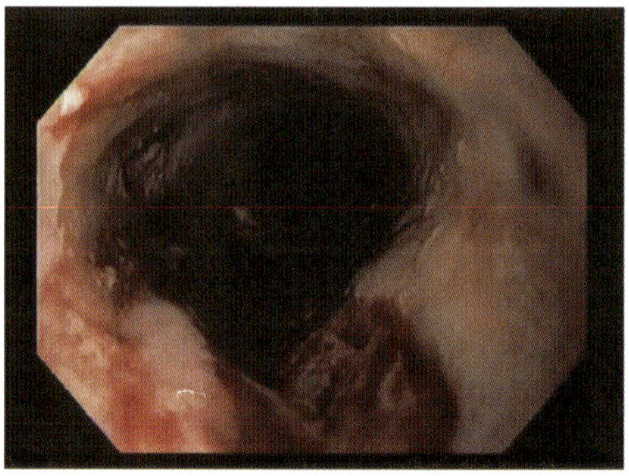

Figure 6: Esophageal mucosal tear after dilatation procedure occurring late in the patient's course highlighting the potential increased risk of complications with further endoscopic interventions.

inhaled swallowed fluticasone propionate 440 mcg twice daily for at one point suspected eosinophilic esophagitis provided no relief. Endoscopic bougie and balloon dilations provided transient improvement but this became less sustained over time. The primary modality of treatment that offered prolonged benefit was recurrent dilations with triamcinolone acetonide injections (10 mg/mL concentration) to strictures though the time interval of relief ultimately decreased as well. A trial of systemic glucocorticoids (40 mg/daily with a tapered course over 10 weeks) was also given for a suspected autoimmune etiology and did not provide any relief.

Seven years after her initial presentation, deep esophageal biopsy specimens were obtained showing severe acute and chronic esophagitis with a lichenoid-like pattern of chronic inflammation with notable features of lymphocytic infiltrate involving the basal layer of the epithelium and scattered apoptotic keratinocytes (Civatte bodies) (Figures 4 and 5) raising strong consideration of ELP. After a multidisciplinary review of these findings along with her consistent history, a diagnosis of ELP was made.

By this time, her symptoms had already become severely debilitating with worsening strictures and narrowing throughout the esophagus, carrying a substantial risk for perforation with continued dilations (Figure 6). The patient ultimately made a decision to undergo a minimally invasive esophagectomy for definitive management with acute and chronic inflammation seen on surgical pathology. Her symptoms significantly improved in the months following her surgery. However, she gradually developed symptoms of dysphagia, abdominal cramping, nausea, emesis, and weight loss. This was felt to be secondary to delayed gastric emptying and a mild anastomotic stricture. She underwent Botox injection into the pylorus along with therapeutic dilation and triamcinolone acetonide injection to stricture. Her symptoms improved after these interventions.

3. Discussion

Similar to our case, the majority of patients with ELP are middle-aged to elderly females (approximately 87% females with a median age of 61.9) [2]. Dysphagia is the most common symptom and was the predominant complaint in this case [3, 5]. Patients often have a history of LP but ELP may be the initial manifestation. Although some autoimmune diseases have been reported to be associated with LP [1], the reported coexisting diseases in ELP are limited in several reports. There has been though a noted increased history of thyroid disorders in ELP cases [2]. Although hepatitis C has been associated with LP, it is infrequent in ELP reports, consistent with our findings [2, 3].

On endoscopic examination, ELP may involve the proximal to distal esophagus; however the proximal esophagus (estimated 89% of cases) is most often affected. This is in contrast to reflux disease with distal involvement [2]. Macroscopic findings are nonspecific but include a friable mucosa, whitish papules, esophageal webs, and strictures that can be multiple in numbers [3, 5, 6].

Histopathology may be nondiagnostic in half of cases with interpretations of esophagitis or chronic inflammation. Findings that help support a diagnosis of ELP include a band-like lymphocytic infiltrate involving the superficial lamina propria and basal epithelium along with the presence of Civatte bodies [7, 8]. Despite multiple biopsies in this case, a diagnosis of ELP was not suggested on histopathology until deep biopsies were performed.

As in our case, reflux esophagitis is often initially suspected with initiation of PPI therapy leading to no improvement in strictures [4]. ELP is often a diagnostic challenge with a large series [3] showing a mean of nearly five years until diagnosis. As a result, multiple endoscopies and dilations are often performed before reaching a diagnosis [3, 4].

Treatment generally starts with oral glucocorticoid therapy. The suggested approach has been doses in the range of 40–60 mg for several weeks (patients usually show response within first couple weeks) with a tapered course [2, 8]. Though the majority of patients often respond to this approach, some may develop symptomatic recurrence during tapering and require longer therapy. In addition, those who had complete response often have recurrence of disease later on highlighting the potential chronic and recurring nature of ELP [4, 5]. Failure to respond is likely to occur for those with strictures at diagnosis as in our case [2]. Fluticasone propionate and intralesional triamcinolone acetate have also been utilized for improving symptoms [9, 10]. Aside from glucocorticoids, limited reports have utilized tacrolimus (including aqueous preparations) and cyclosporine with reported good response [10, 11]. Another aspect of treatment has been dilations for strictures in order to achieve immediate improvement in symptoms [5, 12]. Some cases have demonstrated concern for inducing the Koebner phenomenon at sites of trauma with dilatation [4]. However, dilatations are often necessary in patients and are performed with concurrent therapy aimed at controlling the disease [3]. Moreover, some patients even with prolonged and multiple treatment strategies may not respond sufficiently resulting in frequent dilatation procedures [8]. Our patient had developed poor responses despite aggressive steroid therapies and dilations, ultimately leading to definitive surgical management.

Although it is not certain if LP itself is an independent risk for malignant conversions, there are cases of esophageal squamous cell cancer in those with ELP [3, 5, 13, 14]. Therefore surveillance should be considered. Given the rarity of reported ELP, variable responses to treatment, and reports of malignancy, management may be better served utilizing a multidisciplinary approach. In summary, clinicians should consider ELP in the differential for dysphagia, especially for middle- to elderly-aged females, with refractory stricturing disease and without typical GERD symptoms or failure to respond to antireflux management. Awareness of the clinical history along with improved recognition and reporting of characteristic histopathology of ELP may lead to an earlier diagnosis and optimize outcomes.

References

[1] L. Le Cleach and O. Chosidow, "Clinical practice. Lichen planus," *New England Journal of Medicine*, vol. 366, no. 8, pp. 723–732, 2012.

[2] L. P. Fox, C. J. Lightdale, and M. E. Grossman, "Lichen planus of the esophagus: what dermatologists need to know," *Journal of the American Academy of Dermatology*, vol. 65, no. 1, pp. 175–183, 2011.

[3] D. A. Katzka, T. C. Smyrk, A. J. Bruce, Y. Romero, J. A. Alexander, and J. A. Murray, "Variations in presentations of esophageal involvement in lichen planus," *Clinical Gastroenterology and Hepatology*, vol. 8, no. 9, pp. 777–782, 2010.

[4] G. C. Harewood, J. A. Murray, and A. J. Cameron, "Esophageal lichen planus: the mayo clinic experience," *Diseases of the Esophagus*, vol. 12, no. 4, pp. 309–311, 1999.

[5] A. Chryssostalis, M. Gaudric, B. Terris, R. Coriat, F. Prat, and S. Chaussade, "Esophageal lichen planus: A series of eight cases including a patient with esophageal verrucous carcinoma: a case series," *Endoscopy*, vol. 40, no. 9, pp. 764–768, 2008.

[6] R. Quispel, O. S. Van Boxel, M. E. Schipper et al., "High prevalence of esophageal involvement in lichen planus: a study using magnification chromoendoscopy," *Endoscopy*, vol. 41, no. 3, pp. 187–193, 2009.

[7] V. S. Chandan, J. A. Murray, and S. C. Abraham, "Esophageal lichen planus," *Archives of Pathology & Laboratory Medicine*, vol. 132, no. 6, pp. 1026–1029, 2008.

[8] A. Ukleja, K. R. Devault, M. E. Stark, and S. R. Achem, "Lichen planus involving the esophagus," *Digestive Diseases and Sciences*, vol. 46, no. 10, pp. 2292–2297, 2001.

[9] F. Donnellan, M. P. Swan, G. R. May, G. Kandel, N. E. Marcon, and P. P. Kortan, "Fluticasone propionate for treatment of esophageal lichen planus. A case series," *Diseases of the Esophagus*, vol. 24, no. 4, pp. 211–214, 2011.

[10] R. F. Keate, J. W. Williams, and S. M. Connolly, "Lichen planus esophagitis: report of three patients treated with oral tacrolimus or intraesophageal corticosteroid injections or both," *Diseases of the Esophagus*, vol. 16, no. 1, pp. 47–53, 2003.

[11] M. Chaklader, C. Morris-Larkin, W. Gulliver, and J. McGrath, "Cyclosporine in the management of esophageal lichen planus," *Canadian Journal of Gastroenterology*, vol. 23, no. 10, pp. 686–688, 2009.

[12] D. L. Franco, S. R. Islam, D. M. Lam-Himlin, D. E. Fleischer, and S. F. Pasha, "Presentation, diagnosis, and management of esophageal lichen planus: a series of six cases," *Case Reports in Gastroenterology*, vol. 9, no. 2, pp. 253–260, 2015.

[13] M. P. Schwartz, V. Sigurdsson, W. Vreuls, P. H. W. Lubbert, and A. J. P. M. Smout, "Two siblings with lichen planus and squamous cell carcinoma of the oesophagus," *European Journal of Gastroenterology and Hepatology*, vol. 18, no. 10, pp. 1111–1115, 2006.

[14] C. Calabrese, A. Fabbri, M. Benni et al., "Squamous cell carcinoma arising in esophageal lichen planus," *Gastrointestinal Endoscopy*, vol. 57, no. 4, pp. 596–599, 2003.

Gastrointestinal Involvement of Testicular Germ Cell Tumor: A Case Report and Literature Review

Oluwaseun Shogbesan,[1] Abdullateef Abdulkareem,[1] Asad Jehangir,[2] Sunila Byreddy,[2] Sharon Swierczynski,[3] and Anthony Donato[1]

[1] *Department of Internal Medicine, Reading Health System, Sixth Avenue and Spruce Street, West Reading, PA 19611, USA*
[2] *Hospitalist Services, Reading Health System, Sixth Avenue and Spruce Street, West Reading, PA 19611, USA*
[3] *Department of Pathology, Reading Health System, Sixth Avenue and Spruce Street, West Reading, PA 19611, USA*

Correspondence should be addressed to Oluwaseun Shogbesan; oluwaseun.shogbesan@readinghealth.org

Academic Editor: Yoshihiro Moriwaki

Testicular germ cell tumors (GCT) are the commonest solid tumors in young men. Typical presentation is with painless scrotal swelling; however, symptoms related to complications or metastasis may be the initial presentation. Gastrointestinal (GI) metastasis is seen in about 5% of patients with germ cell tumors and presentation is commonly with GI bleed. It is important to have GCT as a differential diagnosis of GI bleed in young men presenting with unexplained anemia as direct questioning about scrotal swelling and genital examination when appropriate will guide further investigation and facilitate prompt diagnosis. We present a case of a 26-year-old man with testicular germ cell tumor and severe anemia secondary to extension and perforation of duodenum by retroperitoneal metastasis and a review of the literature on the gastrointestinal manifestations of testicular germ cell tumors.

1. Introduction

Testicular germ cell tumors (GCT) make up 95% of testicular cancers and are the commonest solid malignancies in young men [1]. Classic presentation is as a painless testicular swelling; however, in 10% of patients, presentation is variable and related to site of metastasis and complications. Gastrointestinal (GI) metastasis is seen in 5% of germ cell tumors and rare presentation with hemodynamically significant gastrointestinal bleed or as occult bleed have been reported [2, 3].

2. Case Report

A 26-year-old previously healthy man presented to the emergency department (ED) after an outpatient computed tomography (CT) of the chest showed large burden pulmonary embolus and a 13 mm left lower lobe nodule. He had previously presented at his primary care physician's office with complaints of low back pain, shortness of breath, chest pain, and bilateral leg swelling that had prompted the imaging. The patient reported severe low back pain for 2 weeks with limitation of movement due to pain prior to onset of shortness of breath, chest pain, and bilateral leg swelling. There was no associated cough or hemoptysis. History was otherwise unremarkable including no prior history of personal or family history of cancers or thrombotic conditions, recent surgery, or trauma. He had a 6-pack-year history of tobacco use.

On presentation in the ED, vital signs were significant for tachycardia (pulse rate of 107 beats/minutes), blood pressure of 121/62 mmHg, temperature of 36.9°C, and 99% oxygen saturation on room air.

Physical examination revealed a pale patient with bilateral lower extremity edema without tenderness or erythema. Other examinations including abdominal examination were unremarkable; testicular examination was not documented.

Laboratory data showed significant anemia with hemoglobin of 5.6 g/dl (normal: 14.0–17.5 g/dl; last known hemoglobin from 9 years earlier was 15.7 g/dl), white blood

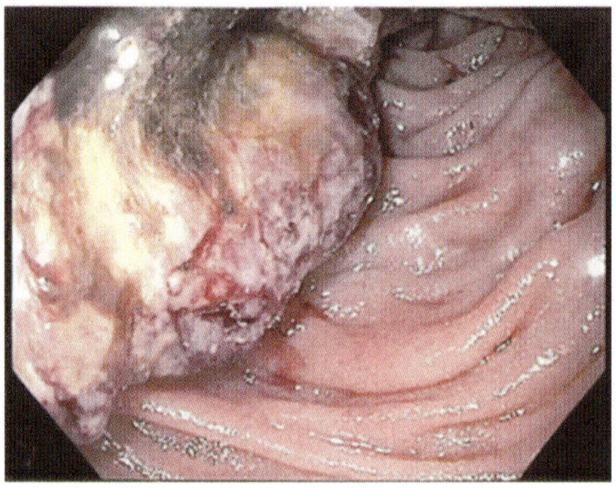

Figure 1: Ulcerated friable duodenal mass noted on esophagogastroduodenoscopy.

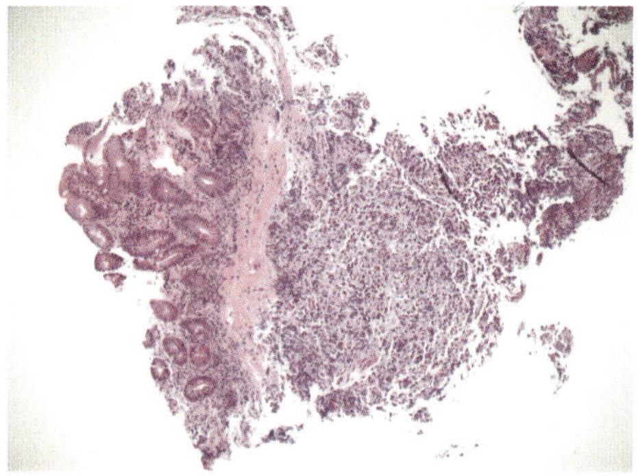

Figure 2: Duodenal mass, metastatic seminoma (H&E stain, magnification ×40).

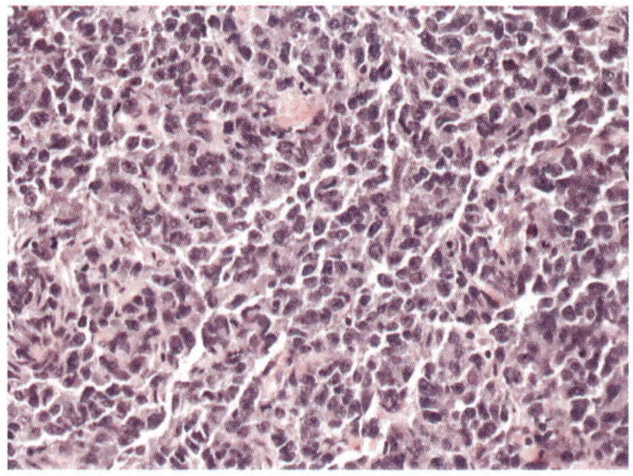

Figure 3: Duodenal mass, metastatic seminoma (H&E stain, magnification ×400).

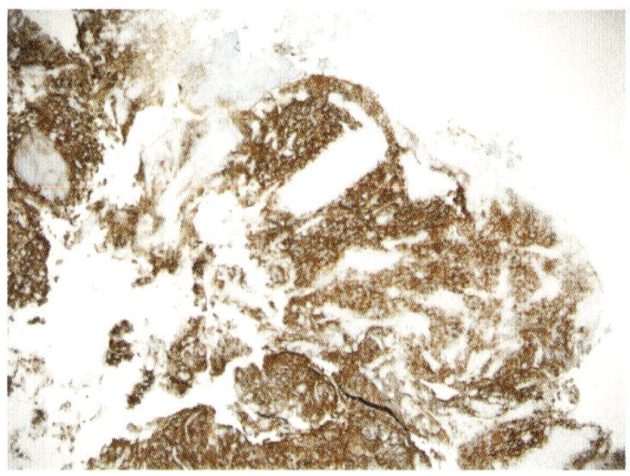

Figure 4: Duodenal mass with metastatic seminoma (PLAP IHC stain, magnification ×200).

count of 6200/μL (normal: 4800–10800/μL), platelet count 264,000/μL (normal: 130,000–400,000 μL), mean corpuscular volume 82.7 fL (normal: 80.0–99.9 fL), and mean corpuscular hemoglobin 27.5 pg (normal: 27–34 pg). Iron studies were consistent with iron deficiency anemia with ferritin of 18 ng/ml (normal: 27–300 ng/ml), iron of <10 mcg/dL (normal: 50–212 mcg/dL), iron saturation < 3% (normal: 20–50%), and high normal TIBC of 390 ug/dL (normal: 250–425 ug/dL). Electrolytes and hepatic function were within normal limits. Troponin was negative and BNP was 27 pg/ml (0–100 pg/ml). Patient admitted to taking Ibuprofen 400 mg twice a day for back pain for 2 weeks but denied hematochezia, melena, or bleeding from any site. He declined a digital rectal examination.

Esophagogastroduodenoscopy (EGD) to further investigate his anemia revealed an ulcerated, friable mass within the mid second to third portion of the duodenum (Figure 1). Multiple biopsies were taken with a recommendation for further work-up for duodenal mass.

A CT scan of abdomen and pelvis found a large soft tissue density mass-like structure in the right retroperitoneal space measuring up to 13.4 cm × 9.2 cm extending into the second and third portion of the duodenum with a contained perforation of the duodenum. In addition, a 3.4 × 2.7 cm enlarged para-aortic lymph node and thrombosis of the IVC extending to the right renal vein was also noted. Magnetic resonance imaging of the brain was normal.

Given findings on EGD and CT scan, additional history was obtained which revealed a history of testicular trauma many years priorly when he was hit by a baseball in the right testicle with persistent scrotal swelling; however, the swelling had progressively worsened in the past 1 year. Testicular exam showed a firm right scrotal swelling, twice the size of the left testicle. Scrotal ultrasound revealed 4 separate masses. B-HCG was elevated to 1468 mIU/mL (normal 0–4 mIU/mL), LDH was 367 IU/L (normal 140–271 IU/L), and alpha fetoprotein (AFP) was normal (0.9 ng/mL).

Histopathology of the duodenal mass showed a poorly differentiated malignant neoplasm strongly positive for placenta alkaline phosphatase (PLAP), consistent with a malignant germ cell tumor (Figures 2–4).

He underwent a right radical orchiectomy. Gross examination of the right testis revealed four distinct tumor nodules in the testis (Figure 5).

Two of the nodules showed reactivity for beta-HCG. Sporadic CK7 immunoreactivity was seen in the nodules expressing beta-HCG. All four nodules showed immunoreactivity for PLAP (Figure 6).

The pathologic findings were consistent with a seminoma. He was staged as Stage IIIA, pT1N3M1aS1 given the metastases to the retroperitoneum and lungs.

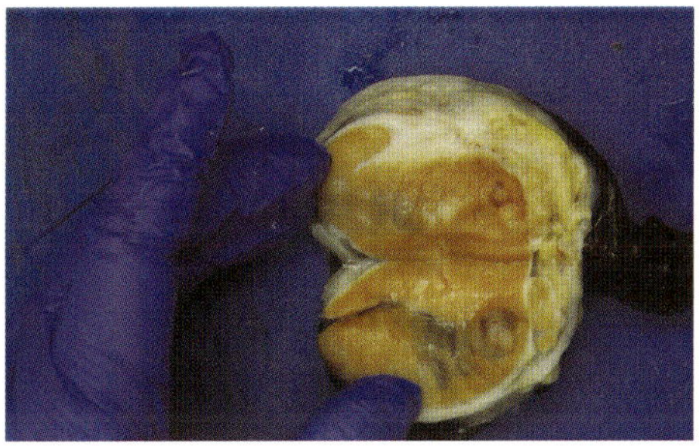

FIGURE 5: Gross right testis, bisected, showing nodules within the testis.

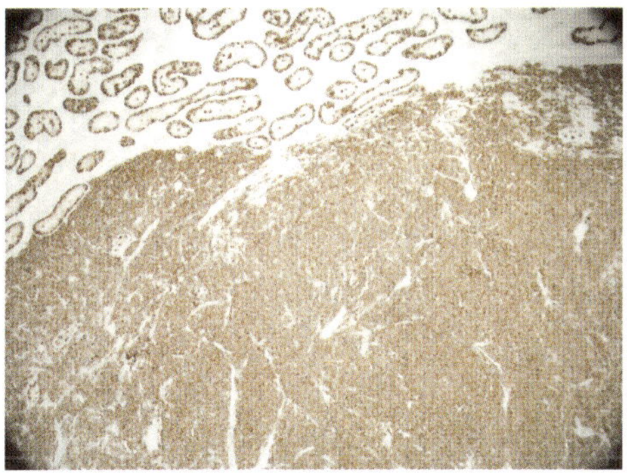

FIGURE 6: Testicular seminoma (PLAP IHC stain, magnification ×40).

Lower extremity Doppler was negative for DVT. Given burden of blood clot and severe anemia with occult gastrointestinal bleed, an inferior vena cava (IVC) filter was urgently placed. During IVC placement, occlusion of the infrarenal IVC with filling defects extending into the right renal vein was noted. He was subsequently started on anticoagulant given extensive clot burden and underlying malignancy.

He initially received standard chemotherapy with bleomycin, etoposide, and cisplatin, but bleomycin was discontinued after the first cycle when surveillance PFT showed diffusion abnormalities. Patient completed 4 cycles of chemotherapy (etoposide and cisplatin). Imaging following completion of chemotherapy showed complete resolution of lung nodule but greater than 3 cm residual retroperitoneal mass with undetectable HCG, but LDH remained elevated at 314 IU/L. Patient is scheduled for a 6-week follow-up PET scan per NCCN clinical guidelines.

3. Discussion

Our patient presented primarily with shortness of breath related to pulmonary embolism and severe anemia. Additionally, extensive thrombosis with bilateral pulmonary embolism, inferior vena cava (IVC), and right renal vein thrombosis were also found. This patient's symptoms related to metastasis included debilitating back pain from retroperitoneal metastasis with extension and perforation of the duodenum, likely resulting in gastrointestinal bleeding and severe anemia. Interestingly, our patient did not report hematochezia or melena.

GI manifestation of GCT is uncommon (5%) with duodenal involvement seen in 1.4% of cases [2]. Gastrointestinal bleeding from site of metastasis following chemotherapy has also been reported [4–6]. Mechanisms include GI perforation following chemotherapy-induced tumor necrosis and shrinking of metastatic gastrointestinal tumor following chemotherapy [7]. Other chemotherapy-related complications involving the GI tract include cases of neutropenic colitis following salvage therapy for refractory nonseminomatous GCT of the testis [8, 9].

There is also an increased risk of stomach cancer following radiotherapy among survivors [10–12]. Overall, gastrointestinal second cancers were higher in seminomas compared to nonseminomas in a review of 5533 survivors in Swedish cancer database [13]. Gastrointestinal symptoms can also be the first symptom of recurrence in patients with previously treated GCT. GCT presenting as abdominal pain with finding of polypoid masses in the gastrointestinal tract within 2 years of orchiectomy and chemotherapy have been reported [14, 15].

Because gastrointestinal presentations of GCT are unusual, they are often not suspected on presentation. A complete physical examination including a scrotal exam may provide the initial clues as to the potential etiology and should not be overlooked, especially since testicular cancers are generally quite curable [16]. Of the estimated 8720 new testicular cancer diagnoses of 2016, less than 400 deaths were anticipated [1]. However, correctly classifying patient and accurate diagnosis play a vital role in achieving good outcomes.

There have been reports of "burnt-out" testicular cancer with presentation related to sites of metastasis in the absence of testicular findings on physical examination or ultrasound. Stokes and Perkins reported a 22-year-old male with metastatic testicular choriocarcinoma with metastasis to the stomach, lungs, liver, kidney, and brain, however, with grossly normal testis with autopsy findings of foci area of scarring and calcification within the testis [17]. Similarly, Altamar et al. reported a 20-year-old with metastatic testicular seminoma with pure seminoma of right testis and concurrent embryonal carcinoma in duodenal mass. A finding of 0.6 cm focus of scarring with calcification likely representing burnt-out primary embryonal tumor versus differentiation at the site of metastasis was a possible explanation [18]. Balogun-Ojuri et al. reported a case of possible primary seminoma of the small bowel with mesenteric nodal involvement. A primary small bowel seminoma was made given normal AFP, normal HCG, and ultrasonographically normal testis. The patient however had a history of undescended testis with orchidopexy and the possibility of jejunal metastasis from an occult primary testicular lesion was entertained [19]. These findings are important as these patients are more likely to present with metastatic symptoms including GI symptoms than testicular mass or swelling.

In a review of patients with GCT with GI symptoms at first presentation, we found 24 publications totaling 25 patients (see Supplementary Table 1 in Supplementary Material

Table 1: Summary table showing studies reporting gastrointestinal involvement of testicular germ cell tumor.

Total N	*25 patients*
Mean age	30.44 years
Range age	16–56 years
	N (%)
Type of GCT	
Seminoma	5 (20%)
NSGCT	15 (60%)
Mixed	5 (20%)
	N (%)
Range of GI symptoms	
Melena	11/25 (44%)
Abdominal pain	9/25 (36%)
Abdominal mass	4/25 (16%)
Hematochezia	2/25 (8%)
Hematemesis	4/25 (16%)
Vomiting, nonbloody	3/25 (12%)
Others (abdominal distension, rigid abdomen)	2/25 (8%)
Mean hemoglobin at presentation (g/dl)	6.8
EGD done (%)	21/24 (84%)
	N
Laterality of testis involved	
Right	14
Left	5
Diffuse scrotal swelling	1
NA	3
Normal testis on Ultrasound	2
Testicular symptoms (swelling or pain) as initial presenting complaint (%)	6/25 (24%)
Outcome	
Survived *N* (%)	Mean follow up (months) 13.2 Survived 15/21 (71%)
Deaths *N* (%)	Mean days to death 25 Death 6/21 (28%)
Choriocarcinoma	4/6 (66%)
Seminoma	1/6 (17%)
Mixed GCT	1/6 (17%)

GCT: germ cell tumor; NSGCT: non seminomatous germ cell tumor; GI: gastrointestinal; EGD: esophagogastroduodenoscopy.

available online at https://doi.org/10.1155/2017/4789259). Mean age was 30.44 years. Sixty percent of patients had NSGCT with the number increasing to 80% when combined with mixed GCT which is treated similarly to NSGCT (Table 1). Prior reviews have demonstrated that NSGCT are more likely to have GI involvement [20, 21]. The commonest GI manifestations were abdominal pain (46%) and melena (44%). Other presentation of GI bleeding including hematemesis and hematochezia accounted for 24% of initial presentation. Mean hemoglobin was 6.8 g/dl with patients requiring large volume transfusion to maintain hemodynamic stability. Other GI presentations including nonbloody vomiting, abdominal mass, and distension were less common. Testicular symptoms as an initial presenting symptom was much less and seen in only 24% of patients.

Six of the 21 patients with follow-up information died, with a mean time to death of 25 days. Four of deaths were in patients diagnosed with choriocarcinoma, a more aggressive GCT associated with extensive metastasis and varied complication including massive hemorrhage [5, 22].

In conclusion, testicular GCT is a malignancy of the young. Young men presenting with evidence of GI bleed with suggestions of underlying malignancy may not offer information on testicular swelling, even if present. A review of systems that includes scrotal/testicular swelling should be conducted and a genital examination done if appropriate.

Acknowledgments

The authors would like to thank Valerie Schaeffer for retrieving articles.

References

[1] R. L. Siegel, K. D. Miller, and A. Jemal, "Cancer statistics, 2016," *CA: A Cancer Journal for Clinicians*, vol. 66, no. 1, pp. 7–30, 2016.

[2] G. S. Rosenblatt, C. J. Walsh, and S. Chung, "Metastatic testis tumor presenting as gastrointestinal hemorrhage," *Journal of Urology*, vol. 164, no. 5, p. 1655, 2000.

[3] C. Nord, S. D. Fossa, and K. E. Giercksky, "Gastrointestinal presentation of germ cell malignancy," *European Urology*, vol. 38, no. 6, pp. 721–724, 2000.

[4] A. Gadodia, I. Ghosh, G. Prakash, S. Thulkar, and V. Raina, "Massive gastro-intestinal haemorrhage in metastatic germ cell tumor from duodenal invasion: a report of two cases," *Tropical Gastroenterology*, vol. 32, no. 3, pp. 232–234, 2011.

[5] K. Komori, D. Takahari, K. Kimura et al., "Recovery from choriocarcinoma syndrome associated with a metastatic extragonadal germ cell tumor hemorrhage," *Case Reports in Gastroenterology*, vol. 10, no. 1, pp. 193–198, 2016.

[6] I. Cicin, F. Ozyilmaz, H. Karagol, F. Yalcin, S. Uzunoglu, and M. Kaplan, "Massive upper gastrointestinal bleeding from pure metastatic choriocarcinoma in patient with mixed germ cell tumor with subclinical intestinal metastasis," *Urology*, vol. 73, no. 2, pp. 443.e15–443.e17, 2009.

[7] J. T. Plukker, H. S. Koops, D. T. Sleijfer, J. W. Oosterhuis, and E. D. Van Jagt, "Intestinal hemorrhages in patients with a nonseminomatous testicular tumor," *Cancer*, vol. 68, no. 12, pp. 2630–2632, 1991.

[8] E.-I. Takaoka, K. Kawai, S. Ando, T. Shimazui, and H. Akaza, "Neutropenic colitis during standard dose combination chemotherapy with nedaplatin and irinotecan for testicular

cancer," *Japanese Journal of Clinical Oncology*, vol. 36, no. 1, pp. 60–63, 2006.

[9] K. Kawai, S. Imada, K. Iida, S. Tsukamoto, N. Miyanaga, and H. Akaza, "Neutropenic colitis as a complication of high-dose chemotherapy for refractory testicular cancer," *Japanese Journal of Clinical Oncology*, vol. 28, no. 9, pp. 571–573, 1998.

[10] M. Hauptmann, S. D. Fossa, M. Stovall et al., "Increased stomach cancer risk following radiotherapy for testicular cancer," *British Journal of Cancer*, vol. 112, no. 1, pp. 44–51, 2015.

[11] L. B. Travis, S. D. Fossa, S. J. Schonfeld et al., "Second cancers among 40,576 testicular cancer patients: focus on long-term survivors," *Journal of the National Cancer Institute*, vol. 97, no. 18, pp. 1354–1365, 2005.

[12] A. Horwich, S. D. Fossa, R. Huddart et al., "Second cancer risk and mortality in men treated with radiotherapy for stage I seminoma," *British Journal of Cancer*, vol. 110, no. 1, pp. 256–263, 2014.

[13] K. Hemminki, H. Liu, and J. Sundquist, "Second cancers after testicular cancer diagnosed after 1980 in Sweden," *Annals of Oncology*, vol. 21, no. 7, pp. 1546–1551, 2009.

[14] S. C. Kadakia, A. Parker, and L. Canales, "Metastatic tumors to the upper gastrointestinal tract: endoscopic experience," *The American Journal of Gastroenterology*, vol. 87, no. 10, pp. 1418–1423, 1992.

[15] A. O. Laiyemo, M. Jack, F. W. Dawkins, and D. T. Smoot, "Upper gastrointestinal bleeding from metastatic testicular cancer," *Journal of the National Medical Association*, vol. 101, no. 8, pp. 808-809, 2009.

[16] R. Hoffmann, I. Plug, M. McKee et al., "Innovations in health care and mortality trends from five cancers in seven European countries between 1970 and 2005," *International Journal of Public Health*, vol. 59, no. 2, pp. 341–350, 2014.

[17] E. W. Stokes and C. Perkins, "Testicular choriocarcinoma. An unusual presentation as occult gastrointestinal blood loss," *Journal of Adolescent Health Care*, vol. 10, no. 2, pp. 146–150, 1989.

[18] H. O. Altamar, G. W. Middleton, T. A. Capozza, B. K. Auge, and C. L. Amling, "Profound anemia from duodenal invasion of metastatic testicular seminoma," *Journal of Urology*, vol. 171, no. 1, pp. 344-345, 2004.

[19] B. Balogun-Ojuri, Y.-M. Lee, V. Save, A. Ibrahim, A. Y. Warren, and N. S. Fearnhead, "A rare case of primary seminoma of the small bowel with lymph node involvement," *Journal of Gastrointestinal Cancer*, vol. 42, no. 3, pp. 183–185, 2011.

[20] M. M. Chait, R. C. Kurtz, and S. I. Hajdu, "Gastrointestinal tract metastasis in patients with germ-cell tumor of the testis," *The American Journal of Digestive Diseases*, vol. 23, no. 10, pp. 925–928, 1978.

[21] J. W. Sweetenham, J. M. Whitehouse, C. J. Williams, and G. M. Mead, "Involvement of the gastrointestinal tract by metastases from germ cell tumors of the testis," *Cancer*, vol. 61, no. 12, pp. 2566–2570, 1988.

[22] M. J. Reilley and L. C. Pagliaro, "Testicular choriocarcinoma: a rare variant that requires a unique treatment approach," *Current Oncology Reports*, vol. 17, no. 2, pp. 2–9, 2015.

25

Primary Mucosal Melanoma of the Stomach

O. Phillips,[1] A. Higdon,[2] R. Colaco,[2] and H. Fish[3]

[1] *St. George's University School of Medicine, West Indies, Grenada*
[2] *Department of Surgery, Trinitas Regional Medical Center, Elizabeth, NJ, USA*
[3] *Division of Surgical Pathology, Trinitas Regional Medical Center, Elizabeth, NJ, USA*

Correspondence should be addressed to O. Phillips; ophillip@sgu.edu

Academic Editor: Yoshihiro Moriwaki

Considered to be rare, mucosal melanomas are rare type of melanoma that are found on mucosal surfaces and are primary or metastatic in origin. We report a case of a 66-year-old Hispanic female who presented with vague abdominal pain and upon further endoscopic work-up revealed 2 gastric lesions. Endoscopic biopsy results revealed gastric melanoma in the distal lesion. A PET/CT scan indicated it to be suspicious for the primary site of metastasis but was ultimately diagnosed as a benign nevus on biopsy. An extensive clinical exam showed no other probable sites of origin. The patient underwent a subtotal Billroth II gastrectomy and enterostomy tube placement for temporary feeding. Primary melanoma of the stomach is an exceptionally rare occurrence with limited cases that can be accounted for in literature; thus we report this case for review.

1. Introduction

Melanoma is the 6th most common cancer in North America [1]. The incidence of cutaneous melanomas continues to increases in the United States and is correlated with exposure to ultraviolet radiation in non-Hispanic whites [2]. However, exposure to ultraviolet light is not seen as a risk factor in mucosal melanomas since the mucosa is not exposed to UV light. No other risk factor for mucosal melanomas has been clearly identified except for those originating from the oral cavity that has been associated with cigarette smoking [3, 4]. Even though melanocytes are predominately cutaneous, they can be found in various other locations such as the oral pharynx, vulvovaginal, and anorectum [3].

As stated, mucosal melanomas are found to be primary or secondary in nature. Primary mucosal melanomas are usually seen in older populations with an average age of 70 years and accounts for one percent of all melanomas [5–7]. Primary sites of mucosal melanomas can also occur along the gastrointestinal tract, however; they are more commonly in the oropharynx [32.8%], anal canal [31.4%], and rectum [22.2%] [3, 8]. They are more rarely found in esophagus [5.9%], stomach [2.7%], and small bowel [2.3%] [3, 8]. Most lesions found along the gastrointestinal tract are metastatic, with the most frequent locations of metastasis being the small intestine, followed by the colon and stomach at the time of presentation [9, 10]. It is rare to find primary gastric melanomas and specific diagnostic criteria are needed in order to be conclusive [11]. The pathogenesis and etiology of mucosal melanomas have not been clearly identified as melanocytes are not part of the innate cellular constitution of the stomach epithelium [12]. To date, the knowledge of any contributing risk factors continues to be elusive [8]. In general mucosal melanomas are considered to have a poor prognosis with a five-year survival of twenty-five percent [5].

2. Case Report

A 66-year-old Hispanic female presented with vague abdominal pain and exertional chest pain. She had a ten-year history of worsening epigastric pain attributed to gastritis that was treated with Dexilant. A general physical exam was done and did not reveal any significant abnormalities; she also denied any fevers, chills, weight loss/gain, or change in bowel habits. Environmental history was noncontributory as she denied extensive sun-exposure or use of tanning beds and reported that she regularly would use sunscreen with a 30 SPF. Still, there was an extensive past medical history for anemia, diabetes mellitus type II, coronary artery disease, asthma,

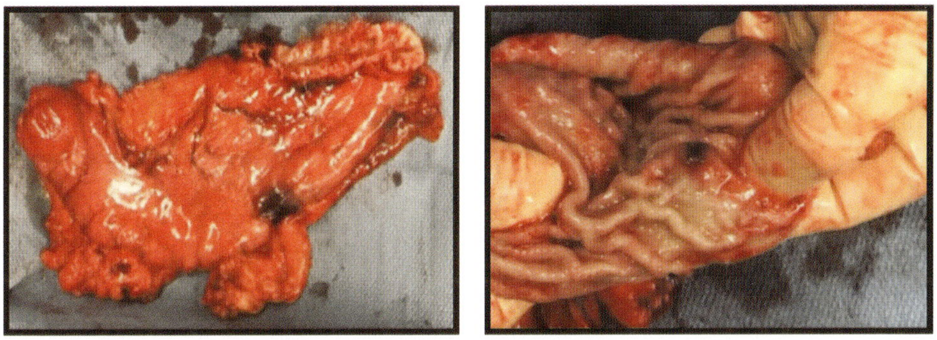

FIGURE 1: Left: gross whole specimen of the subtotal gastrectomy specimen, 14 cm in length. Preoperatively marked on endoscopy with ink along the greater curvature. Right: proximal lesion near the serosa measured to be 1.1cm x 1 cm was found to be normal gastric mucosa. Distal and proximal margins of the resection were found to be negative.

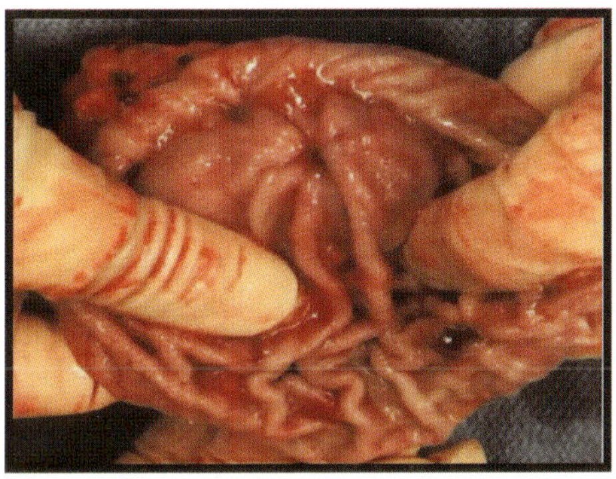

FIGURE 2: Subtotal gastrectomy distal lesion measuring 0.7 cm x 0.7 cm x 0.5 cm. The lesion was found to be malignant melanoma of the stomach that is invasive into the submucosa. No lymphovascular invasion was identified. Six negative lymph nodes appreciated with the specimen.

hypertension, hyperlipidemia, hemorrhoids, and osteoarthritis. She also had a broad surgical history, involving a coronary artery stent in the left anterior descending artery [2016], percutaneous transluminal coronary angioplasty [2016], tubal ligation [1985], cholecystectomy [2007], bladder prolapse repair [2012], rectal prolapse repair [2012], hysterectomy [2012], and total right knee replacement [2013].

There is no report of primary tobacco use; however, she does report an extensive second-hand smoke exposure as a result of her biological father. Her family history is significant for multiple cancers, with her father dying of cancer related complications from a head and neck malignancy at the age of 65. The patient's sister died of breast cancer at the age of 44 and half paternal sister also died of breast cancer at the age of 38. Lastly, her brother died of colon cancer at the age of 70 and her mother's death at the age of 67 was due to a myocardial infarction unrelated to cancer. Interestingly, her eldest daughter was diagnosed with melanoma found in a cutaneous lesion, in 2016. Her physical exam did not reveal any concerning skin lesions or palpable abdominal lesions and her vitals were stable.

A near total gastrectomy was performed and multiple adhesions from prior surgeries were divided at the beginning of the procedure. A thorough surgical exploration of the abdomen demonstrated no lesions of the liver. The gastric lesions, having been preoperatively marked on endoscopy, were inspected. The proximal lesion was near the GE junction and another was located more distally closer to the antrum. Figure 1 demonstrates the proximal lesion that was located near the greater curvature of the stomach. Figure 2 displays the distal lesion marked preoperatively located near the antrum of the stomach with no surrounding necrosis or bleeding but was significant for raised mucosal margins in a wheel pattern.

Reconstruction was performed with a Billroth II anastomosis. Due to the almost complete removal of the stomach, a pouch was created via a jejunojejunostomy. A temporary feeding tube was placed distal to the anastomosis. No blood was transfused through this procedure and the estimated blood loss was 200 ml. The pathology associated with the gross specimens is seen in Figures 3 and 4. They are associated with the second lesion as the first was found to have normal gastric mucosa. The lesions were positive for three significant immunological markers for melanoma, Melanin A, HMB-45, and S100 [13]. Though S100 has been found to have higher sensitivity but much lower specificity for melanoma [13].

Her immediate postoperative course was unremarkable except for a fever of 101 F during the first 24 hours after surgery, which returned to 98.7°F about 9 hours after the initial fever spike in temperature. She remained afebrile for the remainder of her hospital stay. Overall, the patient progressed as expected postoperatively and tolerated her temporary tube feedings well. An upper GI series on postoperative day 5 showed no anastomosis leakage; thus a postgastrectomy diet was started soon thereafter. After a continued unremarkable postoperative course she was discharged on postoperative day 7 to a subacute rehab.

3. Discussion

Mucosal melanomas are a very rare type of melanoma and their etiology and pathogenesis continue to remain elusive. Current literature does not have specific staging for primary mucosal melanomas, though the American Joint Committee on Cancer consider mucosal melanomas of any origin are

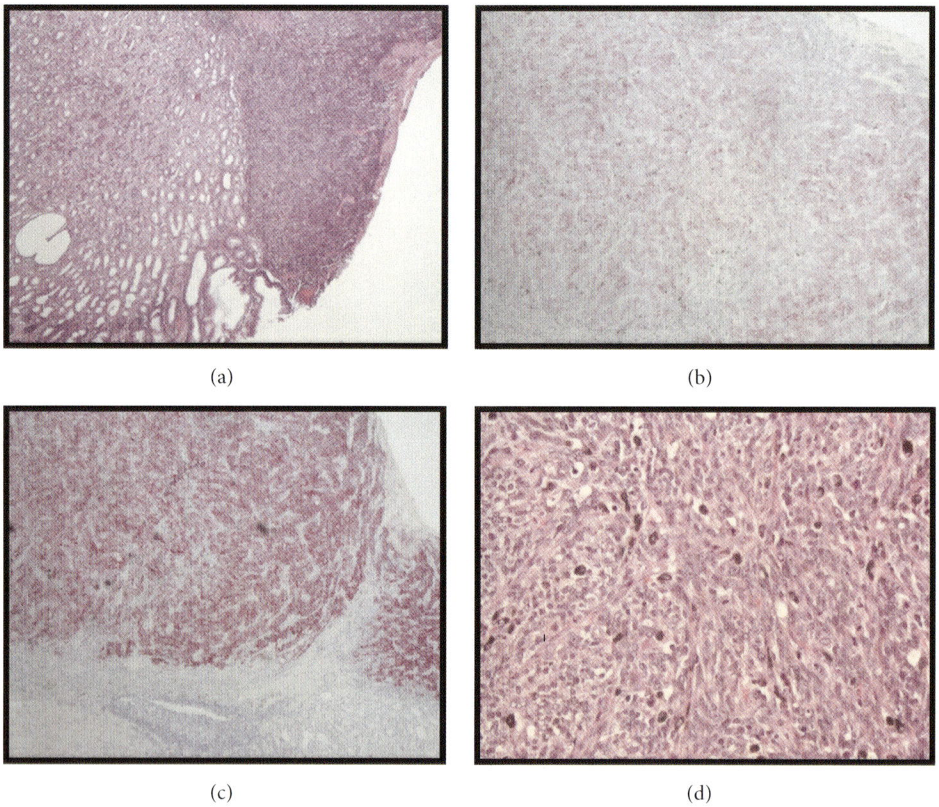

FIGURE 3: *Histological Specimens of Gastric Melanoma.* Histological sections of gastrectomy specimen demonstrating primary gastric melanoma. (a) Right side of the image depicts neoplastic cells that do not invade past the submucosa that still retains normal gastric architecture (H&E x100). (b) Primary gastric melanoma positive stain for Melanin A (H&E x100). (c) Primary gastric melanoma positive stain for HMB-45 (H&E x100). (d) Malignant melanocytic neoplasm producing brown melanin pigment with a cherry red nucleoli and mitotic figures (H&E x 400).

TABLE 1: Basic Classification System of Mucosal Melanoma. AJCC_TNM Classification for Mucosal Melanoma.

Primary Tumor	
T3	Mucosal Disease
T4a	Moderately advanced disease. Tumor involving deep soft tissue
T4b	Very advanced disease
Regional Lymph Node Involvement	
NX	Regional Lymph nodes cannot be assessed
N0	No regional lymph node metastasis
N1	Regional lymph node metastases present
Distant Metastasis	
M0	No distant metastasis present
M1	Distant metastasis

applicable to the current guidelines used for the following mucosal melanomas: head, neck, and vulva (11). This classification system is depicted in Table 1(11).

Lagoudianakis et al. established specific diagnostic criteria for primary malignant melanoma of the gastrointestinal tract [11]. The criteria consist of a lack of any primary sites of melanoma; the patient should have no history or concurrent skin or any other organ removal of a melanocytic lesion, a lack of any adjacent organ involvement, and finally disease free survival for at least 12 months after surgical resection [11]. The last criterion is of critical importance in order to clearly distinguish between primary and metastatic lesions since "50% of patients with stage IV melanoma or visceral disease from unknown primary will have died at 12 months from diagnosis" [11]. This further confirms our diagnosis since at this point in time the patient is currently thirteen months postop.

Additionally, our patient's lack of physical exam findings with a positive histopathology for S100, Melanin A, and HMB-45 suggests that this patient has a true primary gastric

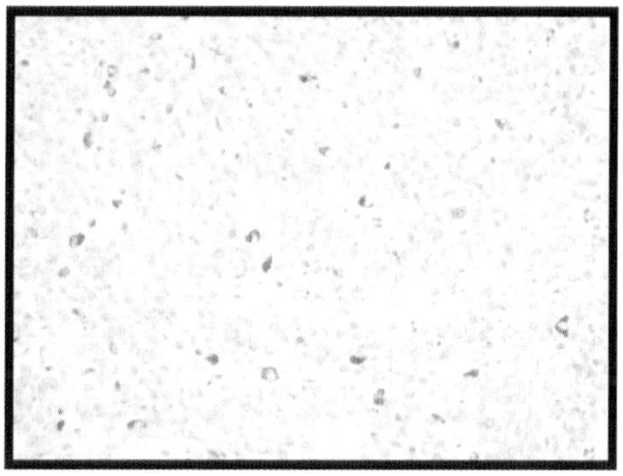

FIGURE 4: *Histological Specimens of Gastric Melanoma.* Primary gastric melanoma positive stain for S100. Weak and high intensity staining are seen throughout the section (H&E x100).

melanoma. Overall, even without clear indication of metastasis, the treatment of choice for mucosal melanomas is surgical resection with clear margins [3, 14]. Current literature states that patients with primary gastric melanomas might benefit from additional adjuvant therapy after the initial surgical resection if anatomically possible [5]. It is imperative that we investigate genetic factors in order to further advance chemotherapies combined with surgical resection in order to give patients the best chance for survival. The poor prognosis that is seen with mucosal melanomas is mostly associated due to its late presentation. However, in patients that present early, without invasion through the basement membrane, as in our patient, or possibly even patients who present late, combined chemotherapy with surgical resection could extend survival.

Moreover, the patient's family history of head and neck, breast, and colon cancer as well as cutaneous melanoma implores us to explore possible genetic elements that may have played a role in the development of her disease. For example, CDKN2A is a cyclin dependent kinase inhibitor and encodes for specific tumor suppressor proteins [15–17]. Early onset cutaneous melanomas have been found to have a familial component involving the CDKN2A gene which also has strong associations with "hereditary nonpolyposis colon cancer, familial adenomatous colon cancer, and familial breast cancer" as well as both cutaneous melanoma and mucosal melanomas [16, 18, 19]. Interestingly, mucosal melanomas show even higher rates of CDKN2A mutations than cutaneous melanomas [3, 15–17]. This suggests that loss of function of the CDKN2A gene has an even higher genetic correlation with mucosal melanoma than cutaneous melanoma. Research has indicated that CDKN2A mutations along with KIT oncogene mutations that are seen in about 39% of mucosal melanomas are more common than other mutations that have a strong association with melanomas such as BRAF [3, 16, 20]. BRAF is one of the most significant gene mutations in cutaneous melanoma but is rare in mucosal melanomas and is only seen in about 10% of patients [3]. Though BRAF inhibition has been shown to be advantageous in patients with cutaneous melanoma its potential as an adjuvant therapy in mucosal melanomas patients that do carry the mutation has not been investigated [3]. It has been suggested that the tumor suppressor gene CDKN2A and KIT protooncogene could be key regulators in the pathogenesis of mucosal melanomas [3, 21]. That being said the CDKN2A and KIT gene would be excellent target for further research as potential adjunct dual-targeted chemotherapy for mucosal melanomas.

4. Conclusions

Given the fact that there are very few cases regarding primary mucosal melanomas of gastric origin reported in literature, primary gastric melanomas can be considered to be rare malignancies that can present in a number of different ways [8]. Most often it has many nonspecific characteristics in its presentation. According to Anupama Ravi the most common presenting symptoms involve upper gastrointestinal bleeding, anemia, and weight loss [12]. Due to high occurrence of metastatic melanoma to the GI tract, it is paramount that a thorough physical examination is performed as well as other diagnostic criteria before the diagnosis of primary gastric melanoma is given. In the end, early detection of primary gastric melanoma and surgical resection are the initial approaches to a patient who is suspected of having a primary gastric melanoma.

5. Limitations

The limitations to this study are mostly concerned with the proper physical examination to confirm the lack of primary lesion. The patient was thoroughly evaluated to confirm the lack of any skin lesions that could have been a primary site of metastasis and none were found. However, the patient had not been evaluated by an ophthalmologist. Therefore, an ocular melanoma at this time has not been ruled out.

References

[1] R. Siegel, D. Naishadham, and A. Jemal, "Cancer statistics," *CA: A Cancer Journal for Clinicians*, vol. 63, no. 1, pp. 11–30, 2013.

[2] M. J. Eide and M. A. Weinstock, "Association of UV index, latitude, and melanoma incidence in nonwhite populations - US Surveillance, Epidemiology, and End Results (SEER) program, 1992 to 2001," *JAMA Dermatology*, vol. 141, no. 4, pp. 477–481, 2005.

[3] K. R. Spencer and J. M. Mehnert, "Mucosal melanoma: epidemiology, biology and treatment," *Melanoma Cancer Treatment and Research*, pp. 295–320, 2015.

[4] T. Axeix and C. A. Hedin, "Epidemiologic study of excessive oral melanin pigmentation with special reference to the influence of tobacco habits," *European Journal of Oral Sciences*, vol. 90, no. 6, pp. 434–442, 1982.

[5] A. E. Chang, L. H. Karnell, and H. R. Menck, "The national cancer data base report on cutaneous and noncutaneous

melanoma: a summary of 84,836 cases from the past decade," *Cancer*, vol. 83, no. 8, pp. 1664–1678, 1998.

[6] M. Meleti, C. R. Leemans, R. De Bree, P. Vescovi, E. Sesenna, and I. Van Der Waal, "Head and neck mucosal melanoma: experience with 42 patients, with emphasis on the role of postoperative radiotherapy," *Head & Neck*, vol. 30, no. 12, pp. 1543–1551, 2008.

[7] R. P. Rapini, L. E. Golitz, R. O. Greer, E. A. Krekorian, and T. Poulson, "Primary malignant melanoma of the oral cavity. A review of 177 cases," *Cancer*, vol. 55, no. 7, pp. 1543–1551, 1985.

[8] M. Mihajlovic, S. Vlajkovic, P. Jovanovic, and V. Stefanovic, "Primary mucosal melanomas: a comprehensive review," *International Journal of Clinical and Experimental Pathology*, vol. 5, no. 8, pp. 739–753, 2012.

[9] D. W. Ollila, R. Essner, L. A. Wanek, and D. L. Morton, "Surgical resection for melanoma metastatic to the gastrointestinal tract," *JAMA Surgery*, vol. 131, no. 9, pp. 975–980, 1996.

[10] P. J. Capizzi and J. H. Donohue, "Metastatic melanoma of the gastrointestinal tract: a review of the literature," *Comprehensive Therapy*, vol. 1, pp. 20–23, 20.

[11] E. E. Lagoudianakis, E. Genetzakis, and M. Tsekouras, "Primary gastric melanoma: A case report," *World Journal of Gastroenterology*, vol. 12, no. 27, p. 4425, 2006.

[12] A. Ravi, "Primary gastric melanoma: A rare cause of upper gastrointestinal bleeding," *Journal of Gastroenterology and Hepatology*, vol. 4, no. 11, pp. 795–797, 2008.

[13] M. Shinohara, H. Deubner, and Z. B. Argenyi, "S100, HMB-45, and melan-A negative primary melanoma," *Dermatology Online Journal*, vol. 15, no. 9, article no. 7, 2009.

[14] E. Hanna, F. Demonte, S. Ibrahim, D. Roberts, N. Levine, and M. Kupferman, "Endoscopic resection of sinonasal cancers with and without craniotomy," *Archives of Otolaryngology–Head & Neck Surgery*, vol. 135, no. 12, p. 1219, 2009.

[15] L. Ai, K. K. Stephenson, W. Ling et al., "The p16 (CDKN2a/INK4a) tumor-suppressor gene in head and neck squamous cell carcinoma: A promoter methylation and protein expression study in 100 cases," *Modern Pathology*, vol. 16, no. 9, pp. 944–950, 2003.

[16] L. Si, X. Wang, and J. Guo, "Genotyping of mucosal melanoma," *Chinese Clinical Oncology*, vol. 3, no. 3, pp. 33-34, 2014.

[17] J. A. Curtin, J. Fridlyand, T. Kageshita et al., "Distinct sets of genetic alterations in melanoma," *The New England Journal of Medicine*, vol. 353, no. 20, pp. 2135–2147, 2005.

[18] A. M. Goldstein, M. C. Fraser, W. H. Clark, and M. A. Tucker, "Age at diagnosis and transmission of invasive melanoma in 23 families with cutaneous malignat melanoma/dysplastic nevi," *Journal of the National Cancer Institute*, vol. 86, no. 18, pp. 1385–1390, 1994.

[19] M. Simons, J. Ferreira, R. Meunier, and S. Moss, "Primary versus metastatic gastrointestinal melanoma: a rare case and review of current literature," *Case Reports in Gastrointestinal Medicine*, vol. 2016, Article ID 2306180, 3 pages, 2016.

[20] J. A. Curtin, K. Busam, D. Pinkel, and B. C. Bastian, "Somatic activation of KIT in distinct subtypes of melanoma," *Journal of Clinical Oncology*, vol. 24, no. 26, pp. 4340–4346, 2006.

[21] F. G. Haluska, H. Tsao, H. Wu, F. S. Haluska, A. Lazar, and V. Goel, "Genetic alterations in signaling pathways in melanoma," *Clinical Cancer Research*, vol. 12, no. 7, 2006.

A Case of Complete Remission from Advanced Gastric Adenocarcinoma with Synchronous Liver Metastasis in Response to EOX Chemotherapy

Zhi-jun Yan,[1] Jia-xin Wang,[1] You-yi Liu,[1] Zhen-hui Li,[2] Li-juan Zhang,[3] Ping Gan,[1] Xiao Han,[1] Li-kun Luan,[1] and You-guo Dai[1]

[1]*Department of Abdominal Surgery, Third Affiliated Hospital of Kunming Medical University, Kunming, Yunnan 650118, China*
[2]*Department of Radiology, Third Affiliated Hospital of Kunming Medical University, Kunming, Yunnan 650118, China*
[3]*Department of Pathology, Third Affiliated Hospital of Kunming Medical University, Kunming, Yunnan 650118, China*

Correspondence should be addressed to You-guo Dai; daiyouguo@126.com

Academic Editor: Shiro Kikuchi

Gastric cancer is a malignant tumor with a high degree of malignancy. Multiple liver metastases from gastric cancer (LMGCs) are common. However, the treatment of LMGCs is very difficult. It is rare to achieve complete remission (CR) and long-term survival after treatment. We present the case of a patient with gastric adenocarcinoma and multiple liver metastases who showed CR for more than 33 months after perioperative EOX (epirubicin, oxaliplatin, and capecitabine) combination chemotherapy with radical distal gastrectomy and resection of liver metastases. The patient is still in follow-up without tumor recurrence. These findings suggest that LMGC does not necessarily mean a poor prognosis; preoperative chemotherapy combined with surgery may be a good treatment option for LMGC in selected patients. Further studies are needed to support this treatment approach.

1. Introduction

Gastric cancer is a common gastrointestinal malignancy originating from the epithelium and considered the fifth most commonly occurring cancer and the second leading cause of cancer-related deaths worldwide [1]. Gastric cancer incidence rates have been declining in most parts of the world in recent decades. However, in 2012, gastric cancer caused more than 320,000 deaths in China, accounting for approximately 45% of stomach cancer-related deaths worldwide, representing a heavy disease burden of stomach cancer in the country [2]. The main reason is that 80% of gastric cancer is in advanced stage when diagnosed; thus, the 5-year survival rate is low. According to statistics from 2010 to 2014, the 5-year survival rate of gastric cancer in China is only 35.9%. In contrast, survival was remarkably high in South Korea (68.9%) and Japan (60.3%) during the same period [3].

Liver metastases from gastric cancer (LMGCs) predict poor prognosis and are present in 40% of patients dying from this disease [4]. There are few surgical opportunities for patients with LMGCs because of polycentric or extraliver disease [5]. However, data from retrospective studies with a relatively small number of subjects suggest that surgical resection for some patients with LMGCs is feasible and beneficial to long-term survival [6]. With the development of chemotherapeutic research for gastric cancer, it has been reported that some patients with LMGC received R0 resection with long-term survival after preoperative chemotherapy [7]. Unfortunately, only rare reports have presented good therapeutic results for LMGC treated with chemotherapy and/or surgical treatment.

The objective of this case report is to explore the role of preoperative chemotherapy combined with surgical resection in the selected patients of LMGC. Here, we report a case of LMGC that showed CR for more than 33 months after having preoperative treatment with EOX (epirubicin, oxaliplatin, and capecitabine) combination chemotherapy followed by radical distal gastrectomy and resection of metastases to the liver.

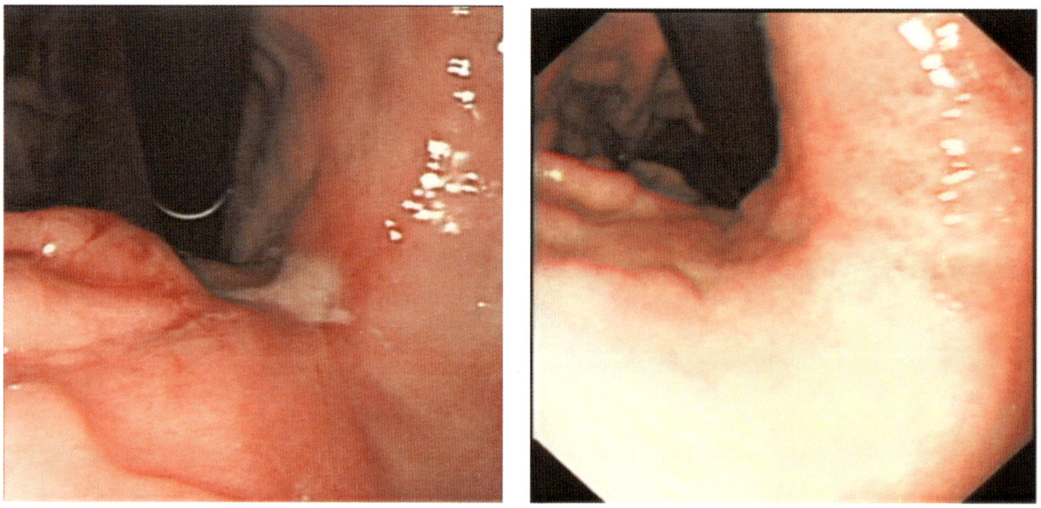

(a) (b)

FIGURE 1: **Initial (a) and follow-up (b) endoscopic findings after six cycles of EOX chemotherapy**. (a) A large ulceroinfiltrative mass at the anterior wall of the lesser antral curvature, covered with whitish fur, and no apparent active bleeding; (b) ulcer lesion disappeared and replaced by scar.

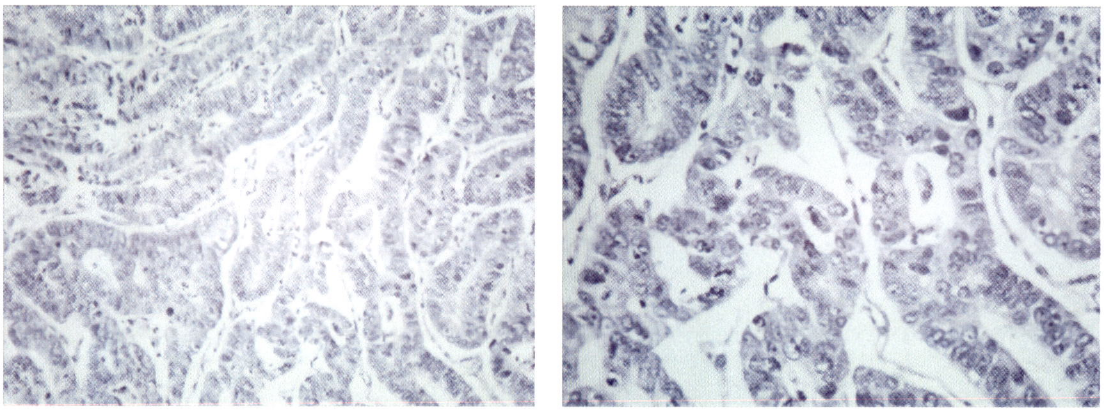

(a) (b)

FIGURE 2: **Microscopic findings at the time of diagnosis. Well differentiated tubular adenocarcinoma** ((a) H&E, ×100; (b) H&E, ×200).

2. Case Report

A 52-year-old man presented with upper abdominal pain for more than 3 months and weight loss of 3 kg in 10 days in July 2015. His performance status was 1 according to the criteria of the Eastern Cooperative Oncology Group (ECOG). The blood count analysis results were as follows: white blood cell (WBC) 23.99 ×10^9/L, neutrophil (NEUT) 86.1%, and absolute neutrophil count (ANC) 20.64 ×10^9/L. The tumor marker test results were as follows: serum carcinoembryonic antigen (CEA) 177 ng/dl, carbohydrate antigen-724 (CA-724) 20.34 IU/ml, and carbohydrate antigen-153 (CA-153) 31.59 IU/ml. Bone marrow biopsy of the granulocyte series demonstrated obvious active hyperplasia, and megakaryocytic and erythrocytic series were active and proliferous. There was no evidence of bone marrow metastasis.

Upper gastrointestinal endoscopic findings showed 3 cm × 2 cm ulcers at the anterior wall of the lesser antral curvature with no apparent active bleeding (Figures 1(a) and 1(b)). Histopathological examination revealed a well differentiated tubular adenocarcinoma (Figure 2). An abdominal computed tomography (CT) scan demonstrated irregular wall thickening on the lesser curvature side of the gastric antrum with mass formation with a large ulceroinfiltration as well as multiple metastases to neighboring lymph nodes (Figures 3(a)–3(c)). The CT scan also revealed metastatic lesions in liver segment 4 (Figure 4(a)) and evidence of hypodense liver metastatic lesions in the left lobe of the liver (Figure 4(b)). The CT scan also showed multiple liver metastases lesions that ranged in size from 1.0 to 4.3 cm over the entire liver (Figures 4(a) and 4(b)).

A clinical diagnosis of stage IV (cT3NxM1) advanced gastric cancer was made according to the 7th American

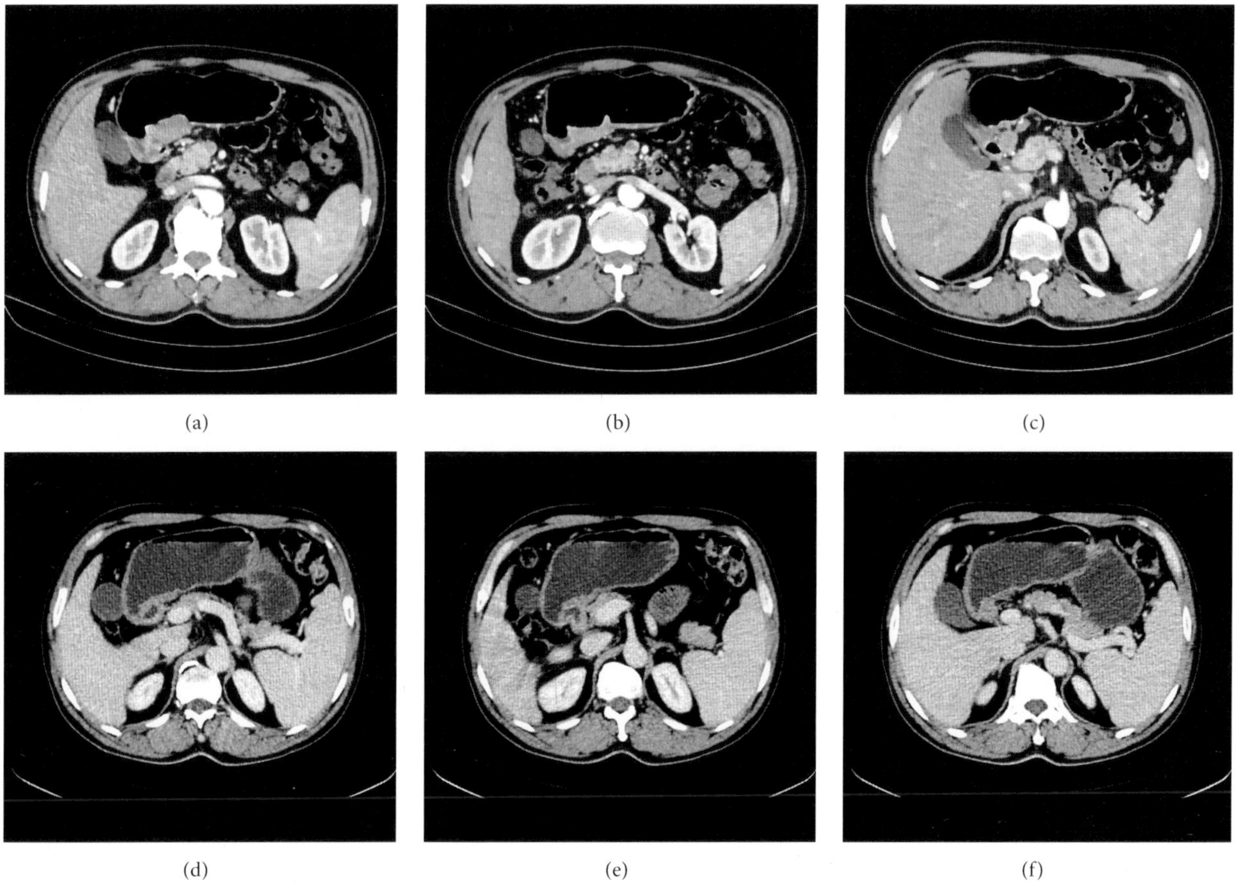

FIGURE 3: **Initial abdominal computed tomography scan (a~c) and follow-up scan after three cycles of EOX chemotherapy (d~f).** (a, b, and c) Irregular wall thickening on the lesser curvature side of the gastric antrum with mass formation, large ulceroinfiltrative, and multiple metastases to neighboring lymph nodes; (d, e) scan shows that the mass of the gastric antrum decreased in range from approximately 7 cm to less than 3.3 cm; (f) disappearance of metastatic lesion of neighboring lymph nodes that had been previously observed.

Joint Committee on Cancer (AJCC) system. Trastuzumab plus cisplatin-based chemotherapy has been recommended as the first-line standard treatment regimen for the patients with HER2-positive advanced gastric cancer according to the 2015.V3 gastric cancer guidelines of the National Comprehensive Cancer Network (NCCN). Since the result of HER2 status testing in this case was negative, it was not necessary to use the drugs targeting HER2, such as trastuzumab, for this patient.

On the basis of the abovementioned findings, we administered EOX combination chemotherapy. For each cycle, intravenous infusion epirubicin (50 mg/m^2) was administered on day 1, followed by an intravenous drip of oxaliplatin (130 mg/m^2) for 2 hours on day 1. Oral capecitabine (625 mg/m^2) was administered twice daily for 3 weeks. This regimen was repeated every 3 weeks.

In October 2015, after completion of three cycles of chemotherapy, an abdominal CT scan showed that the mass of the gastric antrum had decreased to less than 3.3 cm (Figures 3(d) and 3(e)), and metastatic lesions of neighboring lymph nodes that had been previously observed had disappeared (Figure 3(f)). The scan showed that the liver metastatic lesions had almost disappeared, with the exception of lesions in the left lobe of the liver, which measured less than 1.5 cm in size (Figures 4(c) and 4(d)). After an additional three cycles of chemotherapy, another abdominal CT scan was performed in December 2015. In December 2015, after completion of six cycles of chemotherapy, endoscopic findings showed improvement in the gastric antrum mass. This result showed that the liver metastatic nodules that had been previously observed were no longer present (Figures 5(a) and 5(b)). The scan showed that the gastric mass had almost disappeared (Figure 5(c)). Follow-up endoscopy showed that the ulcer lesion had disappeared and was replaced by scar tissue (Figure 1(b)).

Radical distal gastrectomy with Roux-en-Y with a residual stomach and jejunum anastomosis, as well as a D2 lymphadenectomy, combined with obvious metastatic liver lesions resection was performed in January 2016, resulting in complete removal of the primary tumor and any suspicious lymph nodes. Pathological findings after surgery showed no tumor cells detected in the gastric primary lesion. Metastases to perigastric lymph nodes were observed in none of 18 resected lymph nodes, suggesting pathological complete

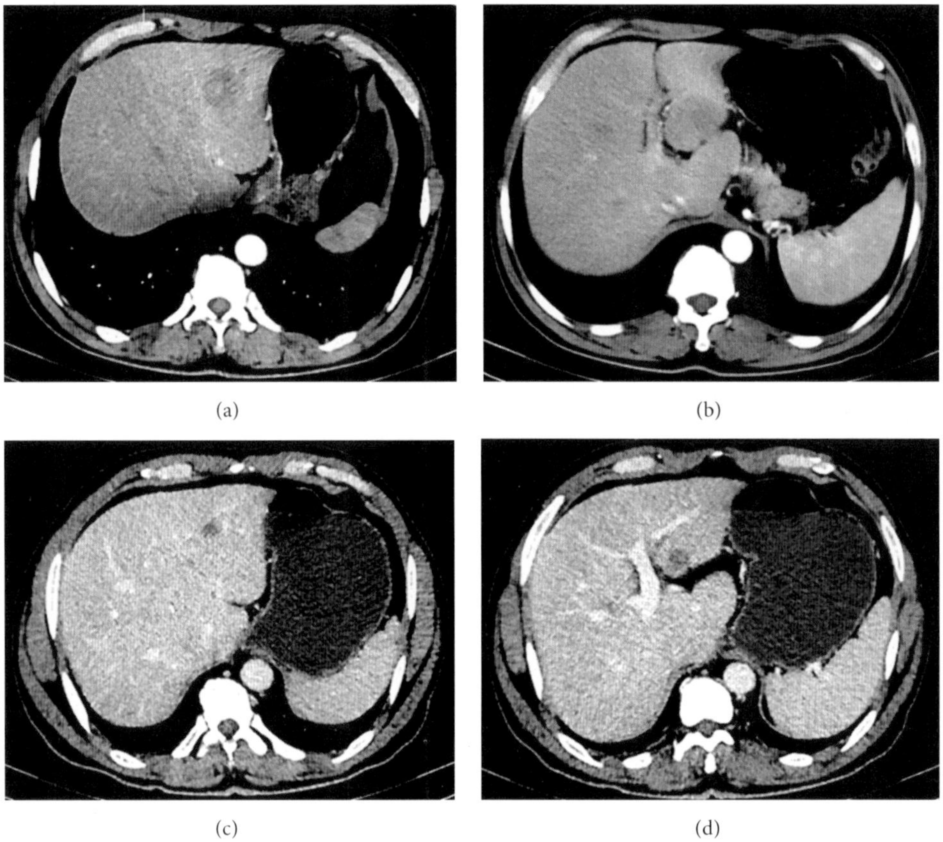

FIGURE 4: **Initial abdominal computed tomography scan (a, b) and follow-up scan after three cycles of EOX chemotherapy (c, d).** (a) Scan shows that the metastatic lesion in liver segment 4; (b) hypodense metastatic lesions in the left lobe of liver; (c) scan shows that the metastatic lesion in liver segment 4 has decreased in size from 2.8 cm to less than 0.9 cm; (d) scan shows that the metastatic lesion in the left lobe of liver has decreased in size from 4.3 cm to less than 1.5 cm.

remission. The final pathological stage was ypT0N0M0. Following the operation, we planned to administer postoperative adjuvant chemotherapy with another two cycles of EOX regimen again.

The side effects and toxicities were evaluated every regimen cycle. During EOX treatment, the patient presented some adverse events such as mild gastrointestinal reaction, grade 1 neuritis, and grades 1-2 hematological toxicities that were considered tolerable. Mild gastrointestinal reactions, including grade 1-2 nausea and vomiting, were the most common EOX-related toxic effects.

Every 3 months, an abdominal CT scan was performed. There was no evidence of recurrent tumor up to February 2018. The patient had maintained CR for more than 27 months after surgery, with a 33-month overall survival (Figures 5(d) and 5(e)). The patient still had no tumor recurrence up to the time of this case history article submission.

3. Discussion

The liver is the most common site for metastases in patients with gastric cancer. It has been reported that approximately 14% of gastric cancer patients have developed synchronous liver metastasis and 25% to 30% of gastric cancer patients have developed metachronous liver metastasis after surgical resection of the primary gastric cancer [8, 9]. There were no effective treatments for patients of LMGCs, and the prognosis of these patients remains very poor [10]. The existing literature suggests that the 5-year survival of gastric cancer patients with liver metastasis is less than 10% [11] and that the median survival rate of patients treated with gastrectomy alone has been reported to range from 3.4 to 5.7 months [10]. There is no significant difference in survival between synchronous and metachronous metastasis [12].

The value of liver resection for LMGC remains controversial. Obviously, the number of liver metastases is a considerable prognostic factor for survival after surgery, and patients with a solitary metastasis of gastric cancer are good candidates for surgical resection [13]. Unfortunately, most LMGCs are multiple, bilateral, and combined with peritoneal or lymph node metastases that directly invade adjacent organs; as a result, hepatectomy was found to be indicated in only 0.4-1.0% of patients with LMGCs [14]. Therefore, surgical resection requires good indications; otherwise, it is difficult to achieve satisfactory results for LMGCs.

Recently, in addition to postoperative chemotherapy [15], preoperative chemotherapy has also been used as a standard treatment for advanced gastric cancer [16]. However, since it

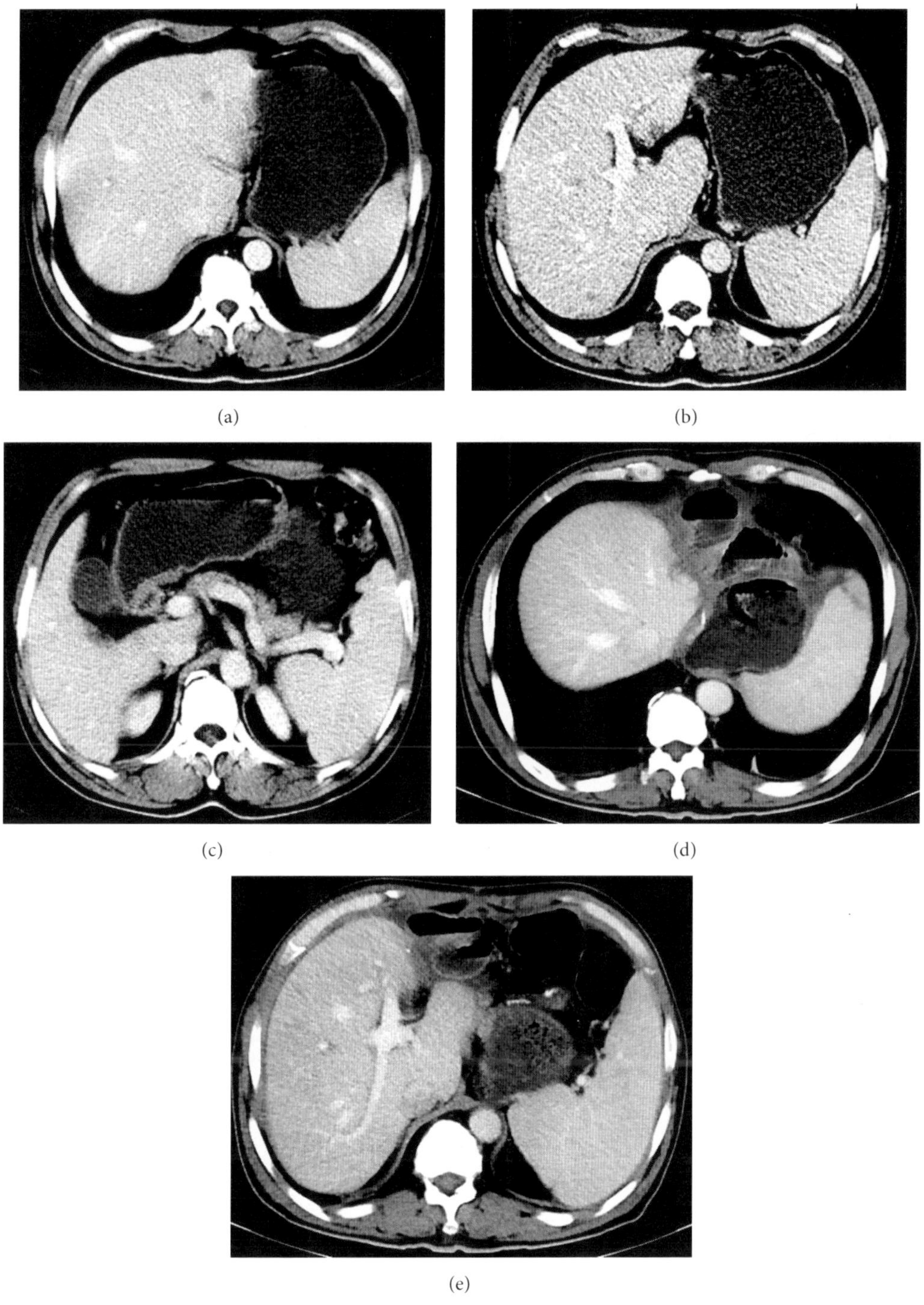

FIGURE 5: **Follow-up abdominal computed tomography scans after six of EOX chemotherapy (a, b, c) and 27 months after surgery (d, e).** (a) The liver metastatic nodules in liver segment 4 that had been previously observed have almost disappeared; (b) the liver metastatic lesion in the left lobe of liver that had been previously observed has evidently been reduced; (c) the gastric mass has almost disappeared; (d) postradical distal gastrectomy with Roux-en-Y with residual stomach and jejunum anastomosis and D2 lymphadenectomy combined with liver metastatic lesions resection, with no evidence of tumor recurrence 27 months after surgery; (e) no recurrence of metastatic lesions after 27 months.

is very difficult to achieve CR in metastatic gastric cancer, palliative chemotherapy is the main treatment option [17]. In a review of the literature, preoperative chemotherapy has been recommended as the preferred treatment pathway for advanced gastric cancer because of the advantages of tumor downstaging, increased tumor resection rate, and improved survival rate [18–20]. The MAGIC study of resectable gastroesophageal cancer showed that ECF (epirubicin, cisplatin, and fluorouracil/leucovorin) perioperative chemotherapy significantly improved progression free survival (PFS) and OS compared with surgery alone [18]. Furthermore, the REAL-2 study found that perioperative EOX chemotherapy was noninferior to perioperative epirubicin, cisplatin, and 5-FU/CF (ECF) chemotherapy in efficacy and median survival of patients suffering gastroesophageal cancer [21]. Inspired by these results, we used EOX in preoperative chemotherapy for the patients of LMGC who had a better performance status.

We have presented a case of a patient with advanced gastric adenocarcinoma with synchronous and multiple liver metastases who was treated with preoperative EOX combination chemotherapy followed by radical distal gastrectomy and resection of metastatic liver lesions resulting in a CR of more than 33 months.. This case suggests that preoperative EOX chemotherapy combined with surgery may be a good treatment option for LMGC. However, to achieve better results, patients with LMGC should have a good ECOG score, and the number of liver metastases should preferably be less than 3. Indeed, there are many problems that need to be further explored after preoperative chemotherapy for LMGC. For example, there is still lack of evidence as to whether patients with CR need to continue chemotherapy after surgery. According to the current consensus of some experts [22], it is recommended to continue the original chemotherapy program after surgery. However, it is difficult for most patients to tolerate the 3-drug chemotherapy because of a relatively poor performance status after surgery. Therefore, dosage adjustment or reduction in drug administration should be considered after surgery. In addition, liver metastases reduced or disappeared after preoperative chemotherapy. At this time, how to determine the extent of hepatectomy and how to determine the extent of the original lesions are also urgent problems to be solved. Recently, a study of the German AIO study group investigating a perioperative FLOT regimen (fluorouracil, leucovorin, oxaliplatin, and docetaxel) versus ECF/X demonstrated higher rates of pathological response for FLOT (15.6% versus 5.8%) and lower rates of one serious adverse event involving a perioperative medical or surgical complication (25% versus 40%) [23]. Based on these results, in the future, we will also consider the use of FLOT chemotherapy in the preoperative chemotherapy of LMGCs.

4. Conclusion

This case suggests that preoperative chemotherapy combined with surgery may be a good treatment option for LMGC in selected patients. However, further clinical trials are required to evaluate the survival benefit, efficacy, and side effects of this therapeutic regimen.

Consent

Informed patient consent for publication of case details was obtained.

Authors' Contributions

Yan ZJ, Dai YG, and Gan P reviewed the case and designed the report; Luan LK, Wang JX, and Liu YY collected the patient clinical data; Gan P and Han X participated in the surgery and analysis of the postoperative status; and Yan ZJ, Dai YG, Li ZH, and Zhang LJ performed the data analyses and wrote the paper.

Acknowledgments

The present study was supported by grants from the Yunnan Cancer Hospital Doctoral Research Fund (no. BSKY201707) and the Joint Special Fund of Yunnan Provincial Science and Technology Department and Kunming Medical University (no. 2018FE001-(064)).

References

[1] M. Venerito, A. Link, T. Rokkas, and P. Malfertheiner, "Gastric cancer – clinical and epidemiological aspects," *Helicobacter*, vol. 21, pp. 39–44, 2016.

[2] International Agency for Research on Cancer, "Cancer Today," http://gco.iarc.fr/today/.

[3] L. Yang, R. Zheng, N. Wang et al., "Incidence and mortality of stomach cancer in China, 2014," *Chinese Journal of Cancer Research*, vol. 30, no. 3, pp. 291–298, 2018.

[4] L. de Mestier, S. Lardière-Deguelte, J. Volet, R. Kianmanesh, and O. Bouché, "Recent insights in the therapeutic management of patients with gastric cancer," *Digestive and Liver Disease*, vol. 48, no. 9, pp. 984–994, 2016.

[5] T. Waddell, M. Verheij, W. Allum, D. Cunningham, A. Cervantes, and D. Arnold, "Gastric cancer: ESMO-ESSO-ESTRO clinical practice guidelines for diagnosis, treatment and follow-up," *Annals of Oncology*, vol. 24, supplement 6, pp. vi57–vi63, 2013.

[6] A. Song, X. Zhang, F. Yu, D. Li, W. Shao, and Y. Zhou, "Surgical resection for hepatic metastasis from gastric cancer: A multi-institution study," *Oncotarget* , vol. 8, no. 41, pp. 71147–71153, 2017.

[7] C. Rim, J.-A. Lee, S. Gong et al., "A case of long-term complete remission of advanced gastric adenocarcinoma with liver metastasis," *Gastric Cancer*, vol. 16, no. 2, pp. 115–119, 2016.

[8] S. P. Kerkar, C. D. Kemp, and I. Avital, "Liver resections in metastatic gastric cancer," *HPB*, vol. 12, no. 9, pp. 589–596, 2010.

[9] A. Mastoraki, C. Benetou, S. Mastoraki et al., "The role of surgery in the therapeutic approach of gastric cancer liver metastases," *Indian Journal of Gastroenterology*, vol. 35, no. 5, pp. 331–336, 2016.

[10] K. Okuyama, K. Isono, I. Juan et al., "Evaluation of treatment for gastric cancer with liver metastasis," *Cancer*, vol. 55, no. 10, pp. 2498–2505, 1985.

[11] S. A. Hundahl, J. L. Phillips, and H. R. Menck, "The National Cancer Data Base report on poor survival of U.S. gastric carcinoma patients treated with gastrectomy: fifth edition American Joint Committee on Cancer staging, proximal disease, and the different diseas hypothesis," *Cancer*, vol. 88, no. 4, pp. 921–932, 2000.

[12] K. Okano, T. Maeba, K. Ishimura et al., "Hepatic resection for metastatic tumors from gastric cancer," *Annals of Surgery*, vol. 235, no. 1, pp. 86–91, 2002.

[13] K. Ueda, M. Iwahashi, M. Nakamori et al., "Analysis of the prognostic factors and evaluation of surgical treatment for synchronous liver metastases from gastric cancer," *Langenbeck's Archives of Surgery*, vol. 394, no. 4, pp. 647–653, 2009.

[14] N. Grimes, J. Devlin, D. F. J. Dunne, G. Poston, S. Fenwick, and H. Malik, "The role of hepatectomy in the management of metastatic gastric adenocarcinoma: A systematic review," *Surgical Oncology*, vol. 23, no. 4, pp. 177–185, 2014.

[15] Y.-J. Bang, Y.-W. Kim, H.-K. Yang et al., "Adjuvant capecitabine and oxaliplatin for gastric cancer after D2 gastrectomy (CLASSIC): a phase 3 open-label, randomised controlled trial," *The Lancet*, vol. 379, no. 9813, pp. 315–321, 2012.

[16] Z. Li, L. Tang, L. Zhang et al., "Weekly docetaxel and cisplatin plus fluorouracil as a preoperative treatment for gastric cancer patients with synchronous multiple hepatic metastases: a pilot study," *Medical Oncology*, vol. 27, no. 4, pp. 1314–1318, 2010.

[17] S. Ochenduszko, M. Puskulluoglu, K. Konopka et al., "Comparison of efficacy and safety of first-line palliative chemotherapy with EOX and mDCF regimens in patients with locally advanced inoperable or metastatic HER2-negative gastric or gastroesophageal junction adenocarcinoma: a randomized phase 3 trial," *Medical Oncology*, vol. 32, no. 10, article 242, 2015.

[18] D. Cunningham, W. H. Allum, S. P. Stenning et al., "Perioperative chemotherapy versus surgery alone for resectable gastroesophageal cancer," *The New England Journal of Medicine*, vol. 355, no. 1, pp. 11–20, 2006.

[19] C. Schuhmacher, S. Gretschel, F. Lordick et al., "Neoadjuvant chemotherapy compared with surgery alone for locally advanced cancer of the stomach and cardia: European organisation for research and treatment of cancer randomized trial 40954," *Journal of Clinical Oncology*, vol. 28, no. 35, pp. 5210–5218, 2010.

[20] M. Ychou, V. Boige, J. Pignon et al., "Perioperative chemotherapy compared with surgery alone for resectable gastroesophageal adenocarcinoma: an FNCLCC and FFCD multicenter phase III trial," *Journal of Clinical Oncology*, vol. 29, no. 13, pp. 1715–1721, 2011.

[21] D. Cunningham, N. Starling, S. Rao et al., "Capecitabine and oxaliplatin for advanced esophagogastric cancer," *The New England Journal of Medicine*, vol. 358, no. 1, pp. 36–46, 2008.

[22] E. C. Smyth, M. Verheij, W. Allum et al., "Gastric cancer: ESMO clinical practice guidelines for diagnosis, treatment and follow-up," *Annals of Oncology*, vol. 27, pp. v38–v49, 2016.

[23] S.-E. Al-Batran, R. D. Hofheinz, C. Pauligk et al., "Histopathological regression after neoadjuvant docetaxel, oxaliplatin, fluorouracil, and leucovorin versus epirubicin, cisplatin, and fluorouracil or capecitabine in patients with resectable gastric or gastro-oesophageal junction adenocarcinoma (FLOT4-AIO): results from the phase 2 part of a multicentre, open-label, randomised phase 2/3 trial," *The Lancet Oncology*, vol. 17, no. 12, pp. 1697–1708, 2016.

27

Colonoscopic Splenic Injury: A Simplified Radiologic Approach

Tara Chen, Qiu Tong, and Alexander Kurchin

Department of Surgery, Rochester General Hospital, Rochester, NY, USA

Correspondence should be addressed to Qiu Tong; tongq6@gmail.com

Academic Editor: Tetsuo Hirata

Colonoscopy is a commonly performed procedure for diagnosis and treatment of large bowel diseases. Recognized complications include bleeding and perforation. Splenic injury during colonoscopy is a rare complication. We report a case of a 73-year-old woman who presented with left-sided abdominal pain after colonoscopy with finding of splenic injury on CT scan. She was managed conservatively. We discuss the diagnostic and therapeutic approach to colonoscopic splenic injury.

1. Introduction

Approximately 14 million colonoscopies are performed in the US every year [1]. It is a safe procedure, with the main complications being bleeding (1-2%) and colonic perforation (0.1-0.2%) [2]. A rare and potentially fatal complication is splenic injury due to manipulation of the colonoscope through the large bowel.

When a patient presents with abdominal pain following colonoscopy, the main concern is that of colonic perforation [3]. CT scan of the abdomen and pelvis is highly sensitive for diagnosing colonic perforation [3]. Splenic injury is usually an unexpected finding of the test. Treatment is based on the hemodynamic status of the patient and on the degree of splenic injury seen on the CT scan [4].

2. Case Presentation

A 73-year-old woman underwent a screening colonoscopy that was initially reported as uneventful. Her medical history included atrial fibrillation treated successfully with radioablation. She was not on anticoagulation at the time of her exam. In her late 40s she underwent a total hysterectomy. Her medications included aspirin 81 mg daily.

Colonoscopy was done under moderate sedation with 75 mcg of fentanyl and 5 mg of midazolam given intravenously. The colonoscope was advanced to the cecum without difficulty. The exam was normal except for pandiverticulosis. The nurses' notes indicated that the patient had mild left-sided abdominal pain shortly after the procedure. This improved after passing gas and she was considered suitable for discharge.

Five hours after the procedure she called the endoscopist reporting increasing left-sided abdominal pain. There was no associated nausea, vomiting, fever, chills, dyspnea, or left shoulder pain. She was reevaluated in the endoscopist's office. On exam her vital signs were normal and there was moderate left-sided abdominal tenderness. There was no rebound or guarding. Concern for colonic perforation prompted a CT scan of the abdomen and pelvis, done without intravenous contrast. The study revealed high density perisplenic fluid consistent with blood, tracking in the left paracolic gutter (Figure 1), with no evidence of parenchymal damage. These findings indicated a grade 1 splenic injury (Table 1) and the patient was admitted for observation. She was managed conservatively with intravenous fluids. A modest overnight drop in hematocrit from 41% to 35% was noted, presumed to be partially related to hemodilution caused by the IV fluids. The next morning, the patient remained hemodynamically stable and her abdominal tenderness was much improved. She was discharged and seen in the office the following day with no further complaints of abdominal pain and no tenderness upon abdominal exam.

3. Discussion

Splenic injury is a rare complication of colonoscopy and is usually not a diagnostic consideration in patients who present

Table 1: The American Association of Surgeons for Trauma (AAST). Splenic Injury Grading Scale (2008).

Grade	Injury	Criteria
I	Hematoma	Subcapsular, <10% of surface area
	Laceration	Capsular tear, <1 cm parenchymal depth
II	Hematoma	Subcapsular, 10–50% of surface area; intraparenchymal, <5 cm diameter
	Laceration	Subcapsular, 1 cm to 3 cm parenchymal depth that does not involve a trabecular vessel
III	Hematoma	Subcapsular, >50% of surface area or expanding; ruptured subcapsular or parenchymal hematoma; intraparenchymal hematoma, ≥5 cm diameter or expanding
	Laceration	>3 cm parenchymal depth or involving trabecular vessels
IV	Laceration	Laceration involving segmental or hilar vessels producing major devascularization of >25% of the spleen
V	Hematoma	Completely shattered spleen
	Laceration	Hilar vascular injury that devascularizes the spleen

*Advance one grade for multiple injuries, up to grade III.
Reprinted from [4], with permission from Elsevier.
License number 3917700781230.
Source: http://www.sciencedirect.com/science/article/pii/S1072751508011010.

with abdominal pain after the procedure. Since the first case report by Wherry et al., in 1974, around 100 cases have been reported [5–7]. The incidence has been estimated to be in the range of 0.00005% to 0.017% [8]. A review of ICD-9 coding for the combination of colonoscopy and splenic injury showed 437 cases out of 2,654,456 colonoscopies performed between the years 2000 and 2007, yielding a rate of 0.016% or about 1 out of 6000 [8]. The true incidence is likely higher due to underreporting resulting from a reluctance to publish information on procedural complications and lack of clear definition of colonoscopic splenic injury [7, 8]. Furthermore, mild cases may resolve before a diagnosis is made or may be misdiagnosed as nonspecific postcolonoscopy discomfort [7]. This complication has a female preponderance, with approximately 75% of cases being diagnosed in women [7, 9].

The mechanism of injury is presumably due to downwards traction on the splenocolic ligament or on adhesions around the spleen during colonoscopic manipulation causing a tear in the splenic capsule [2, 6, 8–10]. Capsular tear or parenchymal injury may also result from direct trauma inflicted on the spleen as the colonoscope passes through the splenic flexure [2, 8–10]. While anticoagulation and antiplatelet therapy do not, per se, cause splenic injury, they are likely to increase the degree of bleeding to a level that will be symptomatic enough to lead to a diagnosis [7]. The presence of splenomegaly has not been described as a contributing factor, but we may assume that an enlarged spleen will be more prone to injury, as reported in the trauma literature [11].

Patients with splenic injury during colonoscopy usually present within 24 to 48 hours, but presentation can be delayed for up to 10 days after the procedure [2, 7, 8, 10]. The most common complaint is left upper quadrant abdominal pain [8]. Additional symptoms include dizziness, palpitations, referred left shoulder pain from diaphragm irritation (Kehr's sign), and diffuse abdominal discomfort [8]. On physical examination patients may have localized left upper quadrant tenderness with or without signs of peritoneal irritation including guarding and rebound [12]. However, these signs and symptoms are nonspecific and the diagnosis of splenic injury is almost never made based on history and exam alone.

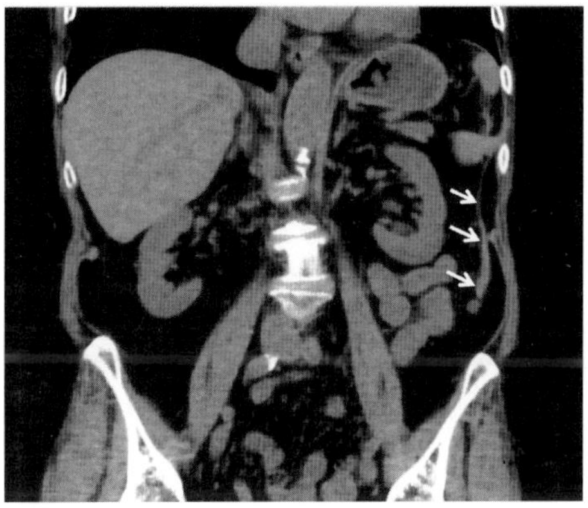

Figure 1: CT abdomen and pelvis without contrast. Coronal view showing small amount of high density perisplenic fluid (white arrows) tracking in the left paracolic gutter and extending into the pelvis.

The majority of cases are diagnosed by CT scan or at the time of laparotomy [7, 9, 13].

CT of the abdomen is the most reliable diagnostic tool for stable patients [4, 9, 13]. Findings suggestive of splenic injury include hemoperitoneum, hypodensity of the spleen, and contrast blush indicating extravasation of blood [13]. Although CT scan without intravenous contrast does not demonstrate parenchymal injury as well as a study with contrast, it is still quite sensitive. A retrospective analysis concluded that CT without contrast has a sensitivity of 93% in detecting splenic injury based on findings of a perisplenic hematoma or free abdominal fluid and strong clinical suspicion [13]. Furthermore, CT scan without contrast will quickly and accurately diagnose colonic perforation, which is the main concern when evaluating postcolonoscopy pain. The advantages of a study without contrast include the rapidity of the procedure and the ease of performing the test in an outpatient facility. It eliminates the need for IV access, checking creatinine, the risk of contrast induced nephropathy, and the concern for contrast allergy. We recommend, as injury is diagnosed on a CT scan without contrast, usually as an unexpected finding, not to repeat the test with contrast on a routine basis. In the few patients in whom more anatomic detail or evaluation of active bleeding is needed, the study can be repeated with contrast [13].

The American Association of Surgeons for Trauma (AAST) Splenic Injury Grading Scale is used to grade splenic injuries based on CT scan findings (Table 1) [4]. Treatment is based on the patient's clinical condition and the extent of splenic injury. There are three treatment options described in the literature: nonoperative management with fluid resuscitation and hemodynamic monitoring, interventional radiologic splenic artery embolization, and surgery [2, 6–8, 10]. Nonoperative treatment is the preferred choice, avoiding major surgery and preserving splenic immune function [12, 14]. Nonoperative management of splenic injury with fluid resuscitation, bed rest, and hemodynamic monitoring is more likely to succeed in patients with AAST grade I or II injury who are hemodynamically stable, lack peritoneal findings on exam, are younger than 55 years of age, and require little to no transfusion [12, 15, 16].

An estimated 85% of patients with blunt splenic injury in the past decade were managed nonoperatively [15]. In patients who fail this initial management and have ongoing bleeding but are hemodynamically stable, splenic artery embolization, which is highly successful in patients in blunt trauma, is the next step [16, 17]. The procedure has decreased the failure rate of nonoperative management from 12-13% to 2-3% [15]. The procedure appears to be safe, both in the elderly population with comorbidities and in patients who take medication that increases the risk of bleeding [15].

Surgical management is indicated in patients who fail conservative treatment and splenic artery embolization. The standard approach is open exploration. Laparoscopic surgery, which may be technically more demanding and more time consuming, is reserved for select patients with minimal hemorrhage and who are hemodynamically stable [18, 19]. Attempts at splenic salvage include splenorrhaphy and partial splenectomy. Splenectomy is indicated when all other management procedures have failed. Mortality from spleen injury is reported to be 5%, with a worse prognosis in patients who are diagnosed later [12].

4. Conclusion

In patients presenting with abdominal pain following colonoscopy, perforation is the primary concern. CT without contrast is recommended as the first diagnostic test. Splenic injury is so rare that it is almost never considered until diagnosis by CT imaging or laparotomy. This test, done without contrast, is sufficient to rule out colonic perforation and for evaluation of most splenic injuries. The scan can be repeated with IV contrast if necessary to obtain more anatomic information or to document active bleeding. Management is initially nonsurgical, which is successful in most patients. If it fails and the patient is hemodynamically stable, splenic artery embolization is the next step. Surgery is indicated, usually by open technique, when the patient is unstable or if bleeding continues after embolization attempt.

Authors' Contributions

Both Tara Chen and Qiu Tong contributed to drafting and revising this paper and performing a search of literature. Alexander Kurchin was active in management of the patient and provided case information and thorough guidance in writing this paper.

References

[1] L. C. Seeff, T. B. Richards, J. A. Shapiro et al., "How many endoscopies are performed for colorectal cancer screening? Results from CDC's survey of endoscopic capacity," *Gastroenterology*, vol. 127, no. 6, pp. 1670–1677, 2004.

[2] M. Sarhan, A. Ramcharan, and S. Ponnapalli, "Splenic injury after elective colonoscopy," *JSLS*, vol. 4, article 616, 2009.

[3] S. M. Kavic and M. D. Basson, "Management of complications of colonoscopy," in *Surgical Treatment: Evidence-Based and Problem-Oriented*, R. G. Holzheimer and J. A. Mannick, Eds., Zuckschwerdt, Munich, Germany, 2001, https://www.ncbi.nlm.nih.gov/books/NBK6945/.

[4] G. Tinkoff, T. J. Esposito, J. Reed et al., "American association for the surgery of trauma organ injury scale I: spleen, liver, and kidney, validation based on the national trauma data bank," *Journal of the American College of Surgeons*, vol. 207, no. 5, pp. 646–655, 2008.

[5] D. C. Wherry and H. Zehner Jr., "Colonoscopy—fiberoptic endoscopic approach to the colon and polypectomy," *The Medical Annals of the District of Columbia*, vol. 43, no. 4, pp. 189–192, 1974.

[6] I. M. Brennan, S. Faintuch, and B. Sacks, "Superselective splenic artery embolization for the management of splenic laceration following colonoscopy," *Acta Radiologica Short Reports*, vol. 3, no. 3, pp. 1–5, 2014.

[7] G. Piccolo, M. Di Vita, A. Cavallaro et al., "Presentation and management of splenic injury after colonoscopy: a systematic review," *Surgical Laparoscopy, Endoscopy and Percutaneous Techniques*, vol. 24, no. 2, pp. 95–102, 2014.

[8] S. Singla, D. Keller, P. Thirunavukarasu et al., "Splenic injury during colonoscopy—a complication that warrants urgent attention," *Journal of Gastrointestinal Surgery*, vol. 16, no. 6, pp. 1225–1234, 2012.

[9] J. R. A. Skipworth, D. A. Raptis, J. S. Rawal et al., "Splenic injury following colonoscopy—an underdiagnosed, but soon to increase, phenomenon?" *Annals of the Royal College of Surgeons of England*, vol. 91, no. 4, pp. W6–W11, 2009.

[10] M. A. Zappa, A. Aiolfi, I. Antonini, C. D. Musolino, and A. Porta, "Splenic rupture following colonoscopy: case report and literature review," *International Journal of Surgery Case Reports*, vol. 21, pp. 118–120, 2016.

[11] J. J. Hallman, K. J. Brasel, N. Yoganandan, and F. A. Pintar, "Splenic trauma as an adverse effect of torso-protecting side airbags: biomechanical and case evidence," *Annals of Advances in Automotive Medicine*, vol. 53, pp. 13–24, 2009.

[12] M. Beuran, I. Gheju, M. D. Venter, R. C. Marian, and R. Smarandache, "Non-operative management of splenic trauma," *Journal of Medicine and Life*, vol. 5, no. 1, pp. 47–58, 2012.

[13] D. R. Murken, J. J. Weis, G. C. Hill et al., "Radiographic assessment of splenic injury without contrast: is contrast truly needed?" *Surgery*, vol. 152, no. 4, pp. 676–684, 2012.

[14] A. Boscak and K. Shanmuganathan, "Splenic trauma: what is new?" *Radiologic Clinics of North America*, vol. 50, no. 1, pp. 105–122, 2012.

[15] A. Corcillo, S. Aellen, T. Zingg, P. Bize, N. Demartines, and A. Denys, "Endovascular treatment of active splenic bleeding after colonoscopy: a systematic review of the literature," *CardioVascular and Interventional Radiology*, vol. 36, no. 5, pp. 1270–1279, 2013.

[16] A. Raikhlin, M. O. Baerlocher, M. R. Asch, and A. Myers, "Imaging and transcatheter arterial embolization for traumatic splenic injuries: review of the literature," *Canadian Journal of Surgery*, vol. 51, no. 6, article 464, 2008.

[17] C. H. Van Der Vlies, J. Hoekstra, K. J. Ponsen, J. A. Reekers, O. M. Van Delden, and J. C. Goslings, "Impact of splenic artery embolization on the success rate of nonoperative management for blunt splenic injury," *CardioVascular and Interventional Radiology*, vol. 35, no. 1, pp. 76–81, 2012.

[18] S. Abunnaja, L. Panait, J. A. Palesty, and S. Macaron, "Laparoscopic splenectomy for traumatic splenic injury after screening colonoscopy," *Case Reports in Gastroenterology*, vol. 6, no. 3, pp. 624–628, 2012.

[19] A. Carobbi, F. Romagnani, G. Antonelli, and M. Bianchini, "Laparoscopic splenectomy for severe blunt trauma: initial experience of ten consecutive cases with a fast hemostatic technique," *Surgical Endoscopy*, vol. 24, no. 6, pp. 1325–1330, 2010.

Salivary Gland Heterotopia in the Gastroesophageal Junction: A Case Series and Review of the Literature

Lina Abdul Karim, Dong Hyang Kwon, and Metin Ozdemirli

Medstar Georgetown University Hospital, Washington, DC, USA

Correspondence should be addressed to Lina Abdul Karim; labdulkarim00@gmail.com

Academic Editor: Gregory Kouraklis

Heterotopia is defined as the presence of mature, histologically normal, tissue in unusual anatomic sites. When this heterotopic tissue forms a mass, it is called a choristoma. This case series describes 3 cases of gastroesophageal junction (GEJ) salivary heterotopias. While heterotopias are usually incidental findings, choristomas can clinically and endoscopically mimic carcinomas and might lead to unnecessary procedures for the patients. Clinicians should therefore be aware of this entity. Literature search, however, failed to show any reports of salivary gland heterotopias in the GEJ. In fact, literature review revealed only 6 reported cases of salivary gland choristoma in the gastrointestinal tract, none at the GEJ. In this case series, we report 2 cases of salivary gland heterotopia and one case of salivary gland choristoma arising at the GE junction. To our knowledge, this is the first series of its kind in the literature.

1. Introduction

Heterotopia is defined as the presence of mature, histologically normal, tissue found in unusual anatomic sites. A mass formed by heterotopic tissue is called a choristoma. Salivary gland choristoma was recognized as early as 1967 by Youngs and Scofield in lower neck [1]. Subsequently more cases of salivary choristoma have been reported mainly in the head and neck region, including the tonsil [2], periparotid and cervical lymph nodes [3], pituitary [4], external auditory canal, thyroglossal duct cyst, mastoid bone, middle ear, tongue, sternoclavicular joint, thyroid and parathyroid glands, and the upper and lower neck regions [5].

Despite common occurrence in the head and neck, reports of salivary gland heterotopia or choristoma in the gastrointestinal tract are scarce. Salivary gland choristoma found in conjunction with gastric heterotopia was first described by Shindo et al. in 1972 [6]. Our literature search revealed only five additional reported cases in the GI since then. The reported anatomic sites include rectal and perianal regions [6–8], descending colon [9], jejunum [10], and esophagus [11]. In this case series, we report 2 cases of salivary gland heterotopia and one case of salivary gland choristoma arising at the GE junction (Table 1). To our knowledge, this is the first series of its kind in the literature.

2. Case Report

2.1. Case 1. A 44-year-old Caucasian male presented with an 8-month history of reflux and heart burn, which was relieved by Esomeprazole. Endoscopic evaluation showed a polypoid shaped mass measuring 1 cm in size at the gastroesophageal junction. Ultrasonic evaluation revealed a hypoechoic lesion that was confined to the deep mucosa and submucosa with no deèper layer involvement. The nodule was resected via the endoscopic mucosal resection technique (EMR). Grossly, the specimen was a 1 cm GEJ nodule. It was a single irregular fragment of tan-pink soft tissue that was bisected and entirely processed for microscopy. Microscopic evaluation showed squamous mucosa with oxyntic-type mucosa with moderate chronic inflammation, ectatic vessels, congestion in the mucosa, and a few lymphoid aggregates. In addition, there were prominent mucus glands with chronic inflammation consistent with heterotopic salivary glands, surrounded by

TABLE 1: Location, clinical features, endoscopic findings, and histopathology of salivary gland heterotopias at the gastroesophageal junction.

	Age/Sex	Location	Clinical	Endoscopy	Histopathology
Case 1	44m	GE Junction	8 month history of gastro-esophageal reflux disease (GERD).	Polypoid shaped, hypoechoic mass measuring 1 cm in size and confined to the deep mucosa and submucosa	Prominent mucus glands with chronic inflammation consistent with heterotopic salivary glands surrounded by prominent adipose tissue and congested vessels in the submucosa (Figures 1 and 2).
Case 2	62 m	GE Junction	History of hypothyroidism, Sjogren's syndrome, Raynaud syndrome, chronic GERD and grade 3 esophagitis	Dilated esophagus with an irregular z-line and 2 small islands of salmon colored mucosa immediately proximal to the GE junction	Focal mild acute erosive esophagitis and basal hyperplasia that was consistent with reflux and detached fragment of salivary gland type glandular tissue with chronic inflammation consistent with heterotopic salivary gland tissue (Figures 3 and 4)
Case 3	72 m	GE Junction	Past medical history of Barrett's esophagus and high-grade dysplasia presented to rule out invasive carcinoma	Concerning focal area of ulceration which was removed via EMR	Focal high-grade dysplasia, cavernous and ectatic venous channels as well as a few prominent lobules of minor salivary glands with cystification (Figures 5 and 6)

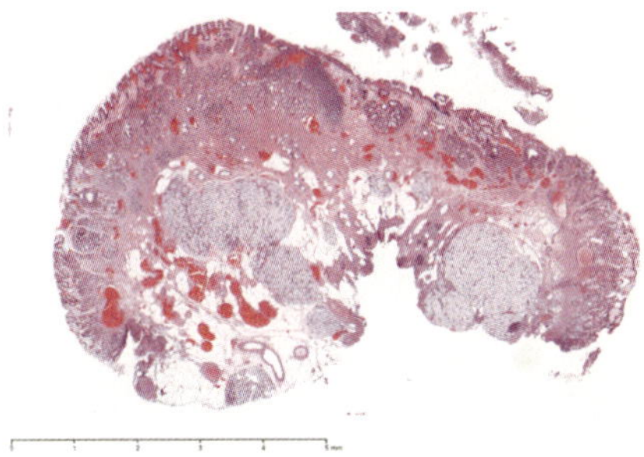

FIGURE 1: Low-magnification appearance of the heterotopic salivary glands demonstrating their submucosal location surrounded by prominent adipose tissue and congested vessels. This case is classified as a salivary gland choristoma since the heterotopic tissue formed a mass.

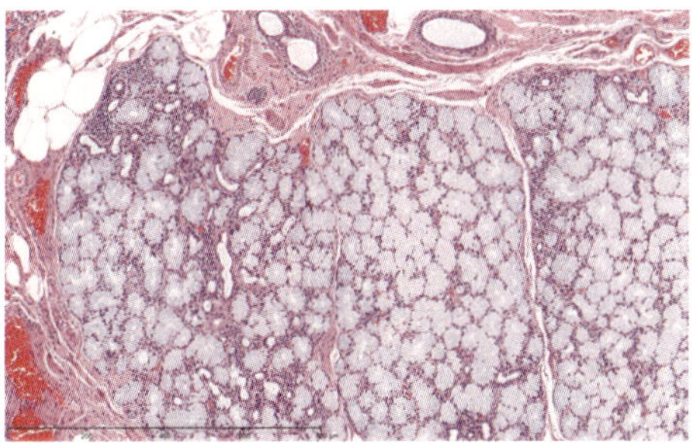

FIGURE 2: High-magnification appearance of the heterotopic salivary glands demonstrating prominent mucus glands with chronic inflammation.

prominent adipose tissue and congested vessels in the submucosa (Figures 1 and 2).

2.2. Case 2. A 62-year-old Caucasian male with a history of hypothyroidism, Sjogren's syndrome, Raynaud syndrome, chronic GERD, and grade 3 esophagitis presented for an upper endoscopy for the evaluation of suspected Barrett's esophagus. Endoscopic evaluation and barium swallow showed a dilated esophagus. The z-line appeared slightly irregular and there were 2 small islands of salmon colored mucosal lesions immediately proximal to the GE junction.

Grossly, the specimen consisted of one piece of tan-white soft tissue, measuring < 1cm. Microscopic evaluation showed fragments of squamous mucosa with focal mild acute erosive esophagitis and basal hyperplasia that was consistent with reflux. In addition, detached fragments of salivary gland type glandular tissue with chronic inflammation, consistent with heterotopic salivary gland tissue, were seen (Figures 3 and 4).

2.3. Case 3. A 72-year-old Caucasian male with past medical history of Barrett's esophagus and high-grade dysplasia presented for EGD and biopsy in order to rule out invasive carcinoma. Endoscopic evaluation revealed a large hiatal hernia and an approximate 3 cm segment of Barrett's esophagus. There was a concerning focal area of ulceration which was removed via EMR.

Grossly, the specimen was one piece of tan-white soft tissue, measuring 0.7 x 0.4 x 0.2 cm. Microscopic evaluation revealed focal high-grade dysplasia adjacent to squamous epithelium in the middle portion of the specimen. In the deeper aspect of the tissue, there were cavernous and ectatic venous channels as well as a few prominent lobules of minor salivary glands with cystification in the ducts (Figures 5 and 6). The patient was treated with radiofrequency ablation.

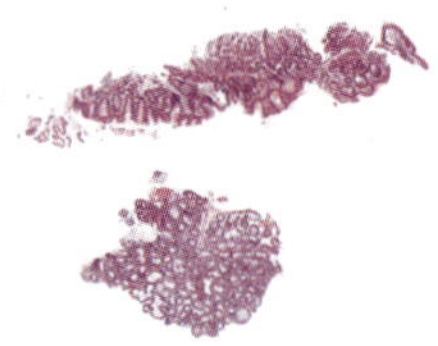

FIGURE 3: Low-magnification appearance of the heterotopic salivary gland tissue that was received as detached fragments.

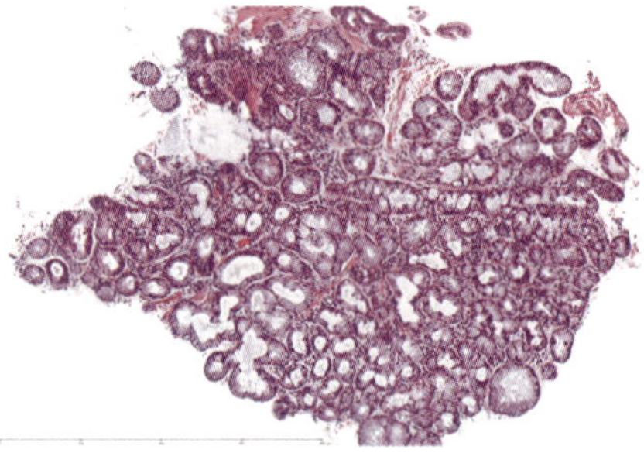

FIGURE 4: High-magnification appearance of the salivary gland type glandular tissue showing chronic inflammation.

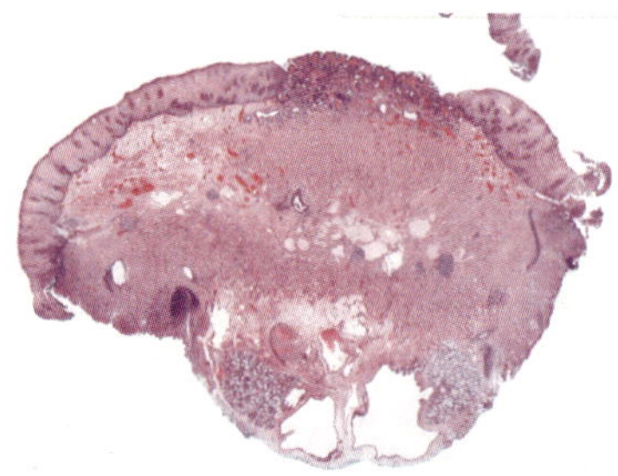

FIGURE 5: Low-magnification image showing focal high-grade dysplasia on the surface with ectatic venous channels and heterotopic minor salivary gland tissue in the deeper aspect.

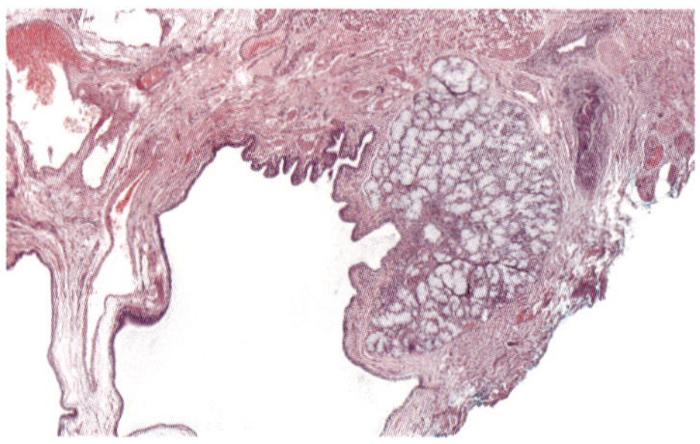

FIGURE 6: Higher magnification image showing the ectatic venous channels as well as a lobule of heterotopic minor salivary gland.

3. Discussion

Salivary gland heterotopia in the GI tract is a rare entity. The heterotopic tissue can form a mass, choristoma, which can present as a mass on imaging or as a hypoechoic mucosal or submucosal lesion on EUS, mimicking the presentation of carcinoma. Other possible differential diagnosis includes gastrointestinal stromal tumor (GIST), schwannoma, leiomyoma, ectopic pancreas, cyst, lipoma, and carcinoid. This review will focus on the clinical features, endoscopic/sigmoidoscopic findings, histopathology, ancillary studies, pathogenesis, treatment, and prognosis of salivary gland heterotopias/choristoma based on the 6 cases published in the literature (Table 2) with the addition of the 3 cases reported here for a total of 9 cases.

Salivary gland choristoma in gastrointestinal tract occurs mainly in adults but has been identified in an age range from 5 to 61 years. It occurs more often in males than it does in females, with 7 cases (78%) occurring in males. The race of the patients was not reported in most cases. It can occur in any location in the GI tract with reports of occurrence in the rectal area, rectal diverticulum, jejunum, esophagus, and, now, gastroesophageal junction. The clinical presentation depends on the location. Rectal cases can present as a rectal protrusion/mass, rectal bleeding, anal pain, and sphincter spasm. Cases in the GE junction either present with chronic reflux or are asymptomatic. One case presented in the esophagus with symptoms of belching, regurgitation, and abdominal pain. The youngest reported case was a 5-year-old girl who presented with severe, intermittent abdominal pain and postprandial vomiting due to a salivary choristoma in the jejunum.

The gross appearance is usually that of a single, tan-pink mucosal to subserosal nodule or pedunculated mass, ranging from 1 to 2 cm in size. Microscopically, mixed serous and mucinous glands with salivary ducts resembling submaxillary or sublingual salivary glands are seen.

All the reported cases were treated with either sigmoidoscopic or endoscopic resection, except for the case of the 5-year-old Nigerian girl who underwent exploratory laparotomy and wedge resection due to the unavailability of endoscopic procedures. There were no reports of complications or recurrences. However, the follow-up intervals varied. There was only one report of malignant transformation in the GI. However, this phenomenon has been described in multiple cases of salivary gland heterotopias in the head and neck.

Salivary gland choristoma in the GI tract can form a mass, which can present as a mass on imaging or as a hypoechoic mucosal or submucosal lesion on EUS, mimicking the presentation of a carcinoma. The authors do not suggest that it should be on top of the differential list, however, clinicians should be aware of its occurrence to prevent delay in diagnosis and inappropriate procedures and treatments for the patient.

TABLE 2: Location, clinical features, endoscopic/sigmoidoscopic findings, histopathology, and treatment of 6 cases of gastrointestinal salivary gland choristomas reported in the literature.

Source	Age/ Sex	Location	Clinical	Endoscopy/ Sigmoidoscopy	Histopathology/ IHC	Treatment
Shindo et al, 1972 [6].	24 m	Hemorrhoid	Severe bleeding by rectum of sudden onset, protrusion, and anal pain, large external and internal hemorrhoids and considerable spasm of the sphincter.	N/A	Ectopic gastric mucosa is of the acid-secreting type normally found lining the corpus and fundus of the stomach. This type of mucosa covers dilated hemorrhoidal veins in this specimen. In another area, proximal to the gastric mucosa, there is a microfocus of mixed serous and mucous glands such as are found normally in the submaxillary salivary glands or in the mucosal glands of the tracheobronchial tree.	Resection
Weitzner et al, 1983 [7].	61 m	Hemorrhoid	1x1 cm anal verge polyp	N/A	Lobules of serous and mucous glands and ducts typical of submaxillary glands with and adjacent hyperplastic polyp	Simoidoscopic removal
Downs-Kelly et al, 2003 [8].	31 m	Rectal diverticulum	Intermittent rectal bleeding, small mass on the rectal wall. An ultrasound of the rectum revealed a 2 cm mass.	Sigmoidoscopy revealed a single diverticulum and an extramucosal mass in the lower rectal segment	In the submucosal region, multiple foci of serous and mucinous glands and ducts resembling salivary gland tissue were present. Some of these foci were associated with a chronic inflammatory cell infiltrate consisting primarily of lymphocytes.	The patient underwent local rectal excision of the 2x 2x 0.8 cm polypoid mass.
Maffini et al, 2012 [9].	55f	Large bowel	Colorectal carcinoma screening	A pedunculated polypoid lesion of 1 cm situated at 19 cm from the anal verge, resembling a submucosal lipoma without other mucosal alterations	A small aggregate of acinar glands with mixed mucous–serous features in the submucosa and an intercalated duct composed of a double layer of cells – epithelial and myoepithelial – that reached the mucosal surface. The glands were positive for lysozyme antibody and negative for pancreatic amylase, S-100 protein, chromogranin, and synaptophysin	Endoscopic resection
Olajide, 2013 [10].	5f	Jejunum	Severe, intermittent abdominal pain with occasional postprandial vomiting	A pale yellow subserosal lesion was seen in the antimesenteric border of the jejunum about 45 cm from the duodeno-jejunal junction.	Submucosal tissue with lobules of serous glands with central lumen, reminiscent of salivary glands. The glands are composed of benign epithelial cells with regular nuclei and ample eosinophilic cytoplasm.	Wedge resection
Wang et al, 2014 [11].	60 m	Esophagus	Belch, regurgitation, and abdominal pain	1.2×1.0 cm mucosal protuberant lesion situated 38 cm from the incisors	Salivary gland tumor, partly basal cell adenoma, partly with the structure of adenoid cystic carcinoma, the glands were positive for CD117, P63, PDGFR, P53, Ki-67, CEA, P-CK, Vimentin, PAS, S-100, Calponin, and CK5/6.	Endoscopic resection

References

[1] L. A. Youngs and H. H. Scofield, "Heterotopic salivary gland tissue in the lower neck," *Arch Pathol*, vol. 83, no. 5, pp. 550-6, 1967.

[2] A. R. Banerjee, J. V. Soames, J. P. Birchall, C. Reid, and R. J. Bray, "Ectopic salivary gland tissue in the palatine and lingual tonsil," *International Journal of Pediatric Otorhinolaryngology*, vol. 27, no. 2, pp. 159–162, 1993.

[3] D. F. Wilson and M. I. MacEntee, "Papillary cystadenoma of ectopic minor salivary gland origin," *Oral Surgery, Oral Medicine, Oral Pathology, Oral Radiology, and Endodontology*, vol. 37, no. 6, pp. 915–918, 1974.

[4] V. Ranucci, A. Coli, and E. Marrucci, "Ectopic salivary gland tissue in a Rathke's cleft cyst," *Int J Clin Exp Pathol*, vol. 6, no. 7, pp. 1437-40, 2013.

[5] A. Ferlito, G. Bertino, A. Rinaldo, G. M. Mannarà, and K. O. Devaney, "A review of heterotopia and associated salivary gland neoplasms of the head and neck," *The Journal of Laryngology & Otology*, vol. 113, no. 4, pp. 299–303, 1999.

[6] K. Shindo, E. E. Bacon, and E. J. Holmes, "Ectopic gastric mucosa and glandular tissue of a salivary type in the anal canal concomitant with a diverticulum in hemorrhoidal tissue: Report of a case," *Diseases of the Colon & Rectum*, vol. 15, no. 1, pp. 57–62, 1972.

[7] S. Weitzner, "Ectopic salivary gland tissue in submucosa of rectum," *Diseases of the Colon & Rectum*, vol. 26, no. 12, pp. 814–817, 1983.

[8] E. Downs-Kelly, A. P. Hoschar, and R. A. Prayson, "Salivary gland heterotopia in the rectum," *Annals of Diagnostic Pathology*, vol. 7, no. 2, pp. 124–126, 2003.

[9] F. Maffini, A. Vingiani, D. Lepanto, G. Fiori, and G. Viale, "Salivary gland choristoma in large bowel," *Endoscopy*, vol. 44, no. 2, pp. E13–E14, 2012.

[10] T. A. Olajide, S. O. Agodirin, R. W. Ojewola et al., "Jejunal Choristoma: A Very Rare Cause of Abdominal Pain in Children," *Case Reports in Surgery*, vol. 2014, Article ID 863647, 3 pages, 2014.

[11] C. Wang, L. Chen, W. Guo, X. Zhu, and Z. Liu, "Salivary gland choriostoma in the esophagus," *Endoscopy*, vol. 46, pp. E658–E659, 2014.

Hemorrhage from Extra-Antral Gastric Antral Vascular Ectasia in a Patient with Duodenal Heterotopic Gastric Mucosa

John Gubatan,[1] Nathan Raines,[1] Hasan Khosravi,[1] Tracy L. Challies,[2] and Tyler M. Berzin[3]

[1]*Department of Medicine, Beth Israel Deaconess Medical Center, Harvard Medical School, Boston, MA, USA*
[2]*Department of Pathology, Beth Israel Deaconess Medical Center, Harvard Medical School, Boston, MA, USA*
[3]*Division of Gastroenterology and Hepatology, Beth Israel Deaconess Medical Center, Harvard Medical School, Boston, MA, USA*

Correspondence should be addressed to John Gubatan; jgubatan@bidmc.harvard.edu

Academic Editor: Hideto Kawaratani

Gastric antral vascular ectasias (GAVE) have been increasingly recognized as an uncommon cause of chronic gastrointestinal bleeding and anemia, although their underlying pathogenesis is not completely well understood. Heterotopic gastric mucosa (HGM) has been reported to occur at various sites along the gastrointestinal tract and although relatively common, it is often asymptomatic. We report a case of a 60-year-old woman with a prior history of GAVE who developed melena and symptomatic anemia during her hospitalization following cardiac catheterization. Initial EGD demonstrated nonbleeding antral GAVE and a newly discovered duodenal mass. Duodenal mass biopsies were ultimately notable for HGM along with histologic features of extra-antral GAVE. The patient required blood transfusions and consequently had a small bowel endoscopy notable for fresh blood in the proximal small bowel. The patient underwent a small bowel push enteroscopy which demonstrated active bleeding of the duodenal mass and overlying oozing GAVE, which was cauterized with Argon-Plasma Coagulation with adequate hemostasis. We present for the first time a novel association between GAVE and HGM. Our case illustrates that extra-antral GAVE may occur with HGM in the duodenum. We explore potential mechanisms by which HGM may be involved in the pathogenesis of GAVE.

1. Introduction

Gastric antral vascular ectasia (GAVE) is a rare disorder characterized by its distinctive endoscopic appearance consisting of red, tortuous ectatic blood vessels arranged in a longitudinal array localized in the gastric antrum converging on the pylorus [1]. Prominent histological features of GAVE include fibromuscular hyperplasia of the lamina propria, capillary ectasia, presence of intravascular fibrin thrombi, and mucosal architectural distortion [2]. GAVE occurs in about a third of patients with cirrhosis and portal hypertension [3]. In noncirrhotic patients, GAVE has been associated with autoimmune disorders, connective tissue disorders, chronic kidney disease, and ectopic pancreas [4–7]. Although GAVE is rare, it accounts for up to 4% of nonvariceal upper gastrointestinal bleeding [8]. Heterotopic gastric mucosa (HGM), gastric tissue found outside the stomach, is found to occur anywhere along the gastrointestinal tract and has been estimated to have a prevalence of 0.1% to 3% [9]. HGM is often asymptomatic and found incidentally on endoscopic studies. In particular, duodenal HGM has been shown to not be associated with significant GI symptoms in previous studies [10, 11]. Although previous cases of duodenal HGM have been described, we report for the first time an unusual case of a patient with known GAVE who presented with melena and was found to have a bleeding duodenal mass with histology consistent with HGM and features of extra-antral GAVE.

2. Case Presentation

A 60-year-old woman with a prior history of GAVE was referred from an outside hospital with exertional dyspnea and further workup of echocardiogram abnormalities. The patient's medical history was most notable for hypertension, diabetes mellitus, coronary artery disease, chronic obstructive pulmonary disease, and diastolic heart failure, but no history of known cirrhosis, connective tissue disorder, or

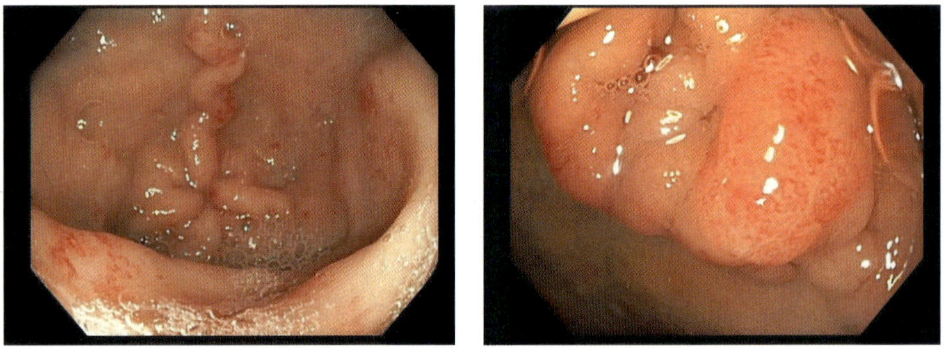

(a) (b)

Figure 1: Initial esophagogastroduodenoscopy (EGD) demonstrating gastric antral vascular ectasias (GAVE) without evidence of active oozing (a) and frond-like mass in the duodenal bulb with no active bleeding or stigmata of recent bleed (b).

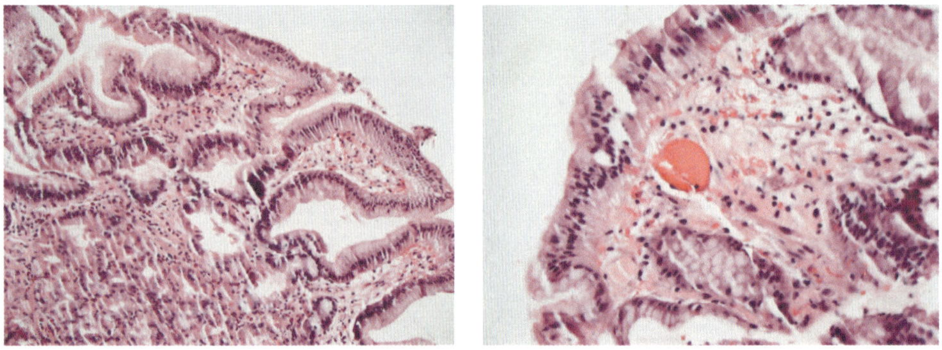

(a) (b)

Figure 2: Duodenal biopsies demonstrating oxyntic gastric glandular cells (specialized acid secreting) underlying gastric foveolar epithelium on the surface, no goblet cells or enterocytes to identify it as intestinal (a), and presence of dilated and ectatic blood vessels with mild vascular congestion, features characteristic of GAVE (b).

autoimmune disease. The patient's GAVE was diagnosed one year prior to presentation. At that time, she presented with melena that required intermittent blood transfusions for symptomatic anemia. She had an esophagogastroduodenoscopy (EGD) which was notable for GAVE. Argon-Plasma Coagulation (APC) was applied to these angioectasias with successful hemostasis.

On admission, the patient was hemodynamically stable, hemoglobin and hematocrit were at baseline, and the patient denied melena. The patient's echocardiogram demonstrated inferoposterolateral wall hypokinesis. The patient subsequently underwent left cardiac catheterization which demonstrated a lesion along the right marginal artery which was stented. The catheterization was complicated by a right coronary artery dissection and ST elevation myocardial infarction (STEMI) requiring three drug-eluting stents. The patient was started on dual antiplatelet therapy with Ticagrelor and aspirin and managed in the cardiac intensive care unit (CCU). In the CCU, the patient experienced significant melena with drop in hemoglobin (from 8.5 g/dL to 6.0 g/dL), requiring blood transfusions. Abdominal CT did not demonstrate a retroperitoneal hematoma or any other source of bleeding. The patient remained hemodynamically stable and hemoglobin increased appropriately with blood transfusions.

The patient underwent further evaluation with colonoscopy and EGD. Colonoscopy was unremarkable. EGD demonstrated small angioectasias in the antrum consistent with known GAVE without evidence of oozing (Figure 1(a)). EGD was most notable for a 2 cm frond-like mass in the duodenal bulb with no active bleeding (Figure 1(b)). Biopsies were obtained from this duodenal mass with histology consistent with heterotopic gastric mucosa (Figure 2(a)) and dilated and ectatic blood vessels with mild vascular congestion, features suggestive of GAVE. On histology, there was no evidence of atrophic gastritis and *Helicobacter pylori* staining was negative. The patient was managed on an oral proton pump inhibitor twice daily. On the medical floor, the patient continued to experience intermittent exertional dyspnea and chest pain. The patient was managed with intravenous diuretics for diastolic heart failure exacerbation and started on oral nitrates for anginal pain from her recent STEMI with improvement in her symptoms. The patient continued to experience melena with worsening anemia and consequently required intermittent blood transfusions.

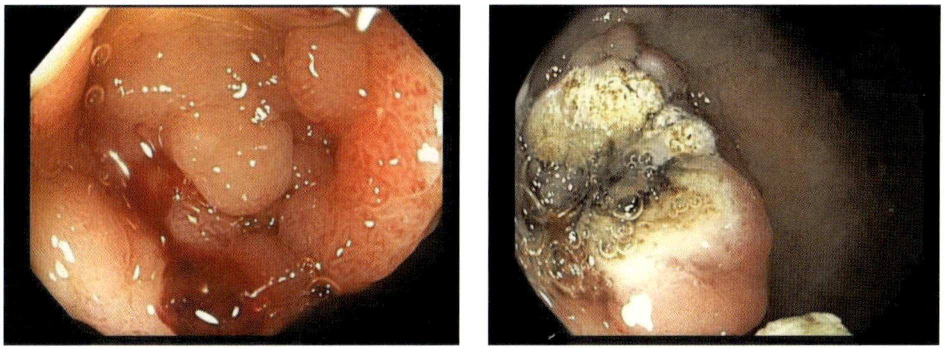

(a) (b)

FIGURE 3: Small bowel push enteroscopy: gastric heterotopia in duodenal bulb with overlying oozing extra-antral GAVE (a) and duodenal mass after Argon-Plasma Coagulation (APC) was applied for successful hemostasis (b).

In the setting of continued gastrointestinal bleeding, the patient had a capsule endoscopy which demonstrated fresh blood in the duodenum and proximal small bowel with no clear source of bleeding. The patient subsequently underwent a small bowel push enteroscopy which demonstrated bleeding from the previously visualized duodenal mass, with overlying oozing extra-antral GAVE (Figure 3(a)). The duodenal mass composed of gastric heterotopia was cauterized with Argon-Plasma Coagulation with successful hemostasis (Figure 3(b)). After the endoscopic procedure, the patient had less episodes of melena and repeat hemoglobin/hematocrit levels were robustly stable. She was discharged home with close follow-up with gastroenterology and plan for regular surveillance of her hemoglobin.

3. Discussion

In the current case, we present a patient with a history of GAVE who presented with melena and symptomatic anemia and was not found to have bleeding GAVE as expected but rather duodenal HGM with histologic features of extra-antral GAVE as an etiology of the patient's gastrointestinal bleeding. The patient was successfully treated with a proton pump inhibitor, blood transfusions, and endoscopic APC to duodenal mass.

Most cases of gastric antral vascular ectasia (GAVE) have been reported to occur in the gastric antrum. One study by Stotzer et al. [12] reported that ectatic lesions are also common in the gastric cardia. However, GAVE has not previously been reported to occur in the duodenum. This is the first reported case in the literature to demonstrate that GAVE may occur in the duodenum with associated HGM. Our finding challenges the paradigm that GAVE only occurs within the gastric antrum and raises some interesting aspects regarding the pathogenesis of GAVE.

The temporality between GAVE and duodenal HGM in our patient is an interesting point. The patient had GAVE visualized by endoscopy one year prior to her current presentation. At that time, the 2 cm duodenal mass was not seen. Heterotopic gastric mucosa in the duodenum is usually congenital, representing a developmental anomaly [11]. The duodenal mass was unlikely from metaplastic change as the patient had no chronic inflammation or peptic ulcer disease in the surrounding area. The patient's duodenal HGM was likely congenital and may have been missed by endoscopic visualization during her last EGD. The fact that the patient's duodenal HGM likely preceded her antral GAVE raises the possibility that HGM may be a risk factor for the development of GAVE. Although ectopic pancreas has been previously described in a patient with associated GAVE [7], heterotopic gastric mucosa in a patient with GAVE has not been reported in the literature.

One hypothesis is that GAVE arises from mechanical stress due to increased gastric peristalsis. Charneau et al. demonstrated [13] that patients with GAVE had abnormal antral motility. Demonstrating extra-antral GAVE in the duodenum suggests that gastric peristalsis and abnormal antral motility are not necessary in the development of GAVE. However, mechanical stress may still play a role in the formation of GAVE as duodenal contractions do occur, although they differ from antral contractions with regard to amplitude and frequency [14]. It is unclear if duodenal motility plays a role in the development of extra-antral duodenal GAVE.

Hypergastrinemia has been previously implicated in the pathogenesis of GAVE [15]. One study demonstrated that patients with gastric oxyntic heterotopia found in the duodenum had increased serum gastrin levels [16]. Our patient's duodenal mass histology indeed demonstrated oxyntic gastric glandular cells. Although we did not measure serum gastrin in our patient, it is possible that our patient also had elevated serum gastrin levels. Hypergastrinemia may have predisposed our patient to developing antral GAVE and extra-antral GAVE in the setting of heterotopic gastric mucosa.

It is interesting to note that GAVE has been described in patients with atrophic gastritis [17, 18]. Patients with atrophic gastritis are known to develop hypergastrinemia. Destruction of parietal cells in atrophic gastritis leads to profound hypochlorhydria which induces G-cell (gastrin-producing) hyperplasia and consequently hypergastrinemia [19, 20]. Hypergastrinemia from underlying atrophic gastritis may be a possible mechanistic link in the association of GAVE with atrophic gastritis. Histology of the duodenal

HGM mass in our patient did not demonstrate any features of atrophic gastritis and was negative for *Helicobacter pylori* on staining. Although we did not obtain gastric mucosal biopsies for histologic evaluation, clinical suspicion in our patient for atrophic gastritis was low. Our patient did not have any symptoms (nausea, vomiting, anorexia, weight loss, and abdominal pain) and labs were not suggestive of iron deficiency or megaloblastic anemia. Thus, atrophic gastritis as a mechanism for the development of GAVE in our patient was unlikely.

Another potential mechanism in the pathogenesis of GAVE involves the local proliferation of neuroendocrine cells which in turn produce high levels of vasoactive substances such as vasoactive intestinal polypeptide and serotonin which result in vascular dilation [21]. Neuroendocrine cells were not visualized on histology from our duodenal specimen; thus this particular pathogenic mechanism is unlikely in our patient.

In conclusion, heterotopic gastric mucosa is associated with the development of GAVE, possibly through increased serum gastrin production owing to ectopic gastric mucosa. Our case report suggests that HGM may be associated with GAVE and that extra-antral GAVE may develop beyond the gastric antrum. Bleeding extra-antral GAVE in the duodenum appears to be responsive to proton pump inhibitor and endoscopic thermal ablation therapy.

Abbreviations

GAVE: Gastric antral vascular ectasia
HGM: Heterotopic gastric mucosa
EGD: Esophagogastroduodenoscopy
APC: Argon-Plasma Coagulation
STEMI: ST elevation myocardial infarction
CCU: Cardiac intensive care unit
CT: Computed tomography.

Consent

Written informed consent was obtained from the patient for publication of this case report and any accompanying images.

Authors' Contributions

J. Gubatan, N. Raines, and H. Koshravi were involved in the clinical care of the patient during her hospitalization. N. Raines and H. Koshravi obtained patient consent and drafted the clinical case presentation section. J. Gubatan designed the conceptual framework of the manuscript, performed the literature review, and drafted the manuscript. Tracy L. Challies was the GI pathology attending involved in the case and provided the histology slides. Tyler M. Berzin was the endoscopy attending of the case and provided guidance in drafting manuscript. All authors contributed to critical review of the manuscript; J. Gubatan had full access to all of the data and takes responsibility for the integrity of the case presentation.

References

[1] C. P. Selinger and Y. S. Ang, "Gastric antral vascular ectasia (GAVE): an update on clinical presentation, pathophysiology and treatment," *Digestion*, vol. 77, no. 2, pp. 131–137, 2008.

[2] P. F. Suit, R. E. Petras, T. W. Bauer, and J. L. Petrini Jr., "Gastric antral vascular ectasia: A Histologic and Morphometric Study of 'The Watermelon Stomach'," *The American Journal of Surgical Pathology*, vol. 11, no. 10, pp. 750–757, 1987.

[3] E. M. Ward, M. Raimondo, B. G. Rosser, M. B. Wallace, and R. D. Dickson, "Prevalence and natural history of gastric antral vascular ectasia in patients undergoing orthotopic liver transplantation," *Journal of Clinical Gastroenterology*, vol. 38, no. 10, pp. 898–900, 2004.

[4] C. J. Gostout, T. R. Viggiano, D. A. Ahlquist, K. K. Wang, M. V. Larson, and R. Balm, "The clinical and endoscopic spectrum of the watermelon stomach," *Journal of Clinical Gastroenterology*, vol. 15, no. 3, pp. 256–263, 1992.

[5] B. C. Valdez, D. Henning, R. K. Busch et al., "A nucleolar RNA helicase recognized by autoimmune antibodies from a patient with watermelon stomach disease," *Nucleic Acids Research*, vol. 24, no. 7, pp. 1220–1224, 1996.

[6] M. Krstić, T. Alempijević, S. Andrejević et al., "Watermelon stomach in a patient with primary Sjögren's syndrome," *Vojnosanitetski Pregled*, vol. 67, no. 3, pp. 256–258, 2010.

[7] B. Yildiz, C. Sokmensuer, and V. Kaynaroglu, "Chronic anemia due to watermelon stomach," *Annals of Saudi Medicine*, vol. 30, no. 2, pp. 156–158, 2010.

[8] G. S. Dulai, D. M. Jensen, T. O. G. Kovacs, I. M. Gralnek, and R. Jutabha, "Endoscopic treatment outcomes in watermelon stomach patients with and without portal hypertension," *Endoscopy*, vol. 36, no. 1, pp. 68–72, 2004.

[9] N. Akbayir, C. Alkim, L. Erdem et al., "Heterotopic gastric mucosa in the cervical esophagus (inlet patch): endoscopic prevalence, histological and clinical characteristics," *Journal of Gastroenterology and Hepatology*, vol. 19, no. 8, pp. 891–896, 2004.

[10] L. Yu, Y. Yang, L. Cui, L. Peng, and G. Sun, "Heterotopic gastric mucosa of the gastrointestinal tract: prevalence, histological features, and clinical characteristics," *Scandinavian Journal of Gastroenterology*, vol. 49, no. 2, pp. 138–144, 2014.

[11] A. M. Lessells and D. F. Martin, "Heterotopic gastric mucosa in the duodenum," *Journal of Clinical Pathology*, vol. 35, no. 6, pp. 591–595, 1982.

[12] P.-O. Stotzer, R. Willén, and A. F. Kilander, "Watermelon stomach: not only an antral disease," *Gastrointestinal Endoscopy*, vol. 55, no. 7, pp. 897–900, 2002.

[13] J. Charneau, R. Petit, P. Cales, A. Dauver, and J. Boyer, "Antral motility in patients with cirrhosis with or without gastric antral vascular ectasia," *Gut*, vol. 37, no. 4, pp. 488–492, 1995.

[14] A. Shafik, O. El Sibai, and A. A. Shafik, "Study of the duodenal contractile activity during antral contractions," *World Journal of Gastroenterology*, vol. 13, no. 18, pp. 2600–2603, 2007.

[15] E. Quintero, J. M. Pique, J. A. Bombi et al., "Gastric mucosal vascular ectasias causing bleeding in cirrhosis. A distinct entity associated with hypergastrinemia and low serum levels of pepsinogen I," *Gastroenterology*, vol. 93, no. 5, pp. 1054–1061, 1987.

[16] E. Kohan, D. Oh, H. Wang, S. Hazany, G. Ohning, and J. R. Pisegna, "Duodenal bulb mucosa with hypertrophic gastric oxyntic heterotopia in patients with Zollinger Ellison syndrome," *Diagnostic and Therapeutic Endoscopy*, vol. 2009, Article ID 298381, 6 pages, 2009.

[17] T. Berk, J. R. Slemmer, and L. S. Friedman, "Gastric antral vascular ectasia associated with gastric carcinoma," *American Journal of Gastroenterology*, vol. 86, no. 6, pp. 768–770, 1991.

[18] S. F. Moss, P. Ghosh, D. M. Thomas, J. E. Jackson, and J. Calam, "Gastric antral vascular ectasia: maintenance treatment with oestrogen-progesterone," *Gut*, vol. 33, no. 5, pp. 715–717, 1992.

[19] J. D. Reinhardt, R. M. McCloy, and C. F. Blackwell, "Autoimmune atrophic gastritis with hypergastrinemia," *Southern Medical Journal*, vol. 69, no. 12, pp. 1551–1553, 1976.

[20] S. Dacha, M. Razvi, J. Massaad, Q. Cai, and M. Wehbi, "Hypergastrinemia," *Gastroenterology Report*, vol. 3, no. 3, pp. 201–208, 2015.

[21] J. R. Lowes and J. Rode, "Neuroendocrine cell proliferations in gastric antral vascular ectasia," *Gastroenterology*, vol. 97, no. 1, pp. 207–212, 1989.

A Calcium Enterolith in a Patient with Crohn's Disease and Its In Vitro Dissolubility in Citric Acid

Masaya Iwamuro,[1,2] Haruo Urata,[3] Sakiko Hiraoka,[1] Masayasu Ohmori,[1] Yoshitaka Kondo,[4] Yoshiro Kawahara,[5] and Hiroyuki Okada[1]

[1]*Department of Gastroenterology and Hepatology, Okayama University Graduate School of Medicine, Dentistry, and Pharmaceutical Sciences, 2-5-1 Shikata-cho, Kita-ku, Okayama 700-8558, Japan*
[2]*Department of General Medicine, Okayama University Graduate School of Medicine, Dentistry, and Pharmaceutical Sciences, 2-5-1 Shikata-cho, Kita-ku, Okayama 700-8558, Japan*
[3]*Central Research Laboratory, Okayama University Medical School, 2-5-1 Shikata-cho, Kita-ku, Okayama 700-8558, Japan*
[4]*Department of Gastroenterological Surgery, Okayama University Graduate School of Medicine, Dentistry, and Pharmaceutical Sciences, 2-5-1 Shikata-cho, Kita-ku, Okayama 700-8558, Japan*
[5]*Department of Endoscopy, Okayama University Hospital, 2-5-1 Shikata-cho, Kita-ku, Okayama 700-8558, Japan*

Correspondence should be addressed to Masaya Iwamuro; iwamuromasaya@yahoo.co.jp

Academic Editor: Warwick S. Selby

The microstructure and dissolubility of a calcified enterolith and enterolith pieces removed from a 26-year-old Japanese woman with Crohn's disease were analyzed using scanning electron microscopy and energy dispersive X-ray spectroscopy. The enterolith showed a multilayered structure with fatty acid calcium and magnesium phosphate. The amount of calcium, magnesium, and phosphate decreased after they were immersed in a citric acid solution, suggesting a potential contribution of acidic aqueous solution to elute inorganic substances contained in calcified enteroliths. This is the first study to investigate the in vitro dissolubility of calcified enteroliths induced by citric acid solution.

1. Introduction

An enterolith is a mass found in the small or large intestine. False enteroliths are formed from indigestible substances trapped in the intestinal tract such as bezoars, gallstones, or foreign objects, whereas true enteroliths are formed from the precipitation of enteric contents [1, 2]. Formation of true enteroliths is generally caused by bowel stasis due to strictures or diverticula, followed by precipitation of inorganic substances or bile acids. Such precipitation of materials contained in intestinal juice is thought to be facilitated by an acid-base imbalance and bacterial overgrowth [3–8]. Most cases with enteroliths were asymptomatic and did not require specific treatment. In symptomatic cases with impacted enteroliths causing ileus or inflammation, endoscopic treatment such as dilation for the stricture of the bowel and fragmentation will be attempted in some cases [9]. If the enterolith is inaccessible via endoscopy devices or refractory for endoscopic treatment, surgical treatment is generally inevitable since enteroliths are unresponsive to medical treatment and successful chemical dissolution of enteroliths has never been reported.

Recently, we removed a calcified enterolith from a patient with Crohn's disease. This paper will discuss how we performed two basic studies to reveal the microstructure and dissolubility of the calcified enterolith by using citric acid solution.

2. Materials and Methods

2.1. Patient History. A 26-year-old Japanese woman presented with abdominal pain, fever, and watery diarrhea. The patient was diagnosed as having Turner syndrome at the age of six years and had been treated for Crohn's disease since the

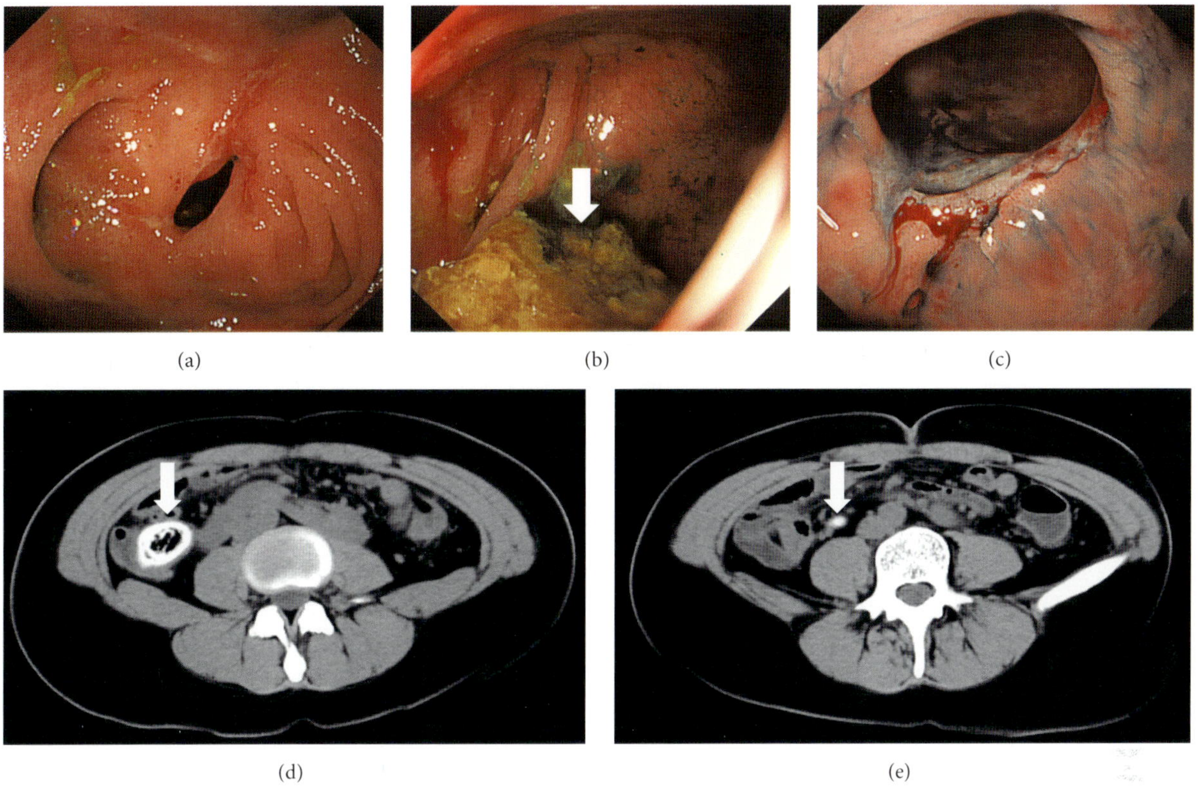

Figure 1: Endoscopic and radiologic images. Colonoscopy performed 15 months previously shows ulceration and stenosis (a) and a mass trapped in the semi-closed lumen in the cecum ((b), arrow). Another ulceration is observed in the anastomotic site (c). CT shows a calcified mass in the cecum ((d), arrow) and fecalomas within the appendix ((e), arrow).

age of 18 years. She underwent left hemicolectomy at the age of 20 years due to complete obstruction of the descending colon. Adalimumab was administered previously, but it was discontinued due to hair loss as a side effect of the drug. The patient had been treated with 10 mg/day of prednisone on admission. A colonoscopy performed 15 months prior to her admission revealed ulceration and stenosis of the cecum (Figure 1(a)). A mass that appeared to be feces was observed in the semi-closed lumen in the cecum (Figure 1(b)). Ulceration was also observed in the anastomotic site (Figure 1(c)). She had a bowel movement once every day. On admission, computed tomography scanning demonstrated a calcified mass that was impacted in the cecum (Figure 1(d)) and fecalomas within the appendix (Figure 1(e)). Laboratory testing revealed slightly elevated levels of C-reactive protein (0.36 mg/dL), whereas the white blood cell count was within the normal ranges (7070/μL). An ileocecal resection was performed under the diagnosis of impacted cecal enterolith. Although appendiceal wall thickening was not noted, infiltration of neutrophils within the mucosa and lymphocytes and eosinophils within the subserosa and adipose tissue were confirmed microscopically. Thus, the final diagnosis of an enterolith impacted in the cecum and acute appendicitis was made. Her abdominal pain, fever, and diarrhea disappeared after the surgery. Since inflammation was pathologically noted in the appendix, we speculate that the impacted cecal enterolith induced appendicitis.

2.2. Structure and Dissolubility Analysis of an Enterolith. Figure 2 shows the surgically removed enterolith of 3×2 cm in size (Figure 2(a)). Multiple-layered structures were seen in the cut surface, resembling annual rings of a tree (Figure 2(b)). The enterolith was cut into four pieces, and one piece was used in an infrared spectroscopy analysis. Infrared spectroscopy revealed that the enterolith was mainly composed of two components: fatty acid calcium and magnesium phosphate. Two enterolith pieces were placed in cell strainers with 40 μm pores (Corning Inc., Corning, NY, USA). The cell strainers were set in 50 mL conical polystyrene tubes. A citric acid solution was prepared by dissolving citric acid powder for food additives (Kenei Pharmaceutical Co., Osaka, Japan) in double-distilled water. One piece (Figure 3(a)) was completely immersed in double-distilled water, and the other (Figure 3(b)) was immersed in a 2% citric acid solution. After 120 hours of immersion at room temperature (25°C) without stirring, the enterolith pieces were removed from the cell strainers and air dried for 30 minutes. The color of the enterolith piece immersed in citric acid solution turned black in color and appeared to have shrunken (Figure 3(d)), compared with the piece immersed in water (Figure 3(c)). The percentage of lysis was calculated by comparing the weight of preimmersion with that of postimmersion. The weight was 1.717 g at preimmersion and 0.842 g at postimmersion in double-distilled water, indicating a 51.0% decrease in weight. Meanwhile, the weight changed from 1.330 g to 0.440 g after

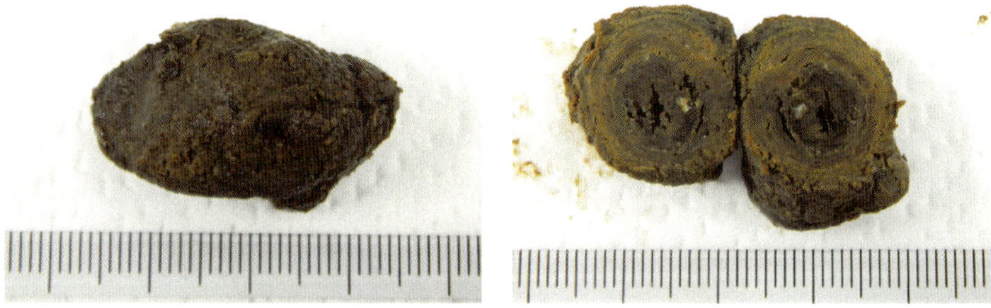

(a) (b)

Figure 2: Photographs of the enterolith. Enterolith of 3 × 2 cm in size was surgically removed (a). The cut surface shows a multilayered structure (b).

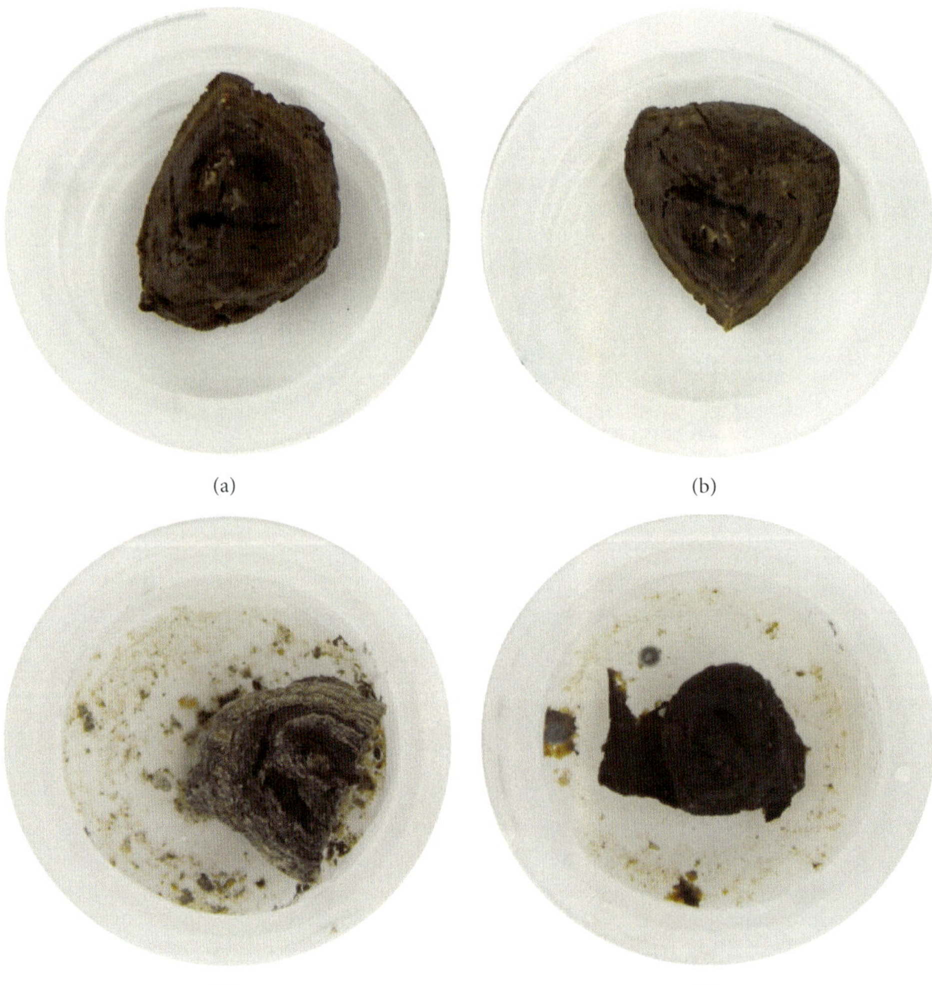

(a) (b) (c) (d)

Figure 3: Photographs of the enterolith pieces. A piece before immersing in double distilled water (a) and a piece before immersing in 2% citric acid solution (b). After 120 hours of immersion and 30 minutes of air-drying, the color of the enterolith piece immersed in citric acid solution turned to black and appeared to have shrunken (d), compared with the piece immersed in water (c).

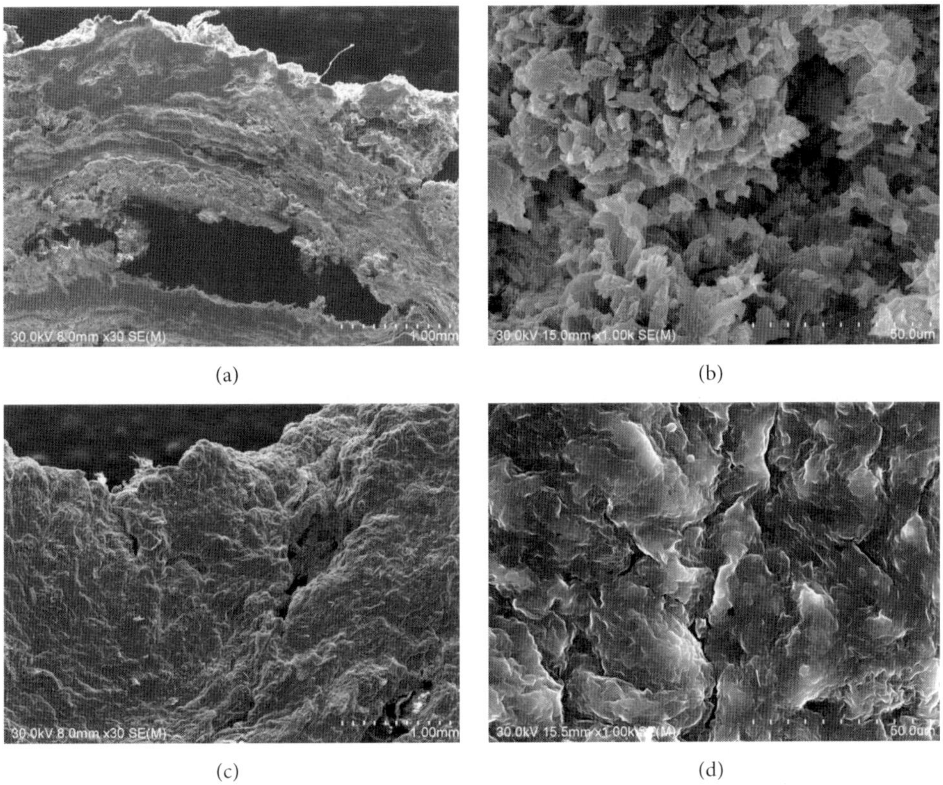

FIGURE 4: Scanning electron microscopy images. The enterolith piece immersed in water revealed a multilayered structure (a), containing crystalloid microparticles (b). In the enterolith piece immersed in citric acid solution, crystalloid microparticles were absent (c, d).

immersing in 2% citric acid solution, indicating a 66.9% decrease in weight.

Subsequently, we investigated the microstructure and elemental composition of the enterolith samples immersed in water and of those in the citric acid solution. We used S4800 scanning electron microscopy (Hitachi, Tokyo, Japan) and an EDAX Genesis APEX2 system (Ametek, Paoli, PA, USA). Elemental mapping of iron was also performed with S4800 scanning electron microscopy and EDAX Genesis APEX2 energy-dispersive X-ray spectroscopy. Scanning electron microscopy analysis of the enterolith piece immersed in water revealed a multilayered structure (Figure 4(a)), which was partly composed of crystalloid microparticles (Figure 4(b)). In the enterolith piece immersed in citric acid solution, crystalloid microparticles were absent (Figures 4(c) and 4(d)). Elemental mapping revealed that the enterolith piece immersed in water contained calcium (Figure 5(a)), magnesium (Figure 5(b)), and phosphate (Figure 5(c)). It was noteworthy that the magnesium and phosphate were deposited in approximately the same areas, whereas the calcium was deposited in different areas from magnesium and phosphate. A photograph merged with scanning electron microscopy image (Figure 5(d)) and mapping images of calcium and magnesium clearly showed that the enterolith piece was composed of two kinds of layers (Figure 5(e)). Spectra obtained with energy-dispersive X-ray spectroscopy showed that calcium, magnesium, and phosphate existed in the enterolith piece immersed in water (Figure 6(a)), whereas the amount of these elements was decreased in the piece immersed in citric acid solution (Figure 6(b)).

3. Discussion

This report focused on the microstructure and dissolution of an enterolith removed from a patient with Crohn's disease. True enteroliths are mainly subdivided into two types: bile acid enteroliths and calcified enteroliths [10]. Primary bile acids (i.e., cholic acid and chenodeoxycholic acid) are metabolized into secondary bile acids (i.e., deoxycholic acid and lithocholic acid) by anaerobic bacteria. These bile acids are relatively insoluble in the acidic milieu, leading to the formation of bile acid enteroliths in the proximal small bowel [7, 11–13]. Meanwhile, calcified enteroliths are reportedly composed of calcium phosphate, calcium oxalate, and calcium carbonate. These salts are insoluble in alkaline environments and thus can precipitate and form calcified enteroliths most often in the terminal ileum [4, 8, 10, 14]. As described previously, precipitation of substances is generally induced by bowel stasis followed by acid-base imbalance and bacterial overgrowth. Diverticular disease of the bowel is the most common etiology to lead enterolith formation, followed by stricture and narrowing of the intestine because of tuberculosis or Crohn's disease and postsurgical alteration of the alimentary tract [10]. The presented patient had a calcified enterolith in the cecum where stricture existed due to Crohn's disease. These features are in concordance with findings reported in earlier reports.

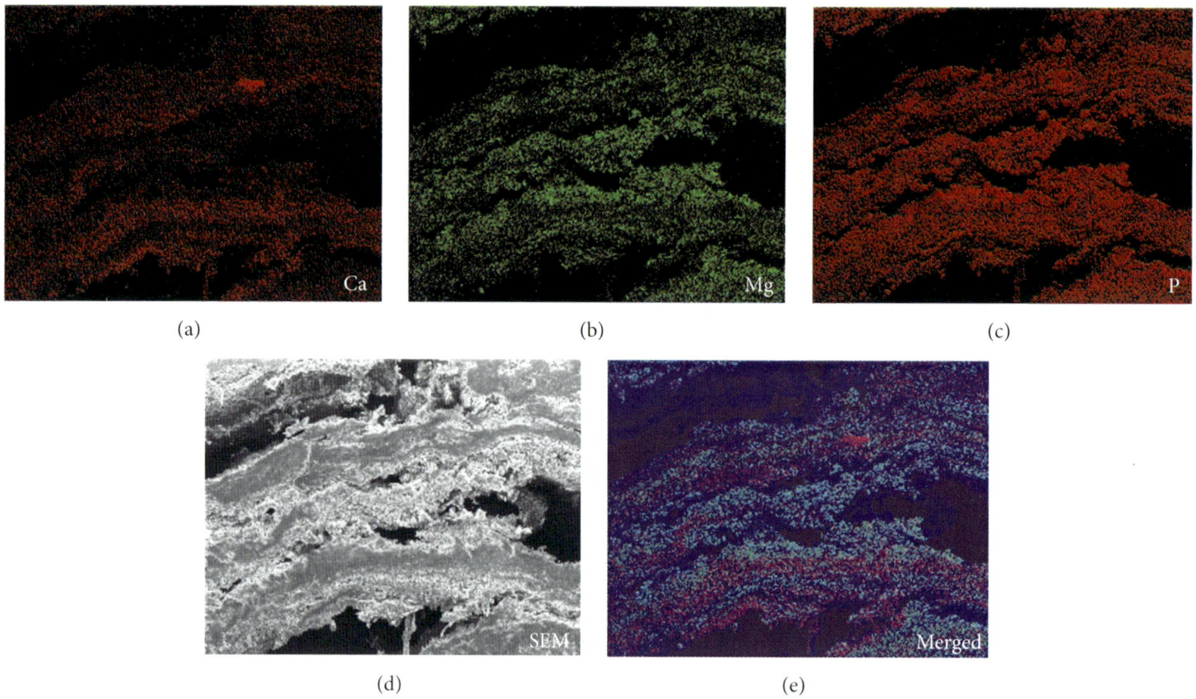

Figure 5: Elemental mapping images. The enterolith piece immersed in water contained calcium (a), magnesium (b), and phosphate (c). A photograph merged with a scanning electron microscopy image (d) and mapping images of calcium and magnesium showed that the enterolith piece was composed of two kinds of layers (e).

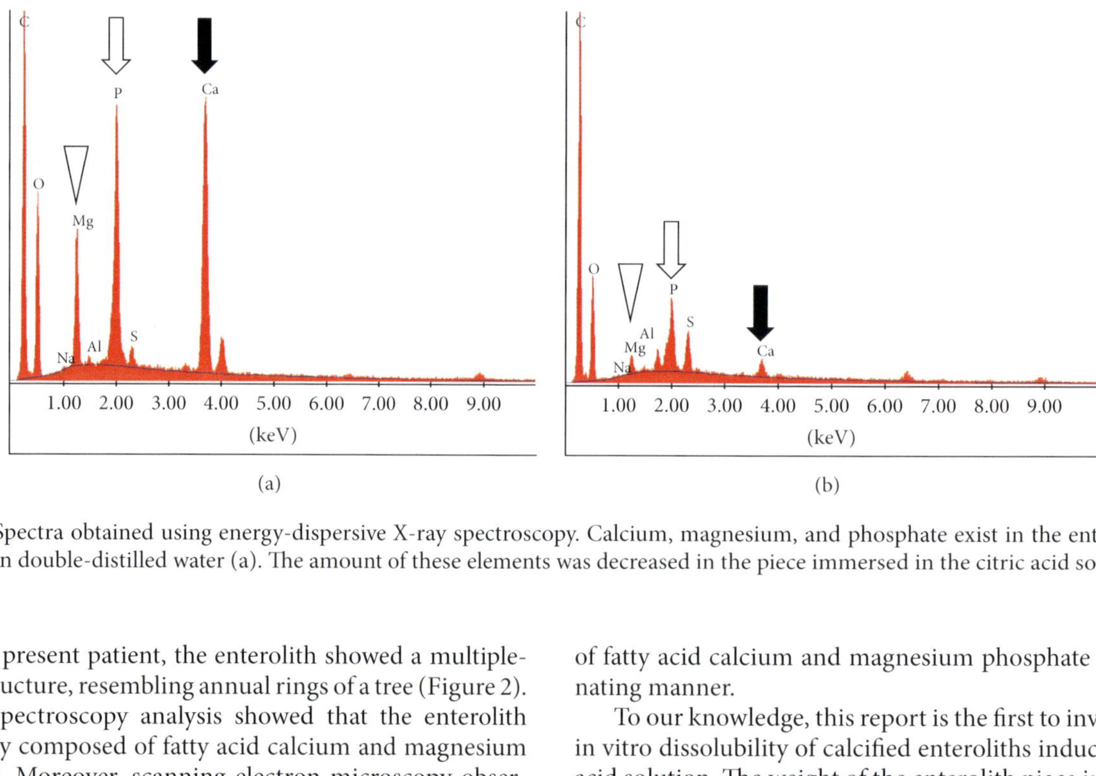

Figure 6: Spectra obtained using energy-dispersive X-ray spectroscopy. Calcium, magnesium, and phosphate exist in the enterolith piece immersed in double-distilled water (a). The amount of these elements was decreased in the piece immersed in the citric acid solution (b).

In the present patient, the enterolith showed a multiple-layered structure, resembling annual rings of a tree (Figure 2). Infrared spectroscopy analysis showed that the enterolith was mainly composed of fatty acid calcium and magnesium phosphate. Moreover, scanning electron microscopy observation of the enterolith piece immersed in water revealed that calcium-containing layers and magnesium phosphate-containing layers constitute the multilayered structure of the enterolith (Figure 5). Consequently, we speculate that the enterolith gradually increased diameter because of deposition of fatty acid calcium and magnesium phosphate in an alternating manner.

To our knowledge, this report is the first to investigate the in vitro dissolubility of calcified enteroliths induced by citric acid solution. The weight of the enterolith piece immersed in double-distilled water for 120 h showed a 51.0% decrease. We speculate that evaporation of water from the enterolith by air-drying is the main cause of the weight change, although some amount of substances might have been liquated from the cut surface into water. Meanwhile, the enterolith piece immersed in the 2% citric acid solution showed a 66.9% decrease in weight. Energy-dispersive X-ray spectroscopy revealed that the amount of calcium, magnesium, and phosphate was lower in the enterolith piece immersed in the citric acid solution, compared with that in water. These results suggest that calcium, magnesium, and phosphate were eluted by the citric acid solution. Moreover, based on the results obtained using energy-dispersive X-ray spectroscopy, we consider that crystalloid microparticles in the enterolith piece immersed in water (Figure 4(b)) were inorganic substances such as calcium, magnesium, and phosphate.

As described above, calcified enteroliths are considered to be formed in alkaline environments. An in vivo equine study revealed that horses with enteroliths had higher calcium, magnesium, phosphorus, and sulfur concentrations and higher pH in colonic contents than control horses [15, 16]. Conversely, calcified enteroliths may partly dissolve in lower pH, as shown in the present study. We also speculate that the residue that remained after immersion in the citric acid solution (Figure 3(d)) was organic substances, since the enterolith piece contained fatty acid and a higher amount of carbon was detected (Figure 6(b)).

This study has several limitations. First, because of the small size of the removed enterolith, only two pieces were used in the dissolution experiment. Therefore, statistical analysis was inapplicable to compare weight changes between the enterolith piece immersed in double-distilled water and that in citric acid solution. Second, the composition of calcified enteroliths is probably diverse in each patient [1, 17], so an acidic aqueous solution may not be useful in dissolving all calcified enteroliths. Lastly, because we examined dissolubility of enteroliths in vitro, further study is required prior to the introduction of a citric acid solution into clinical practice. For example, although a citric acid solution can be ingested in patients without intestinal obstruction, the degree of acidity or alkalinity will be altered under the influence of digestive juices such as gastric acid, bile acid, and a mucus-rich, bicarbonate-containing, alkaline juice produced by Brunner's glands. A possible approach is infusing acidic solution into the diseased bowel via an ileus tube or endoscopy. Investigations with regard to the utility and safety of a citric acid solution for the treatment of enteroliths in clinical settings are required as well.

In summary, we investigated the microstructure of the enterolith removed from the patient with Crohn's disease. This study revealed that inorganic substances constituting the enterolith were eluted and the weight of the enterolith piece was decreased after immersing it in a citric acid solution in vitro. We believe that an acidic aqueous solution has potential for the treatment of enteroliths.

References

[1] M. W. Jones, B. Koper, and W. F. Weatherhead, "Crohn's disease with enterolith treated laparoscopically.," *JSLS : Journal of the Society of Laparoendoscopic Surgeons / Society of Laparoendoscopic Surgeons*, vol. 9, no. 3, pp. 339–341, 2005.

[2] T. Monchal, E. Hornez, S. Bourgouin et al., "Enterolith ileus due to jejunal diverticulosis," *The American Journal of Surgery*, vol. 199, no. 4, pp. e45–e47, 2010.

[3] B. Kirshtein, Z. H. Perry, J. Klein, L. Laufer, and N. Sion-Vardi, "Giant enterolith in ileal diverticulum following ileoplastic bladder augmentation," *International Journal of Surgery Case Reports*, vol. 4, no. 4, pp. 385–387, 2013.

[4] A. Tewari, J. Weiden, and J.-O. Johnson, "Small-bowel obstruction associated with Crohn's enterolith," *Emergency Radiology*, vol. 20, no. 4, pp. 341–344, 2013.

[5] H.-C. Lai, "Intestinal obstruction due to meckel's enterolith," *Pediatrics and Neonatology*, vol. 51, no. 2, pp. 139-140, 2010.

[6] C. Cartanese, G. Campanella, E. Milano, and M. Saccò, "Enterolith causing acute afferent loop syndrome after Billroth ii gastrectomy: A case report," *Giornale di Chirurgia*, vol. 34, no. 5-6, pp. 164–166, 2013.

[7] C.-H. Liu, K.-W. Huang, Y.-H. Mo, and P.-M. Yang, "Enterolith ileus in a patient with jejunal diverticulosis: Sonographic findings," *Journal of Clinical Ultrasound*, vol. 35, no. 3, pp. 169–173, 2007.

[8] M. L. Paige, G. G. Ghahremani, and J. J. Brosnan, "Laminated radiopaque enteroliths: diagnostic clues to intestinal pathology," *American Journal of Gastroenterology*, vol. 82, no. 5, pp. 432–437, 1987.

[9] T. Nishikawa, T. Tsuyuguchi, H. Ohyama et al., "Endoscopy-guided laser lithotripsy for a difficult-to-crush enterolith," *Gastrointestinal Endoscopy*, vol. 80, no. 4, pp. 729-730, 2014.

[10] G. E. Gurvits and G. Lan, "Enterolithiasis," *World Journal of Gastroenterology*, vol. 20, no. 47, pp. 17819–17829, 2014.

[11] A. F. Hofmann and K. J. Mysels, "Bile acid solubility and precipitation in vitro and in vivo: The role of conjugation, pH, and Ca2+ ions," *Journal of Lipid Research*, vol. 33, no. 5, pp. 617–626, 1992.

[12] D. J. Garnet, L. Scalcione, A. Barkan, and D. S. Katz, "Enterolith ileus: Liberated large jejunal diverticulum enterolith causing small bowel obstruction in the setting of jejunal diverticulitis," *British Journal of Radiology*, vol. 84, no. 1004, pp. e154–e157, 2011.

[13] M. Iwamuro, Y. Miyashima, T. Yoshioka et al., "Ultrastructural analysis of an enterolith composed of Deoxycholic acid," *Acta Medica Okayama*, vol. 68, no. 6, pp. 369–374, 2014.

[14] J. G. Yuan, D. B. Sachar, K. Koganei, and A. J. Greenstein, "Enterolithiasis, refractory anemia, and strictures of crohn's disease," *Journal of Clinical Gastroenterology*, vol. 18, no. 2, pp. 105–108, 1994.

[15] D. M. Hassel, S. J. Spier, B. M. Aldridge, M. Watnick, R. A. Argenzio, and J. R. Snyder, "Influence of diet and water supply on mineral content and pH within the large intestine of horses with enterolithiasis," *Veterinary Journal*, vol. 182, no. 1, pp. 44–49, 2009.

[16] D. M. Hassel, P. C. Rakestraw, I. A. Gardner, S. J. Spier, and J. R. Snyder, "Dietary risk factors and colonic pH and mineral concentrations in horses with enterolithiasis," *Journal of Veterinary Internal Medicine*, vol. 18, no. 3, pp. 346–349, 2004.

[17] G. Yadav, S. Husain, R. Shukla, R. Patidar, and R. Luthra, "A Rare Case of Calcified Enterolith Presenting As Subacute Intestinal Obstruction," *Indian Journal of Surgery*, vol. 77, no. 4, pp. 327-328, 2015.

31

Deep Venous Thrombosis and Bilateral Pulmonary Embolism Revealing Silent Celiac Disease: Case Report and Review of the Literature

Igor Dumic,[1,2] Scott Martin,[3] Nadim Salfiti,[4] Robert Watson,[5] and Tamara Alempijevic[6,7]

[1]*Department of Hospital Medicine, Mayo Clinic Health System, Eau Claire, WI, USA*
[2]*Mayo Clinic College of Medicine and Science, Rochester, MN, USA*
[3]*Department of Pathology, Mayo Clinic Health System, Eau Claire, WI, USA*
[4]*Department of Gastroenterology and Hepatology, Mayo Clinic Health System, Eau Claire, WI, USA*
[5]*Department of Family Medicine, Mayo Clinic Health System, Eau Claire, WI, USA*
[6]*Department of Gastroenterology and Hepatology, Clinical Center of Serbia, Belgrade, Serbia*
[7]*School of Medicine, Belgrade University, Belgrade, Serbia*

Correspondence should be addressed to Igor Dumic; dumic.igor@mayo.edu

Academic Editor: Warwick S. Selby

Celiac disease (CD) is a systemic, chronic autoimmune disease that occurs in genetically predisposed individuals following dietary gluten exposure. CD can present with a wide range of gastrointestinal and extraintestinal manifestations and requires lifelong adherence to a gluten-free diet [GFD]. Venous thromboembolism (VTE) as a presentation of celiac disease is unusual and rarely reported. We present a case of a 46-year-old man who was admitted for shortness of breath and pleuritic chest pain and was found to have iron deficiency anemia, deep venous thrombosis, and bilateral pulmonary emboli (PE). After work-up for his anemia, the patient was diagnosed with CD. Comprehensive investigation for inherited or acquired prothrombotic disorders was negative. It is becoming increasingly recognized that CD is associated with an increased risk for VTE. PE, however, as a presentation of CD is exceedingly rare and to the best of our knowledge this is the third case report of such an occurrence and the only case report of a patient from North America. It is important to recognize that the first symptoms or signs of celiac disease might be extraintestinal. Furthermore, VTE as a presentation of CD is rare but life-threatening.

1. Introduction

Celiac disease (CD), or gluten sensitive enteropathy, is a common, systemic autoimmune disease that occurs in genetically predisposed individuals secondary to exposure to dietary protein gluten and requires lifelong dietary treatment [1]. The prevalence of celiac disease worldwide is about 1% with wide geographical variations. It affects about 0.3% of the population in Germany and up to 2.4% in Finland for reasons that are not completely understood [2, 3]. The classic form of CD manifests as a malabsorption syndrome associated with chronic diarrhea, mineral deficiencies, failure to thrive, and weight loss. Not all patients with celiac disease have these classic symptoms. In fact, many patients who suffer from celiac disease have only extraintestinal manifestations or even no symptoms at all; these forms are termed atypical and silent celiac disease, respectively [4].

Hematologic abnormalities are frequently found in CD patients, with iron deficiency anemia (IDA) being the most common. Apart from IDA, other hematologic abnormalities seen in patients with CD are thrombocytosis, splenic hypofunction, leukopenia, IgA deficiency, enteropathy-associated T cell lymphoma (EATL), and rarely venous thromboembolism (VTE), including deep venous thrombosis (DVT) and pulmonary embolism (PE). Osteoporosis, elevated transaminases, aphthous stomatitis, and chronic fatigue are other nonhematologic extra intestinal manifestations of CD [4–6]. PE has rarely been reported as a presentation of celiac disease [7, 8]. Here we report a case of pulmonary embolism that

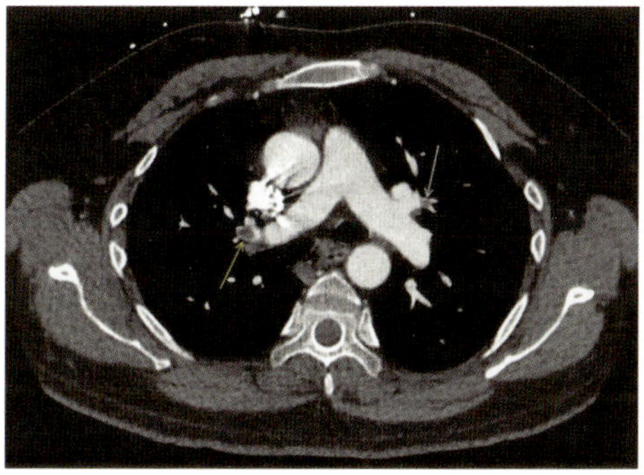

Figure 1: Axial CT image of the chest at the level of the main pulmonary artery bifurcation. Arrows denote two of the multiple pulmonary artery emboli (filling defects) which were observed bilaterally in this patient within both lobar and segmental pulmonary arteries.

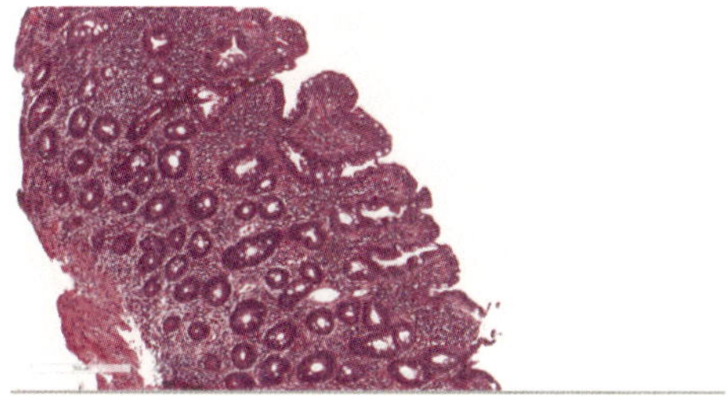

Figure 2: Duodenal biopsy demonstrating partial villous atrophy with crypt hyperplasia.

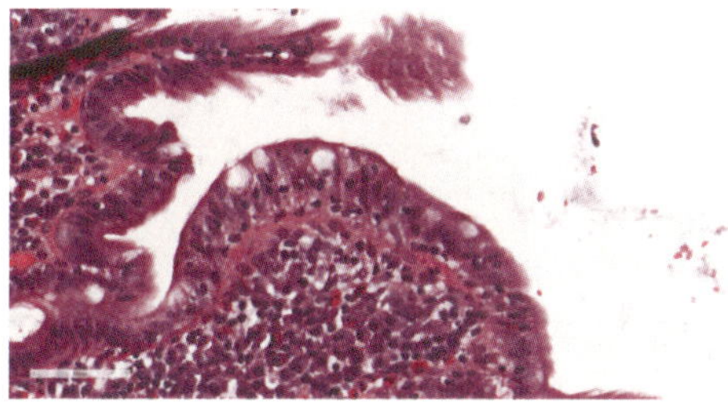

Figure 3: Higher power view highlighting a marked increase in intraepithelial lymphocytes.

was the presenting feature of celiac disease and review of the literature.

2. Case Presentation

A 48-year-old Caucasian man from Wisconsin, USA, was referred to our hospital for further evaluation of iron deficiency anemia, palpitations, dizziness, and right calf discomfort. His symptoms progressively developed over a period of two weeks before presentation. Apart from a history of intermittent heartburn relieved by calcium carbonate, he had no other major medical problems and was not on any prescription medications. He was not a smoker and did not drink alcohol or use any illicit drugs. He denied a previous history of malignancy or venous thromboembolism. His parents and siblings were healthy and there was no history of VTE in any first-degree relatives. He was complaining of mild dizziness and intermittent mild shortness of breath that started on the day of presentation. He denied any chest pain, syncope, bloody stools, or fevers.

Physical exam revealed a well appearing male in no distress. He was afebrile, normotensive, and tachycardic with a heart rate of 103 beats per minute. Laboratory studies showed severe iron deficiency anemia (Hgb: 91 g/dL, MCV: 60 fL, iron: 14 mcg/dL, iron saturation: 4%, TIBC: 369 mcg/dL, and ferritin: 7 mcg/dL). Other laboratory studies included WBC: 5.8, Plt: 269, and INR: 1.1. Fecal occult blood testing was negative. He had no microscopic hematuria and liver function tests were normal. Troponin I was undetectable.

Doppler of the right lower extremity showed extensive DVT, occlusive in the calf veins, popliteal and lower segments of right femoral vein and nonocclusive thrombosis in the mid and upper segments of the femoral vein. CT scan of the chest with IV contrast showed bilateral pulmonary emboli, greater on the right, most prominently seen within the distal right main pulmonary artery and to a lesser degree on the left within segmental and subsegmental branches (Figure 1). There was some flattening of the interventricular septum suggesting right heart strain. Echocardiogram was subsequently performed and demonstrated normal left ventricular ejection function, mild decrease in right ventricular ejection function, and no wall motion abnormalities. He received IV heparin initially and was transitioned to apixaban for long term anticoagulation. Extensive work-up for hypercoagulability revealed no abnormalities. It included Factor V Leiden, protein C and S levels, prothrombin mutation, antithrombin deficiency, antiphospholipid antibodies, and homocysteine levels. CT scan of abdomen and pelvis with and without IV contrast showed no masses suspicious for malignancy.

Serologic studies for celiac disease revealed positive and significantly elevated antibodies: anti-gliadin IgA (>150 units, normal range < 20 units), anti-gliadin IgG (81.5 units, normal range < 20 units), anti-tissue transglutaminase IgA (127.3 units, normal range < 15 units), anti-tissue transglutaminase IgG (60.1, normal range < 15 units), and positive IgA endomysial antibodies (1:80 titer). Celiac associated HLA-DQ typing revealed a permissive genotype with positive HLA-DQ2 and HLA-DQ8. Esophagogastroduodenoscopy (EGD) showed nearly complete absence of duodenal folds along with flattened duodenal mucosa. Biopsies were taken and histology showed partial villous atrophy (villous : crypt ratio 1:3) with crypt hyperplasia and a marked increase in intraepithelial lymphocytes (80 lymphocytes per 100 epithelial cells) consistent with celiac sprue, Marsh classification 3B (Figures 2 and 3). Colonoscopy showed normal mucosa throughout the colon. He was started on a gluten-free diet and was prescribed iron supplements for 3 months. For his pulmonary embolism, he has been placed on long term anticoagulation using apixaban. Three months following the diagnosis, his hemoglobin, iron, and ferritin levels have normalized. He continues to follow a gluten-free diet and has experienced no adverse effects from anticoagulation.

3. Discussion

The majority of patients with celiac disease present with typical symptoms such as chronic diarrhea, failure to thrive, and weight loss. However, atypical and silent forms of the disease are being increasingly recognized, most likely due to better diagnostics, increased screening, and increased awareness of atypical presentations. In its atypical form, symptoms and findings of celiac disease are predominantly extraintestinal, while in its silent form symptoms and signs are completely absent [1, 4].

The most common hematologic manifestations of celiac disease are iron deficiency and megaloblastic anemia. Thrombocytosis or thrombocytopenia, IgA deficiency, and hyposplenism have also been described. Rare manifestations include venous thromboembolism, dermatitis herpetiformis, gluten ataxia, and celiac crisis syndrome [4, 5, 25]. The most feared, but thankfully rare, complications of untreated CD are enteropathy-associated T cell lymphoma and small bowel adenocarcinoma [1]. The diagnosis of celiac disease requires a high index of suspicion followed by screening for IgA anti-tissue transglutaminase antibodies (unless the patient has selective IgA deficiency in which case IgG anti-tissue transglutaminase antibodies should be measured) and is confirmed by small bowel biopsy [1, 26]. The prevalence of anemia in patients with celiac disease is estimated to be up to 20% [27]. Iron deficiency anemia is explained by decreased absorption of iron which is not surprising since the majority of iron is reabsorbed in the duodenum. IDA refractory to iron supplementation in the absence of bleeding should raise concern for CD [28, 29]. Folic acid is reabsorbed in the jejunum and folic acid deficiency is common in CD. Anemia secondary to folic acid deficiency is usually macrocytic. However, due to frequent and concomitant presence of IDA in patients with CD, macrocytosis is unusual [4]. Megaloblastic anemia due to deficiency of vitamin B12 is rare as vitamin B12 is mostly absorbed in the terminal ileum, which is usually spared in CD [30].

Several studies have investigated the association between CD and VTE [31–34]. These studies have yielded different and conflicting results. A cross-sectional study by Miehsler et al. [31] did not show increased risk of VTE among patients with CD; however, this study likely had low power since it was primarily designed to investigate risk of VTE among patients with inflammatory bowel disease, not CD. Two retrospective cohort studies by Ramagopalan et al. [32] and Zöller et al. [33] both showed statistically significant increased risk of VTE in patients with autoimmune disease, including celiac disease. A case control study from Denmark by Johannesdottir et al. [34] found significant risk of VTE only within 90 days from the diagnosis of celiac disease. Ludvigsson et al. [35] found a modest increase in risk of VTE in patients with celiac disease but that was restricted to individuals that were diagnosed in adulthood. They explained their findings based on a combination of surveillance bias and chronic inflammation. In an effort to summarize data and further investigate a potential association between celiac disease and the risk for VTE Ungprasert and colleagues from Mayo Clinic [36] conducted a meta-analysis that demonstrated significantly increased risk of VTE in patients with CD.

Over the last 30 years several case reports have been published suggesting a connection between CD and an increased risk of thrombosis and thromboembolism. We performed a literature search using PubMed for full articles, case reports, and case series published in English, involving adult patients, and using the following keywords, alone and in combination: "celiac disease", "coeliac disease", "gluten sensitive enteropathy", "venous thromboembolism", "deep venous thrombosis", "pulmonary embolism", "thromboembolism and celiac disease", and "thrombosis and celiac disease". Additionally, we added relevant studies and case reports from the reference list of selected articles. Cases without biopsy proven celiac disease were excluded. Our search yielded 19 cases (Table 1).

As we can see from Table 1 the most commonly reported location of thrombosis is in the hepatic veins (6/19) followed by DVT (5/19). Mesenteric vein thrombosis, portal vein thrombosis, and PE were reported in 3 cases each. Splenic vein thrombosis was reported in one case. Unusual places of thrombosis have been described such as LV thrombus in one case, central retinal vein thrombosis in one case, and two cases of cerebral vein thrombosis [7–24]. Among reported cases, patient median age was 33.1 years (range 18–53), with the majority of patients in the 4th decade of life (8/19). Of reported cases, 57% (11/19) were female patients. Most of the cases were reported from North Africa and the Middle East (9/19). The only case described from North America had central retinal vein thrombosis associated with celiac disease [14]

Three cases of pulmonary embolism have been described [7–9]. Interestingly, in the first case [9] the patient had celiac disease complicated by mesenteric vein thrombosis requiring surgery for mesenteric ischemia. Pulmonary embolism developed postoperatively; hence, CD alone cannot be solely responsible for the VTE and possibly perioperative risk was a contributing factor. The other two cases [7, 8] had elevated homocysteine levels, unlike in our patient, so it might be that hyperhomocysteinemia was the primary risk factor for VTE. Our patient interestingly did not have any of the traditionally recognized risk factors for VTE including elevated homocysteine level. In our case we argue that severe inflammation associated with celiac disease and evident by markedly elevated antibodies and biopsy findings were responsible for a procoagulant state and development of thrombosis.

DVT in patients with celiac disease has been described in 5 cases [7, 8, 18, 19, 22]. As mentioned above, in two of those cases the patients had elevated homocysteine levels; one case was associated with protein S deficiency; and in two cases [19, 22] similar to our case there were no other identifiable risk factors for thromboembolism apart from celiac disease. In 13 of 19 reported cases thromboses preceded the diagnosis of celiac disease and only in 7 of 19 cases did the patients present with classic symptoms of celiac disease. These are consistent with the previous statements suggesting that a significant number of patients with celiac disease have atypical or silent forms of the disease.

The mechanism by which celiac disease increases the risk of venous thromboembolism is unclear. However, several theories have been proposed:

(i) *Elevated homocysteine levels* secondary to folic acid deficiency due to malabsorption seen in celiac disease [37].

TABLE 1: Summary of published case reports on thrombosis associated with celiac disease.

Case [ref]	Year of publication	Age	Sex	Country	Site of thrombosis	Admission Hgb	Admission MCV	Admission Plt	GI symptoms on admission	Thrombosis risk factors	Order of occurrence	Comment	Treatment	Outcome
1 [9]	1987	37	F	UK	Mesenteric vein, PE	n/a	n/a	654	Yes	Surgery	Thrombosis first	IgA deficiency + RF	GFD	Improved, without recurrence
2 [10]	1994	26	F	Algeria	Hepatic vein	126	85	153	Yes	None	CD first	Noncompliant with GFD	GFD	Lost in follow-up
3 [10]	1994	40	F	Algeria	Hepatic vein, PVT	120	69	450	Yes	OCP use, MPD	Thrombosis first	Interruption of GFD followed by thrombosis	GFD Long term Warfarin	Thrombosis reoccurred after stopping GFD despite anticoagulation
4 [11]	1995	46	F	Algeria	Hepatic vein, PVT	105	107	300	No	MPD	Thrombosis first	Low levels of folic acid and vit B12	GFD	Improved
5 [7]	1999	35	M	Australia	DVT, PE	n/a	n/a	n/a	No	Elevated homocysteine level, MTHFR mutation	Thrombosis first	Low folic acid	GFD Heparin Warfarin Folic acid	n/a Plan to stop warfarin if homocysteine level normalizes
6 [12]	2002	33	M	Israel	LV thrombus	10	71	n/a	Yes	Elevated homocysteine level, low folic acid level	Thrombosis first	Recurrent strokes in the setting of LV thrombus	GFD Warfarin Folic acid	Improved
7 [8]	2003	53	M	Italy	DVT, PE	108	n/a	n/a	No	Elevated homocysteine level, low folic acid level	Thrombosis first	Before DVT multiple prior episodes of thrombophlebitis	GFD Warfarin for 3 months	No recurrence in 1-year follow-up
8 [13]	2003	19	M	Spain	Hepatic vein	142	n/a	158	Yes	None	Thrombosis first	Had significant ascites, low folic acid	GFD Warfarin	No recurrence in 2-year follow-up
9 [14]	2005	33	F	USA	Central retinal vein	n/a	n/a	n/a	No	Pregnancy dehydration	CD first	Postpartum	Clopidogrel	n/a

Table 1: Continued.

Case [ref]	Year of publication	Age	Sex	Country	Site of thrombosis	Admission Hgb	MCV	Plt	GI symptoms on admission	Thrombosis risk factors	Order of occurrence	Comment	Treatment	Outcome
10 [15]	2006	40	M	UK	Mesenteric veins	n/a	n/a	481	Yes	Protein S deficiency	CD first	Coexisting Crohn's disease	GFD	Improved
11 [16]	2006	30	F	Saudi Arabia	SMV, PVT, splenic vein thrombosis	73	n/a	518	No	Elevated homocysteine level	Thrombosis first	Failed iron supplementation	GFD Heparin Warfarin	Improved in 6 months' follow-up
12 [17]	2008	39	F	India	Splenic vein	11	n/a	170	No	Elevated homocysteine level	Thrombosis first	n/a	GFD LMWH	Improved in 6 months' follow-up
13 [18]	2009	18	M	Tunisia	DVT	135	n/a	440	No	Protein S deficiency	Thrombosis first	Significant weight gain with GFD	GFD Warfarin	Improved, symptom-free 4 years after diagnosis
14 [19]	2009	44	M	Turkey	DVT	11.7	n/a	n/a	Yes	None	CD first	n/a	LMWH Warfarin	Improvement
15 [20]	2009	19	M	India	Hepatic vein	6	n/a	175	No	Protein C and S deficiency	Thrombosis first	N/a	LMWH Warfarin	Improvement in 10 months' follow-up
16 [21]	2010	26	F	UK	Cerebral vein thrombosis	n/a	n/a	n/a	No	None	CD first	Lane Hamilton syndrome	UFH	Improvement
17 [22]	2012	30	F	Iraq	DVT	5	n/a	950	No	None	Thrombosis first	n/a	GFD Warfarin	Improvement
18 [23]	2016	27	F	Jordan	Hepatic vein	n/a	n/a	145	No	None	CD first	Thrombosis occurred despite compliance with GFD	Warfarin portocaval shunt for ascites	Improved
19 [24]	2017	35	F	Tunisia	Cerebral vein thrombosis	9.4	n/a	n/a	No	OCP use	Thrombosis first	Recurrent cerebral vein thrombosis upon cessation of AC	Warfarin	Improvement

Hgb: hemoglobin (g/L), MCV: mean corpuscular volume, PLT: platelets (10^9/L), CD: celiac disease, DVT: deep venous thrombosis, OCP: oral contraceptive, GFD: gluten-free diet, PVT: portal vein thrombosis, AC: anticoagulation, SMV: superior mesenteric vein, LV: left ventricle, LMWH: low molecular weight heparin, and MTHFR: methyl-tetrahydrofolate reductase.

Saibeni et al. showed that the degree of intestinal injury correlates with homocysteine levels. However, this does not apply to our patient who had normal folic acid and homocysteine levels

(ii) *Elevated levels of thrombin-activatable fibrinolysis inhibitor (TAFI)* [38]

(iii) *Ongoing inflammation and provocative effect of inflammatory cytokines* secondary to the autoimmune nature of CD. It would be similar to other autoimmune diseases with well recognized increased risk for thrombosis (such as Crohn's disease and ulcerative colitis) [31]

(iv) *Protein C and S deficiency* secondary to vitamin K malabsorption [39]

(v) *Thrombocytosis leading to hyperviscosity of the blood* [9]. Thrombocytosis in celiac disease is likely secondary to IDA and/or hyposplenism. However, it cannot be solely responsible since not all patients with celiac disease have thrombocytosis. In reviewing the literature only 4 out of 12 patients who had a reported platelet value on admission had thrombocytosis

(vi) *Hyperviscosity secondary to high levels of circulating antibodies* including antiphospholipid antibodies [40]

(vii) *Genetic/environmental causes* since the majority of initial case reports were from North Africa and the Middle East (9 out of 19) [10, 23].

Extensive hypercoagulability work-up including screening for congenital or acquired prothrombotic disorders as well as malignancy in our patient failed to reveal any hypercoagulable disorders. Similarly, reviewing available cases published so far, only 6 cases out of 19 published had no other identifiable risk factor apart from celiac disease.

While there are clear guidelines on how to treat first and recurrent episodes of venous thromboembolism in the setting of provoked or idiopathic VTE, there are no guidelines for how long patients with celiac disease who develop VTE should be anticoagulated. Should we consider celiac disease a provoking factor that will disappear once GFD is started?

The majority of cases were treated with anticoagulation and all with GFD. However, duration of anticoagulation was not specified in many cases and greatly varied among those reported. For patients with recurrent thrombosis (cases 3, 19) lifelong warfarin was given. Cases with thrombosis despite GFD suggest that just GFD is not enough to completely eliminate the risk of thrombosis [23]. It is further supported by the study of Lee et al., who showed that the intestinal mucosa does not recover completely and inflammation does not completely resolve despite strict GFD up to 2 years following the diagnosis [41]. Interestingly, in one case [10] thrombosis reoccurred after stopping GFD despite anticoagulation which exemplifies the severity of inflammation in patients with CD who do not adhere to a gluten-free diet. Some authors suggest stopping anticoagulation once homocysteine levels return to normal [7]. It seems like a plausible solution in those cases where there is documented hyperhomocysteinemia, which might be a direct cause of VTE. However, in cases like ours, when levels of homocysteine are normal, it cannot be applied. Furthermore, the clinical trial by Den Heijer et al. [42] showed that homocysteine lowering by vitamin B and folic acid supplementation had no protective effect on the development of VTE.

We decided to anticoagulate our patient for 6 months using the direct oral anticoagulant apixaban, which has not been used before in this setting. We consider untreated celiac disease to be a provoking risk factor. We believe that even when adhering to a gluten-free diet, the inflammation and risk for VTE will not completely disappear; hence, following completion of anticoagulation we are planning on starting long term aspirin 81 mg daily. Should he experience recurrent DVT, he would need lifelong anticoagulation. At this moment it remains unclear whether we should use aspirin to prevent thrombotic complications in patients who are diagnosed with celiac disease, or at least shortly after the initial diagnosis when risk of VTE appears to be at its highest.

4. Conclusion

Here, we present a patient who developed extensive DVT and bilateral PE in the setting of untreated, silent celiac disease. Additionally, we summarized all similar case reports and reviewed the available literature on this topic. Due to better appreciation for atypical presentations of both celiac disease and venous thromboembolism, we expect that we will see more of these cases in the future. We will need more studies to determine the optimal duration of anticoagulation and more studies to determine the degree of VTE risk elevation in patients with CD.

References

[1] A. Fasano and C. Catassi, "Clinical practice. Celiac disease," *The New England Journal of Medicine*, vol. 367, no. 25, pp. 2419–2426, 2012.

[2] A. Fasano, I. Berti, T. Gerarduzzi et al., "Prevalence of Celiac disease in at-risk and not-at-risk groups in the United States: a large multicenter study," *Archives of Internal Medicine*, vol. 163, no. 3, pp. 286–292, 2003.

[3] K. Mustalahti, C. Catassi, A. Reunanen et al., "The prevalence of celiac disease in Europe: results of a centralized, international mass screening project," *Annals of Medicine*, vol. 42, no. 8, pp. 587–595, 2010.

[4] T. R. Halfdanarson, M. R. Litzow, and J. A. Murray, "Hematologic manifestations of celiac disease," *Blood*, vol. 109, no. 2, pp. 412–421, 2007.

[5] A. Baydoun, J. E. Maakaron, H. Halawi, J. Abou Rahal, and A. T. Taher, "Hematological manifestations of celiac disease," *Scandinavian Journal of Gastroenterology*, vol. 47, no. 12, pp. 1401–1411, 2012.

[6] P. H. R. Green and B. Jabri, "Coeliac disease," *The Lancet*, vol. 362, no. 9381, pp. 383–391, 2003.

[7] A. P. Grigg, "Deep venous thrombosis as the presenting feature in a patient with coeliac disease and homocysteinaemia," *Australian and New Zealand Journal of Medicine*, vol. 29, no. 4, pp. 566-567, 1999.

[8] M. Gabrielli, A. Santoliquido, G. Gasbarrini, P. Pola, and A. Gasbarrini, "Latent coeliac disease, hyperhomocysteinemia and

pulmonary thromboembolism: a close link?" *Thrombosis and Haemostasis*, vol. 89, no. 1, pp. 203-204, 2003.

[9] R. Upadhyay, R. H. Park, R. I. Russell, B. J. Danesh, and F. D. Lee, "Acute mesenteric ischaemia: a presenting feature of coeliac disease?" *British Medical Journal*, vol. 295, no. 6604, pp. 958-959, 1987.

[10] P. Marteau, J.-F. Cadranel, B. Messing, D. Gargot, D. Valla, and J.-C. Rambaud, "Association of hepatic vein obstruction and coeliac disease in North African subjects," *Journal of Hepatology*, vol. 20, no. 5, pp. 650–653, 1994.

[11] T. Zenjari, A. Boruchowicz, P. Desreumaux et al., "Association of coeliac disease and portal venous thrombosis," *Gastroentérologie Clinique et Biologique*, vol. 19, no. 11, pp. 953-954, 1995.

[12] D. Gefel, M. Doncheva, E. Ben-Valid et al., "Recurrent stroke in a young patient with celiac disease and hyperhomocysteinemia," *The Israel Medical Association Journal*, vol. 4, no. 3, pp. 222-223, 2002.

[13] F. Martínez, M. Berenguer, M. Prieto, H. Montes, M. Rayón, and J. Berenguer, "Budd-Chiari syndrome caused by membranous obstruction of the inferior vena cava associated with coeliac disease," *Digestive and Liver Disease*, vol. 36, no. 2, pp. 157–162, 2004.

[14] E. S. Lee and J. S. Pulido, "Nonischemic central retinal vein occlusion associated with celiac disease," *Mayo Clinic Proceedings*, vol. 80, no. 2, p. 157, 2005.

[15] A. McNeill, F. Duthie, and D. J. Galloway, "Small bowel infarction in a patient with coeliac disease," *Journal of Clinical Pathology*, vol. 59, no. 2, pp. 216–218, 2006.

[16] N. Ali Azzam, H. Al Ashgar, M. Dababo, N. Al Kahtani, and M. Shahid, "Mesentric vein thrombosis as a presentation of subclinical celiac disease," *Annals of Saudi Medicine*, vol. 26, no. 6, pp. 471–473, 2006.

[17] S. Khanna, D. Chaudhary, and P. Kumar, "Occult celiac disease presenting as splenic vein thrombosis," *Indian Journal of Gastroenterology*, vol. 27, no. 1, pp. 38-39, 2008.

[18] L. Kallel, S. Matri, S. Karoui, M. Fekih, J. Boubaker, and A. Filali, "Deep venous thrombosis related to protein s deficiency revealing celiac disease," *American Journal of Gastroenterology*, vol. 104, no. 1, pp. 256-257, 2009.

[19] E. Beyan, M. Pamukcuoglu, and C. Beyan, "Deep vein thrombosis associated with celiac disease," *Bratislavske Lekarske Listy*, vol. 110, no. 4, pp. 263-264, 2009.

[20] R. Kochhar, I. Masoodi, U. Dutta et al., "Celiac disease and Budd Chiari syndrome: Report of a case with review of literature," *European Journal of Gastroenterology & Hepatology*, vol. 21, no. 9, pp. 1092–1094, 2009.

[21] P. J. Grover, R. Jayaram, and H. Madder, "Management of cerebral venous thrombosis in a patient with Lane-Hamilton syndrome and coeliac disease, epilepsy and cerebral calcification syndrome," *British Journal of Neurosurgery*, vol. 24, no. 6, pp. 684-685, 2010.

[22] Z. T. Mezalek, B. A. Habiba, H. Hicham et al., "C0396 Venous thrombosis revealing celiac disease. Three cases," *Thrombosis Research*, vol. 130, pp. S154–S155, 2012.

[23] R. Beyrouti, M. Mansour, A. Kacem, H. Derbali, and R. Mrissa, "Recurrent cerebral venous thrombosis revealing celiac disease: an exceptional case report," *Acta Neurologica Belgica*, vol. 117, no. 1, pp. 341–343, 2017.

[24] K. A. Jadallah, E. W. Sarsak, Y. M. Khazaleh, and R. M. Barakat, "Budd-Chiari syndrome associated with coeliac disease: case report and literature review," *Gastroenterology Report*, gow030, 2016.

[25] M. Hadjivassiliou, D. S. Sanders, N. Woodroofe, C. Williamson, and R. A. Grünewald, "Gluten ataxia," *The Cerebellum*, vol. 7, no. 3, pp. 494–498, 2008.

[26] T. T. Salmi, P. Collin, I. R. Korponay-Szabó et al., "Endomysial antibody-negative coeliac disease: clinical characteristics and intestinal autoantibody deposits," *Gut*, vol. 55, no. 12, pp. 1746–1753, 2006.

[27] J. W. Harper, S. F. Holleran, R. Ramakrishnan, G. Bhagat, and P. H. R. Green, "Anemia in celiac disease is multifactorial in etiology," *American Journal of Hematology*, vol. 82, no. 11, pp. 996–1000, 2007.

[28] B. Annibale, C. Severi, A. Chistolini et al., "Efficacy of gluten-free diet alone on recovery from iron deficiency anemia in adult celiac patients," *American Journal of Gastroenterology*, vol. 96, no. 1, pp. 132–137, 2001.

[29] C. Hershko and J. Patz, "Ironing out the mechanism of anemia in celiac disease," *Haematologica*, vol. 93, no. 12, pp. 1761–1765, 2008.

[30] A. Dahele and S. Ghosh, "Vitamin B12 deficiency in untreated celiac disease," *American Journal of Gastroenterology*, vol. 96, no. 3, pp. 745–750, 2001.

[31] W. Miehsler, W. Reinisch, E. Valic et al., "Is inflammatory bowel disease an independent and disease specific risk factor for thromboembolism?" *Gut*, vol. 53, no. 4, pp. 542–548, 2004.

[32] S. V. Ramagopalan, C. J. Wotton, A. E. Handel, D. Yeates, and M. J. Goldacre, "Risk of venous thromboembolism in people admitted to hospital with selected immune-mediated diseases: record-linkage study," *BMC Medicine*, vol. 9, article 1, 2011.

[33] B. Zöller, X. Li, J. Sundquist, and K. Sundquist, "Risk of pulmonary embolism in patients with autoimmune disorders: A nationwide follow-up study from Sweden," *The Lancet*, vol. 379, no. 9812, pp. 244–249, 2012.

[34] S. A. Johannesdottir, R. Erichsen, E. Horváth-Puhó, M. Schmidt, and H. T. Sørensen, "Coeliac disease and risk of venous thromboembolism: A nationwide population-based case-control study," *British Journal of Haematology*, vol. 157, no. 4, pp. 499–501, 2012.

[35] J. F. Ludvigsson, A. Welander, R. Lassila, A. Ekbom, and S. M. Montgomery, "Risk of thromboembolism in 14,000 individuals with coeliac disease," *British Journal of Haematology*, vol. 139, no. 1, pp. 121–127, 2007.

[36] P. Ungprasert, K. Wijarnpreecha, and P. Tanratana, "Risk of venous thromboembolism in patients with celiac disease: A systematic review and meta-analysis," *Journal of Gastroenterology and Hepatology*, vol. 31, no. 7, pp. 1240–1245, 2016.

[37] S. Saibeni, A. Lecchi, G. Meucci et al., "Prevalence of hyperhomocysteinemia in adult gluten-sensitive enteropathy at diagnosis: Role of B12, folate, and genetics," *Clinical Gastroenterology and Hepatology*, vol. 3, no. 6, pp. 574–580, 2005.

[38] N. H. van Tilburg, F. R. Rosendaal, and R. M. Bertina, "Thrombin activatable fibrinolysis inhibitor and the risk for deep vein thrombosis," *Blood*, vol. 95, no. 9, pp. 2855–2859, 2000.

[39] D. Thorburn, A. J. Stanley, A. Foulis, and R. Campbell Tait, "Coeliac disease presenting as variceal haemorrhage," *Gut*, vol. 52, no. 5, p. 758, 2003.

[40] A. Lerner, N. Agmon-Levin, Y. Shapira et al., "The thrombophilic network of autoantibodies in celiac disease," *BMC Medicine*, vol. 11, no. 1, article 89, 2013.

[41] S. K. Lee, W. Lo, L. Memeo, H. Rotterdam, and P. H. R. Green, "Duodenal histology in patients with celiac disease after treatment with a gluten-free diet," *Gastrointestinal Endoscopy*, vol. 57, no. 2, pp. 187–191, 2003.

[42] M. Den Heijer, H. P. J. Willems, H. J. Blom et al., "Homocysteine lowering by B vitamins and the secondary prevention of deep vein thrombosis and pulmonary embolism: A randomized, placebo-controlled, double-blind trial," *Blood*, vol. 109, no. 1, pp. 139–144, 2007.

32

Yogi Detox Tea: A Potential Cause of Acute Liver Failure

Keerthana Kesavarapu,[1] Mitchell Kang,[1] Jaewook James Shin,[2] and Kenneth Rothstein[3,4]

[1] *Department of Internal Medicine, Drexel University Hospital, Philadelphia, PA, USA*
[2] *Drexel School of Medicine, Philadelphia, PA, USA*
[3] *Department of Gastroenterology, Drexel University Hospital, Philadelphia, PA, USA*
[4] *Department of Hepatology, Drexel University Hospital, Philadelphia, PA, USA*

Correspondence should be addressed to Keerthana Kesavarapu; kkesavarapu@gmail.com

Academic Editor: Hideto Kawaratani

We present a case of acute fulminant liver failure from a liver detoxification tea. We present a 60-year-old female with weakness, lethargy, scleral icterus, jaundice, and worsening mental status. She drank herbal tea three times a day for 14 days prior to symptom development. Liver tests were elevated. Remaining laboratory tests and imaging were negative for other etiologies. An ultrasound-guided liver biopsy showed submassive necrosis. A literature search on the ingredients shows six ingredients as having hepatotoxic effects and remaining ingredients as having very sparse hepatoprotective data. Healthcare professionals should discuss herbal medication and tea use and report adverse effects.

1. Introduction

The American Association for the Study of Liver Diseases (AASLD) defines acute fulminant liver failure as an acute deterioration of function resulting in altered mentation and coagulopathy without any known preexisting disease [1]. In 308 patients from 17 tertiary care centers participating in US Acute Liver Failure Study Group, drug reactions including acetaminophen overdose were the presumptive cause in 52% of cases [2]. Prevalent medication offenders include acetaminophen, mushrooms, and antiepileptics (phenytoin and valproic acid); however herbal supplement induced hepatotoxicity is gaining prevalence. According to the Drug-Induced Liver Injury Network (DILIN), causes of acute liver failure (ALF) from herbal supplements have increased from 7% to 20% over their study period from 2007 to 2013 [3]. This number is probably a gross underestimation as patients do not report use to their physicians and physicians do not report side effects to the Food and Drug Association (FDA) and might not be identified by DILIN. Here we report a case of ALF after the use of an herbal detoxification tea marketed to be hepatoprotective.

2. Case Report

A 60-year-old female with past medical history of hypertension presented with new-onset generalized weakness and lethargy worsening over the past two weeks. She denied any fevers, chills, changes in stool, changes in mental status, sick contacts, or recent travel. Her past medical history was significantly only for obesity. Her social history included no tobacco use, frequent alcohol consumption (3 glasses of wine every night), no IV drug use, no acetaminophen use, and no high risk sexual activity. Her alcohol use has been stable since she started drinking ten years ago. Previous laboratory testing showed normal liver function. She was fully vaccinated with no history of hepatitis. Her only home medication was hydrochlorothiazide, which she had been taking for years. She had no preexisting liver disease with normal liver function tests prior to this admission. She reported drinking Yogi Detox herbal tea three times a day for 14 days prior to symptom development. As per the patient, she was consuming this tea as a cleanse.

Physical examination demonstrated a normotensive and afebrile patient in mild distress. the patient was jaundiced

Table 1: Hepatic function panel on day of admission, 1 week and 2 weeks later.

Laboratory testing	On admission	1 week	2 weeks
Aspartate aminotransferase (5–35 U/L)	450	1864	51
Alanine aminotransferase (4–35 U/L)	583	2162	82
Alkaline phosphatase (30–99 U/L)	202	143	72
Total bilirubin (0.2–1.2 mg/dl)	27	43	30
Direct bilirubin (0.01–0.19 mg/dl)	20	33	21
INR (0.9–1.2)	4	2.7	7.8

Table 2: Roussel Uclaf Causality Assessment Method, an assessment of the causality of drug-induced liver injury.

Items for mixed liver injury	Score in our patient
Time to onset from cessation of drug/herb: <15 days	+2
Course of ALT after cessation of drug/herb: decrease ≥ 50% within 180 days	+2
Risk factors: alcohol use (>2 drinks/d for women) and Age ≥ 55	+1
Concomitant drug/herbs: none	0
Alternative causes: all causes ruled out	+2
Previous hepatotoxicity of the drug/herb: reaction published but unlabeled	+1
Response to unintentional reexposure: none	0
Total score	8

with scleral icterus. Examination demonstrated a soft and nondistended abdomen with moderate right upper quadrant tenderness. Mental status was intact on admission; however, on the ninth day of the admission she became lethargic and developed asterixis. Initial laboratory tests are depicted in Table 1. Radiological examinations performed consisted of an abdominal ultrasound with Doppler's and triple-phase computerized tomography (CT) with contrast of the abdomen, which were normal. Extensive laboratory testing was ordered to determine the etiology of her liver failure. Serological markers including those for autoimmune hepatitis (Anti-KLM antibodies, ANA, and AMA), viral hepatitis (A, B, C, and D), Wilson's disease (ceruloplasmin), and alpha-1-antitrypsin deficiency were analyzed and found to be negative. In addition, CMV, EBV, VZV, and HSV were negative. HEV testing was not performed as there is no approved test in the United States [4].

There was concern that the cause of her liver injury might have been due to her Yogi detox herbal tea consumption. Using the 2016 Roussel Uclaf Causality Assessment Method (RUCAM) score as highlighted in Table 2, the relationship between this herbal tea and liver injury was determined [26].

The *R* ratio, which is the initial step in the RUCAM assessment, was 8.16 indicating a hepatocellular pattern of

Table 3: 18-ingredient list contained in the Yogi Detox Tea and the articles published in PubMed highlighting their hepatotoxicity.

Ingredient	Number of hepatotoxic articles/case reports
Sarsaparilla root	0
Cinnamon bark	1 [5]
Ginger root	0
Licorice root	0
Dandelion root	0
Cardamom seed	0
Clove bud	0
Black pepper	1 [6]
Juniper berry	1 [7]
Long pepper berry	0
Phellodendron bark	0
Rhubarb root	4 [8–11]
Skullcap root	7 [12–18]
Coptis root	0
Forsythia fruit	0
Gardenia fruit	7 [19–25]
Honeysuckle	0
Winter melon	0

injury. In our patient, her RUCAM score was 7 (2 points for time from drug intake < 15 days, 2 points for ≥50% reduction of ALT after herb cessation, 1 point for risk factors of alcohol use, 2 points for other causes being ruled out, and 1 point for previous reaction to herb but unlabeled), which indicates that the detox tea is the probable offending agent of her hepatic injury. Given the worsening clinical picture, an ultrasound-guided liver biopsy was performed. The liver histology was notable for submassive necrosis with portal, periportal, and panlobular inflammation with lymphocytes, numerous neutrophils, plasma cells, and few eosinophils (Figures 1(a) and 1(b)). Hepatocyte ballooning, Mallory hyaline, and single cell apoptosis were also noted. Her lethargy progressed to somnolence requiring intubation. She was placed on the transplant list on day 15 and passed away on day 17.

3. Discussion

The prevalence of herbal supplementation intake has been increasing; however, their use is unregulated by the Food and Drug Administration and unsupervised by medical professionals [27]. The patient discussed in this case consumed Yogi Detoxification tea, an American produced tea that is an amalgamation of eighteen herbs marketed to be hepatoprotective. The Ingredients of this tea are listed in Table 3. Literature review of these ingredients in PubMed showed that all had articles endorsing hepatoprotection. The basis behind protection is hypothesized and demonstrated to be through their antioxidant and anti-inflammatory properties. However, literature search of these ingredients showed that less than 10% were done with human or liver-injury cell

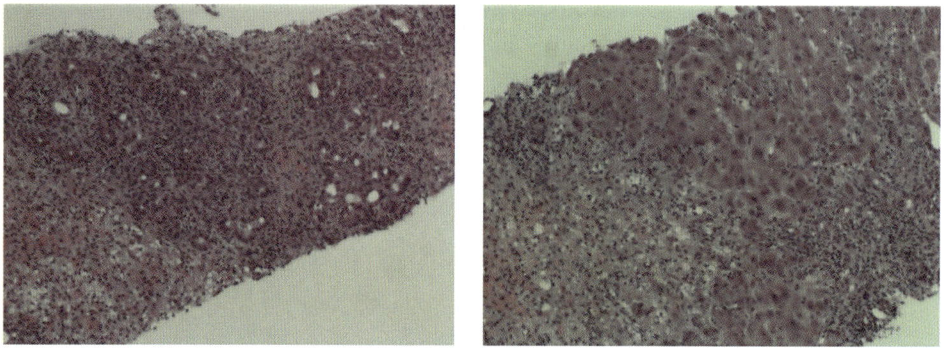

(a) (b)

FIGURE 1: US-guided liver biopsy showing submassive necrosis.

models. Animal studies may not be able to mimic the complex process of herb-induced inflammatory response of human physiology and progress. Therefore, the safety and efficacy may not be translatable to human trials. Not only is more basic research needed to understand the pathophysiology of hepatotoxicity, but more human trials are necessary to elucidate potential effects.

Six ingredients had one or more published studies associating it with hepatotoxicity. Hepatic toxicity caused by Gardenia has been demonstrated to cause oxidative stress-induced hepatocyte necrosis and apoptosis in murine models. Seven different articles attributed Gardenia's component geniposide to its hepatotoxic effect [19–25]. Yang described liver biopsy findings in rats exposed to geniposides that showed swollen and necrotic cells and an inflammatory infiltrate similar to the biopsy of our patient [25]. Similarly, skullcap root, another ingredient, was shown in a two-year retrospective study of 1169 hospitalized patients to be a common cause of hepatotoxicity [12]. Four case reports featuring seven patients show complications can range from mild hepatitis to acute hepatic failure requiring transplantation [13–16]. Cinnamon bark, black pepper, juniper berry, and rhubarb root, other ingredients of this tea, have all been associated with liver dysfunction [5–7].

While evidence suggests that the patient's acute change is associated with tea consumption, the exact toxicity-inducing agent of this tea is unclear. Preexisting alcohol consumption in combination with the herbal supplementation may have hastened the progression of hepatotoxicity. In addition to the 19 ingredients, herbal products are contaminated with other toxins or added adulterants that are not advertised on the packaging. In addition, ingestion of multiple substances may increase the risk of hepatotoxicity. This "cluster" effect of herbal supplements has not been elucidated in the literature; however, it has been known that risk factors such as alcohol ingestion are susceptible to drug toxicity from alterations in drug metabolism. Regardless, herbal tea consumption must be monitored by healthcare professionals, and any side effects should be reported to specific organizations in order to take regulatory measures and control usage of such products.

Consent

Informed consent was obtained from the patient involved.

Disclosure

The author guarantor is Keerthana Kesavarapu. The remaining authors aided in caring for and editing the content of this case report. An earlier version of this work was presented as a poster at the Annual Scientific Meeting of the American College of Gastroenterology being held October 14–19, 2016.

References

[1] W. M. Lee, A. M. Larson, and R. T. Stravitz, "AASLD position paper: the management of acute liver failure," in *Hepatology*, vol. 55, pp. 965–967, 2012.

[2] G. Ostapowicz, R. J. Fontana, F. V. Schioødt et al., "Results of a prospective study of acute liver failure at 17 tertiary care centers in the United States," *Annals of Internal Medicine*, vol. 137, no. 12, pp. 947–954, 2002.

[3] V. J. Navarro, H. Barnhart, H. L. Bonkovsky et al., "Liver injury from herbals and dietary supplements in the U.S. drug-induced liver injury network," *Hepatology*, vol. 60, no. 4, pp. 1399–1408, 2014.

[4] Centers for Disease Control and Prevention, "Hepatitis E for Health Professionals," 2017, https://www.cdc.gov/hepatitis/hev/hevfaq.htm.

[5] N. Iwata, M. Kainuma, D. Kobayashi et al., "The relation between hepatotoxicity and the total coumarin intake from traditional Japanese medicines containing cinnamon bark," *Frontiers in Pharmacology*, vol. 7, article no. 174, 2016.

[6] P. J. Rao, S. D. Kolla, F. Elshaari et al., "Effect of piperine on liver function of CF-1 albino mice," *Infectious Disorders—Drug Targets*, vol. 15, no. 2, pp. 131–134, 2015.

[7] Y. Liu, T. J. Flynn, M. S. Ferguson, E. M. Hoagland, and L. L. Yu, "Effects of dietary phenolics and botanical extracts on hepatotoxicity-related endpoints in human and rat hepatoma cells and statistical models for prediction of hepatotoxicity," *Food and Chemical Toxicology*, vol. 49, no. 8, pp. 1820–1827, 2011.

[8] L.-N. He, A.-H. Yang, T.-Y. Cui et al., "Reactive metabolite activation by CYP2C19-mediated rhein hepatotoxicity," *Xenobiotica*, vol. 45, no. 4, pp. 361–372, 2015.

[9] J.-B. Wang, W.-J. Kong, H.-J. Wang et al., "Toxic effects caused by rhubarb (*Rheum palmatum* L.) are reversed on immature and aged rats," *Journal of Ethnopharmacology*, vol. 134, no. 2, pp. 216–220, 2011.

[10] J. B. Wang, M. a. YG, P. Zhang, and C. Jin, "Effect of processing on the chemical contents and hepatic and renal toxicity of rhubarb studied by canonical correlation analysis," *Yao Xue Xue Bai*, vol. 44, no. 8, pp. 885–890, 2009.

[11] J. Wang, Y. Zhao, X. Xiao et al., "Assessment of the renal protection and hepatotoxicity of rhubarb extract in rats," *Journal of Ethnopharmacology*, vol. 124, no. 1, pp. 18–25, 2009.

[12] H. J. Woo, H. Y. Kim, E. S. Choi et al., "Drug-induced liver injury: a 2-year retrospective study of 1169 hospitalized patients in a single medical center," *Phytomedicine*, vol. 22, no. 13, pp. 1201–1205, 2015.

[13] R. Dhanasekaran, V. Owens, and W. Sanchez, "Chinese skullcap in move free arthritis supplement causes drug induced liver injury and pulmonary infiltrates," *Case Reports in Hepatology*, vol. 2013, Article ID 965092, 4 pages, 2013.

[14] L. Yang, A. Aronsohn, J. Hart, and D. Jensen, "Herbal hepatoxicity from Chinese skullcap: a case report," *World Journal of Hepatology*, vol. 4, no. 7, pp. 231–233, 2012.

[15] S. A. Linnebur, O. C. Rapacchietta, and M. Vejar, "Hepatotoxicity associated with Chinese skullcap contained in move free advanced dietary supplement: two case reports and review of the literature," *Pharmacotherapy*, vol. 30, no. 7, 2010.

[16] O. A. Jorge and A. D. Jorge, "Hepatotoxicity associated with the ingestion of Centella asiatica," *Revista Española de Enfermedades Digestivas*, vol. 97, no. 2, pp. 115–124, 2005.

[17] J.-Y. Wang, C.-Y. Lee, P.-J. Pan et al., "Herb-induced autoimmune-like hepatitis in C57BL/6J mice," *Liver International*, vol. 34, no. 4, pp. 583–593, 2014.

[18] C. Bunchorntavakul and K. R. Reddy, "Review article: herbal and dietary supplement hepatotoxicity," *Alimentary Pharmacology & Therapeutics*, vol. 37, no. 1, pp. 3–17, 2013.

[19] K. Wang, R.-M. Jin, and C.-X. Chen, "Comparative study on hepatic toxicity of gardeniae fructus and Huanglian Diedu decoction," *Zhongguo Zhongyao Zazhi*, vol. 38, no. 14, pp. 2365–2368, 2013.

[20] J. Wei, F. Zhang, Y. Zhang et al., "Proteomic investigation of signatures for geniposide-induced hepatotoxicity," *Journal of Proteome Research*, vol. 13, no. 12, pp. 5724–5733, 2014.

[21] Y. Ding, T. Zhang, J.-S. Tao, L.-Y. Zhang, J.-R. Shi, and G. Ji, "Potential hepatotoxicity of geniposide, the major iridoid glycoside in dried ripe fruits of Gardenia jasminoides (Zhi-zi)," *Natural Product Research (Formerly Natural Product Letters)*, vol. 27, no. 10, pp. 929–933, 2013.

[22] H. Zhang, W. Wu, F. Li, W. Song, Y. He, and M. Yang, "Study on liver protection, cholagogic effect and hepatotoxicity of Gardeniae fructus," *Zhongguo Zhongyao Zazhi*, vol. 36, no. 19, pp. 2610–2614, 2011.

[23] T. Nuanyai, R. Sappapan, T. Teerawatananond, N. Muangsin, and K. Pudhom, "Cytotoxic 3,4-seco-cycloartane triterpenes from Gardenia sootepensis," *Journal of Natural Products*, vol. 72, no. 6, pp. 1161–1164, 2009.

[24] Y. Tetsuo, T. Yuji, N. Tsutomu et al., "Hepatotoxicity of gardenia yellow color in rats," *Toxicology Letters*, vol. 44, no. 1-2, pp. 177–182, 1988.

[25] H. J. Yang, F. u. MH, W. u. ZL, and R. X. Liang, "Experimental studies on hepatotoxicity on rats induced by fructus Gardeniae," *Zhongguo Zhong Yao Za Zhi*, vol. 31, no. 13, pp. 1091–1093, 2006.

[26] G. Danan and R. Teschke, "RUCAM in drug and herb induced liver injury: the update," *International Journal of Molecular Sciences*, vol. 17, no. 1, 14 pages, 2016.

[27] C. Wu, C. Wang, M. Tsai, W. Huang, and J. Kennedy, "Trend and pattern of herb and supplement use in the United States: results from the 2002, 2007, and 2012 national health interview surveys," *Evidence-Based Complementary and Alternative Medicine*, vol. 2014, Article ID 872320, 7 pages, 2014.

33

A Severe Case of Tuberculosis Radiologically and Endoscopically Mimicking Colorectal Cancer with Peritoneal Carcinomatosis

Timo Rath,[1] Raja Atreya,[1] Walter Geißdörfer,[2] Roland Lang,[2] Andreas Nägel,[1] and Markus F. Neurath[1]

[1] *Department of Medicine 1, Friedrich-Alexander University Erlangen-Nuremberg, Division of Gastroenterology, Endocrinology and Pneumology, Ludwig Demling Endoscopy Center of Excellence, Ulmenweg 18, 91054 Erlangen, Germany*
[2] *Institute of Clinical Microbiology, Immunology and Hygiene, University Hospital of Erlangen, Friedrich-Alexander University Erlangen-Nuremberg, Wasserturmstrasse 3-5, 91054 Erlangen, Germany*

Correspondence should be addressed to Markus F. Neurath; markus.neurath@uk-erlangen.de

Academic Editor: Tetsuo Hirata

Although generally rising in incidence, intestinal tuberculosis is still rare in western countries and due to unspecific manifestations mainly as ulcerations on endoscopy, diagnosis of intestinal tuberculosis is challenging. Within this report, we describe a case of severe intestinal tuberculosis radiologically and endoscopically masquerading as colorectal cancer with peritoneal carcinomatosis. Our case exemplifies that intestinal tuberculosis needs to be considered as a differential diagnosis in patients at risk and that undelayed and sensitive diagnosis of intestinal tuberculosis is of central importance for avoiding unfavorable disease outcome.

1. Introduction

Tuberculosis (TB) represents a major health problem in developing countries and while also many developed countries face a resurgence of TB, intestinal tuberculosis is still rare in western countries [1, 2]. Due to unspecific manifestations mainly as ulcerations on endoscopy [1–3], diagnosis of intestinal tuberculosis is challenging, especially when pulmonary infection is absent [4, 5]. Further, intestinal tuberculosis can mimic various abdominal pathologies including Crohn's disease, periappendiceal abscess, ischemic colitis, tumors, or intestinal infections other than TB [6, 7]. Although colonoscopy with biopsies is the procedure of choice for the diagnosis of intestinal TB, even histopathologic diagnosis can be difficult especially when granulomas are absent.

Herein, we report about intestinal tuberculosis radiologically and endoscopically masquerading as colorectal cancer with peritoneal carcinomatosis. Our case exemplifies that a high level of suspicion for intestinal tuberculosis is critical in patients at risk and that rapid and sensitive diagnosis is important to avoid unfavorable disease outcome.

2. Case Report

A 51-year-old kidney transplanted patient was admitted to the department of nephrology with abdominal pain and significant weight loss for several weeks. CT scan showed multiple contrast-enhancing peritoneal nodules and large intraperitoneal soft-tissue masses radiologically impressing as severe peritoneal carcinomatosis (Figure 1), a hypodense lesion within the right adrenal gland radiologically appearing as a metastasis as well as enlarged retroperitoneal lymph nodes, while the lung was unremarkable on CT scan. The patient was then referred to our endoscopy unit for tumor screening. Colonoscopy with virtual chromoendoscopy (i-scan) revealed a polypoid lesion at the hepatic flexure with irregular mucosa, hemorrhages, contact bleeding, and a central ulceration (Figure 2). On histopathology, no dysplasia or cancer was found. Importantly, histopathology was also negative for the presence of granulomas. A second colonoscopy for targeted biopsies was initiated and histopathology was again negative for cancer; however, subsequently performed Ziehl-Neelsen stain revealed acid-fast bacteria. In a third colonoscopy,

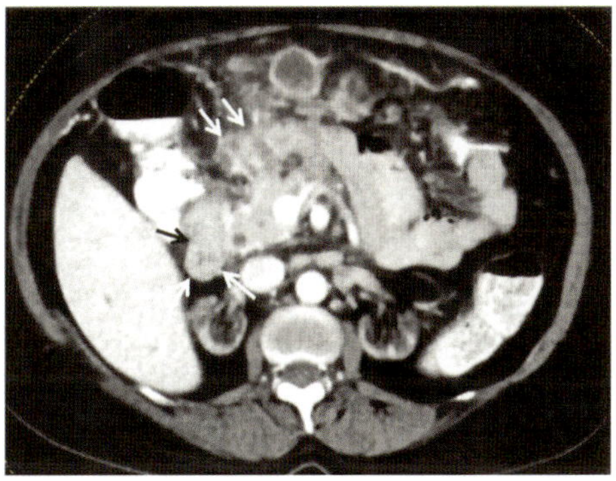

Figure 1: CT scan with multiple contrast-enhancing peritoneal nodules and large intraperitoneal soft-tissue masses (arrows), radiologically impressing as severe peritoneal carcinomatosis.

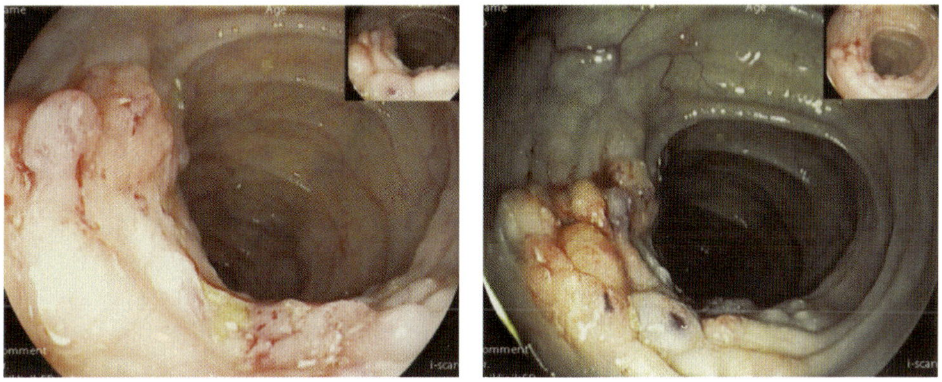

Figure 2: Polypoid-tumorous lesion with irregular mucosa, superficial hemorrhages, contact bleeding, and a central ulceration at the hepatic flexure on virtual chromoendoscopy with i-scan.

biopsies for microbiological analysis and resistance testing were obtained and DNA of rifampicin-sensitive *M. tuberculosis* complex was detected using the Xpert MTB/RIF assay on the GeneXpert Dx System (Cepheid, Sunnyvale, CA) on the same day. Immediately thereafter, first-line antituberculostatic treatment was initiated. Liquid culture (BACTEC™ MGIT™, Becton Dickinson, Franklin Lakes, NJ) was positive after 4 days. The strain was identified as *M. tuberculosis* based on *gyrB* sequence analysis [8] and phenotypically susceptible to all first-line tuberculostatic drugs. The subsequent course of disease was complicated by episodes of epileptic seizures with aphasia and hemiparesis. Cranial CT and MRI showed bilateral ischemic lesions and contrast-enhancing lesions directly adjacent to the dura, radiologically consistent with multiple septic emboli and tuberculosis manifestation within the CNS (Figure 3). Under tuberculostatic therapy, neurological symptoms slowly ameliorated; however, organic brain syndrome persisted.

3. Discussion

The incidence of abdominal TB has been steadily increasing in the past 20 years [6, 9, 10]. At the same time, diagnosis of intestinal tuberculosis remains challenging, especially when active pulmonary infection is absent. The current hurdles in the diagnosis of intestinal TB are mainly based on its unspecific clinical and endoscopic presentation and histopathology that frequently misses the pathognomonic lesions. As a result, time to diagnosis can range from 2 days to 11 months with a median time to diagnosis of 50 days, as indicated by data from a North American hospital [11]. In light of this, diagnosing intestinal tuberculosis requires a high index of suspicion especially in countries in which tuberculosis is not endemic and an increased awareness of intestinal tuberculosis as a severe differential diagnosis seems critical especially in patients at risk in order to warrant undelayed treatment initiation.

Intestinal TB is predominantly located in the ileocecal region and the presence of lymphoid tissue within the ileum and a physiologic stasis facilitating prolonged contact between bacteria and the mucosa have been discussed as reasons for the ileum and cecum being the most common sites of disease manifestation [1–3, 6].

Endoscopically, intestinal tuberculosis typically appears as ulcerations, nodules, or luminal narrowing [1–3] and the clinical presentation is usually nonspecific with fever, weight loss, abdominal pain, and changes of bowel habits as the most commonly observed symptoms [2, 7].

To date, endoscopy with biopsies is considered the procedure of choice for the diagnosis of intestinal TB. In addition

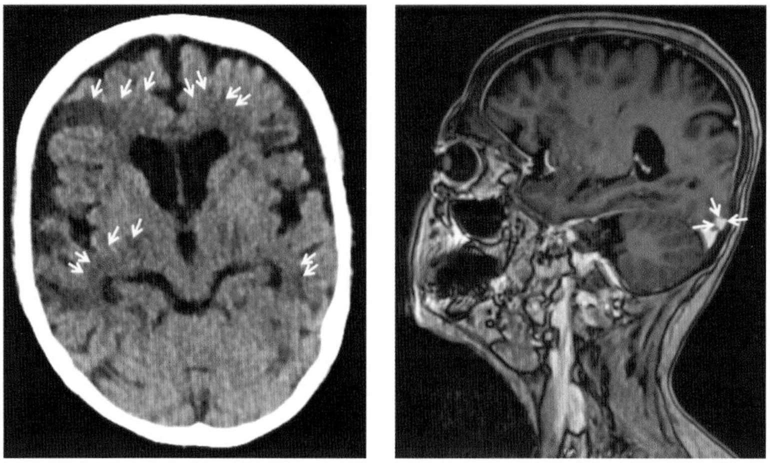

(a) (b)

Figure 3: Bilateral ischemic lesions (CT, (a) arrows) and contrast-enhancing lesions directly adjacent to the dura mater (MRI, (b) arrows), radiologically consistent with multiple septic emboli and tuberculosis manifestation within the CNS.

to the diagnostic dilemma of rather unspecific appearance on endoscopy and eventually vague clinical symptoms as outlined above, the pathognomonic features of epithelioid granulomas with Langhans giant cells, central caseous necrosis, and presence of acid-fast bacilli are identified only in a minority of biopsy specimens [12, 13]. In fact, granulomas with or without caseation are present in less than 50% of patients [7, 14, 15], while clusters of epithelioid cells without well-formed granulomas are only observed in 20–30% of the biopsies [14, 15]. In contrast, a large percentage of patients with colonic tuberculosis histology reveals only chronic nonspecific changes in the form of chronic inflammatory cells in the lamina propria [2, 13]. This diagnostic dilemma is very well reflected in our patient, in which the biopsies obtained during the first colonoscopy did not exhibit pathognomonic features of intestinal TB. Therefore, a second colonoscopy was necessary in which the presence of acid-fast bacteria confirmed mycobacterial infection.

Culture of biopsy material remains the gold standard for the diagnosis of intestinal tuberculosis but usually requires 4 to 6 weeks until results are obtained [6, 7]. Furthermore, studies in patients with colonic tuberculosis indicate that positive culture can be found in only one-third of patients or even less [15, 16].

In contrast, PCR for *M. tuberculosis* from biopsies provides rapid diagnosis of TB and positive predictive values up to 100% have been reported [17]. Although more sensitive than culture and acid-fast stains in diagnosing intestinal TB [18], recent data reported lower negative prediction and variable specificity in extrapulmonary TB [19, 20]. Nevertheless, the possibility of obtaining results within 48 hours by itself confers a major advantage over histopathology and thus should be considered in patients at risk for intestinal TB such as HIV-infected individuals and immunosuppressed or immunocompromised patients.

In summary, this case exemplifies the fact that intestinal tuberculosis can radiologically and endoscopically mimic colorectal cancer. Further, as illustrated within this case, a high level of suspicion is necessary in patients at risk in which PCR analysis of a colonic biopsy might be considered initially and in parallel to conventional histopathology for sensitive and fast differential diagnosis and undelayed treatment initiation in order to avoid unfavorable disease outcome.

Consent

Informed patient consent was obtained for case publication.

Authors' Contributions

Timo Rath and Andreas Nägel performed the endoscopies. Walter Geißdörfer and Roland Lang performed microbiological analyses. Timo Rath, Raja Atreya, and Markus Neurath wrote the manuscript.

References

[1] S. Mukewar, R. Ravi, and A. Prasad, "Colon tuberculosis: endoscopic features and prospective endoscopic follow-up after anti-tuberculosis treatment," *Clinical and Translational Gastroenterology*, vol. 3, 24 pages, 2012.

[2] J. F. Alvares, H. Devarbhavi, P. Makhija, S. Rao, and R. Kottoor, "Clinical, colonoscopic, and histological profile of colonic tuberculosis in a tertiary hospital," *Endoscopy*, vol. 37, no. 4, pp. 351–356, 2005.

[3] S. Sato, K. Yao, T. Yao et al., "Colonoscopy in the diagnosis of intestinal tuberculosis in asymptomatic patients," *Gastrointestinal Endoscopy*, vol. 59, no. 3, pp. 362–368, 2004.

[4] O. Giouleme, P. Paschos, M. Katsaros et al., "Intestinal tuberculosis: a diagnostic challenge - Case report and review of the literature," *European Journal of Gastroenterology and Hepatology*, vol. 23, no. 11, pp. 1074–1077, 2011.

[5] P. Martínez Tirado, M. López de Hierro Ruiz, R. Martínez García, J. G. Martínez Cara, M. M. Martín Rodríguez, and M. M.

Castilla Castellano, "Intestinal tuberculosis. A diagnostic challenge," *Gastroenterol Hepatol*, vol. 26, no. 6, pp. 351–354, 2003.

[6] K. D. Horvath and R. L. Whelan, "Intestinal tuberculosis: return of an old disease," *The American Journal of Gastroenterology*, vol. 93, no. 5, pp. 692–696, 1998.

[7] J. B. Marshall, "Tuberculosis of the gastrointestinal tract and peritoneum," *The American Journal of Gastroenterology*, vol. 88, no. 7, pp. 989–999, 1993.

[8] H. Kasai, T. Ezaki, and S. Harayama, "Differentiation of phylogenetically related slowly growing mycobacteria by their gyrB sequences," *Journal of Clinical Microbiology*, vol. 38, no. 1, pp. 301–308, 2000.

[9] H. D. Donoghue and J. Holton, "Intestinal tuberculosis," *Current Opinion in Infectious Diseases*, vol. 22, no. 5, pp. 490–496, 2009.

[10] D. E. Snider Jr. and W. L. Roper, "The new tuberculosis," *The New England Journal of Medicine*, vol. 326, no. 10, pp. 703–705, 1992.

[11] J. S. Bernhard, G. Bhatia, and C. M. Knauer, "Gastrointestinal tuberculosis: an eighteen-patient experience and review," *Journal of Clinical Gastroenterology*, vol. 30, no. 4, pp. 397–402, 2000.

[12] R. Kirsch, M. Pentecost, P. D. M. Hall, D. P. Epstein, G. Watermeyer, and P. W. Friederich, "Role of colonoscopic biopsy in distinguishing between Crohn's disease and intestinal tuberculosis," *Journal of Clinical Pathology*, vol. 59, no. 8, pp. 840–844, 2006.

[13] S. P. Misra, V. Misra, M. Dwivedi, and S. C. Gupta, "Colonic tuberculosis: clinical features, endoscopic appearance and management," *Journal of Gastroenterology and Hepatology*, vol. 14, no. 7, pp. 723–729, 1999.

[14] S. Shah, V. Thomas, M. Mathan et al., "Colonoscopic study of 50 patients with colonic tuberculosis," *Gut*, vol. 33, no. 3, pp. 347–351, 1992.

[15] V. Singh, P. Kumar, J. Kamal, V. Prakash, K. Vaiphei, and K. Singh, "Clinicocolonoscopic profile of colonic tuberculosis," *The American Journal of Gastroenterology*, vol. 91, no. 3, pp. 565–568, 1996.

[16] R. Balamurugan, S. Venkataraman, K. R. John, and B. S. Ramakrishna, "PCR amplification of the IS6110 insertion element of Mycobacterium tuberculosis in fecal samples from patients with intestinal tuberculosis," *Journal of Clinical Microbiology*, vol. 44, no. 5, pp. 1884–1886, 2006.

[17] R. S. Wiener, P. Della-Latta, and N. W. Schluger, "Effect of nucleic acid amplification for Mycobacterium tuberculosis on clinical decision making in suspected extrapulmonary tuberculosis," *Chest*, vol. 128, no. 1, pp. 102–107, 2005.

[18] B. S. Anand, F. E. Schneider, F. A. El-Zaatari, R. M. Shawar, J. E. Clarridge, and D. Y. Graham, "Diagnosis of intestinal tuberculosis by polymerase chain reaction on endoscopic biopsy specimens," *The American journal of gastroenterology*, vol. 89, no. 12, pp. 2248-2249, 1994.

[19] P. K. Mehta, A. Raj, N. Singh, and G. K. Khuller, "Diagnosis of extrapulmonary tuberculosis by PCR," *FEMS Immunology and Medical Microbiology*, vol. 66, no. 1, pp. 20–36, 2012.

[20] M. Pai, J. Minion, K. Steingart, and A. Ramsay, "New and improved tuberculosis diagnostics: evidence, policy, practice, and impact," *Current Opinion in Pulmonary Medicine*, vol. 16, no. 3, pp. 271–284, 2010.

Medical Treatment of Postendoscopic Submucosal Dissection Phlegmonous Gastritis in an Elderly Diabetic Woman with Myelodysplastic Syndrome

Ko Matsuura, Shinsuke Hiramatsu, Rika Taketani, Kohei Ishibashi, Masanao Uraoka, Shinichi Baba, Akihiro Nakamura, Hiroshi Takihara, Chie Ueda, and Taro Inoue

Department of Gastroenterology, Kishiwada Tokushukai Hospital, 4-27-1 Kamori-cho, Kishiwada, Osaka 596-0042, Japan

Correspondence should be addressed to Ko Matsuura; matuurac90@gmail.com

Academic Editor: Chia-Tung Shun

Phlegmonous gastritis is a rare, suppurative disease characterized by full-thickness exudative changes, infiltration of inflammatory cells, and edema primarily in the submucosal layer. A 76-year-old woman with type 2 diabetes and myelodysplastic syndrome underwent endoscopic submucosal dissection (ESD) for early gastric cancer. Postoperatively, she developed persistent fever and computed tomography displayed full-circumference thickening of the gastric wall and increased levels of fat stranding. Endoscopy showed post-ESD ulcer floor expansion, formation of a false lumen between the ulcer floor and surrounding folds, and adhesion of purulent matter. *Klebsiella pneumoniae*, *Pseudomonas aeruginosa*, and *Candida albicans* were detected from pus culture and *Klebsiella pneumoniae* from blood culture, leading to a diagnosis of phlegmonous gastritis. Contrast examination showed no leakage outside the gastric wall; therefore, the patient fasted and was given antibiotics. She was successfully treated with medical therapy, as demonstrated by repeat endoscopy. Based on our experience, we recommend antibiotics before and after ESD in patients thought to be at high risk of infection, as well as careful postoperative management including postoperative endoscopy.

1. Introduction

Phlegmonous gastritis is a rare, suppurative disease characterized by full-thickness exudative changes, infiltration of inflammatory cells, and edema primarily in the submucosal layer. Herein, we report a case of phlegmonous gastritis that occurred after endoscopic submucosal dissection (ESD) for early gastric cancer in an elderly diabetic woman with myelodysplastic syndrome (MDS), treated successfully with medical therapy.

Gastrointestinal phlegmon is common in the appendix but, in rare cases, can affect the esophagus, stomach, duodenum, small intestine, and colon. Phlegmonous gastritis can lead to critical outcomes including sepsis and shock [1]. Phlegmonous gastritis is categorized into 3 groups based on etiology: primary, secondary, and idiopathic [2].

2. Case Presentation

A 76-year-old Japanese woman with type 2 diabetes was referred to our hospital for further investigation of anemia. An upper endoscopy to exclude gastrointestinal bleeding demonstrated an IIc+IIa lesion in the antrum. Tubular adenocarcinoma was diagnosed via biopsy and ESD was planned. Initial blood tests showed pancytopenia with white blood cells (WBC) 1,500/μL, hemoglobin (Hb) 4.6 g/dL, and platelets $5.1\times10^4/\mu$L. Serum biochemistry was normal except for HbA1c 7.0%.

On admission, the patient was diagnosed with MDS by the hematology team. She was given transfusions and follow-up was arranged. After a preoperative transfusion, repeat blood tests showed Hb 8.3 g/dL and platelets $23.4\times10^4/\mu$L. ESD was performed due to this improvement and the patient's desired treatment. The patient was subsequently diagnosed

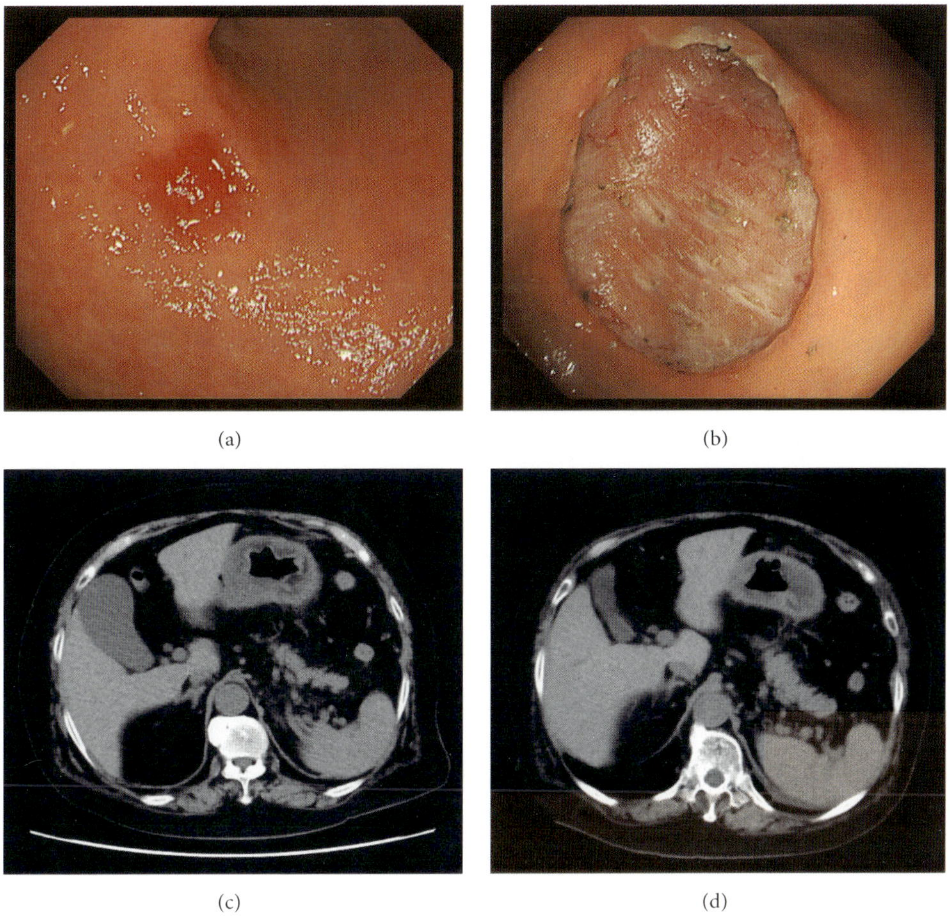

Figure 1: (a, b) ESD. (c) Abdominal CT (day 3 post-ESD). (d) Abdominal CT (day 20 post-ESD).

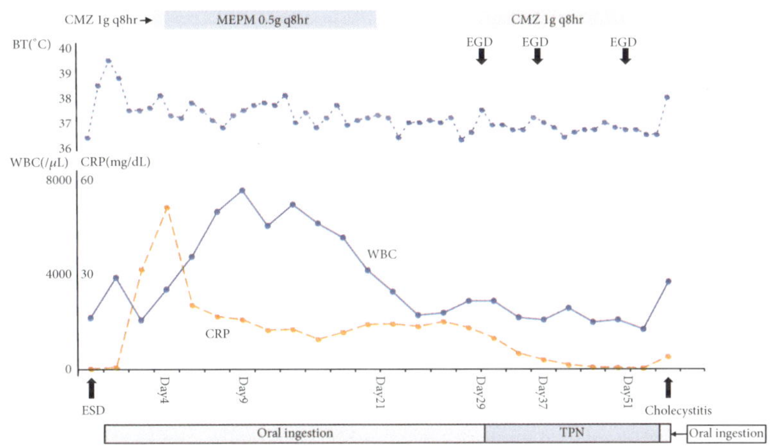

Figure 2: Post-ESD course. Transition of WBC, CRP, body temperature, and course of treatment.

with pseudothrombocytopenia based on repeat platelet count levels.

ESD (Figures 1(a) and 1(b)): There was an IIc+IIa lesion in the antrum. There was only a small amount of intraoperative bleeding and the resection took 80 minutes. The size of the mucosa resected en bloc was 38×34 mm^2 in diameter including 11×10 mm^2 of cancer lesion. No perforation and minimal bleeding were observed after finishing ESD.

Post-ESD course (Figure 2): No bleeding was observed on repeat endoscopy performed the day after ESD; therefore, the patient was allowed to eat. Her temperature spiked to around 38°C that day, and post-ESD abdominal computed tomography (CT) was performed on day 3 (Figure 1(c)),

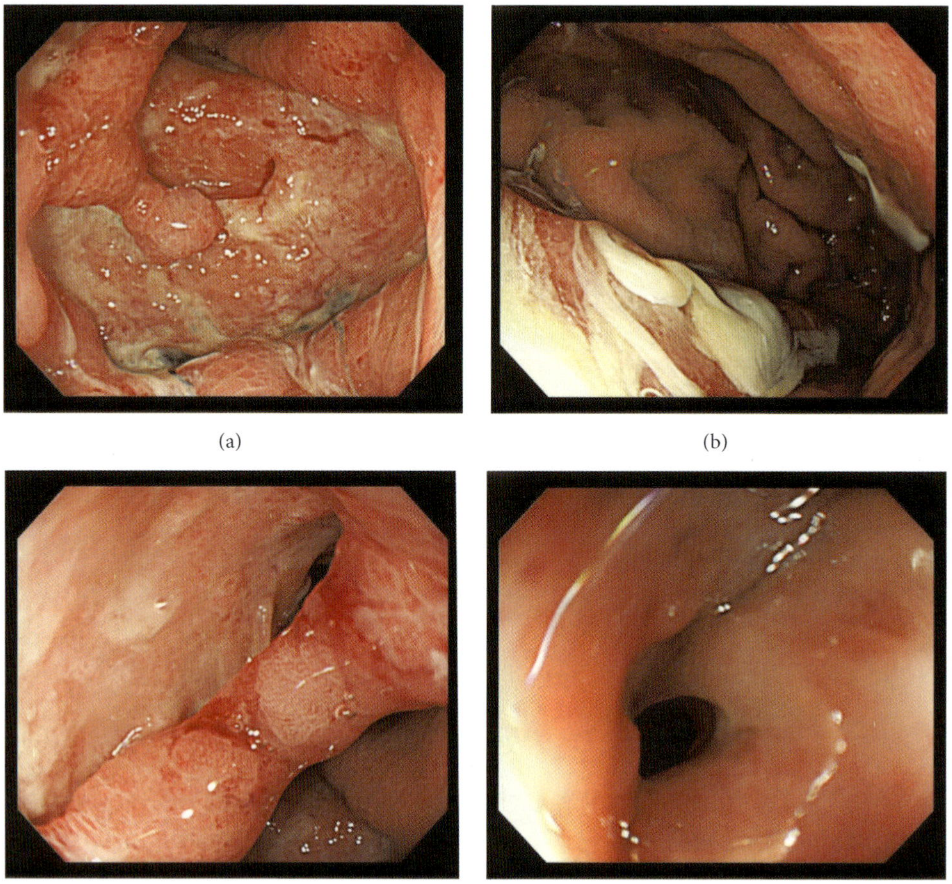

(a) (b) (c) (d)

Figure 3: Upper endoscopy (day 29 post-ESD), (a) ulcer, (b) yellow mucus, and (c, d) ulcer and false lumen.

which showed full-circumference thickening of the gastric wall. However, the patient did not exhibit abdominal pain, so a definitive diagnosis of phlegmonous gastritis could not be concluded. Antibiotic treatment with cefmetazole sodium (CMZ, 3 g/d) was started to cover for *E. coli* urinary tract infection with a positive urine culture. However, after *Klebsiella pneumoniae* was detected in a blood culture, the possibility of a bloodstream infection related to ESD injection was considered. C-reactive protein (CRP) levels increased to 51.5 mg/dL; therefore, antibiotic treatment was switched to meropenem hydrate (MEPM, 1.5 g/d) on day 4 post-ESD, after which the inflammatory reaction gradually improved. Abdominal CT performed on day 20 post-ESD (Figure 1(d)) showed full-circumference thickening of the gastric wall and increased levels of perigastric fat stranding. At this time, the patient had no high fever and abdominal pain; therefore, antibiotic treatment was terminated. On day 29 post-ESD, upper endoscopy was performed (Figure 3) because the patient began experiencing epigastric pain after eating on day 27 post-ESD. In addition to a post-ESD ulcer in the antrum, we observed expansion of the ulcer floor, a false lumen between the ulcer floor and surrounding folds on the lesser curvature side, and yellow mucus thought to be purulent matter adhered to the superior portion of the gastric body. Based on these findings, a diagnosis of phlegmonous gastritis was made. Contrast examination with gastrografin did not show any exudate outside the gastric wall from the false lumen.

Therefore, antibiotic treatment was continued. *Klebsiella pneumoniae*, *Pseudomonas aeruginosa*, and *Candida albicans* were detected from a pus culture. The patient was made nil by mouth, given intravenous hyperalimentation, and was treated with antibiotics (CMZ 3 g/d) and proton-pump inhibitors (PPI). Endoscopy performed on day 37 post-ESD (Figures 4(a) and 4(b)) showed granulation on the ulcer floor. Endoscopy performed on day 51 post-ESD (Figure 4(c)) showed that the ulcer shrunk and the false lumen disappeared and, on the basis of these findings, antibiotic treatment was terminated. The phlegmonous gastritis was considered to have been cured with medical therapy. The patient resumed eating on day 55 post-ESD, and acute cholecystitis occurred the next day. She underwent cholecystectomy which was complicated by a postoperative wound infection and intra-abdominal abscess, which improved with antibiotic therapy. She was discharged from the hospital on week 16. Endoscopy at 4 months post-ESD (Figure 4(d)) showed complete resolution.

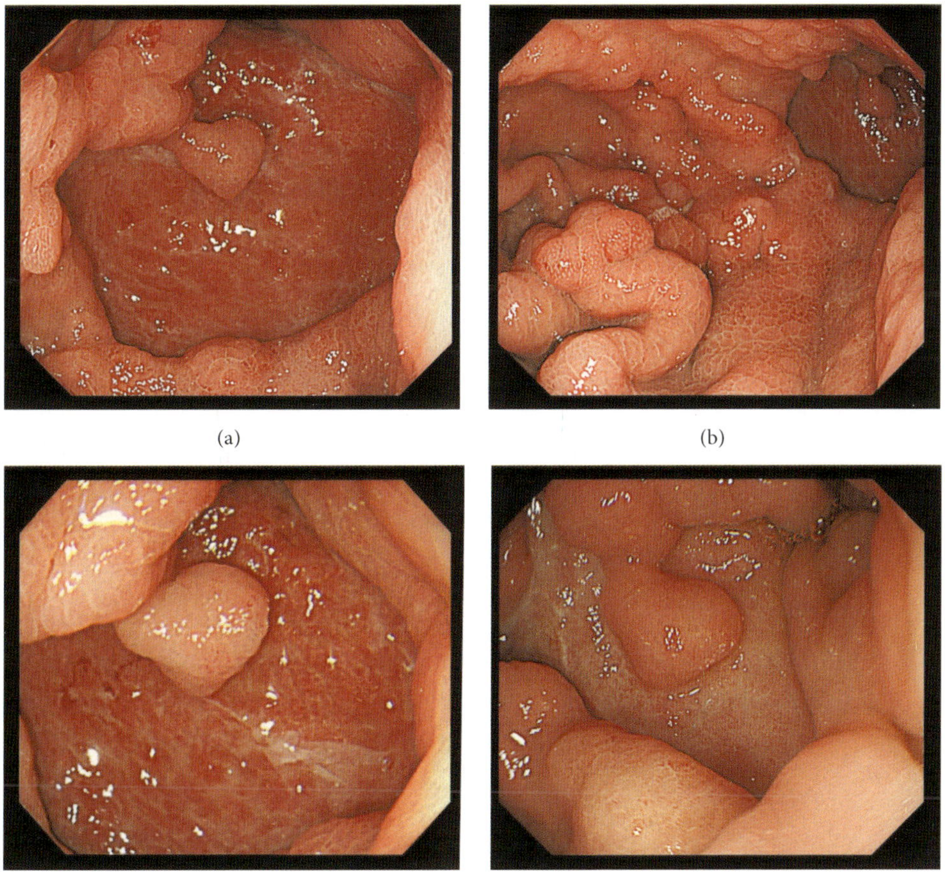

(a) (b) (c) (d)

FIGURE 4: (a) day 37 post-ESD, (b) day 37 post-ESD, (c) day 51 post-ESD, and (d) 4 months post-ESD.

3. Discussion

Herein, we describe a patient with a history of MDS and diabetes who developed phlegmonous gastritis after ESD for early gastric cancer.

Abdominal CT, upper endoscopy, and EUS are considered useful diagnostic tools. CT can be used to observe full-circumference thickening of the gastric wall, which if accompanied by severe inflammatory findings could indicate phlegmonous gastritis, though it is often difficult to reach a definitive diagnosis by CT alone [3]. In the present case, the above findings were observed by CT on days 3 and 20 post-ESD, but because of the absence of abdominal pain, we were unable to confirm a diagnosis of phlegmonous gastritis at this time. Endoscopic findings include rubor, edema, and erosion [4].

Searching PubMed for the keywords "endoscopic submucosal dissection" and "phlegmonous gastritis" in papers published between 1983 and 2017, we identified only 1 case report on post-ESD phlegmonous gastritis [5]. Total gastrectomy was performed in the case, but we treated our patient with medical therapy.

The most common pathogenic bacterium in phlegmonous gastritis is *Streptococcus* at 60-70%, with *Enterococcus, Klebsiella pneumoniae, Staphylococcus, Haemophilus influenzae, and Clostridium* also being reported [1].

Phlegmonous gastritis is caused by reduced immunity because of factors such as habitual alcohol use and diabetes in about half of patients [1]. Our patient also had MDS, which was implicated in the etiology of phlegmonous gastritis. The present case is the only one we could find that occurred post-ESD and which was accompanied by positive blood cultures.

Elevated gastric fluid pH is also said to be a risk factor for phlegmonous gastritis [6]. The patient in the present case had been taking a PPI (lansoprazole 15 mg/d) and was also administered PPI intravenously before and after ESD. It is therefore possible that administration of a strong acid-suppressive agent reduced the stomach's ability to kill bacteria by increasing gastric pH, which contributed to onset of the disease [6]. PPIs are said to be useful in healing post-ESD ulcers [7], but given their association with phlegmonous gastritis, further studies are warranted to investigate whether PPIs or H2-blockers are indicated in immunocompromised patients.

In a 1919 review of 215 cases of phlegmonous gastritis, Sundberg et al. reported a mortality rate of 92% [8], while in a 2014 review of 45 cases of phlegmonous gastritis, Rada-Palomino et al. reported a mortality rate of 27%, showing that prognostication improved over time [1]. It has also been reported that antibiotic therapy can be selected as long as there are no serious complications, such as hemorrhage or perforation [4], and that surgery and antibiotic therapy do not produce significantly different outcomes [1]. The present case was not accompanied by perforation or hemorrhage, and because of the presence of MDS and diabetes, we decided that the patient was susceptible to infection and postoperative suture rupture, so we elected for antibiotic treatment.

Gastric ESD was first reported in 1998 and became eligible for insurance coverage in 2006. This short history and lack of case reports on post-ESD phlegmonous gastritis mean that much remains unclear about its incidence rate, relationship with the techniques used, and other factors [5]. It is thought that this disease can be caused by a variety of pathogenic bacteria, so starting therapy with a broad-spectrum antibiotic then changing to a narrower range based on reliable culture results appears to be a valid approach. Different bacteria are often detected from pus, gastric mucosa biopsies, blood, and other sources, so it must be recognized that culture results are not absolute and there should be no hesitation to use broad-spectrum antibiotics for long periods, depending on the clinical course. Antibiotics are not routinely administered before and after gastric ESD [9], but in patients like ours with high infection risk factors, such as high age, diabetes, and habitual alcohol use, the possibility of postoperative phlegmonous gastritis should be taken into consideration when deciding whether to administer antibiotics before and after surgery. Such patients also require careful postoperative management, including upper gastrointestinal endoscopy.

Consent

Written informed consent was obtained from the patient.

References

[1] A. Rada-Palomino, A. Muñoz-Duyos, N. Pérez-Romero et al., "Phlegmonous gastritis: A rare entity as a differential diagnostic of an acute abdomen. Description of a case and a bibliographic review," *Revista Española de Enfermedades Digestivas*, vol. 106, no. 6, pp. 418–424, 2014.

[2] G. E. Konjetzny, *Entgunclungen des Margens. Handbuch der Speziellen pathologischen Anatomie und Histologie*, vol. 4, Julius Springer Verlag, Berlin, Germany, 1928.

[3] B. Y. Kim and H.-S. Kim, "Phlegmonous gastritis in an ankylosing spondylitis patient treated with infliximab," *Korean Journal of Internal Medicine*, vol. 32, no. 6, pp. 945-946, 2017.

[4] K. Nomura, T. Iizuka, S. Yamashita et al., "Phlegmonous gastritis secondary to superior mesenteric artery syndrome," *SAGE Open Medical Case Reports*, vol. 3, 2015.

[5] H. Ajibe, H. Osawa, M. Yoshizawa et al., "Phlegmonous gastritis after endoscopic submucosal dissection for early gastric cancer," *Therapeutic Advances in Gastroenterology*, vol. 1, no. 2, pp. 91–95, 2008.

[6] I. Fujita, T. Toyokawa, S. Omote et al., "Two cases of phlegmonous gastritis after ESD for early gastric cancer," *Gastroenterological Endoscopy*, vol. 55, no. 6, pp. 1812–1817, 2013.

[7] N. Uedo, Y. Takeuchi, T. Yamada et al., "Effect of a proton pump inhibitor or an H2-receptor antagonist on prevention of bleeding from ulcer after endoscopic submucosal dissection of early gastric cancer: A prospective randomized controlled trial," *American Journal of Gastroenterology*, vol. 102, no. 8, pp. 1610–1616, 2007.

[8] H. Sundberg, "Phlegmonous Gastritis," *JAMA*, vol. 73, p. 802, 1919.

[9] S. Itaba, Y. Iboshi, K. Nakamura et al., "Low-frequency of bacteremia after endoscopic submucosal dissection of the stomach," *Digestive Endoscopy*, vol. 23, no. 1, pp. 69–72, 2011.

35

Association between Oesophageal Diverticula and Leiomyomas: A Report of Two Cases

Muhammad Chowdhry, Christina Spyratou, Bruno Lorenzi, Sritharan Kadirkamanathan, and Alexandros Charalabopoulos

Department of Upper Gastrointestinal Surgery, Broomfield Hospital, Mid Essex Hospital Services NHS Trust, Essex, UK

Correspondence should be addressed to Christina Spyratou; christina.spyratou@meht.nhs.uk

Academic Editor: Naohiko Koide

We report two rare cases of female patients presenting with oesophageal leiomyoma associated with oesophageal diverticulum, both of whom were surgically managed. Oesophageal leiomyoma and oesophageal diverticulum are uncommon as separate entities and rare as combined disease presentation. Clinicians need to be aware of the rare combination of the two entities and need to be able to exclude the presence of a tumour (benign or malignant) within a diverticulum and so plan the optimum treatment. Herein, we present two cases of oesophageal leiomyoma within oesophageal diverticulum and we try to elucidate the association between the two. To date, there is no consensus whether a diverticulum is secondary to a leiomyoma or, on the contrary, a leiomyoma arises within a diverticulum.

1. Introduction

Oesophageal diverticula and oesophageal leiomyomas are infrequent benign conditions of the oesophagus that may render a potentially difficult diagnosis as well as challenging management. Simultaneous existence is even scarcer and there are only a limited number of cases reported in the English published literature [1]. In terms of the pathogenesis of the two synchronous entities, to date it is still unclear which of the two is preexisting and which results in the presence of the first one. Different schools of thought\are in support of each theory (diverticulum leading to leiomyoma or leiomyoma to diverticulum), without a firm favorite so far. Their management varies from conservative to local excision for diverticula and from enucleation to oesophagectomy for leiomyomas [2, 3]. The diagnosis of the two entities preoperatively can be difficult to establish and frequently the discovery of the leiomyoma within the diverticulum is an incidental finding. Clinicians involved in the diagnosis and management of oesophageal conditions need to also bear in mind that there is a low probability of cancerous transformation within the diverticulum [4]. This needs careful consideration regarding best investigations and management of these patients. Most oesophageal conditions, including diverticula and leiomyomas, are nowadays being dealt with in high volume tertiary centers where great expertise and multidisciplinary team effort have provided better results in the management and outcome of these indeed challenging conditions [2]. Therefore, careful history, investigations, and clinician's awareness towards possible synchronous disease is imperative in order to ensure the best outcome for these patients. In the current study we describe two interesting cases of synchronous disease as well as their management and follow-up. Furthermore, alongside a literature review, we provide a description of the two disease entities and we try to elucidate their combination, which complementary could help immensely any clinician dealing with oesophageal conditions.

2. Case Report 1

A 35-year-old woman presented to the upper gastrointestinal clinic with dysphagia, odynophagia, reflux, and persistent bloating after meals. Her abdominal ultrasound did

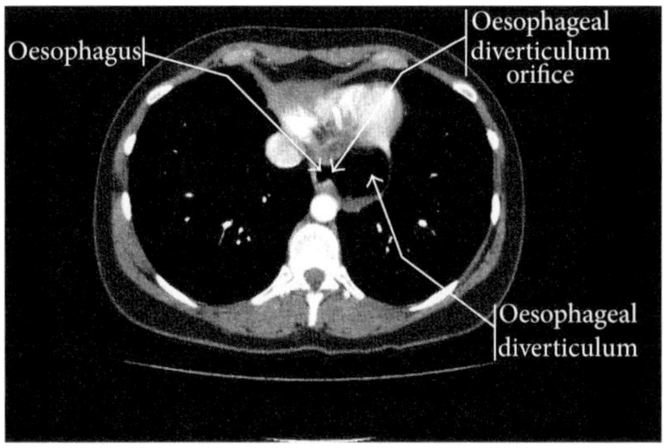

FIGURE 1: Epiphrenic oesophageal diverticulum containing food residue. CT chest with IV contrast.

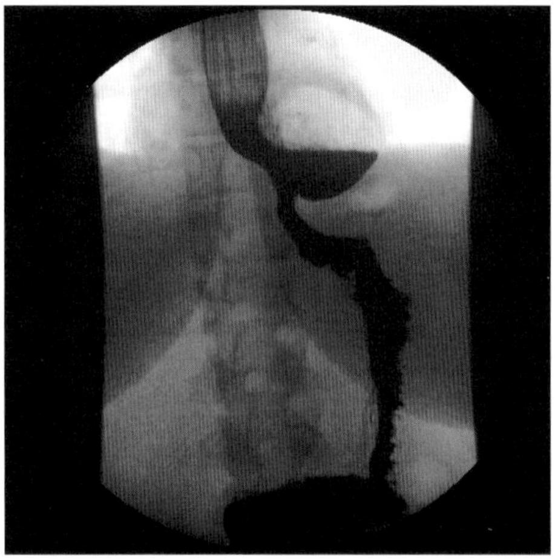

FIGURE 2: Oesophageal diverticulum with air-fluid level. Barium swallow.

not detect any abnormalities. Subsequent oesophagogastroduodenoscopy (OGD) revealed the presence of a paraoesophageal hernia within which two 4 cm cream lesions were apparent. Biopsies of the area showed mild chronic inflammation and intestinal metaplasia consistent with Barrett's oesophagus and no dysplasia. A CT scan revealed that what was thought to be a paraoesophageal hernia in the OGD was in reality a 5.5 × 4.7 cm epiphrenic oesophageal diverticulum containing food residue (Figure 1). Finally, barium swallow revealed gross reflux up to the upper third of the oesophagus and a large distal oesophageal diverticulum (Figure 2).

Due to the severity of symptoms, surgical intervention was planned. Intraoperative findings confirmed an oesophageal diverticulum near the gastrooesophageal junction. Robotic-assisted laparoscopic excision of the epiphrenic diverticulum with distal oesophageal myotomy and hiatal closure with crural repair was performed. Postoperative water-soluble swallow demonstrated no leak from the diverticulectomy site and some narrowing at the gastrooesophageal junction likely due to postoperative oedema. The patient had an uneventful recovery and was discharged home two days later. Histology showed an oesophageal diverticulum of 55×35×20 mm containing a firm lesion of 30 mm. The diverticulum was lined by gastrooesophageal mucosa and the

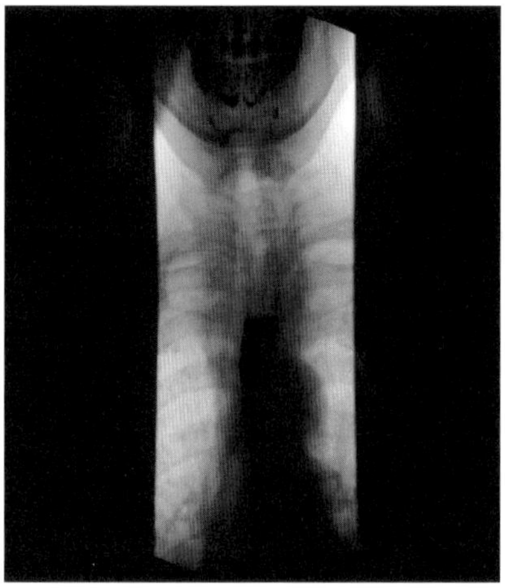

FIGURE 3: Corkscrew oesophagus. Barium swallow.

wall contained a lobulated smooth muscle tumour arising from the muscularis propria. The lesion composed of spindle cells with no evidence of nuclear pleomorphism, necrosis, or increased mitotic figures. Immunohistochemistry found lesion cells positive for SMA and desmin and negative for CD34, CD117, DOG1, and S100 protein and concluding that the appearance was in keeping with leiomyoma with no evidence of malignancy. A year later, a follow-up CT was performed, with no abnormalities detected.

Two years later, she complained of increasing reflux symptoms and mild dysphagia especially after large meals. Barium swallow showed free flow of contrast into stomach. Further filling the stomach with a larger quantity of barium and tilting the fluoroscopy table to a semisupine position demonstrated gross gastrooesophageal reflux into a dilated oesophagus. A year later, she underwent laparoscopic 270-degree posterior fundoplication (modified Toupet) to control her reflux symptoms, with good results to date.

3. Case Repot 2

A 72-year-old woman presented with a 20-year history of dysphagia. She complained of heartburn but no weight loss. She had a barium swallow, which revealed corkscrew oesophagus (Figure 3). Her symptoms were improving with GTN spray.

Station pull-through manometry revealed grossly abnormal oesophageal body motility with very hypertonic contractions in the mid and distal body and concluded on diffuse oesophageal spasm involving at least 15 cm of the distal oesophagus.

She had an OGD where marked tertiary oesophageal contractions were present and the stomach could not be visualized, as it could not be intubated.

After failure of Botox injections (300 Units) to control her symptoms, she underwent a laparoscopic-assisted oesophagogastrectomy for corkscrew oesophagus.

Histology revealed an oesophageal diverticulum 44 mm from the proximal oesophageal resection margin and 27 mm from the gastrooesophageal junction (GOJ) containing small amount of food debris. Also a smaller diverticulum was

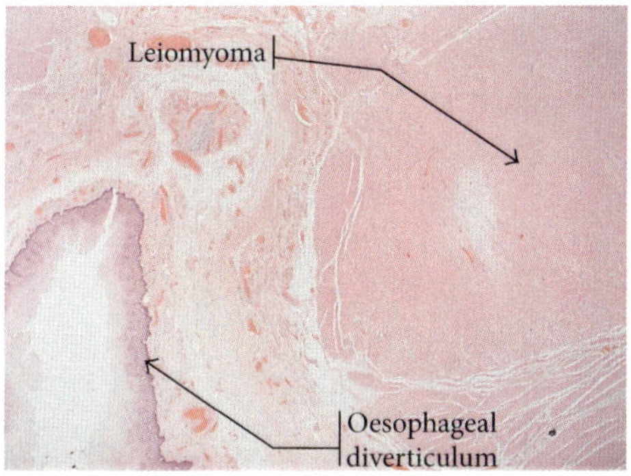

FIGURE 4: Histological view showing leiomyoma and oesophageal diverticulum. Haematoxylin & eosin stain ×10.

present nearby lined with squamous mucosa. The larger diverticulum contained a small fibrous nodule of 9 mm, in the outer layer of the muscularis propria at the proximal end of the diverticulum. It was identified as a benign leiomyoma (Figure 4). Immunohistochemistry was positive for SMA and desmin and negative for CD34 and CD117 and DOG.

She recovered well from the operation, but over the next few months she progressively developed symptoms of delayed gastric emptying. An upper gastrointestinal endoscopy was performed that showed a patent anastomosis and increased food residue within the gastric conduit. A barium swallow showed no anastomotic stricture but hold-up of contrast at the pylorus. Following the OGD, the patient complained of progressive and severe vomiting triggered by meals until not being able to tolerate solids, fluids, or medication.

She was diagnosed with pylorospasm after oesophagectomy (secondary to vagus nerve injury) and underwent endoscopic treatment. She had endoscopic balloon dilation and Botox injection of the pylorus to improve gastric drainage, which relieved her symptoms to date.

4. Discussion

Oesophageal diverticulum is a rare condition that can be managed conservatively when asymptomatic or surgically when symptoms become debilitating. An oesophageal diverticulum is defined as the outpouching or sac of the epithelial lined tissue of the oesophagus. True diverticula involve all the layers of the oesophagus, whereas false diverticula are limited to involving the mucosal or submucosal layers protruding through the circular and longitudinal oesophageal muscle layers [5].

Oesophageal diverticula can be classified by location of occurrence, be it proximally at the pharyngooesophageal area (Zenker diverticulum), the mid oesophagus, or more distal (epiphrenic) diverticula [2]. The mechanism of occurrence is thought to be either traction (due to scaring and conditions following chronic inflammation such as TB) or pulsion (due to motility disorders of the oesophagus such as achalasia) and diverticula can be named accordingly. Rarer causes include retained foreign bodies [6, 7] and iatrogenic causes (oesophageal stents [8], gastric bands [9], and tracheostomy tubes [10]). Malignant lesions such as squamous cell carcinoma have also been described as possible cause of oesophageal diverticula [11, 12].

Oesophageal leiomyomas on the other hand are rare accounting for about 1% of all oesophageal neoplasms; however, they are the most common benign tumours of the oesophagus [13]. It is more common in men and usually arises from the inner circular muscle layer at the distal oesophagus. They are similar to classic endometrial leiomyoma as originally described consisting of a circumscribed lesion of muscularis propria or muscularis mucosae composed of intersecting fascicles of bland spindle cells with abundant cytoplasm and may show calcification. They stain positive for desmin, SMA (alpha smooth muscle actin), and high molecular weight caldesmon and negative for CD34, CD117, S100, and DOG1/ANO1. Oesophageal leiomyomas are typically treated with enucleation (open or thoracoscopic) for small tumours and oesophagectomy for large tumours [14, 15].

Oesophageal diverticula associated with leiomyomas although considered to be rare are reported in the literature since 1958 [16]. Several cases have been described since then but the etiology has not been clear yet. It is possible that the mechanism of diverticulum formation involves pulsion due to motility disorders caused by the leiomyoma itself (especially if it is bulky). In most of the cases the diverticula associated with leiomyoma are in the lower part of oesophagus (epiphrenic), which are typically considered to be pulsion diverticula. In our series, both cases had oesophageal motility disorder. However, recently a case of epiphrenic diverticulum associated with leiomyoma in a patient with no primary motor disorder has been described [1]. Therefore, other causes like traction due to surrounding tissue inflammation must be considered as well. Furthermore, for reasons that are not very well understood, there is a thought that leiomyomas can develop within a primary oesophageal diverticulum.

The incidence of cancer in a diverticulum is 0.3–7%, 1.8%, and 0.6% for pharyngooesophageal, midoesophageal, and epiphrenic diverticula, respectively [4]. Benign tumours are even rarer. Malignant transformation in a diverticulum is linked to stasis and it should always be taken into consideration when treating a long-standing oesophageal diverticulum.

In our series both patients had epiphrenic diverticula associated with leiomyomas. Both patients had oesophageal motility disorders and leiomyomas were only discovered histopathologically in the resected specimen. In both cases it is unclear if the diverticulum preexisted the leiomyoma or vice versa; however in our opinion given the findings we conclude that most probably these represent pulsion diverticula.

To date, in most of the cases reported, it is not possible to tell which comes first (the diverticulum or the leiomyoma). More studies are needed so as to be able to identify the primary cause in this combined disease.

References

[1] J. H. Conklin, D. Singh, and M. R. Katlic, "Epiphrenic esophageal diverticula: spectrum of symptoms and consequences," *Journal of the American Osteopathic Association*, vol. 109, no. 10, pp. 543–545, 2009.

[2] F. A. M. Herbella and M. G. Patti, "Modern pathophysiology and treatment of esophageal diverticula," *Langenbeck's Archives of Surgery*, vol. 397, no. 1, pp. 29–35, 2012.

[3] P. Glover, T. Westmoreland, R. Roy, D. Sawaya, H. Giles, and M. Nowicki, "Esophageal diverticulum arising from a prolonged retained esophageal foreign body," *Journal of Pediatric Surgery*, vol. 48, no. 2, pp. E9–E12, 2013.

[4] E. Gutkin, A. Shalomov, H. Delshadfar, E. Chorney, and P. Mehta, "Hidden treasure-esophageal diverticulum retained 'foreign' bodies," *Gastrointestinal Endoscopy*, vol. 75, no. 1, pp. 187–189, 2012.

[5] M. R. Kunkala and C. Deschamps, "Delayed esophageal diverticulum formation after stent-based treatment of perforation," *The Journal of Thoracic and Cardiovascular Surgery*, vol. 147, no. 1, pp. e5–e8, 2014.

[6] M. Suhail, A. Smith, A. H. Olivencia-Yurvati, and J. Patel, "Giant esophageal diverticula after laparoscopic band placement," *Annals of Thoracic Surgery*, vol. 94, no. 4, pp. 1330–1332, 2012.

[7] J. H. Jung, J. S. Kim, and Y. K. Kim, "Acquired tracheoesophageal fistula through esophageal diverticulum in patient who had a prolonged tracheostomy tube-a case report," *Annals of Rehabilitation Medicine*, vol. 35, no. 3, pp. 436–440, 2011.

[8] J.-J. Hung, C.-C. Hsieh, S.-C. Lin, and L.-S. Wang, "Squamous cell carcinoma in a large epiphrenic esophageal diverticulum," *Digestive Diseases and Sciences*, vol. 54, no. 6, pp. 1365–1368, 2009.

[9] R. Bagheri, G. Maddah, M. R. Mashhadi et al., "Esophageal diverticula: analysis of 25 cases," *Asian Cardiovascular and Thoracic Annals*, vol. 22, no. 5, pp. 583–587, 2014.

[10] R. W. Postlethwait, "Benign tumors and cysts of the esophagus," *Surgical Clinics of North America*, vol. 63, no. 4, pp. 925–931, 1983.

[11] Y. C. Tay, C. T. Ng, D. Lomanto, and T. K. Ti, "Leiomyoma of the oesophagus managed by thoracoscopic enucleation," *Singapore Medical Journal*, vol. 47, no. 10, pp. 901–903, 2006.

[12] B.-C. Cheng, S. Chang, Z.-F. Mao et al., "Surgical treatment of giant esophageal leiomyoma," *World Journal of Gastroenterology*, vol. 11, no. 27, pp. 4258–4260, 2005.

[13] G. Nese, "Benign tumors and cysts of the esophagus," *Acta chirurgica Scandinavica*, vol. 114, no. 3, pp. 165–171, 1958.

[14] O. Abdel-lah Fernández, A. Alvarez Delgado, F. Carlos Parreño, and A. Rodriguez, "Epiphrenic esophageal diverticulum within a leiomyoma: a rare cause of dysphagia," *Integrative Cancer Science and Therapeutics*, vol. 2, no. 5, pp. 235–238, 2015.

[15] F. A. M. Herbella, A. Dubecz, and M. G. Patti, "Esophageal diverticula and cancer," *Diseases of the Esophagus*, vol. 25, no. 2, pp. 153–158, 2012.

[16] D. Ramos, P. Priego, M. Coll et al., "Comparative study between open and minimally invasive approach in the surgical management of esophageal leiomyoma," *Revista Española de Enfermedades Digestivas*, vol. 108, no. 1, pp. 8–14, 2016.

Atypical Aortoesophageal Fistula with Atypical and Delayed Presentation and Negative Imaging Studies

Seifeldin Hakim,[1] Mihajlo Gjeorgjievski,[1] Lohit Garg,[1] Molly Orosey,[1] and Tusar Desai[2,3]

[1]*Department of Internal Medicine, William Beaumont Hospital, Royal Oak, MI 48073, USA*
[2]*Department of Gastroenterology, William Beaumont Hospital, Royal Oak, MI 48073, USA*
[3]*Oakland University William Beaumont School of Medicine, Royal Oak, MI 48073, USA*

Correspondence should be addressed to Seifeldin Hakim; seifeldinhakim@gmail.com

Academic Editor: Hirotada Akiho

A 59-year-old man with past medical history of thoracic aortic aneurysm treated with thoracic endovascular aortic repair presented with melena for 2 weeks. Initial EGD did not reveal the source of bleeding and showed normal esophagus; abdominal arteriogram did not reveal a fistulous communication and initial CTA showed normal position of the aortic graft stent without endoleak. The sixth EGD revealed a submucosal tumor-like projection in the upper esophagus and stigmata of recent bleeding. Another thoracic endovascular aortic repair with stent was placed over the old graft for presumed aortoesophageal fistula. Poststent upper gastrointestinal series with contrast showed extravasation of the contrast from the esophagus and CTA showed fistulous tract between aorta and esophagus. The patient refused definitive surgical repair despite having infected aortic graft; jejunostomy tube was placed and life-long suppressive antibiotic treatment was given and the patient is doing well at 2-year follow-up.

1. Introduction

Thoracic endovascular aortic repair (TEVAR) has become one of the main therapies for thoracoabdominal aortic diseases including thoracic aortic aneurysm (TAA), traumatic aortic transection, or aortoesophageal fistula (AEF). Although TEVAR is preferred over open surgical repairs for AEF treatment due to better perioperative morbidity and mortality, it is associated with high rate of reintervention due to its complications that occur after TEVAR. TEVAR is performed more frequently despite the lack of randomized controlled trial proving the long-term effectiveness of TEVAR over open surgical repair. AEF is one of the catastrophic complications of TEVAR, although TEVAR itself can be used as a temporary treatment for AEF. In this case, we are presenting AEF that developed as an unusual late complication after an initial TEVAR to treat traumatic thoracic aortic aneurysm; this AEF was treated with another TEVAR and the patient is doing well at 2-year follow-up despite infected old aortic graft that was not removed.

2. Case Presentation

A 59-year-old man with past medical history of repaired saccular descending TAA 5 years ago presented with melanotic stools, progressively worsening epigastric discomfort, low-grade fever, and fatigue for 2 weeks with no episodes of nausea, vomiting, or hematemesis. The patient was taking at least 6 tablets of full-dose aspirin for joint pain daily. Colonoscopy revealed old blood in terminal ileum and esophagogastroduodenoscopy (EGD) revealed gastric petechiae and hiatal hernia. He received proton pump inhibitor for hemorrhagic gastritis and quit taking NSAIDs. After 2 weeks, he presented to our facility with recurrent episodes of melena only without hematemesis. Physical examination revealed stable vital signs, pallor, and soft, nontender abdomen. Laboratory analysis showed hemoglobin = 6.7 g/dL with normal platelet count and normal coagulation profile. Serum parameters of liver and kidney functions were normal. An emergent EGD revealed large adherent blood clot along the greater curvature of the stomach, which could not be removed,

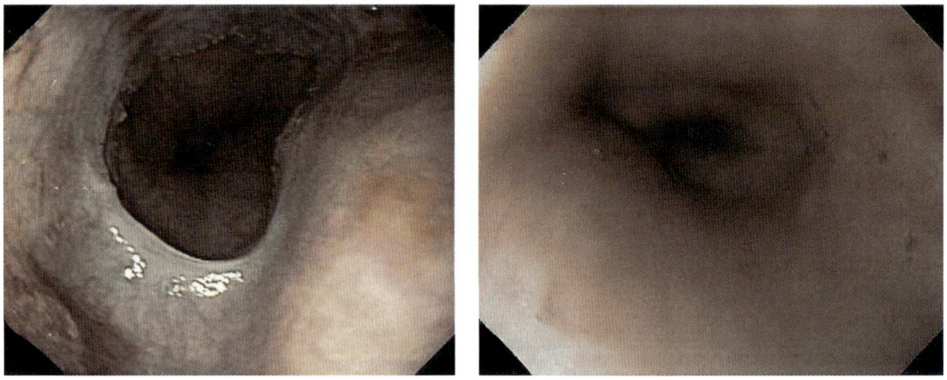

FIGURE 1: Initial EGDs showed normal esophagus with no evidence of aortoesophageal fistula. No evidence of bleeding in the esophagus.

and there was no evidence of active bleeding. The patient was started on proton pump inhibitor continuous infusion for upper gastrointestinal (GI) bleeding from the stomach. Computerized tomography with angiography (CTA) revealed an unchanged position of the aortic graft stent without endoleak.

3. Hospital Course

A follow-up EGD showed more extensive blood clot adherent to the same location that could not be removed. Despite commencement of proton pump inhibitor infusion, the patient continued to have melanotic stool. Abdominal arteriogram revealed no contrast extravasation from the blood vessels, and empiric embolization of the left gastric artery was performed as the source of bleeding was thought to be from a lesion underlying the blood clot along the greater curvature of the stomach. Over the next few days, he continued to have melena and he required transfusion of 12 units of packed red blood cells. Multiple EGDs (Figure 1) were performed, which showed stigmata of recent bleeding with normal esophagus. He developed fever spikes, blood cultures were positive for *Streptococcus* viridans, and the appropriate antibiotics were given. Extensive diagnostic tests were performed including colonoscopy; Technetium-Labeled Red Blood Cell Bleeding Scan and CTA of the abdomen were insignificant. The sixth EGD revealed coagulated blood in the upper one-third of the esophagus overlying a tumor-like submucosal projection secondary to extrinsic compression 5 cm below the upper esophageal sphincter (Figure 2), which was not seen on previous EGDs. TEVAR was performed under fluoroscopic guidance for presumed AEF and a new stent graft was placed over the previous graft with resolution of the GI bleeding. Upper gastrointestinal series (UGIS) with barium revealed extraluminal contrast arising from the esophagus at the level of the aortic arch (Figure 3). A repeat CTA revealed linear high-density tract extending from the left esophageal wall towards the aorta as well as multiple air bubbles adjacent to the aortic graft (Figure 4). These findings confirmed the presence of AEF with closure of aortic side by the recently placed stent. The patient refused to have a definitive open surgical repair. Jejunostomy tube was placed, and life-long suppressive antibiotic treatment is being given as the infected graft is still in place. Follow-up EGD (Figure 5) showed granulation tissue with surrounding inflammation around the fistulous opening with no evidence of recent bleeding and follow-up UGIS showed extravasation of the contrast at the site of the fistula without spillage of the contrast into the aorta. The patient is doing well at 2-year follow-up.

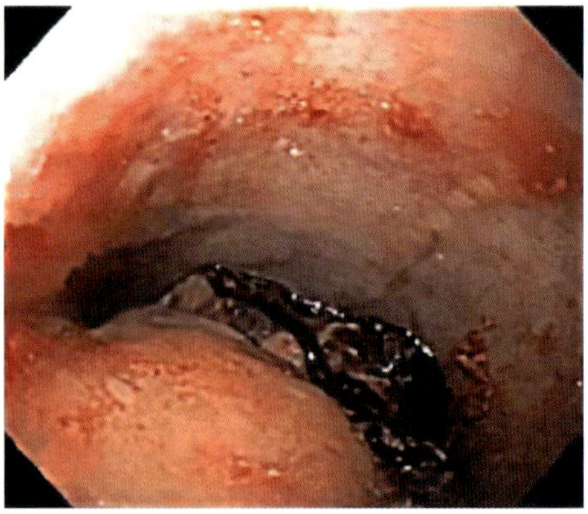

FIGURE 2: Esophagogastroduodenoscopy (EGD) showing submucosal tumor-like projection secondary to extrinsic compression of the upper esophagus with blood clot sitting on top of the compression at 5 cm below the upper esophageal sphincter (UES).

4. Discussion

AEF is a condition that is defined as an abnormal communication between the esophagus and the aorta [1]. AEF occurs primarily due to local disease in the aorta or esophagus including aneurysms, malignancies, and ulcers or secondary to other factors that can cause damage to these organs including presence of foreign bodies, prosthetic grafts, and stents [2, 3]. Hollander and Quick [1] evaluated 500 patients with AEF, revealing that the most common cause of AEF is TAA (256 cases out of 500; 54.2%), followed by foreign body ingestion (93/500; 19.2%) and esophageal malignancy

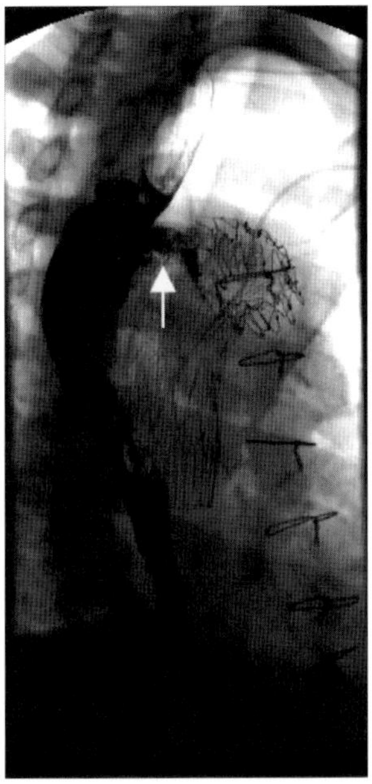

FIGURE 3: Upper gastrointestinal study with barium contrast showing extraluminal contrast seen arising from proximal esophagus extending outward visualizing the fistulous tract.

(85/500; 17%). Prosthetic grafts represented a small number of cases (7/500; 1.4%) with no clear definition whether stents were included or not.

The number of patients undergoing TEVAR has increased significantly in the last 2 decades due to the minimally invasive nature of this technique. AEF is a potential complication of TEVAR that usually occurs within 1–16 months after the procedure and is invariably fatal [4]. Eggebrecht et al.'s [4] study revealed that 6 patients out of 268 developed AEF as a complication of TEVAR (incidence 1.9%). Different mechanisms of AEF development following TEVAR have been postulated including direct erosion of the stent graft into the esophagus, pressure necrosis of the self-expanding prosthesis, ischemic necrosis of the esophagus due to interruption of its vasculature, infection of the stent graft, and the presence of an endoleak [5, 6]. AEF usually occurs within few months after TEVAR, but Kouritas et al. [7] reported one case of AEF that developed 6 years after TEVAR.

Hollander and Quick [1] mentioned in their study that 63% of the patients had sentinel hematemesis, 58% had chest pain, and 42% had dysphagia. Chiari's triad of chest pain and sentinel hematemesis followed by massive hematemesis has been reported in the literature as a common characteristic presentation in patients with AEF [6, 8–12]. Other less frequent presentations include mediastinitis or fever [4, 10]. One case of AEF with positive blood cultures for *Streptococcus* viridans has been reported [3] and this case is the second one. Complications of AEF include mediastinitis, infection of the surgical or endovascular graft, sepsis, and death. Thus, AEF can be a cause or can develop as a complication of graft infection [3].

EGD is the most sensitive and specific modality for diagnosis of AEF [6, 8, 9, 13] and it is the first test used for diagnosis although its sensitivity for detecting AEF is 38% [14]. The most common finding of AEF on EGD is submucosal tumor-like protrusion; however, extrinsic compression, ulcerative lesion, pulsating protrusion with central fistula, and exposure of the aortic stent have been reported as other findings on EGD [11]. CTA might show an extravasation of the contrast material outside the aorta, which is considered a definite sign; however, it is rarely seen [3, 6, 15]. We should suspect AEF when we see the following findings on a CT following TEVAR: mediastinal air, aortic lumen air, persistent or expanding perigraft fluid, soft tissue density beyond 6 months from the date of the procedure, or loss of the aortoesophageal fat plane. An UGIS is an easy way to diagnose AEF as it can visualize an extravasated contrast arising from the esophageal side of the fistula, which is also considered a definite sign [2].

Development of AEF has a very poor prognosis [16] and the condition is generally fatal. The only definitive treatment of AEF is surgical repair and it has to be initiated as soon as possible [8, 9], definitive surgical management includes left thoracotomy with aortic graft replacement, esophageal wall repair, and removal of the fistula, and antibiotics are used as an adjunct to surgery [3]. Using stent graft placement for management of AEF is controversial as there is a theoretical increase in the risk of endoleak after stent placement due to weakening of the aortic wall that already exists by inflammatory changes associated with AEF development [3]. Insertion and inflation of a Blakemore tube can be used to stop bleeding temporarily until patients undergo surgery [17–19]. Xi et al. [20] revealed the advantages of TEVAR over open surgical repair for AEF, which are as follows: it is well tolerated by high risk patients, minimizes risk of cardiovascular disease, reduces mortality, can be performed under sedation and local anesthesia, and is a rapid method to minimize blood loss even in unstable patients, but some studies [3, 20, 21] also suggested that TEVAR should be used as a stop gap measure before definitive surgical repair. Burks Jr. et al. [22] revealed in their case series that TEVAR is a safe method for bleeding control, when it is combined with long-term antibiotic treatment and percutaneous drainage if there is fluid collection or may be combined with esophageal diversion proximal to AEF. Many patients died of coexistent cardiopulmonary disease before infection or aortic degeneration becomes a significant problem; however, it is not a definitive therapy and complete eradication of infection is impossible without debridement of all contaminated prosthetic infected tissues. Antibiotics alone are not recommended as a primary measure to treat AEF because antibiotics alone will not eliminate infection in an infected foreign body [3].

This case had an atypical presentation; he did not present with Chiari's triad. He developed symptoms after 5 years of TEVAR, he underwent 5 EGDs, which showed blood in the stomach without findings suggestive of AEF especially in the setting of a normal esophagus, and the source of bleeding could not be identified until the characteristic tumor-like submucosal protrusion was noticed on the sixth EGD. The normal abdominal arteriogram might be due to the exclusion of the thoracic part of the aorta from the study. Also the initial CTA did not show extravasation of the contrast or other

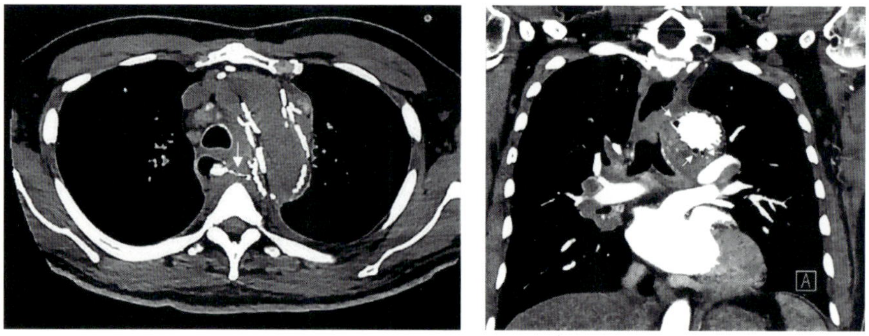

Figure 4: CT angiography axial view showing linear high-density contrast collection extending from esophageal wall towards the aortic graft representing retained barium contrast from the patient's recent upper gastrointestinal series visualizing fistulous tract and the coronal view showing multiple foci of gas or air bubbles adjacent to the patient's aortic stent graft.

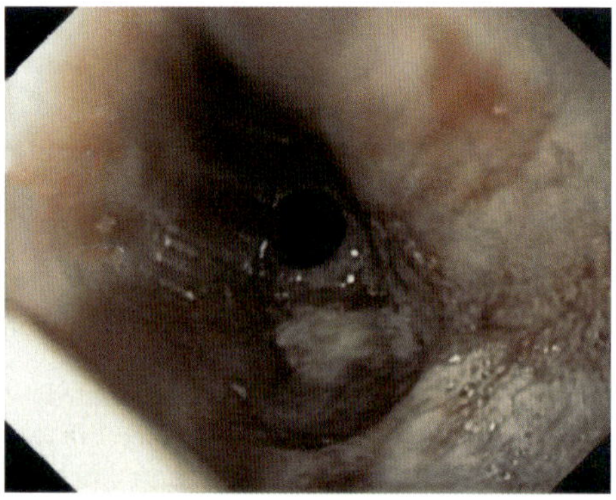

Figure 5: Follow-up EGD showed granulation tissue with inflammation at the site of fistula but no bleeding, no pulsating mass, and no ulcer.

findings suggestive of AEF. The combination of the history of aortic stent graft, upper GI bleeding and endoscopic findings on the sixth EGD, raised the suspicion for AEF and we proceeded with another TEVAR for a presumed AEF and the patient improved after the procedure. UGIS was performed after the second TEVAR, which revealed extraluminal contrast confirming the presumed diagnosis of AEF and the contrast used in UGIS was visualized in the CTA that was performed after TEVAR; this contrast is related to the barium contrast used in UGIS and not the injected contrast of the CTA as the aortic side of the AEF is blocked by the recently placed stent. The patient refused open surgical repair as his symptoms improved after TEVAR, so jejunostomy tube was necessary to avoid continuous food passage into the fistula, which may lead to mediastinitis. Life-long suppressive antibiotics were the only option available although it is not recommended to leave an infected stent without removal especially in the setting of a 59-year-old man who is not old and without comorbid conditions as this will affect his quality of life significantly, but he refused any surgical repairs at least for the meantime. The patient tried to eat soft food, but he developed fever, so he was advised not to swallow anything until definitive surgical repair is performed as it may cause life-threatening mediastinitis. We believe the cause of late AEF formation is either due to delayed infection of the stent or an atypical slow inflammatory changes developed over years. The management was different in this case as the patient refused the recommended definitive treatment. We are presenting this case to share the complicated atypical presentation; despite having negative imaging, the diagnosis of AEF was not ruled out. Diagnosis was confirmed retrospectively after the second TEVAR was performed with UGIS and CTA.

Consent

The patient gave oral consent for publishing his case, endoscopic pictures, and radiological images.

Authors' Contributions

Seifeldin Hakim wrote the whole first draft of the paper and contributed to the edited, final version. Mihajlo Gjeorgjievski contributed to the edited, final version of the paper. Lohit Garg contributed to the edited, final version of the paper. Molly Orosey reviewed the edited, final version. Tusar Desai, Gastroenterology Attendant, performed the consult and the diagnostic esophagogastroduodenoscopy on the reported patient and contributed to the final review of the paper.

References

[1] J. E. Hollander and G. Quick, "Aortoesophageal fistula: a comprehensive review of the literature," *The American Journal of Medicine*, vol. 91, no. 3, pp. 279–287, 1991.

[2] A. R. Bakhshandeh, M. Salehi, H. Radmehr, and G. R. Riahi, "A case of aortoesophageal fistula," *Asian Cardiovascular and Thoracic Annals*, vol. 19, no. 6, pp. 419–421, 2011.

[3] J. D. Christensen and L. E. Heyneman, "Case of the season: aortoesophageal fistula complicating thoracic aortic aneurysm stent graft repair," *Seminars in Roentgenology*, vol. 44, no. 1, pp. 4–7, 2009.

[4] H. Eggebrecht, R. H. Mehta, A. Dechene et al., "Aortoesophageal fistula after thoracic aortic stent-graft placement: a rare but catastrophic complication of a novel emerging technique," *JACC: Cardiovascular Interventions*, vol. 2, no. 6, pp. 570–576, 2009.

[5] A. Morisaki, H. Hirai, Y. Sasaki, K. Hige, Y. Bito, and S. Suehiro, "Aortoesophageal fistula after endovascular repair for aberrant right subclavian artery aneurysm," *Annals of Thoracic and Cardiovascular Surgery*, vol. 20, pp. 790–793, 2014.

[6] E.-P. Xi, J. Zhu, S.-B. Zhu, and Y. Zhang, "Secondary aortoesophageal fistula after thoracic aortic aneurysm endovascular repair: literature review and new insights regarding the hypothesized mechanisms," *International Journal of Clinical and Experimental Medicine*, vol. 7, no. 10, pp. 3244–3252, 2014.

[7] V. K. Kouritas, P. Dedeilias, K. Sotiriou, and S. Klimopoulos, "Delayed presentation of aortoesophageal fistula after endovascular repair," *Asian Cardiovascular and Thoracic Annals*, vol. 24, no. 1, pp. 51–53, 2016.

[8] Y.-H. Fang, X.-L. Zhou, and J.-C. Liu, "Aortoesophageal fistula (AEF): fatal upper gastrointesinal haemorrhage," *The Turkish Journal of Gastroenterology*, vol. 25, supplement 1, pp. 321–323, 2014.

[9] E. D. Genuis and D. J. Kim, "A case of secondary aortoesophageal fistula," *Journal of Emergency Medicine*, vol. 49, no. 6, pp. e193–e194, 2015.

[10] A. Muradi, M. Yamaguchi, A. Kitagawa et al., "Secondary aortoesophageal fistula after thoracic endovascular aortic repair for a huge aneurysm," *Diagnostic and Interventional Radiology*, vol. 19, no. 1, pp. 81–84, 2013.

[11] D. Chiba, N. Hanabata, Y. Araki et al., "Aortoesophageal fistula after thoracic endovascular aortic repair diagnosed and followed with endoscopy," *Internal Medicine*, vol. 52, no. 4, pp. 451–455, 2013.

[12] S. Amin, J. Luketich, and A. Wald, "Aortoesophageal fistula: case report and review of the literature," *Digestive Diseases and Sciences*, vol. 43, no. 8, pp. 1665–1671, 1998.

[13] B. Dołega-Kozierowski, K. Sokratous, K. Dyś et al., "Aortoesophageal fistula as a complication of thoracic aorta aneurism stent grafting—a case report and literature review," *Polish Journal of Radiology*, vol. 77, no. 4, pp. 77–80, 2012.

[14] K. Soga, R. Kitamura, S. Takenaka, K. Kassai, and K. Itani, "Progressive endoscopic findings in a case of aortoesophageal fistula," *Digestive Endoscopy*, vol. 24, no. 4, p. 290, 2012.

[15] K. D. Hagspiel, U. C. Turba, U. Bozlar et al., "Diagnosis of aortoenteric fistulas with CT angiography," *Journal of Vascular and Interventional Radiology*, vol. 18, no. 4, pp. 497–504, 2007.

[16] E. Kieffer, L. Chiche, and D. Gomes, "Aortoesophageal fistula: value of in situ aortic allograft replacement," *Annals of Surgery*, vol. 238, no. 2, pp. 283–290, 2003.

[17] D. M. McFaddin and C. Dang, "Management of aortoesophageal fistula. A case report," *American Surgeon*, vol. 51, no. 9, pp. 548–550, 1985.

[18] B. S. Strug, D. A. Saltzman, M. I. Feldman, and A. H. Sabbagh, "Aorto-esophageal fistula," *Cardiovascular Research Center Bulletin*, vol. 18, no. 1, pp. 34–38, 1979.

[19] A. Gomez-Alonso, F. Lozano, F. Cuadrado, and A. Almazan, "Traumatic aorto-esophageal fistula," *The Journal of Thoracic and Cardiovascular Surgery*, vol. 87, no. 1, pp. 148–149, 1984.

[20] E.-P. Xi, J. Zhu, S.-B. Zhu et al., "Surgical treatment of aortoesophageal fistula induced by a foreign body in the esophagus: 40 years of experience at a single hospital," *Surgical Endoscopy and Other Interventional Techniques*, vol. 27, no. 9, pp. 3412–3416, 2013.

[21] E. L. Verhoeven and G. Vourliotakis, "Thoracic endovascular aortic repair for aortobronchial or aortoesophageal fistulas: permanent or temporary salvage or not an option at all?" *Journal of Endovascular Therapy*, vol. 16, no. 4, pp. 441–442, 2009.

[22] J. A. Burks Jr., P. L. Faries, E. C. Gravereaux, L. H. Hollier, and M. L. Marin, "Endovascular repair of bleeding aortoenteric fistulas: a 5-year experience," *Journal of Vascular Surgery*, vol. 34, no. 6, pp. 1055–1059, 2001.

Pancreaticopleural Fistula: A Review of Imaging Diagnosis and Early Endoscopic Intervention

Ali Kord Valeshabad,[1,2] Jennifer Acostamadiedo,[3] Lekui Xiao,[1] Winnie Mar,[1] and Karen L. Xie[1]

[1]Department of Radiology, University of Illinois at Chicago, USA
[2]Division of Interventional Radiology, University of Illinois at Chicago, USA
[3]Department of Medicine, Mercy Hospital and Medical Center, Chicago, IL, USA

Correspondence should be addressed to Karen L. Xie; karenlin@uic.edu

Academic Editor: Engin Altintas

A 49-year-old male with history of chronic alcohol-induced pancreatitis presented with one month of worsening left pleuritic chest pain and shortness of breath. Chest radiograph demonstrated bilateral pleural effusions. Thoracentesis revealed increased amylase in the pleural fluid. Computed tomography (CT) and magnetic resonance cholangiopancreatography (MRCP) showed a fistula tract between the left pleural cavity and pancreas which was confirmed on endoscopic retrograde cholangiopancreatography (ERCP). Patient was treated with placement of a pancreatic stent with complete resolution of the fistula tract approximately in 9 weeks. A systematic literature search was performed on reported cases with pancreaticopleural fistula (PPF) who underwent early therapeutic endoscopy within the last 10 years. Imaging modalities, particularly CT and MRCP, play essential role in prompt preprocedural diagnosis of PPF. Early therapeutic ERCP is an effective and relatively safe treatment option for PPF, so invasive surgery may be avoided.

1. Introduction

Pancreaticopleural fistula (PPF) is an uncommon complication of chronic pancreatitis, often presenting with recurrent unilateral or bilateral pleural effusions [1, 2]. There is usually an abnormal communication to the pleural space from posterior pancreatic duct disruption or pancreatic pseudocyst extension into the pleural cavity [3]. Minimally invasive endoscopic intervention following medical therapy is usually the first choice before invasive surgical management [2, 3]. To our knowledge, there is no recent comprehensive data available regarding the outcome of early endoscopic treatment in the patients with PPF. In this study, we present a case of PPF treated successfully by endoscopic retrograde cholangiopancreatography (ERCP) and transpapillary pancreatic duct stent placement. In our case imaging played an important role in the investigation of PPF and follow-up after ERCP. We performed a systematic literature search of reported PPF cases who underwent early therapeutic endoscopy within the last 10 years, with a review of the utility of diagnostic imaging and the outcome of endoscopic management of PPF.

2. Methods

A review of the literature was performed using the MEDLINE database with searching of the keywords: pancreaticopleural fistula, pancreatico-pleural fistula, and pancreaticopleural effusion. Inclusion was limited to cases reported in the English or Spanish language between 2007 and 2017 who underwent early ERCP alone or before any operative management. Forty-three patients (including the patient in this study) with PPF were reported during the 2007-2017 period [2, 4–36]. Data is presented as percentage or mean values ± standard deviation (SD). N throughout the manuscript stands for total number of cases with available data for that variable.

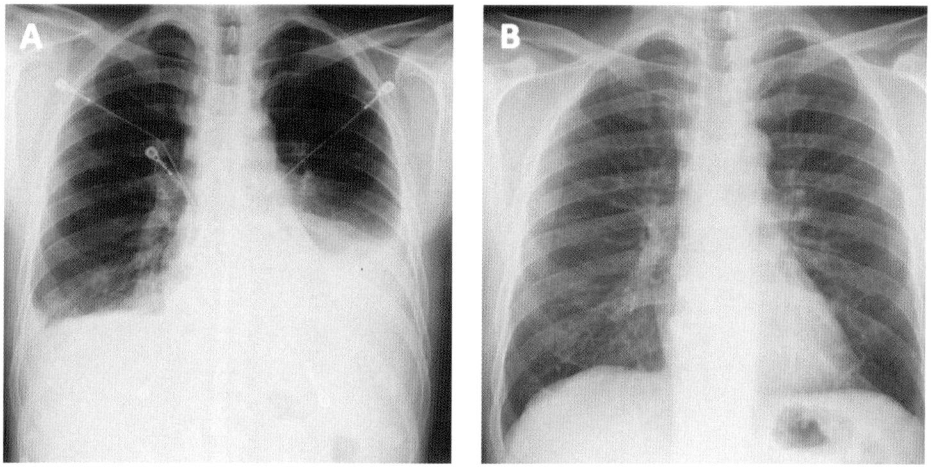

(a) (b)

FIGURE 1: Chest radiograph at admission (a) demonstrates moderate left and trace right pleural effusions with a left retrocardiac opacity. Follow-up chest radiograph shows complete resolution of the abnormalities after treatment (b).

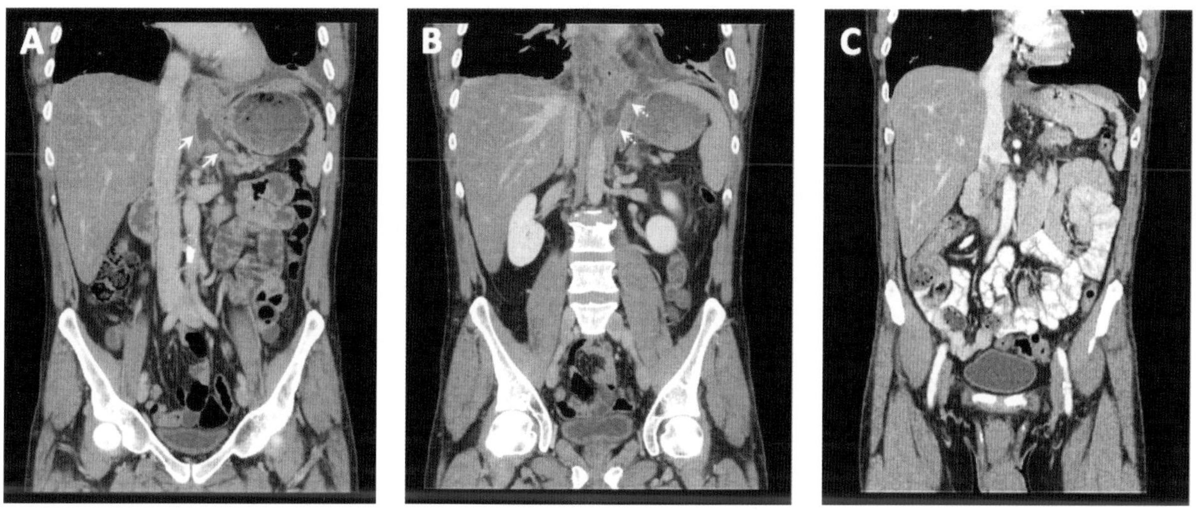

(a) (b) (c)

FIGURE 2: Coronal views of contrast-enhanced CT of the abdomen and pelvis show a fistula tract arising from the tail of the pancreas ((a) white arrows) extending caudally and connecting to the left pleural space ((b) dashed white arrows) with small pleural effusion and overlying atelectasis. A follow-up CT (c) demonstrates resolution of the fistula tract and pleural effusion.

3. Results

3.1. Case Presentation. A 49-year-old male with history of alcohol-induced pancreatitis presented with 1 month of worsening left pleuritic chest pain and shortness of breath. Initial physical exam was unremarkable, and laboratory tests were only remarkable for increased lactate dehydrogenase and borderline-low albumin. Initial chest radiograph showed moderate left and small right pleural effusions with left retrocardiac opacity (Figure 1). Computed tomography (CT) pulmonary angiogram was performed and was negative for pulmonary embolism and showed only small bilateral pleural effusions.

On admission, patient underwent thoracentesis and approximately 1L of brown fluid from the left pleural space was removed. Pleural fluid evaluation demonstrated an exudative effusion with lipase of 2912 IU/L and amylase of 2783 IU/L. CT abdomen and pelvis demonstrated a fluid density tract arising from the pancreatic tail, extending caudally through the diaphragm from the esophageal hiatus, communicating with the left pleural space (Figure 2). The patient was started on medical therapy with octreotide. Magnetic resonance cholangiopancreatography (MRCP) confirmed a PPF tract with irregular, dilated, main pancreatic and common bile ducts (Figure 3). The patient underwent ERCP two days after admission which redemonstrated mild diffuse dilatation of ventral pancreatic duct involving the head, body, and tail of the pancreas with evidence of pancreatic duct leak in the most upstream tail of the pancreas that extended caudally to the left pleural cavity, consistent with PPF. A 5 FR x 10 cm

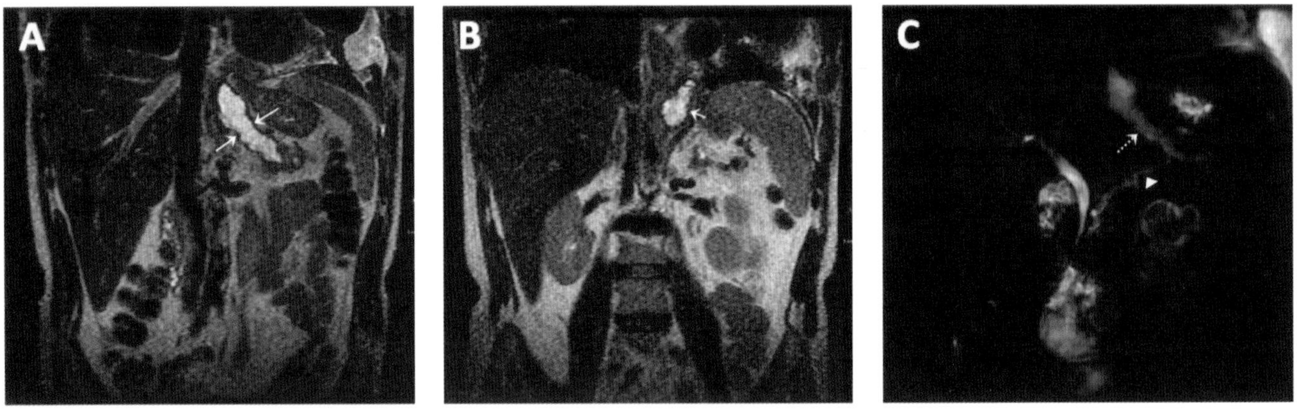

(a) (b) (c)

FIGURE 3: Coronal T2-weighted MRCP images (a, b) demonstrate a hyperintense tract arising from the tail of pancreas ((a) large white arrows), crossing the diaphragm and entering the pleural space ((b) short white arrow). Thick slab 2D MRCP images (c) show an irregular main pancreatic duct (white arrow head) and redemonstrates the fistula tract arising from the tail of pancreas (white dashed arrow).

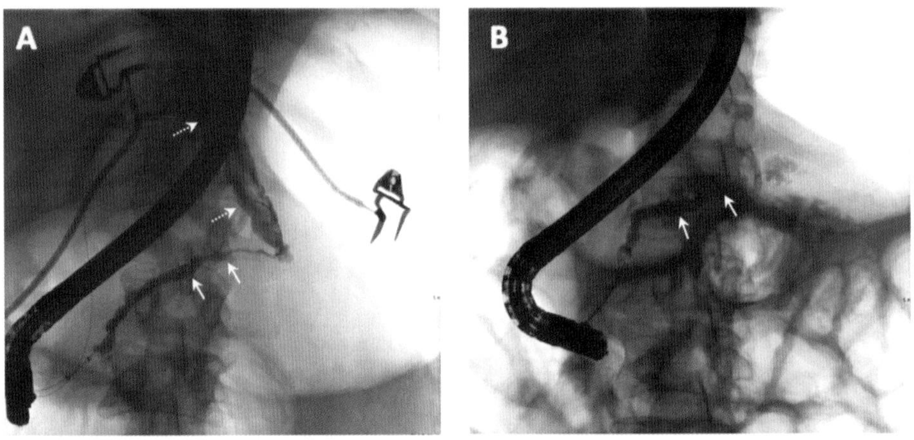

(a) (b)

FIGURE 4: ERCP at admission (a) shows mild diffuse dilatation of ventral pancreatic duct involving the head, body, and tail of the pancreas (white arrows) with pancreatic duct leak in the most upstream tail of the pancreas that extends caudally to the pleural cavity (dashed white arrows). A follow-up ERCP after treatment (b) demonstrates mild diffuse dilatation of the main pancreatic duct with resolution of the fistula tract.

plastic stent was placed in the pancreatic duct and a biliary and pancreatic sphincterotomy was performed to divert the fluid leak.

The hospital course was complicated by post-ERCP acute pancreatitis, which was treated with bowel rest and empiric antibiotics. Postprocedure chest radiograph showed worsening pleural effusions and surgical management including distal pancreatectomy was considered. However, surgery was deferred after the patient improved clinically with medical management, and a repeat chest radiograph revealed improvement of the pleural effusions. The patient improved clinically and was discharged with pain medications.

The patient returned to the emergency department within the first week after discharge with complaints of worsening abdominal and chest pain. Another thoracentesis was performed with removal of 400 mL fluid. The study of pleural fluid specimen demonstrated amylase level > 1000 IU/L which was positive for Klebsiella and enterococcus faecalis. The patient was treated with intravenous antibiotics and the pancreatic stent was upsized to 7Fr.

Approximately 9 weeks following the initial ERCP, repeat ERCP demonstrated no extravasation of contrast from the pancreatic tail, and the stent was downsized to 5Fr. Repeat ERCP 15 weeks after the index procedure showed mild diffuse dilatation of the main pancreatic duct with no extravasation of contrast or stenosis (Figure 4). Therefore, the pancreatic duct stent was removed. Chest radiograph and CT abdomen pelvis showed complete resolution of pleural effusions bilateral as well as the PPF tract (Figures 1 and 2).

3.2. Previous Cases of Pancreaticopleural Fistula. Table 1 summarizes the demographics and clinical data of previously reported cases of PPF. Seventy-nine percent of the cases were male with a mean age of 50 ± 13 years (N = 41, range:

TABLE 1: Demographics and clinical data of previously reported cases of pancreaticopleural fistula between 2007 and 2017. N = total number of cases. n is the number of cases data reported. SD = standard deviation.

Variables	N	n (percentage) or Mean ± SD
Male gender	43	34 (79%)
Mean Age (years)	41	50 ± 13
History of chronic pancreatitis	30	20 (47%)
History of alcohol use	40	31 (78%)
Pleural fluid amylase (IU/L)	43	30021 ± 25410
CT Identified Fistula Tract	40	25 (63%)
MRCP Identified Fistula Tract	24	20 (83%)
ERCP Identified Fistula Tract	43	30 (70%)
Medical treatment	39	33 (85%)
Post-ERCP acute pancreatitis	21	2 (9.5%)
Post-ERCP superinfection of pleural fluid	22	6 (27.0%)
Operative management	43	23 (53%)
Partial/total pancreatectomy		7 (30%)
Thoracostomy/decortication		7 (30%)
Pancreaticojejunostomy		4 (18%)
Exploratory laparoscopy and external drainage		4 (18%)
Surgical sphincterotomy		1 (4%)
Duration of hospital stay (days)		27 ± 16
Mortality	43	1 (2%)

5-78 years). History of alcohol use and chronic pancreatitis was present in 78% (N = 40) and 67% (N = 30) of the patients, respectively. All patients presented with respiratory symptoms including shortness of breath and pleuritic chest pain. The pleural fluid amylase level ranged 1200-138000 IU/L (N = 43).

Chest radiograph was performed in 95% of the patients and showed unilateral or bilateral pleural effusion. Forty (93%) of the patients underwent CT which demonstrated the fistula tract in 25 out of 40 patients (63%). MRCP was performed in 24 patients which revealed the fistula tract in 20 of them (83%). The fistula tract was visualized in 30 patients out of 43 (70%) during the ERCP procedure. In 3 patients the diagnosis was made based on the high amylase level of the pleural fluid.

The majority of the patients (85%, N = 39) received medical therapy before any intervention. The medical therapy included octreotide, somatostatin, total parenteral nutrition, and antibiotics. The time to ERCP after admission was available only in 4 cases and ranged 1-21 days. Post-ERCP acute pancreatitis was reported in 9.5% of cases (N = 21) and superinfection of the pleural fluid occurred in 27.0% of patients (N = 22). Twenty-three out of 43 patients required surgery after the initial ERCP, including distal pancreatectomy (30%), surgical thoracostomy/decortication (30%), pancreaticojejunostomy (18%), exploratory laparoscopy, and external drainage (18%). One patient (4%) underwent surgical sphincterotomy secondary to difficult anatomy for ERCP. ERCP alone and ERCP with surgery were successful in 100% and 96% of patients, respectively. The total duration of the hospital stay was 27 ± 16 days (N = 28). One patient (2%, N = 43) with refractory pleural effusion refused surgical intervention and died.

4. Discussion

4.1. Demographics and Presentations. Pancreatic Pleural Fistula (PPF) is a rare entity with an approximate incident rate of 0.4%. Based on this literature review, PPF usually involves males in their late 40s with chronic pancreatitis mainly from excessive alcohol abuse, consistent with previous studies [1]. A smaller percentage of cases may be due to biliary stones, trauma, and idiopathic pancreatitis [1]. Patients with PPF usually present to the emergency room with respiratory symptoms including shortness of breath [37], as seen in our patient, and less commonly with diffuse upper quadrant abdominal pain, nausea, and vomiting without rebound or guarding [1, 2, 8, 27].

4.2. Diagnosis. History and physical examination are nonspecific for PPF and further evaluation with imaging and laboratory work-up is required. In patients with PPF, chest radiograph usually demonstrates unilateral or bilateral pleural effusion, with the left side being more common. Blood laboratory evaluation may show increased levels of gamma-glutamyl transferase [37]. Thoracentesis is usually required for symptom relief. Laboratory analysis of the pleural fluid shows an amylase level greater than 1000 IU which may be suggestive for PPF in the absence of malignant cells [1]. In our patient, the initial CT imaging showed the fistula communication between the tail of the pancreas and left pleural space which was confirmed by MRCP and ERCP. From our review, CT was performed on majority of patients with PPF (93%) and was able to identify the fistula in 63% of patients which was comparable with ERCP (70%). Compared to ERCP, CT has the advantages of being noninvasive and relatively less expensive and can be completed in a much shorter time with no sedation required. ERCP has the advantages that it can locate the site of ductal leak and perform simultaneous intervention [2, 3, 30, 37]. In old studies CT was reported to identify fistula tract only in 30% of cases with PPF [1]; application of high resolution CT images with multiplanar reconstruction has likely increased the ability to visualize the fistula tract in newer studies. MRCP showed fistula tract in 83% of patients with PPF in this study, which is similar to reported studies [38]. In addition, CT and MRCP are useful in evaluating additional pancreatic parenchyma and ductal structural abnormalities such as pancreatic mass, pseudocysts, or collections [32, 35], which is valuable for surgical or interventional planning [1].

4.3. Management and Outcome. The majority of patients (85%) in the studies we reviewed received medical therapy before any intervention, consistent with previous reports [1]. The medical therapy included octreotide, somatostatin, total parenteral nutrition, and antibiotics. King et al. [1] reported the outcome of early operative management in 63 patients with PPF between 1970 and 2008. In their study, the early operative management had a success rate of 94%. Six patients underwent ERCP which was successful in all cases. ERCP alone and ERCP with surgery was successful in 100% and 96% of patients in our review, which is comparable to king et al. study. The total duration of the hospital stay in this review was 27 ± 16 days which was relatively shorter than reported 40 ± 6 days for patients who received medical therapy and surgery [1]. Postprocedural acute pancreatitis and superinfection of the pleural fluid were the most common complications after ERCP based on our review. Endoscopic pancreatico- or cystogastric plastic stent placement may be helpful to avoid postprocedural acute pancreatitis. Some other less common complications are intra-abdominal infections, wound infections, entrapped lung and in some cases diabetes mellitus after surgery [2]. Only one patient (2%) died after the index endoscopic procedure who had refractory pleural effusion and refused surgical intervention. The mortality rate of patients with PPF who underwent surgical intervention with or without medical therapy has been reported as high as 12-17% [1, 3]. In addition, in patients after ERCP ductal stenting there is a faster transition to feeding and reduction of recovery time. ERCP is both a diagnostic and therapeutic tool which has reduced the hospital stay and mortality rate compared to the traditional operative management [2–4, 37], although further prospective studies are still required to compare the cost-effectiveness and long-term outcome of ERCP with surgery.

5. Conclusion

Imaging modalities, particularly CT and MRCP, play essential role in prompt preprocedural diagnosis of PPF. Early therapeutic ERCP is an effective and relatively safe treatment option for PPF, so invasive surgery may be avoided.

Authors' Contributions

Jennifer Acostamadiedo and Lekui Xiao have equal contribution and ordered alphabetically.

Acknowledgments

The manuscript is supported by the Research Open Access Publishing (ROAAP) Fund of the University of Illinois at Chicago for financial support towards the open access publishing fee for this article.

References

[1] J. C. King, H. A. Reber, S. Shiraga, and O. J. Hines, "Pancreatic-pleural fistula is best managed by early operative intervention," *Surgery*, vol. 147, no. 1, pp. 154–159, 2010.

[2] C. M. Tay and S. K. Y. Chang, "Diagnosis and management of pancreaticopleural fistula," *Singapore Medical Journal*, vol. 54, no. 4, pp. 190–194, 2013.

[3] B. Y. Safadi and J. M. Marks, "Pancreatic-pleural fistula: the role of ERCP in diagnosis and treatment," *Gastrointestinal Endoscopy*, vol. 51, no. 2, pp. 213–215, 2000.

[4] E. Wee, C. Anastassiades, and B. C. Yip, "Endoscopic treatment of a pancreaticopleural fistula associated with a tension hydrothorax," *Journal of Digestive Diseases*, vol. 18, no. 5, pp. 309–312, 2017.

[5] K. Vijaykumar, K. G. Dsouza, and L. Lerner, "Pancreaticopleural Fistula: The Formidable Liaison," *Journal of Bronchology & Interventional Pulmonology*, vol. 24, no. 4, pp. e60–e61, 2017.

[6] K. Dąbkowski, A. Białek, M. Kukla et al., "Mediastinal Pancreatic Pseudocysts," *Clinical Endoscopy*, vol. 50, no. 1, pp. 76–80, 2017.

[7] J. C. Branco, D. V. Horta, and J. Reis, "A rare acute thoracic manifestation of a chronic digestive disease: pancreaticopleural fistula," *Revista Española de Enfermedades Digestivas*, vol. 109, pp. 317-318, 2017.

[8] E. Virgilio, P. Mercantini, F. Catta, M. Grieco, M. Cavallini, and M. Ferri, "Pancreaticopleural fistula," *Surgical Infections*, vol. 17, no. 2, pp. 266-267, 2016.

[9] E. E.-H. Chan and V. G. Shelat, "Pancreaticopleural Fistula Causing Massive Right Hydrothorax and Respiratory Failure," *Case Reports in Surgery*, vol. 2016, Article ID 8294056, 3 pages, 2016.

[10] M. J. Blayney, A. Nguyen, and D. M. Aboulafia, "Diagnosis and Management of a Pancreaticopleural Fistula in a Patient with AIDS and a Large Pleural Effusion," *Journal of the International Association of Providers of AIDS Care*, vol. 15, no. 6, pp. 459–462, 2016.

[11] S. Abdalla, I. Nikolopoulos, and R. Kerwat, "Pancreatic Pseudocyst Pleural Fistula in Gallstone Pancreatitis," *Case Reports in Emergency Medicine*, vol. 2016, Article ID 4269424, 3 pages, 2016.

[12] C. E. Redmond, S. H. McEvoy, A. Cullen, S. J. Skehan, and K. C. Conlon, "Pancreaticopleural fistula as a presentation of a pancreatic neoplasm. A report of a case and review of the literature," *Journal of the Pancreas*, vol. 16, no. 1, pp. 95-96, 2015.

[13] K. Gowrinath, P. Jyothy, and C. Raghavendra, "Unusual cause of bilateral pleural effusion," *Journal of Clinical and Diagnostic Research*, vol. 9, no. 6, pp. OJ02–OJ03, 2015.

[14] E. Francisco, M. Mendes, S. Vale, and J. Ferreira, "Pancreaticopleural fistula: An unusual complication of pancreatitis," *BMJ Case Reports*, vol. 2015, 2015.

[15] L. Vasilieva, S. Adamidi, N. Kittou, K. Papiris, A. Romanos, and S. P. Dourakis, "Right-sided pancreaticopleural fistula," *Annals of Gastroenterology*, vol. 27, no. 4, pp. 436-437, 2014.

[16] M. Jimenez-Fuertes, M. Duran-Poveda, and D. Garcia-Olmo, "Pancreaticopleural fistula: An unusual cause of persistent pleural effusion," *Revista Española de Enfermedades Digestivas*, vol. 106, pp. 428-429, 2014.

[17] I. S. Choe, Y. S. Kim, T. H. Lee et al., "Acute mediastinitis arising from pancreatic mediastinal fistula in recurrent pancreatitis," *World Journal of Gastroenterology*, vol. 20, no. 40, pp. 14997–15000, 2014.

[18] T. Altasan, Y. Aljehani, A. Almalki, S. Algamdi, A. Talag, and K. Alkattan, "Pancreaticopleural fistula: An overlooked entity," *Asian Cardiovascular and Thoracic Annals*, vol. 22, no. 1, pp. 98–101, 2014.

[19] S. Ozbek, M. Gumus, H. A. Yuksekkaya, and A. Batur, "An unexpected cause of pleural effusion in paediatric emergency medicine," *BMJ Case Reports*, vol. 2013, 2013.

[20] A. Okano, M. Ohana, F. Kusumi, and M. Nabeshima, "Hepatobiliary and pancreatic: Pancreaticopleural fistula," *Journal of Gastroenterology and Hepatology*, vol. 28, no. 11, pp. 1692-1692, 2013.

[21] T.-Y. Huang and M.-J. Tsai, "Gastrointestinal: Black pleural effusion induced by pancreaticopleural fistula," *Journal of Gastroenterology and Hepatology*, vol. 28, no. 12, pp. 1798-1798, 2013.

[22] S. Sonoda, M. Taniguchi, T. Sato et al., "Bilateral pleural fluid caused by a pancreaticopleural fistula requiring surgical treatment," *Internal Medicine*, vol. 51, no. 18, pp. 2655–2661, 2012.

[23] D. Shah, A. B. Desai, and B. Salvi, "Pancreaticopleural fistula complicating chronic pancreatitis," *BMJ Case Reports*, vol. 2012, 2012.

[24] M. Kutz Leoz, R. Irisarri Garde, J. J. Vila Costas et al., "Pleural effusion secondary to pancreaticopleural fistula following acute pancreatitis," *Gastroenterología y Hepatología*, vol. 35, no. 2, pp. 70–73, 2012.

[25] J. Giaccotto, D. Curtis, and E. Shore, "Pancreaticopleural fistula: An unusual cause of pleural effusion," *Connecticut Medicine*, vol. 76, no. 4, pp. 201–203, 2012.

[26] H. El-Beialy and I. Fernandez, "Unusual case of persistent unilateral pleural effusion secondary to pancreaticopleural fistula," *International Journal of Surgery Case Reports*, vol. 3, no. 9, pp. 435-436, 2012.

[27] M. Wronski, M. Slodkowski, W. Cebulski, D. Moronczyk, and I. W. Krasnodebski, "Optimizing management of pancreaticopleural fistulas," *World Journal of Gastroenterology*, vol. 17, no. 42, pp. 4696–4703, 2011.

[28] B. Eovaldi and C. Zanetti, "Non-anion gap metabolic acidosis in a patient with a pancreaticopleural fistula," *The Journal of the American Osteopathic Association*, vol. 111, no. 5, pp. 344-345, 2011.

[29] A. Saleem, M. D. Sawyer, and T. H. Baron, "Laparoscopy assisted transjejunal ERCP for treatment of pancreaticopleural fistula," *Journal of the Pancreas*, vol. 11, no. 1, pp. 69–71, 2010.

[30] S. T. Cooper, J. Malick, K. McGrath, A. Slivka, and M. K. Sanders, "EUS-guided rendezvous for the treatment of pancreaticopleural fistula in a patient with chronic pancreatitis and pancreas pseudodivisum," *Gastrointestinal Endoscopy*, vol. 71, no. 3, pp. 652–654, 2010.

[31] A. Cocieru and P. F. Saldinger, "Frey procedure for pancreaticopleural fistula," *Journal of Gastrointestinal Surgery*, vol. 14, no. 5, pp. 929-930, 2010.

[32] S. Vyas, D. Gogoi, S. K. Sinha, P. Singh, T. D. Yadav, and N. Khandelwal, "Pancreaticopleural fistula: an unusual complication of pancreatitis diagnosed with magnetic resonance cholangiopancreatography," *Journal of the Pancreas*, vol. 10, no. 6, pp. 671–673, 2009.

[33] M. Sut, R. Gray, M. Ramachandran, and T. Diamond, "Pancreaticopleural fistula: a rare complication of ERCP—induced pancreatitis," *The Ulster Medical Journal*, vol. 78, no. 3, pp. 185-186, 2009.

[34] A. Kilic, C. Cook, I. Qureshi, R. J. Landreneau, and M. J. Schuchert, "Pancreaticopleural Fistula Presenting as Right-Sided Hemothorax," *The Annals of Thoracic Surgery*, vol. 87, no. 4, pp. 1262–1264, 2009.

[35] J. J. Kiewiet, M. Moret, W. L. Blok, M. F. Gerhards, and L. T. de Wit, "Two Patients with Chronic Pancreatitis Complicated by a Pancreaticopleural Fistula," *Case Reports in Gastroenterology*, vol. 3, no. 1, pp. 36–42, 2009.

[36] M. S. Boudaya, M. Alifano, S. Baccari, and J.-F. Regnard, "Hemothorax as the clinical presentation of a pancreaticopleural fistula: Report of a case," *Surgery Today*, vol. 37, no. 6, pp. 518–520, 2007.

[37] H. Elkaoui, F. Atoini, S. M. Bouchentouf et al., "Pancreatic-pleural fistula in chronic pancreatitis," *Arab Journal of Gastroenterology*, vol. 13, no. 1, pp. 38–40, 2012.

[38] K. Keyashian and J. Buxbaum, "Pleural effusion caused by a pancreatic pleural fistula," *Gastrointestinal Endoscopy*, vol. 76, no. 2, pp. 422–424, 2012.

Seronegative Intestinal Villous Atrophy: A Diagnostic Challenge

Cláudio Martins, Cristina Teixeira, Suzane Ribeiro, Daniel Trabulo, Cláudia Cardoso, João Mangualde, Ricardo Freire, Ana Luísa Alves, Élia Gamito, Isabelle Cremers, and Ana Paula Oliveira

Department of Gastroenterology, Setúbal Hospital Center, São Bernardo Hospital, Setúbal, Portugal

Correspondence should be addressed to Cláudio Martins; cmartinsl@campus.ul.pt

Academic Editor: Maria Teresa Bardella

Celiac disease is the most important cause of intestinal villous atrophy. Seronegative intestinal villous atrophy, including those that are nonresponsive to a gluten-free diet, is a diagnostic challenge. In these cases, before establishing the diagnosis of seronegative celiac disease, alternative etiologies of atrophic enteropathy should be considered. Recently, a new clinical entity responsible for seronegative villous atrophy was described—olmesartan-induced sprue-like enteropathy. Herein, we report two uncommon cases of atrophic enteropathy in patients with arterial hypertension under olmesartan, who presented with severe chronic diarrhea and significant involuntary weight loss. Further investigation revealed intestinal villous atrophy and intraepithelial lymphocytosis. Celiac disease and other causes of villous atrophy were ruled out. Drug-induced enteropathy was suspected and clinical improvement and histologic recovery were verified after olmesartan withdrawal. These cases highlight the importance for clinicians to maintain a high index of suspicion for olmesartan as a precipitant of sprue-like enteropathy.

1. Introduction

The combination of diarrhea, weight loss, and villous atrophy (VA) is usually associated with celiac disease (CD) [1]. The diagnosis of CD is supported by positive serological tests, celiac permissive HLA type, and symptomatic and histologic response to a gluten-free diet (GFD). Although CD is the most common cause of VA, patients with VA and negative celiac serology are encountered, placing a diagnostic and therapeutic dilemma. Testing for other conditions such as *Crohn*'s disease, autoimmune enteropathy, microscopic enterocolitis, and infectious enteritis should be warranted. Another possible cause of VA has recently garnered more attention—drug-induced enteropathy. Reports of damage to the intestinal villi by pharmaceuticals have been described previously with the use of immunosuppressive drugs, in particular azathioprine and methotrexate [2, 3]. Recently, a new drug was linked to sprue-like enteropathy—the oral angiotensin-receptor blocker (ARB) olmesartan. To date, the pathophysiologic mechanisms of olmesartan-induced sprue-like enteropathy (OISLE) remain unknown, although a cell-mediated immune response and a genetic predisposition are suggested.

Herein, we report two uncommon cases of severe OISLE and discuss the natural history of this entity.

2. Case Report 1

A 53-year-old Caucasian female was admitted to our Department with a 6-month clinical picture of diarrhea and significant involuntary weight loss (20% body weight). She reported between 6 and 10 daily episodes of bulky, watery, and nonbloody diarrhea, abdominal bloating, and, more recently, severe asthenia. She denied abdominal pain, fever or other symptoms suggestive of local or systemic infections, recent travels or sick contacts, prior exposure to health care environments, or changes in her diet habits or medications within the last few years. Apart from arterial hypertension treated with olmesartan 40 mg/daily for the last six years, her past medical and surgical history were unremarkable. The patient did not respond to initial therapeutic approach,

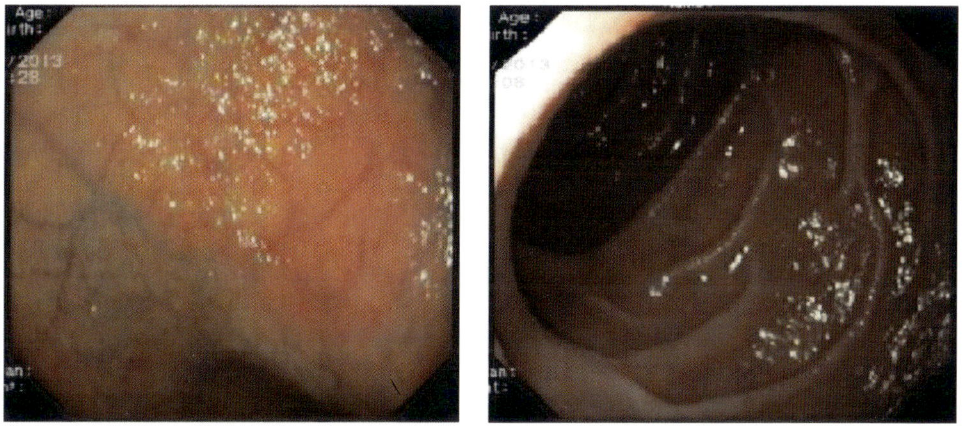

(a) (b)

Figure 1: Endoscopic findings. (a) Visible blood vessels on the duodenal bulb. (b) Attenuation of mucosal folds on the second portion of duodenum.

including probiotics, an opioid-receptor agonist, and gluten- and lactose-free diet, as well a trial of oral antibiotic for possible small bowel bacterial overgrowth.

On admission, physical examination showed pallor and muscle wasting. Initial blood tests showed mild microcytic anemia (11 g/dL; N: 11.5–15.5), leukopenia (3.8×10^9/L; N: 4.5–10), thrombocytopenia (130×10^9/L; N: 150–400), and hypokalemia (2.8 mmol/L; N: 3.5–5). The rest of the laboratory study was unremarkable including erythrocyte sedimentation rate, C-reactive protein, liver and kidney tests, total protein, albumin, and immunoglobulin levels, B12 vitamin, folic acid, thyroid-stimulating hormone, anti-tissue transglutaminase antibodies, and serology for human immunodeficiency virus (HIV) and cytomegalovirus. Stool culture for infectious agents and polymerase chain reaction testing for *C. difficile* toxins A and B were negative.

The subsequent workup included abdominopelvic computed tomography scan which was negative for pancreatic abnormalities or other suspicious lesions for malignancy; total colonoscopy and terminal ileoscopy with random biopsies that were normal and with no evidence of inflammatory bowel disease or microscopic colitis; and upper endoscopy that showed attenuation of duodenal folds (Figure 1) and histopathological examination confirmed a partial villous atrophy and intraepithelial lymphocyte infiltration with no signs of granulomas, microorganisms, or malignancy (Figure 2).

A diagnostic hypothesis of OISLE was placed and, therefore, this drug was withdrawn and switched to lisinopril. Prompt improvement was achieved within 72 h with resolution of diarrhea and normalization of laboratory tests. Upper endoscopy was repeated two months later showing normal duodenal appearance and complete recovery of duodenal villi and no intraepithelial lymphocyte infiltration, on histology. At six-month follow-up, the patient remained asymptomatic with complete recovery of weight loss.

3. Case Report 2

A 65-year-old Caucasian female with arterial hypertension under olmesartan 40 mg/daily in the last four years was admitted to our Department with a 2-month clinical picture of watery and nonbloody diarrhea (7–10 stools/day), diffuse abdominal pain, fatigue, anorexia, and involuntary weight loss (10% body weight). She denied fever and any other relevant epidemiologic context. She was previously evaluated by her family doctor who prescribed empiric antibiotic but with no improvement. On admission, physical examination showed dehydration, hypotension, and tachycardia. Laboratory evaluations revealed normocytic anemia (10.9 g/dL; N: 11.5–15), urea 84 mg/dL (N: 21–43), creatinine 3.63 mg/dL (N: 0.6–1.1), serum potassium (2.5 mmol/L; N: 3.5–5), and albumin 3.1 g/dL (N: 3.4–4.8). Serology for celiac disease and thyroid hormone levels and stool analysis for infectious agents (*C. difficile*, virology, bacteriology, mycobacteriology, and parasitology) and serology for HIV, cytomegalovirus, and herpes simplex virus were all negative. Total colonoscopy revealed normal mucosa without evidence of microscopic colitis or inflammatory bowel disease, on histopathology. Upper endoscopy showed normal gastroduodenal mucosa. Duodenal biopsies highlighted partial villous atrophy with severe intraepithelial lymphocytosis. Given the high suspicion of OISLE, this drug was suspended and switched to lisinopril, with replacement of electrolytes. One week after admission, the patient was discharged without diarrhea or need of nutritional/electrolyte support. Two months later, a complete recovery of weight was seen along with full normalization of laboratory tests and histopathological changes.

4. Discussion

CD is an immunomediated disorder occurring in people genetically susceptible to gluten and results in variable

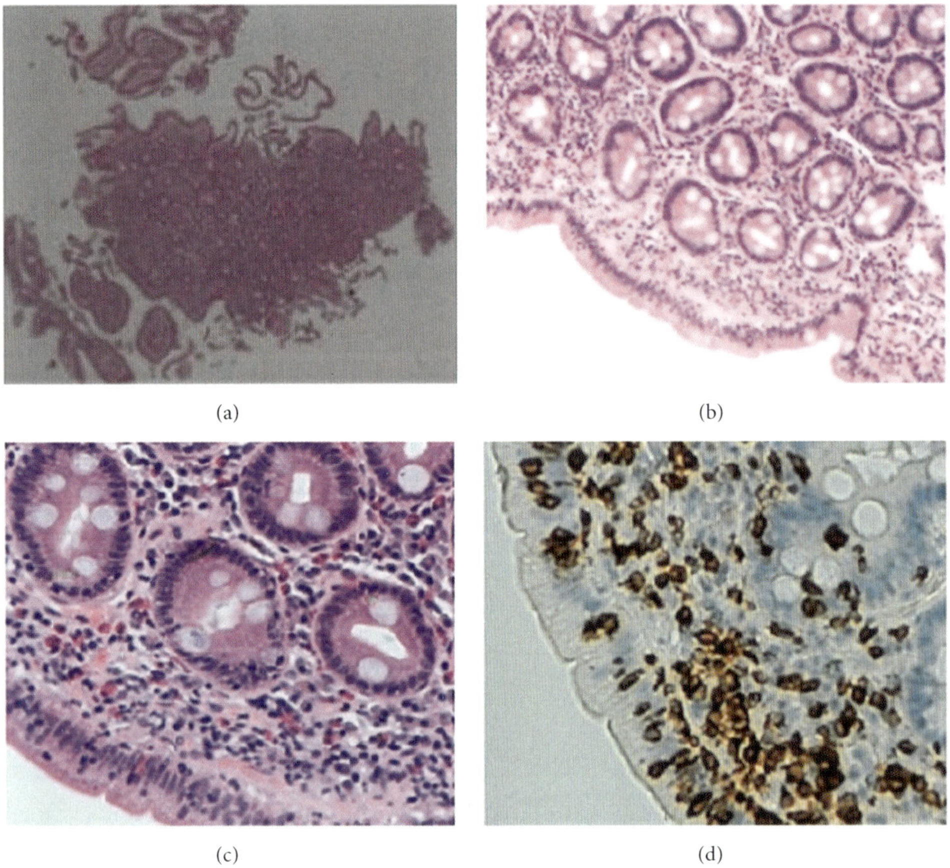

Figure 2: Duodenal histopathological features. (a, b, c) Partial villous atrophy with lymphocytic inflammatory infiltrate in lamina propria and surface intraepithelial lymphocytosis (H&E). (d) CD3 immunostaining shows pathological increase of intraepithelial lymphocytes (IHC ×200).

degrees of VA and an increase in intraepithelial lymphocytes [1]. The diagnosis of CD is supported by positive antibody tests (anti-tissue transglutaminase antibodies) and symptomatic and histologic response to a GFD. When celiac serologies are negative on a gluten-containing diet, alternative etiologies for VA should be considered before diagnosis of seronegative CD to prevent an unnecessary lifelong GFD [4]. Differential diagnosis includes autoimmune enteropathy, *Crohn*'s disease, microscopic enterocolitis, hypogammaglobulinemic sprue, *Whipple*'s disease, tropical sprue, intestinal tuberculosis, HIV-associated enteropathy, infectious enteritis, intestinal malignancies, and drugs-induced enteropathy. DeGaetani et al. [5] studied 72 patients with seronegative VA at a tertiary care center and, interestingly, the two most common diagnoses in these patients were seronegative CD (28%) and drug-induced sprue-like enteropathy (26%).

Olmesartan is one of the several ARBs commonly prescribed for the management of hypertension. The earliest evidence of OISLE was first described in 2012 by Rubio-Tapia et al. [6], and a few reports were published subsequently, leading Food and Drug Administration to institute label changes addressing this adverse event, in July 2013. Based on cases reported to date, this entity most frequently affects older adults (mean age, 68 years; range, 46–91 years) with no gender predominance. Symptoms of OISLE include severe chronic diarrhea (95%), weight loss (89%), fatigue (56%), nausea and vomiting (45%), abdominal pain (37%), bloating (29%), and, less commonly, reflux symptoms and loss of appetite [7]. Laboratory evaluation usually shows evidence of malabsorption with normocytic anemia, hypoalbuminemia, and multiple electrolyte abnormalities. Dehydration and acute renal failure have been reported as the main causes of hospitalization, although a case of colonic perforation has also been documented [8]. Patients can develop signs/symptoms months to years after olmesartan initiation. In the series by Rubio-Tapia et al. [6], the average duration of exposure to olmesartan was 3.1 years (range, 0.5–7 years).

Imaging and endoscopic findings in the gastrointestinal tract may reveal no significant abnormalities. Reported imaging abnormalities include diffuse edema and bowel wall thickening of the small intestine and enlarged abdominal lymph nodes. Reported abnormal endoscopic features of the small bowel include mucosal nodularity, villous atrophy, and ulceration. The most common histopathological findings are variable degrees of intestinal villous atrophy (92%). As in celiac disease, increased intraepithelial lymphocytes, according to the modified Marsh classification, are also commonly seen (61%). In addition, involvements of the stomach and colon with lymphocytic and/or collagenous gastritis and/or colitis were also reported, suggesting that this disease may affect the entire gastrointestinal tract [9]. Discontinuation of olmesartan is the mainstay of treatment. Clinical remission often occurs within a few days of stopping the drug, and almost all of the patients show histological recovery of the duodenum.

Currently, the mechanism of OISLE is unknown. The long latency period between initiation of olmesartan and development of symptoms is suggestive of cell-mediated immune damage and, furthermore, inhibitory effects of ARBs on transforming growth factor beta, an important mediator of gut homeostasis, may play a role. Rubio-Tapia et al. [6] found a prevalence of HLA-DQ2 in 68% of patients with OISLE, significantly higher than what is expected for the general population, suggesting a genetic predisposition. Scialom et al. [10] described extraintestinal autoimmune diseases in three of seven patients with OISLE. Besides this, symptomatic improvement is reported in some patients treated with steroids or other immunosuppressors prior to receiving a diagnosis of OISLE, which is supportive of an autoimmune background.

In this report, we described two uncommon cases of severe sprue-like enteropathy that achieved a remarkable improvement with suspension of olmesartan. Both patients presented with severe chronic diarrhea and significant weight loss complicated with electrolyte imbalance and/or acute renal failure. Duodenal biopsies confirmed villous atrophy and intraepithelial lymphocytosis. CD was excluded by negative conventional serologic tests and, in the first case, by the absence of clinical response to a GFD. Other causes of atrophic enteropathy were excluded and the diagnosis of OISLE was considered. Complete resolution of symptoms and laboratory changes and histological recovery after olmesartan withdrawal without any other therapeutic/dietary measures were verified, supporting the diagnosis of OISLE.

In conclusion, although OISLE is a rare cause of sprue-like enteropathy, we emphasize that this entity should be included in the differential diagnosis of seronegative villous atrophy. Considering the worldwide use of olmesartan as an antihypertensive agent, we aim to alert clinicians to this condition and other drug-induced enteropathies in patients with unexplained severe chronic diarrhea and weight loss, particularly when CD is excluded. A high index of suspicion of OISLE is important because it allows a correct early diagnosis and avoids a frustrating, unnecessary, and often expensive investigation. Up to now, a very few cases have been described and the scarcity of available data does not allow for a correct characterization of this entity, requiring additional investigations.

References

[1] J. F. Ludvigsson, D. A. Leffler, J. C. Bai et al., "The Oslo definitions for coeliac disease and related terms," *Gut*, vol. 62, no. 1, pp. 43–52, 2012.

[2] T. R. Ziegler, C. Fernández-Estívariz, L. H. Gu, M. W. Fried, and L. M. Leader, "Severe villus atrophy and chronic malabsorption induced by azathioprine," *Gastroenterology*, vol. 124, no. 7, pp. 1950–1957, 2003.

[3] M. M. Boscá, R. Añón, E. Mayordomo et al., "Methotrexate induced sprue-like syndrome," *World Journal of Gastroenterology*, vol. 14, no. 45, pp. 7009–7011, 2008.

[4] N. J. Hall, G. Rubin, and A. Charnock, "Systematic review: adherence to a gluten-free diet in adult patients with coeliac disease," *Alimentary Pharmacology and Therapeutics*, vol. 30, no. 4, pp. 315–330, 2009.

[5] M. DeGaetani, C. A. Tennyson, B. Lebwohl et al., "Villous atrophy and negative celiac serology: a diagnostic and therapeutic dilemma," *The American Journal of Gastroenterology*, vol. 108, no. 5, pp. 647–653, 2013.

[6] A. Rubio-Tapia, M. L. Herman, J. F. Ludvigsson et al., "Severe spruelike enteropathy associated with olmesartan," *Mayo Clinic Proceedings*, vol. 87, no. 8, pp. 732–738, 2012.

[7] G. Laniro, S. Bibbo, M. Montalto et al., "Systematic review: sprue-like enteropathy associated with olmesartan," *Alimentary Pharmacology & Therapeutics*, vol. 40, no. 1, pp. 16–23, 2014.

[8] M. Abdelghany, L. Gonzalez III, J. Slater, and C. Begley, "Olmesartan associated sprue-like enteropathy and colon perforation," *Case Reports in Gastrointestinal Medicine*, vol. 2014, Article ID 494098, 3 pages, 2014.

[9] E. Y. Karen Choi and B. McKenn, "Olmesartan-associated enteropathy: a review of clinical and histologic findings," *Archives of Pathology & Laboratory Medicine*, vol. 139, no. 10, pp. 1242–1247, 2015.

[10] S. Scialom, G. Malamut, B. Meresse et al., "Gastrointestinal disorder associated with olmesartan mimics autoimmune enteropathy," *PLoS ONE*, vol. 10, no. 6, article e0125024, 2015.

Two Cases of Leiomyoma in the Colon Masquerading as Other Types of Colonic Pedunculated Polyps

Ailee Ikeda,[1] Masaya Iwamuro,[1] Takehiro Tanaka,[2] Toshihiro Inokuchi,[1] Asuka Nakarai,[1] Yuusaku Sugihara,[3] Keita Harada,[4] Sakiko Hiraoka,[1] Yoshiro Kawahara,[4] and Hiroyuki Okada[1]

[1] *Department of Gastroenterology and Hepatology, Okayama University Graduate School of Medicine, Dentistry and Pharmaceutical Sciences, Okayama 700-8558, Japan*
[2] *Department of Diagnostic Pathology, Okayama University Hospital, Okayama 700-8558, Japan*
[3] *Department of General Medicine, Okayama University Graduate School of Medicine, Dentistry and Pharmaceutical Sciences, Okayama 700-8558, Japan*
[4] *Department of Endoscopy, Okayama University Hospital, Okayama 700-8558, Japan*

Correspondence should be addressed to Ailee Ikeda; p17q5fj9@okayama-u.ac.jp

Academic Editor: R. J. L. F. Loffeld

We describe two cases of leiomyoma in the colon that were diagnosed histologically after endoscopic resection. The first case was a 79-year-old Japanese woman who presented with a pedunculated polyp of 14 mm length at the splenic flexure. Preoperative diagnosis suggested a colonic mucosubmucosal elongated polyp. The second case was a 29-year-old Japanese woman who presented with a pedunculated polyp of 40 mm length at the hepatic flexure and had an ulcer on top of the polyp. Preoperative diagnosis suggested an inflammatory fibroid polyp. A pathological diagnosis of colonic leiomyoma was made after endoscopic resection in both cases. Both tumors were confirmed to originate, not from the proper muscle layer, but from the muscularis mucosae. These cases underscore that although colonic involvement is infrequent, leiomyomas can display pedunculated morphology in the colon rather than the typical gross appearance of gastrointestinal submucosal tumors seen with sessile morphology.

1. Introduction

Today, endoscopic examinations and interventions are extensively performed worldwide to investigate the digestive tract and to treat gastrointestinal diseases. Advances in endoscopic devices and techniques and in the understanding of typical endoscopic features of each disease enable an accurate preoperative diagnosis of various gastrointestinal lesions, even before performing the examination of biopsy samples. However, there are lesions that are not diagnosable by endoscopy.

In this report, we describe two cases of leiomyoma in the colon that were presented as pedunculated polyps. We could not diagnose either case as a leiomyoma preoperatively; the final diagnosis was made after endoscopic resection of the polyps. Differential diagnosis of these two cases and morphology of the colorectal leiomyomas are discussed.

2. Case Report

2.1. Case 1. A 79-year-old Japanese woman was referred to our hospital for further investigation of a positive fecal occult blood test. A blood examination revealed no specific abnormalities. Colonoscopy revealed an oval-shaped pedunculated polyp at the splenic flexure of the transverse colon (Figure 1). The surface of the polyp was covered with intact mucosa; regularly arranged round pits were observed under magnification (Figure 1(a)). A preoperative diagnosis of colonic mucosubmucosal elongated polyp was made, and an endoscopic submucosal dissection was performed on the basis of this diagnosis. The resected polyp was 10 mm in diameter and 14 mm in length (Figure 1(c)). Histologically, dense proliferation of spindle cells was observed in the submucosal layer (Figures 2(a) and 2(b)). Tumor nests were clearly demarcated from the overlying mucosa by fibrous

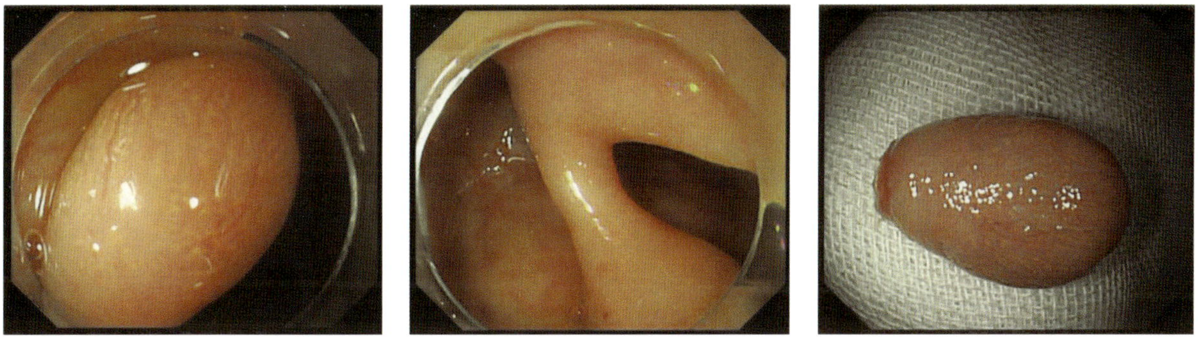

(a) (b) (c)

FIGURE 1: Endoscopic images of Case 1. A pedunculated polyp covered with intact mucosa is observed (a, b). Resected polyp is 10 mm in diameter and 14 mm in length (c).

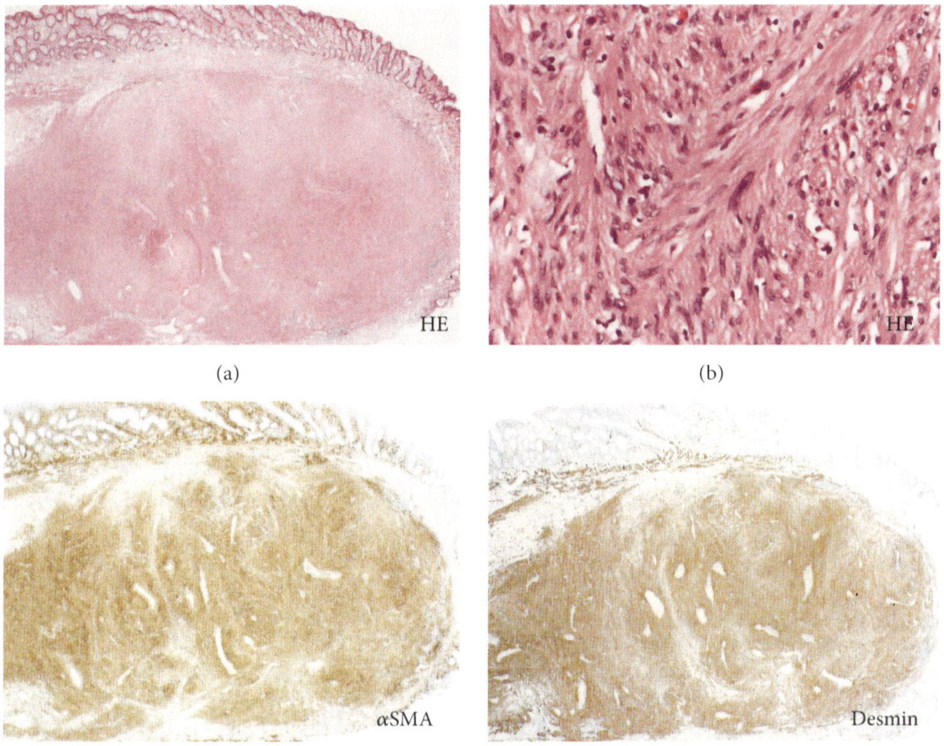

(a) (b) (c) (d)

FIGURE 2: Pathological images of Case 1. A tumor composed of eosinophilic cells is observed. The tumor is covered with normal appearing mucosa ((a), hematoxylin and eosin staining, ×40). The tumor cells have relatively uniform nuclei, abundant cytoplasm, and indistinct cell boundaries. Mitoses are rarely observed ((b), hematoxylin and eosin staining, ×400). The cells are positive for α-SMA ((c), ×40) and desmin ((d), ×40).

connective tissue. Continuity between the tumor and the muscularis mucosae was observed, indicating that the tumor arose from the muscularis mucosae. Mitoses were rarely observed. The cells were positive for α-smooth muscle cell actin (α-SMA, Figure 2(c)) and desmin staining (Figure 2(d)) but were negative for c-kit, S-100, or DOG-1 staining. Consequently, a diagnosis of colonic leiomyoma was made.

2.2. Case 2. A 29-year-old Japanese woman was referred to our hospital for further investigation of abdominal pain and bloody stools. Laboratory investigation revealed microcytic hypochromic anemia with red blood cell count: $3.92 \times 10^6/\text{mm}^3$, hemoglobin: 8.5 g/dL, hematocrit: 29.4%, platelet count: $373 \times 10^3/\text{mm}^3$, and C-reactive protein: 0.53 mg/dL. A pedunculated polyp, 40 mm in diameter and 40 mm in length, was identified at the hepatic flexure of the colon during colonoscopy (Figures 3(a) and 3(b)). The surface of the polyp was ulcerated and covered with a white substance (Figure 3(a)). Although the mucosa of the unulcerated parts of the polyp was partly swollen, the pit structure was

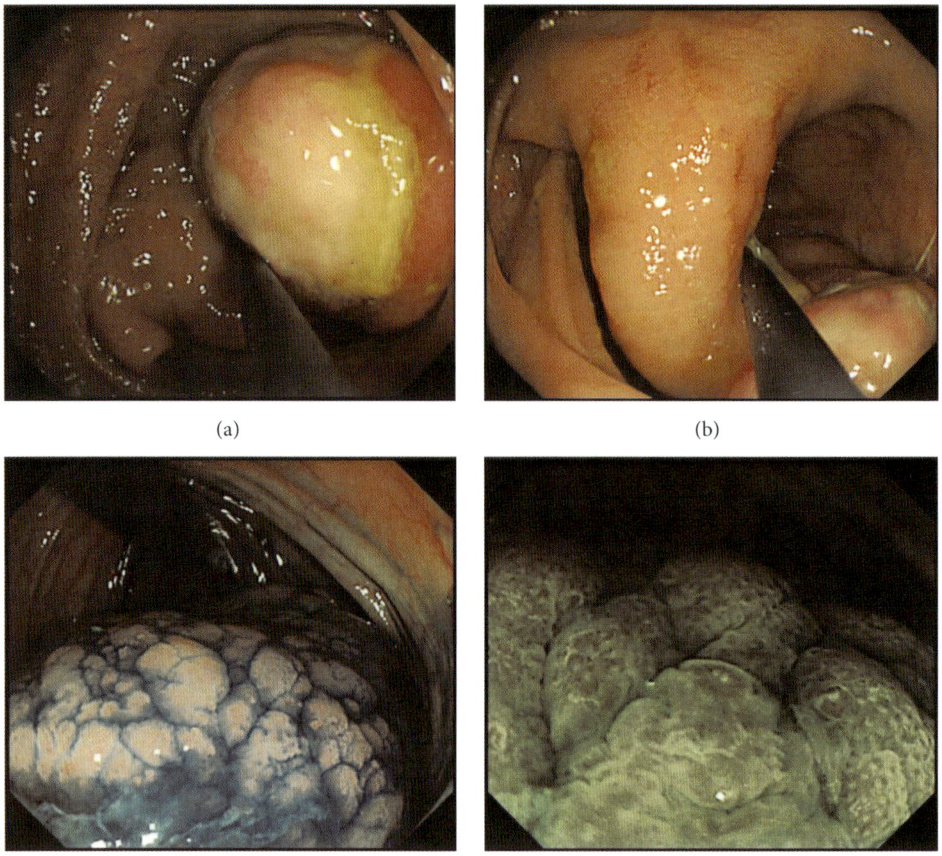

(a) (b) (c) (d)

FIGURE 3: Endoscopic images of Case 2. The surface of the polyp head is ulcerated (a). The polyp is of pedunculated form (b). The unulcerated part of the polyp shows intact pit structure after indigo carmine spraying (c). Narrow-band imaging (d).

mostly normal and round; this was emphasized after indigo carmine spraying (Figure 3(c)). Narrow-band imaging, under magnification, also showed partial swelling of the surface structure (Figure 3(d)). Based on the pedunculated morphology and partial ulceration, our preoperative diagnosis of the polyp suggested an inflammatory fibroid polyp. We removed the polyp using the endoscopic mucosal resection technique. Histological analysis revealed a dense proliferation of spindle cells with round to oval nuclei beneath the thin, normal mucosal epithelium (Figures 4(a) and 4(b)). Mitoses were rarely observed. The stalk of the polyp was composed of muscular tissue. Tumor cells were positive for α-SMA (Figure 4(c)) and desmin (Figure 4(d)) but were negative for c-kit, S-100, or DOG-1. Therefore, we made a pathological diagnosis of leiomyoma.

3. Discussion

According to Japanese clinical practice guidelines for colonic polyps, they are classified into at least eight types: conventional adenomas, serrated polyps, polypoid adenocarcinomas, inflammatory polyps, hamartomatous polyps, stromal polyps, lymphoid polyp, and endocrine (or carcinoid) tumors, as well as others [1]. Although lesions arising from or involving colon mucosa can be easily identified and diagnosed during colonoscopy, based on the morphological structure of the mucosal surface, it is generally difficult to immediately diagnose subepithelial lesions covered with normal mucosa. The two cases under study had pedunculated polyps that we diagnosed as a colonic mucosubmucosal elongated polyp and an inflammatory fibroid polyp, preoperatively.

As pertains to the gastrointestinal tract, leiomyomas occur most frequently in the esophagus while the colorectum is a relatively infrequent site of occurrence, accounting for 3% of all the gastrointestinal leiomyomas [2–5]. Since a majority of esophageal leiomyomas originate from the proper muscle layer, they present as sessile lesions covered with intact esophageal mucosa, that is, the typical appearance of subepithelial tumors. Meanwhile, it has been reported that colonic leiomyomas arise from the muscularis mucosae. Although colonic leiomyomas predominantly appear as sessile lesions, they can form semipedunculated or pedunculated lesions as well [6]. Choi et al. reported 22 cases with leiomyomas arising from the muscularis mucosae in the colon [7]. Seventeen cases showed sessile polyps, while the remaining five cases showed pedunculated morphology. Agaimy and Wünsch reported that all of the 67 colorectal leiomyomas arising from

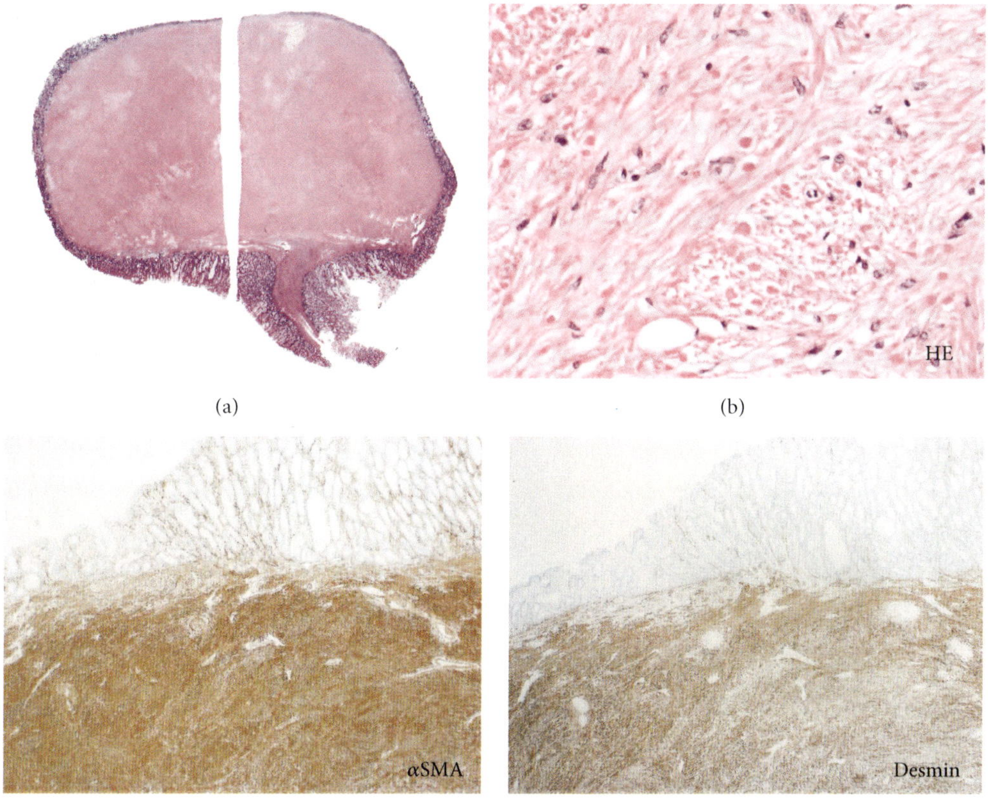

(a) (b) (c) (d)

FIGURE 4: Pathological images of Case 2. Spindle cells with round to oval nuclei are observed in the resected specimen ((a), ×4, (b), ×400). The tumor cells are positive for α-SMA ((c), ×100) and desmin ((d), ×100).

the muscularis mucosae were well-circumscribed, sessile polypoid masses detected incidentally during colonoscopy [6]. Miettinen et al. reviewed 88 patients with leiomyoma of the muscularis mucosae and described that the lesions typically appeared as small sessile polyps [8]. Hence, it is evident that colonic leiomyomas present semipedunculated or pedunculated lesions only in rare instances.

Colonic leiomyomas are often misdiagnosed. Several authors have noted that most colonic leiomyomas with sessile morphology mimic epithelial polyps in their gross appearance during colonoscopy [4, 7]. Choi et al. reported that 45.5% of colorectal leiomyomas (10 of 22 lesions) were accurately diagnosed based on their endoscopic features [7]. However, more than half of colorectal leiomyomas were not correctly diagnosed prior to undergoing resection. We speculate that it is more difficult for gastroenterologists to diagnose pedunculated lesions as leiomyomas preoperatively because of their infrequency and physician's prejudices that leiomyomas form sessile lesions and not pedunculated lesions. In the two cases under study, our preoperative diagnosis for one case was mucosubmucosal elongated polyp and, for the other, inflammatory fibroid polyp.

Colonic mucosubmucosal elongated polyp is a distinct entity that is composed of mucosa and submucosa [9]. Typical endoscopic features have been identified as worm-like, thin projections covered by unremarkable mucosa [10]. Our patient, from Case 1, showed a pedunculated polyp lined with intact mucosa. Although subepithelial tumors rarely display pedunculated morphology, we have considered subepithelial tumors as a differential diagnosis of the polyp identified in Case 1 because the polyp head seemed to be thicker than a typical colonic mucosubmucosal elongated polyp.

The inflammatory fibroid polyp is a rare mesenchymal gastrointestinal tumor found mostly in the stomach (70%) and the small intestine (20%) [11]. Involvement of the colon in this disease is infrequent. However, reports of inflammatory fibroid polyp of the proximal colon, particularly those of the cecum, have increased due to recent advances in and widespread use of colonoscopy examinations [12]. Pathologically, an inflammatory fibroid polyp is characterized by blood vessels, fibroblasts, and an edematous stroma rich in eosinophils [13]. Representative endoscopic features of this entity are a firm, solitary, and often ulcerated polyp with sessile or pedunculated form [14]. We consider that colonic inflammatory fibroid polyp is a reasonable preoperative diagnosis for the patient in Case 2, as it is hard to conceive of the polyp as a leiomyoma.

Unlike the esophageal leiomyoma, colonic leiomyomas can be endoscopically removed because most of them arise from the muscularis mucosa. Choi et al. report that they have removed colorectal leiomyomas using cold forceps biopsy

($N = 10$) and conventional polypectomy or endoscopic mucosal resection ($N = 12$) and have experienced no complications such as bleeding or perforation [7]. Miettinen et al. summarized 88 colorectal leiomyomas and noted that endoscopic snare polypectomy resulted in complete tumor removal in virtually all cases [8]. The overall prognosis is reportedly good, and no recurrence has been documented in literature [15]. Thus, endoscopic resection is a treatment of choice for leiomyomas arising from the muscularis mucosa of the colon. In the two cases under discussion, we could not preoperatively diagnose the polyps as leiomyomas; a final diagnosis was made after endoscopic resection. In such cases, additional treatment is unnecessary, if the leiomyoma arises from the muscularis mucosa.

In conclusion, we treated two cases of colonic leiomyoma presented as pedunculated polyps. Accurate preoperative diagnoses were difficult based solely on their morphology. These cases underscore that although colonic involvement is infrequent, colonic leiomyomas can display the pedunculated form, rather than the typical gross appearance of gastrointestinal submucosal tumors as in the sessile form. In addition, they can be treated with endoscopic resection alone because most of colonic leiomyomas arise from the muscularis mucosa.

References

[1] The Japanese Society of Gastroenterology, "Clinical Question 3-1," in *Evidence-Based Clinical Practice Guidelines for Colonic Polyp*, The Japanese Society of Gastroenterology, Ed., pp. 26-27, Nankodo, Tokyo, Japan, (Japanese) 2014.

[2] S.-J. Tsai, C.-C. Lin, C.-W. Chang et al., "Benign esophageal lesions: endoscopic and pathologic features," *World Journal of Gastroenterology*, vol. 21, no. 4, pp. 1091–1098, 2015.

[3] L. S. Lee, S. Singhal, C. J. Brinster et al., "Current management of esophageal leiomyoma," *Journal of the American College of Surgeons*, vol. 198, no. 1, pp. 136–146, 2004.

[4] K. R. Badipatla, C. Kamireddy, M. Niazi, and S. K. Nayudu, "Cecal leiomyoma: can we attempt endoscopic resection?," *Gastroenterology Research*, vol. 9, no. 6, pp. 105–107, 2016.

[5] H. L. Baker Jr. and C. A. Good, "Smooth muscle tumors of the alimentary tract; their roentgen manifestations," *American Journal of Roentgenology*, vol. 74, no. 2, pp. 246–255, 1955.

[6] A. Agaimy and P. H. Wünsch, "True smooth muscle neoplasms of the gastrointestinal tract: morphological spectrum and classification in a series of 85 cases from a single institute," *Langenbeck's Archives of Surgery*, vol. 392, no. 1, pp. 75–81, 2007.

[7] H. H. Choi, Y. S. Cho, S. K. Choi et al., "Clinical outcomes of endoscopic removal in patients with colorectal polypoid leiomyomas," *The Korean Journal of Gastroenterology*, vol. 68, no. 4, pp. 179–185, 2016.

[8] M. Miettinen, M. Sarlomo-Rikala, and L. H. Sobin, "Mesenchymal tumors of muscularis mucosae of colon and rectum are benign leiomyomas that should be separated from gastrointestinal stromal tumors—a clinicopathologic and immunohistochemical study of eighty-eight cases," *Modern Pathology*, vol. 14, no. 10, pp. 950–956, 2001.

[9] H. Matake, T. Matsui, T. Yao et al., "Long pedunculated colonic polyp composed of mucosa and submucosa: Proposal of a new entity, colonic muco-submucosal elongated polyp," *Diseases of the Colon & Rectum*, vol. 41, no. 12, pp. 1557–1561, 1998.

[10] C. L. Tan, S. H. Tan, J. B. So, and F. Petersson, "Muco-submucosal elongated polyps of the gastrointestinal tract: A case series and a review of the literature," *World Journal of Gastroenterology*, vol. 19, no. 11, pp. 1845–1849, 2013.

[11] A. L. Shrestha and P. Shrestha, "Giant inflammatory fibroid polyp of the hepatic flexure of colon presenting with an acute abdomen," *Case Reports in Gastrointestinal Medicine*, vol. 2016, Article ID 2178639, 4 pages, 2016.

[12] O. Aderemi and A. Nicholas, "Rectal inflammatory fibroid polyp in a Nigerian: Case report & brief review of literature," *African Health Sciences*, vol. 16, no. 3, pp. 873–876, 2016.

[13] A. Kayyali, A. Toumeh, U. Ahmad, L. E. De Las Casas, and A. Nawras, "Giant inflammatory fibroid polyp of the descending colon treated with endoscopic resection," *ACG Case Reports Journal*, vol. 1, no. 1, pp. 36–39, 2013.

[14] K. Tanaka, T. Sakuno, R. Yamada et al., "Gastrointestinal: gastric inflammatory fibroid polyp that was resected after a 10-year follow-up," *Journal of Gastroenterology and Hepatology*, vol. 33, no. 1, 5 pages, 2018.

[15] A. Sagnotta, A. Sparagna, S. Uccini, and P. Mercantini, "Giant extraluminal leiomyoma of the colon: Rare cause of symptomatic pelvic mass," *International Surgery*, vol. 100, no. 5, pp. 805–808, 2015.

40

A Case Report and Literature Review of *Clostridium difficile* Negative Antibiotic Associated Hemorrhagic Colitis Caused by *Klebsiella oxytoca*

Aaron Fisher[1] **and Alexandra Halalau**[2,3]

[1]*Internal Medicine Resident, Beaumont Health, Royal Oak, MI, USA*
[2]*General Internal Medicine Section Head, Beaumont Health, Royal Oak, MI, USA*
[3]*Associate Professor, Oakland University William Beaumont School of Medicine, Rochester, MI, USA*

Correspondence should be addressed to Aaron Fisher; aaronsethfisher@gmail.com

Academic Editor: Hirotada Akiho

Klebsiella oxytoca hemorrhagic colitis is a rare form of antibiotic associated hemorrhagic colitis that is *Clostridium difficile* negative. *Klebsiella oxytoca* colitis has been shown to be triggered by penicillin administration, yet other antibiotics have been implicated as well. It can mimic the appearance of ischemic colitis on endoscopy; however it will generally be found in young, otherwise healthy patients without risk factors. We present a case of a 33-year-old Caucasian female who presented to the emergency room with profuse, bloody diarrhea for 5 days, after a one-week course of ampicillin. Colonoscopy was notable for ulcerated mucosa with erythema and easy friability and the biopsy was suggestive of ischemic colitis. Stool culture was positive for many *Klebsiella oxytoca*. The patient was discharged home with resolution of symptoms after three days in the hospital. She was instructed to avoid penicillin antibiotics and minimize nonsteroidal anti-inflammatory drug use.

1. Introduction

Colitis can originate from a wide range of etiologies including ischemic, infectious, and inflammatory bowel disease. A thorough history is imperative to determine the causative nature of the patient's presenting symptoms. Investigations range from observation and stool analysis, to endoscopy with biopsies, depending upon particular risk factors and severity of symptoms. A growing subset of colitis is antibiotic associated colitis. A majority of these cases are secondary to *Clostridium difficile* infection (CDI), with an estimated 453,000 cases of CDI throughout the United States in 2011 [1]. Within the most common antibiotics used, antibiotic associated diarrhea has been reported in 5-10% of patients taking ampicillin, 10 to 25% of those who are treated with amoxicillin–clavulanate, 15 to 20% of those who receive cefixime, and 2 to 5% of those who are treated with other cephalosporins, fluoroquinolones, azithromycin, clarithromycin, erythromycin, and tetracycline [2]. Yet, in cases of clostridium difficile-negative antibiotic associated hemorrhagic colitis (AAHC), *Klebsiella oxytoca* has been isolated at a significantly high rate [3]. In Hogenauer et al.'s study, 385 healthy patients had stool testing for *Klebsiella oxytoca* and in 1.6% of the patients, the pathogen was isolated [4]. Interestingly, *Klebsiella oxytoca* is found mainly in young healthy individuals compared to patients with CDI who are generally older and with previous hospitalizations [4]. Here we present a case of *Clostridium difficile*-negative AAHC caused by *K. oxytoca* infection after taking ampicillin for a urinary tract infection.

2. Case Presentation

A 33-year-old Caucasian female with significant family history of inflammatory bowel disease (IBD) presents with profuse, bloody diarrhea for 5 days and associated tenesmus and urgency. One day prior to admission, she completed

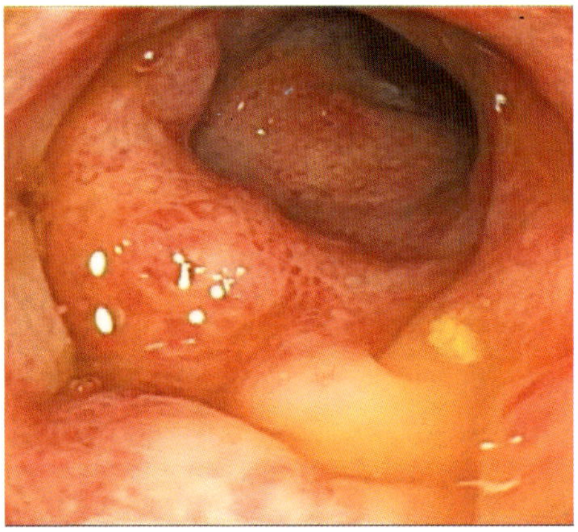

Figure 1: Endoscopic view of ulcerated mucosa with erythema and easy friability, suggestive of moderate colitis.

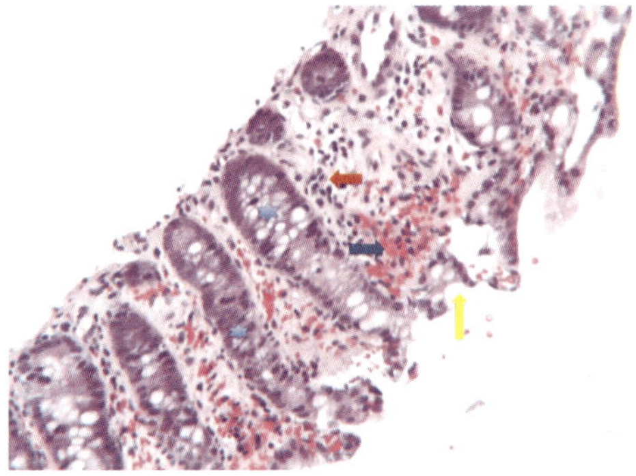

Figure 2: Colonic biopsy. Yellow arrow indicates epithelial surface erosion. Green arrow indicates extravasated red blood cells. Orange arrow indicates lymphocytes. Blue star indicates reactive intestinal glands.

a one-week course of ampicillin for a urinary tract infection and noted that her symptoms began three days after she had initiated treatment. On presentation, patient was hemodynamically stable, afebrile, with mild lower abdominal pain, and a positive guaiac exam. Laboratory findings showed WBC 12.4 bil/L (normal values 3.3–10.7 bil/L), neutrophils 11.0 bil/L (normal values 1.6–7.2 bil/L), Hgb 13.1 g/dL (normal values 12.1–15.0 g/dL), platelets 275 bil/L (normal values 150–400 bil/L), lactic acid 1.4 mmol/L (normal values 0.5–2.2 mmol/L), and liver function tests within normal limits. Initial stool studies that included stool culture, ova and parasite, and *Clostridium difficile* toxin PCR were negative. A colonoscopy was planned as the patient had an extensive family history of IBD and presented with bloody diarrhea. *Klebsiella oxytoca* testing was requested on the stool culture after *Clostridium difficile* PCR came back negative, given her previous use of penicillins. Colonoscopy was notable for ulcerated mucosa with erythema and easy friability, suggestive of moderate colitis throughout the colon with rectosigmoid sparing (Figure 1). Colonic biopsy was remarkable for mucosal congestion and ischemia suggestive of ischemic colitis (Figure 2). Subsequently, requested stool culture was positive for many *Klebsiella oxytoca*. The patient's hematochezia resolved prior to discharge on day 3 of hospitalization, four days after cessation of ampicillin. She was advised to avoid future use of penicillins and minimize nonsteroidal anti-inflammatory drug (NSAID) use.

The patient has continued to follow with her gastroenterologist 10 months after her colonoscopy. She has had epigastric abdominal pain relieved by daily omeprazole. She no longer has documented hematochezia and there has been no repeat colonoscopy.

3. Discussion

Colitis is a well-known complication of treatment with antibiotic agents, yet the cause of antibiotic associated hemorrhagic colitis is not completely understood. Several mechanisms have been proposed including allergic reaction, mucosal ischemia, and *Klebsiella oxytoca* infection. *Klebsiella oxytoca* positive hemorrhagic colitis is a rare form of antibiotic associated hemorrhagic colitis that is *Clostridium difficile* negative [4]. In 1978, Toffler et al. were the first to describe AAHC [5]. It has been described that, in a majority of cases, penicillin and penicillin derivative administration typically precede AAHC; however, quinolones and cephalosporins have been described as well [6].

There appears to be a greater incidence of AAHC secondary to *K. oxytoca* in the Japanese population [13]. *K. oxytoca* has been reported in the United States as well, yet appears to be more rare. A PubMed literature review was conducted in order to consolidate all English written and adult population case reports on *K. oxytoca* hemorrhagic colitis. Search was conducted via the phrases "Klebsiella oxytoca AND colitis AND case report" and "colitis AND Klebsiella oxytoca." A total of 74 articles resulted, 18 of which were case reports: 7 written in English, 8 written in French, and 3 written in Japanese. The English written cases range from the years 1999 to 2017 and total 9 cases. Five of the cases are reported from Japan and 4 from cities throughout the United States. Ages range from 37 years to 85 years with 4 males and 5 females. Eight of the 9 cases reported bloody diarrhea. The types of antibiotics reported were three penicillin derivatives (amoxicillin twice and amoxicillin-clavulanic acid once), one macrolide (clarithromycin), three fluoroquinolones (tosufloxacin, enoxacin, and levofloxacin), and one with metronidazole, and one case only reported perioperative antibiotics yet specifics were unknown. Two of the 9 cases noted prior use of a NSAID. Duration of antibiotic use ranged from 1 to 7 days. Interestingly, there was a delay of 3-4 weeks in symptomatology in patients who had taken fluoroquinolones compared to the other patients in which symptoms began closer to time of antibiotic use. Location of endoscopic findings varied throughout the 9 cases. Of the 9 cases, 2 cases were right sided only, 3 cases were from ascending to descending colon, 2 cases only involved the sigmoid colon, 1 case involved the transverse colon, and 1 patient declined colonoscopy. The duration of time for resolution of symptoms ranged from 4 days to 3 weeks. Seven of the 9 cases were treated supportively (one case was treated

TABLE 1: Literature review of case reports of colitis secondary to *Klebsiella oxytoca*.

Author	Year and Location	Patient Age and Gender	Presenting symptoms	Antibiotic prior to presentation	NSAID use prior to presen- tation	Duration of Abx prior to sx	Endo- scopic location of disease	Time to reso- lution of sx	Treatment
Koga et al. [6]	1999 Japan	37 y/o Female	Bloody diarrhea and abdominal pain	Tosu- floxacin tosylate 450 mg	none	5 days*	Entire colon excluding rectum	2 weeks	Hydration and Loperamide
Koga et al. [6]	1999 Japan	46 y/o Male	Bloody diarrhea and abdominal pain	Enoxacin	none	7 days*	Right sided	3 weeks	Supportive
Koga et al. [6]	1999 Japan	37 y/o Male	Bloody diarrhea	Levo- floxacin 300 mg	none	7 days*	Transverse to sigmoid	3 weeks	Supportive
Chen, Cachay, and Hunt [7]	2004 San Diego, CA	79 y/o Male	Diarrhea, abdominal pain, hemato- chezia	none	Aspirin	none	Sigmoid colon	2 weeks	Cipro- floxacin
Philbrick, Ernst [8]	2007 Iowa	63 y/o Male	Watery diarrhea and BRBPR	Amoxicillin 500 mg q8h	Ibuprofen 800mg q8h	5 days	Ascending to descending colon	1 week	Metro- nidazole and Levo- floxacin
Miyauchi, Kinoshita, Tokuda [9]	2013 Japan	67 y/o Female	Mucobloody diarrhea and abdominal pain	Clarithro- mycin 200 mg q12h	none	5 days	Right sided	Not specified	Supportive
Sweetser, Schroede, Pardi [10]	2009 Rochester, MN	67 y/o Female	Watery diarrhea	Peri- operative abx	none	3 days	Sigmoid colon	4 days	Supportive
Kazuyuki et al. [11]	2017 Japan	65 y/o Female	Abdominal pain and hemato- chezia	Amoxicillin 1500 mg and Metro- nidazole 500 mg	none	1 day	Transverse colon	6 days	Bowel rest and prednisolone
Akanbi et al.[12]	2017 Chicago, IL	85 y/o Female	Abdominal pain and muco- bloody diarrhea	Amoxicillin - clavulanic acid	none	5 days	Declined colon- oscopy	5 days	Supportive care

* Symptoms did not start until ~3-4 weeks after antibiotic cessation.
Q8h, every 8 hours; q12h, every 12 hours; BRBPR, bright red blood per rectum; abx, antibiotics; ASA, aspirin; sx, symptoms; y/o, years old.

with prednisolone as well). Two of the 9 cases were treated with fluoroquinolones (one of the cases with metronidazole as well) with no reported recurrence of symptoms. In all cases, antibiotic course was either completed or terminated early prior to symptomatic improvement (Table 1). The diagnosis of *K. oxytoca* can be established by stool [6, 8–10, 12], tissue [7], or bacterial [11] culture. The priority of which culture is of highest yield is uncertain. Of the 9 cases, the most common past medical history was type 2 diabetes mellitus in 3 of the patients, hypertension in 2 of the patients, and systemic lupus erythematosus in 1 of the patients.

Our case is rare given her Caucasian ethnicity; however, as evident by Table 1, *K. oxytoca* in Caucasians have been reported in the past. The patient's symptomatology, duration of symptoms, and time for resolution of symptoms are consistent with previous reported cases [8, 9, 14]. There have been reports of symptoms manifesting weeks after antibiotic course, yet these were reported after fluoroquinolone use [6]. Her age and lack of risk factors for hemorrhagic colitis are also consistent with previous described cases [4]. Colonic biopsy is generally misinterpreted as ischemic colitis [6–9], just as in this case. Diagnosis is made upon stool culture of *K. oxytoca*, which has to be specifically requested. Stool culture of *K. oxytoca* can result within 24 hours of testing. If suspicion is high enough, and physician is aware of such entity, diagnosis of AAHC secondary to *K. oxytoca* can be made and can possibly prevent unnecessary and risky diagnostic procedures. The disease course is generally self-limited with withdrawal of the offending penicillin. Avoidance of NSAIDs is recommended as well, as this can exacerbate the colitis in these patients [7, 14, 15]. It is unclear at this time if readministration of ampicillin would lead to a similar episode [16]; however, the patient has been advised to avoid all penicillins.

In conclusion, we presented a case of *K. oxytoca* colitis in order to raise awareness of the possible etiology of AAHC to be considered in young patients taking antibiotics in which the simple interruption of antibiotic should improve the symptomatology and potentially avoid unnecessary testing or invasive procedures like colonoscopy to be done.

Acknowledgments

The authors would like to thank Dr. Alia Gupta for providing the histological images.

References

[1] F. C. Lessa et al., "Burden of clostridium difficile infection in the united states," *The New England Journal of Medicine*, vol. 372, pp. 825–843, 2015.

[2] J. G. Bartlett, "Antibiotic-associated diarrhea," *Clinical Infectious Diseases*, vol. 15, no. 4, pp. 573–581, 1992.

[3] L. Beaugerie, M. Metz, F. Barbut et al., "Klebsiella oxytoca as an agent of antibiotic-associated hemorrhagic colitis," *Clinical Gastroenterology and Hepatology*, vol. 1, no. 5, pp. 370–376, 2003.

[4] C. Högenauer, C. Langner, and E. Beubler, "Klebsiella oxytoca as a causative organism of antibiotic-associated hemorrhagic colitis," *The New England Journal of Medicine*, vol. 355, no. 23, pp. 2418–2426, 2006.

[5] R. Toffler et al., "Acute colitis related to penicillin and penicillin derivatives," *The Lancet*, vol. 312, no. 8092, pp. 707–709, 1978.

[6] H. Koga et al., "Can quinolones cause hemorrhagic colitis of late onset?" *Diseases of the Colon and Rectum*, vol. 42, no. 11, pp. 1502–1504, 1999.

[7] J. Chen, E. R. Cachay, and G. C. Hunt, "Klebsiella oxytoca: A rare cause of severe infectious colitis: First North American case report," *Gastrointestinal Endoscopy*, vol. 60, no. 1, pp. 142–145, 2004.

[8] A. M. Philbrick and M. E. Ernst, "Amoxicillin-associated hemorrhagic colitis in the presence of Klebsiella oxytoca," *Pharmacotherapy*, vol. 27, no. 11, pp. 1603–1607, 2007.

[9] R. Miyauchi, K. Kinoshita, and Y. Tokuda, "Clarithromycin-induced haemorrhagic colitis," *BMJ Case Reports*, 2013.

[10] S. Sweetser, K. W. Schroeder, and D. S. Pardi, "Pseudomembranous colitis secondary to klebsiella oxytoca," *American Journal of Gastroenterology*, vol. 104, no. 9, pp. 2366–2368, 2009.

[11] K. Tanaka, M. Fujiya, A. Sakatani et al., "Second-line therapy for Helicobacter pylori eradication causing antibiotic-associated hemorrhagic colitis," *Annals of Clinical Microbiology and Antimicrobials*, vol. 16, no. 1, 2017.

[12] O. Akanbi et al., "Antibiotic-associated haemorrhagic colitis: Not always Clostridium difficile," *BMJ Case Reports*, 2017.

[13] A. M. Miller, M. L. Bassett, J. E. Dahlstrom, and W. F. Doe, "Case report: Antibiotic-associated haemorrhagic colitis," *Journal of Gastroenterology and Hepatology*, vol. 13, no. 11, pp. 1115–1118, 1998.

[14] M. Yilmaz et al., "Prospective observational study on antibiotic-associated bloody diarrhea," *European Journal of Gastroenterology and Hepatology*, vol. 24, no. 6, pp. 688–694, 2012.

[15] G. Gorkiewicz, "Nosocomial and antibiotic-associated diarrhoea caused by organisms other than Clostridium difficile," *International Journal of Antimicrobial Agents*, vol. 33, no. 1, pp. S37–S41, 2009.

[16] H. Moulis and R. J. Vender, "Antibiotic-associated hemorrhagic colitis," *Journal of Clinical Gastroenterology*, vol. 18, no. 3, pp. 227–231, 1994.

Polypoid Dysplasia in Barrett's Esophagus: Diagnosis, Management, and Very Different Outcomes in Two Consecutive Cases

Megan Murphy,[1] Christina Tofani,[2] Kunjal Gandhi,[2] and Anthony Infantolino[2]

[1] *Department of Internal Medicine, Thomas Jefferson University Hospital, Philadelphia, PA 19107, USA*
[2] *Department of Gastroenterology & Hepatology, Thomas Jefferson University Hospital, Philadelphia, PA 19107, USA*

Correspondence should be addressed to Christina Tofani; christina.tofani@gmail.com

Academic Editor: Gregory Kouraklis

Background. Barrett's esophagus is associated with an increased risk of adenocarcinoma. Dysplasia in Barrett's esophagus is a precursor to adenocarcinoma. Rarely, dysplastic polypoid lesions are superimposed on Barrett's esophagus. Most reported cases of polypoid dysplasia in Barrett's esophagus have been advanced on presentation and treated with esophagectomy. We describe two cases of polypoid changes in Barrett's esophagus and treatment with polypectomy followed by radiofrequency ablation. *Cases.* A 75 yo male presented with esophageal polyps, which on biopsy showed gastric cardia/foveolar mucosa with focal intestinal metaplasia without dysplasia. Biopsy of intervening flat mucosa was consistent with nondysplastic Barrett's esophagus. Extensive hot snare polypectomies were performed followed by RFA. One year later, repeat EGD revealed no evidence of Barrett's esophagus. A 61 yo male presented with esophageal polyps, which on biopsy showed gastric cardia/foveolar mucosa with intestinal metaplasia and foci of low-grade dysplasia. Extensive hot snare polypectomies were performed followed by RFA. At repeat EGD, four months later, an esophageal mass was found. Biopsy of the mass showed invasive adenocarcinoma. The patient was referred for esophagectomy. *Conclusion.* This case series shows two outcomes, one with successful eradication of dysplasia and the other with disease progression to invasive adenocarcinoma requiring esophagectomy.

1. Introduction

Barrett's esophagus with dysplasia rarely presents as several polypoid esophageal lesions. To date, the management of this presentation is not standardized. Herein, we report two cases of polypoid dysplastic Barrett's esophagus managed with hot snare polypectomies followed by radiofrequency ablation.

1.1. Patient 1. A 75-year-old male with history of chronic gastroesophageal reflux disease presented with a known history of esophageal polyps. The patient was not felt to be a good surgical candidate due to multiple comorbid medical conditions and the patient was not interested in the surgical option. An esophagogastroduodenoscopy (EGD) (Figure 1) and endoscopic ultrasound (EUS) were performed in October 2013. Barrett's esophagus was noted at 31–40 cm (C9M9) from the incisors along with multiple frond-like, short-stalked polypoid lesions, which were removed by multiple hot snare polypectomies. EUS showed wall layers were intact with no surrounding adenopathy. All pathology specimens were reviewed by an expert gastrointestinal pathologist. Pathology from polypectomies showed gastric cardiac/foveolar type polyps with focal intestinal metaplasia and reactive glands and was negative for dysplasia. Biopsies of the surrounding flat mucosa were consistent with Barrett's esophagus, glandular epithelium with focal metaplasia and negative for dysplasia. The patient returned in January 2014 for repeat EGD. Again, multiple frond-like, short-stalked polypoid lesions were superimposed on Barrett's esophagus (Figure 2). Multiple hot snare polypectomies were performed and sent for histologic evaluation. The pathology at this time showed low-grade dysplasia with focal high-grade dysplasia arising in extensive intestinal metaplasia. Given the extensive nature of the disease and high perioperative risk secondary to medical comorbidities, the patient was not deemed a candidate for endoscopic submucosal dissection (ESD) or

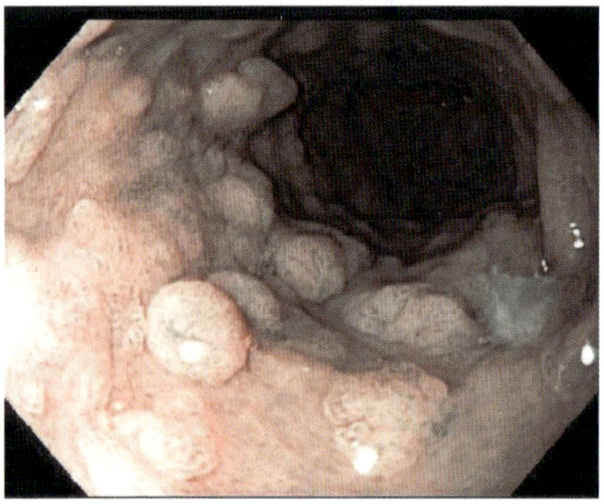

FIGURE 1: Patient 1. Original EGD (NBI). Several short-stalked polypoid lesions in the esophagus.

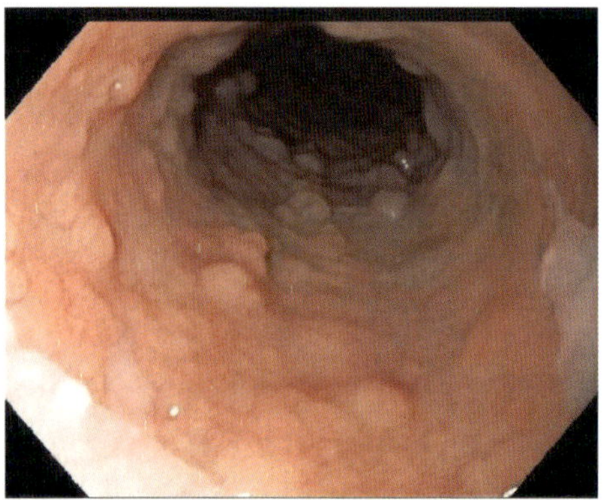

FIGURE 2: Patient 1 (white light endoscopy). Esophagus after multiple hot snare polypectomies, prior to RFA.

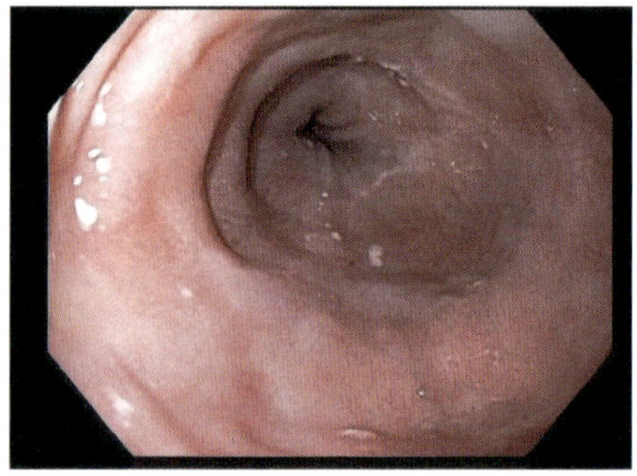

FIGURE 3: Patient 1 (white light endoscopy). Esophagus with squamous-appearing mucosa after RFA.

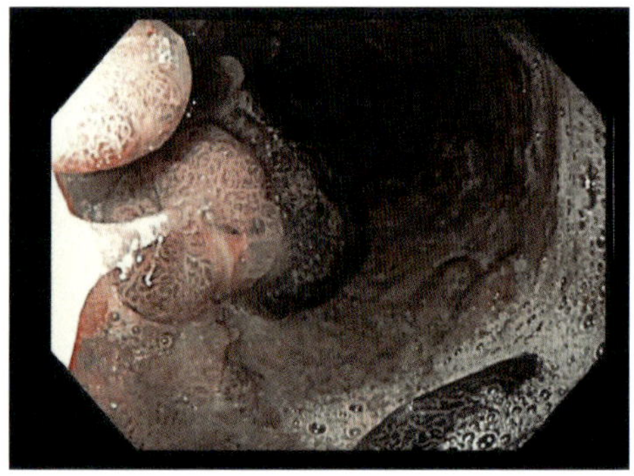

FIGURE 4: Patient 2. Original EGD (NBI). Several short-stalked polypoid lesions in the esophagus.

esophagectomy. The patient returned two months later, in March 2014, for repeat EGD and radiofrequency ablation (RFA) therapy. Subsequent RFA procedures were performed at 3, 6, and 9 months. Pathology from June 2014 showed the esophageal nodule to be consistent with hyperplastic gastric polyp formation and no evidence of adenomatous changes. In June 2015, one year after the last RFA treatment, EGD with esophageal biopsies showed Barrett's esophagus and benign squamous mucosa without pathologic change (Figure 3). No polyps were visualized at that time. A volumetric laser endomicroscopy (Ninepoint®) procedure was also performed and it failed to reveal any evidence of subsquamous Barrett's esophagus. The patient was instructed to follow up for continued close surveillance.

1.2. Patient 2. A 61-year-old man with known long segment Barrett's esophagus and esophageal polyps presented for evaluation. An EGD (Figure 4) and EUS were performed January 2010. Barrett's esophagus was noted at 20–40 cm (C20M20) from the incisors. Two nodules were noted at 22 and 24 cm and were removed by endomucosal resection (EMR). EUS showed nodules to be confined to the mucosa, possible submucosa, and no lymph nodes were identified. All pathology specimens were reviewed by an expert gastrointestinal pathologist. Pathology for both nodules was determined to be inflamed glandular mucosa with intestinal metaplasia negative for dysplasia. Due to the uncertain nature and the extent of the polypoid Barrett's esophagus, after several discussions, the patient was offered an evaluation for esophagectomy but refused at that time. Due to the 20 cm segment length, extensive ESD was not considered an option. Repeat EGD in March 2015 showed a segment from 20 to 40 cm compatible with Barrett's esophagus with multiple frond-like, short-stalked polyps scattered throughout. Many of the polyps were removed by snare cautery and the intervening mucosa was biopsied. Surrounding flat mucosa was confirmed Barrett's esophagus with low-grade dysplasia. Pathology of the polyps showed foci of low-grade dysplasia, foveolar type, arising in gastric cardiac type mucosa with intestinal metaplasia. The patient returned two weeks later in April 2015 for further polypectomies. Ten semipedunculated polyps of multilobular appearance, ranging from 4 to 8 mm in size, in the middle and lower third of the esophagus were removed by snare cautery. Again, foci of low-grade dysplasia were identified on pathology. One month later, the patient underwent his first RFA treatment with no complications (Figure 5). Four months later in September 2015, repeat EGD was performed. An ulcerated, nonbleeding mass was visualized in the middle third of the esophagus at 31–33 cm (Figure 6). Biopsy showed invasive carcinoma with high and low-grade dysplasia. Given these findings, subsequent RFA treatments were cancelled and the patient was referred to surgery for esophagectomy evaluation.

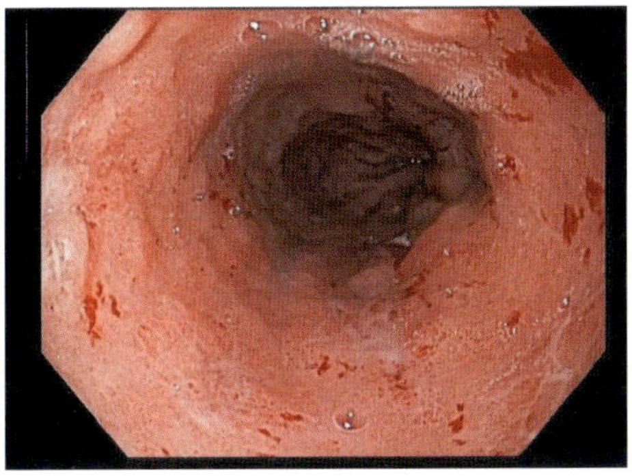

FIGURE 5: Patient 2 (white light endoscopy). Esophagus after multiple hot snare polypectomies and RFA.

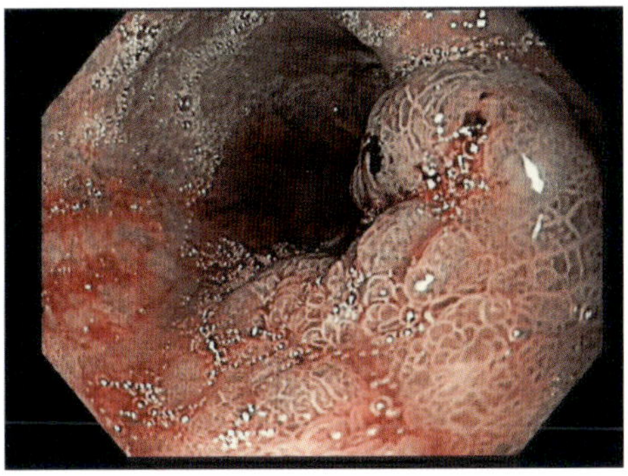

FIGURE 6: Patient 2 (NBI). New esophageal mass.

2. Discussion

Barrett's esophagus is acquired metaplasia of the esophagus and is associated with increased risk of adenocarcinoma, presumably through a metaplasia-dysplasia-carcinoma sequence [1]. The overall prevalence of Barrett's esophagus is 1.6%, with the majority of patients not progressing beyond nondysplastic intestinal metaplasia or low-grade dysplasia [2, 3]. However, in those who advance to high-grade dysplasia, the risk of adenocarcinoma may be as high as 10% per patient-year [4]. Thus, it is important to identify and stratify any dysplastic changes. Typically, dysplasia in Barrett's esophagus occurs as flat or nodular areas. However, it rarely can occur as a stalked, polyp-like lesion. Studies on the few reported cases of polypoid dysplasia have shown that Barrett's esophagus-associated polypoid dysplasia shares similar clinical, pathological, and molecular features as flat dysplasia, including a predisposition to adenocarcinoma [5]. However, optimal management remains unclear.

Radiofrequency ablation (RFA) is a known treatment option that has the potential to eradicate dysplasia and metaplasia in a significant amount of patients with Barrett's esophagus, thus decreasing their risk for adenocarcinoma [6]. However, given the infrequency of polypoid dysplasia of Barrett's esophagus, it has not been reported if the same outcomes are to be expected.

A review of the literature yielded six case studies with polypoid dysplastic lesions within Barrett's esophagus. Five of the cases contained adenocarcinoma and were treated with esophagectomy [6–10]. In one case, piecemeal polypectomies were performed with biopsy forceps and pathology showed tubular adenomas with low-grade dysplasia. However, through close-interval endoscopic surveillance, a recurrence of the lesion with high-grade dysplasia was detected and subsequently treated with esophagectomy [11].

Case 1 presented above is the only reported case of a dysplastic polypoid lesion completely treated with hot snare polypectomy followed by RFA. The patient, as described in the case, did have eradication of the dysplastic pathology, consistent with treatment of flat dysplasia in Barrett's esophagus. Conversely, case 2 represents the aggressive nature of esophageal adenocarcinoma. After one treatment of RFA, the patient progressed from low-grade dysplastic changes to invasive adenocarcinoma over the course of four months. Similar to previously described cases, the histologic changes were too advanced for RFA therapy and esophagectomy was recommended. Both patients were appropriately surveyed during treatment with esophageal biopsies following the Seattle protocol [12]. Currently, a surgical approach to polypoid BE with dysplasia may be the most definitive way to manage this disease. However, as presented in our two cases, endoscopic therapy may be a viable treatment option for those patients that either refuse or are not candidates for surgery. We suggest that, if appropriate, a surgical option always be offered to the patient.

In summary, true polypoid dysplasia, unlike the more common nodular dysplasia, in Barrett's esophagus is quite rare, with very few cases in the literature. However, they appear to share similar clinicopathologic and molecular features as typical dysplasia seen in Barrett's esophagus. In the literature, all cases of polypoid were treated with esophagectomy when adenocarcinoma or high-grade dysplasia was identified. In case 1 presented above, the patient had eradication of low- and high-grade dysplastic tissue after treatment with RFA. However, case 2 had progression of disease to invasive carcinoma in the setting of one RFA treatment and esophagectomy was recommended. Further studies of dysplastic polypoid changes are warranted to determine the efficacy of RFA therapy in this setting and to elucidate the disease course of these lesions. However, in the setting of Barrett's esophagus with dysplastic polypoid lesions in nonsurgical candidates or those who refuse surgery, we suggest considering EMR/polypectomy to achieve flat mucosa and RFA therapy in concert with close endoscopic surveillance as a treatment option. At centers capable of ESD, ESD for less extensive Barrett's esophagus is also an option, although the complication risk may be higher.

References

[1] R. C. Haggitt, J. Tryzelaar, F. H. Ellis, and H. Colcher, "Adenocarcinoma complicating columnar epithelium-lined (Barrett's) esophagus," *American Journal of Clinical Pathology*, vol. 70, no. 1, pp. 1–5, 1978.

[2] D. J. Drewitz, R. E. Sampliner, and H. S. Garewal, "The incidence of adenocarcinoma in Barrett's esophagus: a prospective study of 170 patients followed 4.8 years," *American Journal of Gastroenterology*, vol. 92, no. 2, pp. 212–215, 1997.

[3] P. Sharma, G. W. Falk, A. P. Weston, D. Reker, M. Johnston, and R. E. Sampliner, "Dysplasia and cancer in a large multicenter cohort of patients with Barrett's esophagus," *Clinical Gastroenterology and Hepatology*, vol. 4, no. 5, pp. 566–572, 2006.

[4] A. Rastogi, S. Puli, H. B. El-Serag, A. Bansal, S. Wani, and P. Sharma, "Incidence of esophageal adenocarcinoma in patients with Barrett's esophagus and high-grade dysplasia: a meta-analysis," *Gastrointestinal Endoscopy*, vol. 67, no. 3, pp. 394–398, 2008.

[5] B. L. Thurberg, P. H. Duray, and R. D. Odze, "Polypoid dysplasia in Barrett's esophagus: a clinicopathologic, immunohistochemical, and molecular study of five cases," *Human Pathology*, vol. 30, no. 7, pp. 745–752, 1999.

[6] G. B. McDonald, D. L. Brand, and D. R. Thorning, "Multiple adenomatous neoplasms arising in columnar lined (Barrett's) esophagus," *Gastroenterology*, vol. 72, no. 6, pp. 1317–1321, 1977.

[7] J. J. Thompson, K. R. Zinsser, and H. T. Enterline, "Barrett's metaplasia and adenocarcinoma of the esophagus and gastroesophageal junction," *Human Pathology*, vol. 14, no. 1, pp. 42–61, 1983.

[8] D. G. Cavanaugh, L. D. Crandall, L. P. Harrison, J. H. Layer, and R. K. Waits Jr., "Malignant gastroesophageal polyp: a case report," *Wisconsin Medical Journal*, vol. 94, no. 8, pp. 443–445, 1995.

[9] R. G. Lee, "Dysplasia in Barrett's esophagus: a clinicopathologic study of six patients," *American Journal of Surgical Pathology*, vol. 9, no. 12, pp. 845–852, 1985.

[10] A. E. Stillman and J. I. Selwyn, "Primary adenocarcinoma of the esophagus arising in a columnar-lined esophagus," *The American Journal of Digestive Diseases*, vol. 20, no. 6, pp. 577–582, 1975.

[11] G. L. Arnold and H. E. Mardini, "Barrett's esophagus-associated polypoid dysplasia: a case report and review of the literature," *Digestive Diseases and Sciences*, vol. 47, no. 8, pp. 1897–1900, 2002.

[12] D. S. Levine, R. C. Haggitt, P. L. Blount, P. S. Rabinovitch, V. W. Rusch, and B. J. Reid, "An endoscopic biopsy protocol can differentiate high-grade dysplasia from early adenocarcinoma in Barrett's esophagus," *Gastroenterology*, vol. 105, no. 1, pp. 40–50, 1993.

Two Cases of White Globe Appearance in Autoimmune Atrophic Gastritis

Masaya Iwamuro,[1] Takehiro Tanaka,[2] Hiromitsu Kanzaki,[1] Seiji Kawano,[1] Yoshiro Kawahara,[3] and Hiroyuki Okada[1]

[1]*Department of Gastroenterology and Hepatology, Okayama University Graduate School of Medicine, Dentistry, and Pharmaceutical Sciences, 2-5-1 Shikata-cho, Kita-ku, Okayama 700-8558, Japan*
[2]*Department of Pathology, Okayama University Hospital, Okayama 700-8558, Japan*
[3]*Department of Endoscopy, Okayama University Hospital, Okayama 700-8558, Japan*

Correspondence should be addressed to Masaya Iwamuro; pr145h2k@okayama-u.ac.jp

Academic Editor: Shiro Kikuchi

In this report, we described two patients with white globe appearance in autoimmune atrophic gastritis. Endoscopy revealed multiple white substances in the stomach in both cases. Biopsied specimens from the lesions contained dilated glands and showed a decrease in parietal cells. Intraglandular necrotic debris and carcinoma were absent. These results confirmed that white globe appearance can be observed in autoimmune atrophic gastritis. Moreover, microscopic features for white globe appearance observed in these cases were different from those reported previously in gastric cancer lesions and were similar to those observed for noncancerous stomach.

1. Introduction

White globe appearance has been reported to be characterized by a small (<1 mm) white lesion with a globular shape and microvessels overlying the white substance, reflecting the white substance existing underneath the gastric epithelium and subepithelial microvessels [1–3]. Detection of white globe appearance during esophagogastroduodenoscopy is clinically significant because this endoscopic feature is reportedly found within the margin of the cancerous gastric epithelium.

Although the white globe appearance is generally associated with the presence of gastric cancer, it can be rarely found in the noncancerous mucosa of the stomach. We have recently reported endoscopic pictures and detailed pathological features of white globe appearance in two patients without gastric cancer [4]. Herein, we reported white globe appearance detected in two cases of autoimmune atrophic gastritis, mainly focusing on the differences in pathological features between the two present cases and previously reported cases.

2. Case Report

2.1. Case 1. A 66-year-old Japanese woman was referred to the Department of Neurology for investigation of aphasia. The patient had no previous disease history and does not take any medications. Laboratory testing revealed decreased levels of vitamin B_{12} at 107 pg/mL (normal range: 257-989 pg/mL), for which she underwent esophagogastroduodenoscopy. Increased levels of rheumatoid factor at 38.9 IU/mL, hemoglobin A1c at 6.5%, and gastrin at 1,016 pg/mL were also noted. The number of red blood cells and the hemoglobin levels were within the normal ranges. She was positive for anti-intrinsic factor antibody and antiparietal cell antibody.

Esophagogastroduodenoscopy revealed gastric atrophy predominantly in the fornix (Figure 1(a)) and in the body (Figure 1(b)), whereas atrophic changes were not evident in the antrum endoscopically (Figure 1(c)). Close-up observation of the gastric fornix showed multiple, slightly elevated, round, white substances (Figure 1(d)). Magnified observation with narrow-band imaging revealed microvasculature on its

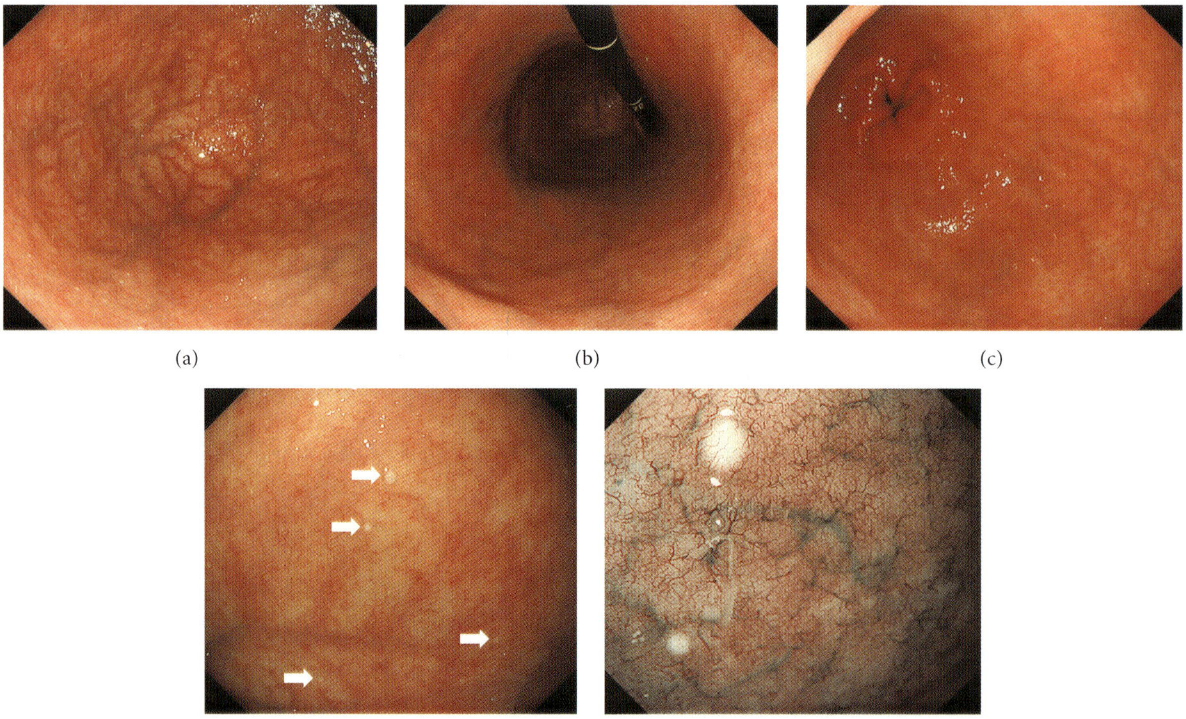

(a) (b) (c)

(d) (e)

Figure 1: Esophagogastroduodenoscopy images of Case 1. Atrophy is predominantly observed in the gastric fornix (a) and body (b), while it is not evident in the antrum (c). Close-up observation of the gastric fornix shows multiple white substances (d). Magnifying observation with narrow-band imaging reveals microvasculature on its surface (e).

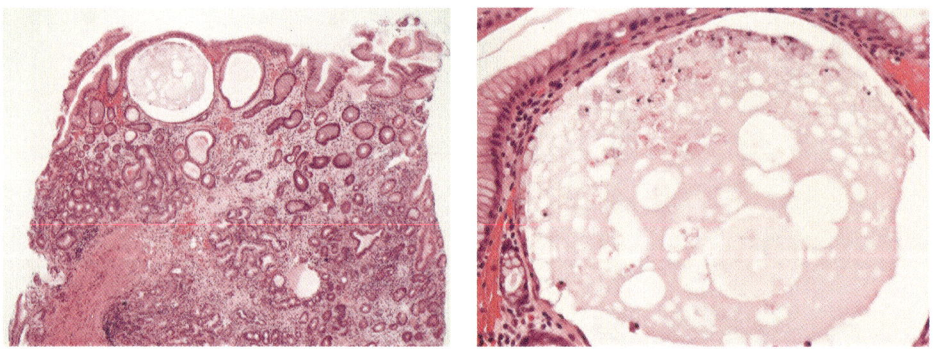

(a) (b)

Figure 2: Pathology images of Case 1. Biopsy specimens taken from the gastric mucosa with white globe appearance show cystic dilatation of the gastric glands (hematoxylin and eosin staining, (a): ×4.2, (b): ×20).

surface, suggesting deposition of the white substance within the mucosa (Figure 1(e)). Two biopsy samples were endoscopically taken from the fornix mucosa with the white substance. Three additional biopsies were done on the mucosa of the middle body, the lower body, and the antrum of the stomach, where the white substance was absent. Two biopsy specimens taken from the gastric mucosa that contained white substance revealed cystic dilatation of the gastric glands (Figure 2). In contrast to this, there was no cystic dilatation in the glands of the gastric mucosa specimens where the white globe appearance was not observed. A prominent decrease in parietal cells was also noted. Parietal cell protrusion was absent. There were no *Helicobacter pylori* pathologically. We diagnosed autoimmune atrophic gastritis based on the serology, endoscopy, and pathology results.

2.2. Case 2. An 81-year-old Japanese woman underwent esophagogastroduodenoscopy for annual screening purposes. The patient had been taking amlodipine for hypertension. Although she had undergone appendectomy at 30 years of age, she had no other history of abdominal diseases. Esophagogastroduodenoscopy showed diffuse gastric

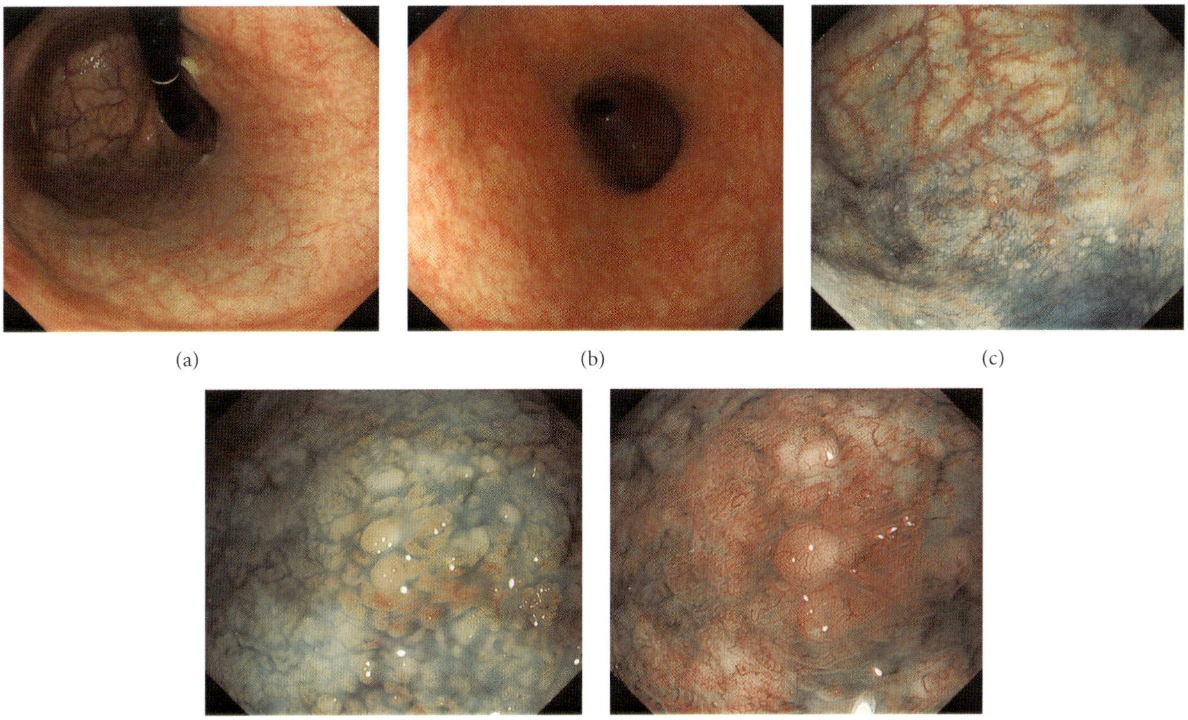

(a) (b) (c) (d) (e)

FIGURE 3: Esophagogastroduodenoscopy images of Case 2. Atrophy is more prominent in the fornix (a), compared to the antrum (b). Multiple white substances are seen in the gastric fornix and in the body after indigo carmine spraying (c, d). Microvasculature is also observed on magnified observation with narrow-band imaging (e).

atrophy; the atrophic changes were more prominent in the fornix (Figure 3(a)) than in the antrum (Figure 3(b)). After indigo carmine spraying, we noticed multiple, slightly elevated, round, white substances in the gastric fornix and body (Figures 3(c) and 3(d)). Microvasculature was also noted on its surface as seen on the magnified observation with narrow-band imaging (Figure 3(e)). Biopsy from the gastric mucosa showed cystically dilated gastric glands (Figures 4(a)–4(c)). Immunohistochemically, pepsinogen-positive cells were present (Figure 4(d)), whereas H+/K+ ATPase-positive cells were absent (Figure 4(e)).

Laboratory testing revealed normocytic anemia: hemoglobin was 10.2 g/dL, mean corpuscular volume was 92.5 fL, and mean corpuscular hemoglobin was 29.7 pg. Gastrin level was elevated at 392 pg/mL. Although the level of folic acid was decreased at 2.8 ng/mL, vitamin B_{12} level was within the normal range. The patient was positive for antiparietal cell antibody, while anti-intrinsic factor antibody was negative. She tested negative for urea breath test and *H. pylori* IgG antibody. Consequently, we diagnosed her as autoimmune atrophic gastritis.

The patient underwent esophagogastroduodenoscopy 12 months later. White substances were not detected in the gastric mucosa, even in the gastric fornix and body (Figure 5).

3. Discussion

Autoimmune atrophic gastritis, also known as type A gastritis, is an inflammatory disease affecting the gastric mucosa, wherein the parietal cells are destroyed by the patient's immune system. The progressive damage to the parietal cells decreases the ability to absorb iron and vitamin B_{12}, which in turn causes pernicious anemia and neurological problems [5–7]. Since the diagnostic criteria have not yet been established, diagnosis of autoimmune atrophic gastritis is made based on laboratory testing, endoscopic examination, and biopsy results. Serologically, anti-intrinsic factor antibodies are highly specific for the disease, while the sensitivity is low. Conversely, antiparietal cell antibodies have high sensitivity but low specificity [8]. On esophagogastroduodenoscopy, atrophic changes are predominantly positive in the fornix and in the gastric body. On biopsy, chronic inflammation and oxyntic gland destruction are the most common histologic findings. We diagnosed the two patients with autoimmune atrophic gastritis, since they had these serological, endoscopic, and pathological features.

To our knowledge, this report is the first to describe the presence of white globe appearance in autoimmune atrophic gastritis. It was noteworthy that cystic dilatation of the gland was identified in the specimens of the gastric mucosa with white globe appearance in Case 1. Conversely, no cystic dilatation was present in the glands of the gastric mucosa specimens where the white globe appearance was not observed. This observation indicates that cystically dilated glands correspond to the endoscopically observed white globe appearance in the gastric mucosa. Another interesting observation from Case 2 is that white globe appearance was

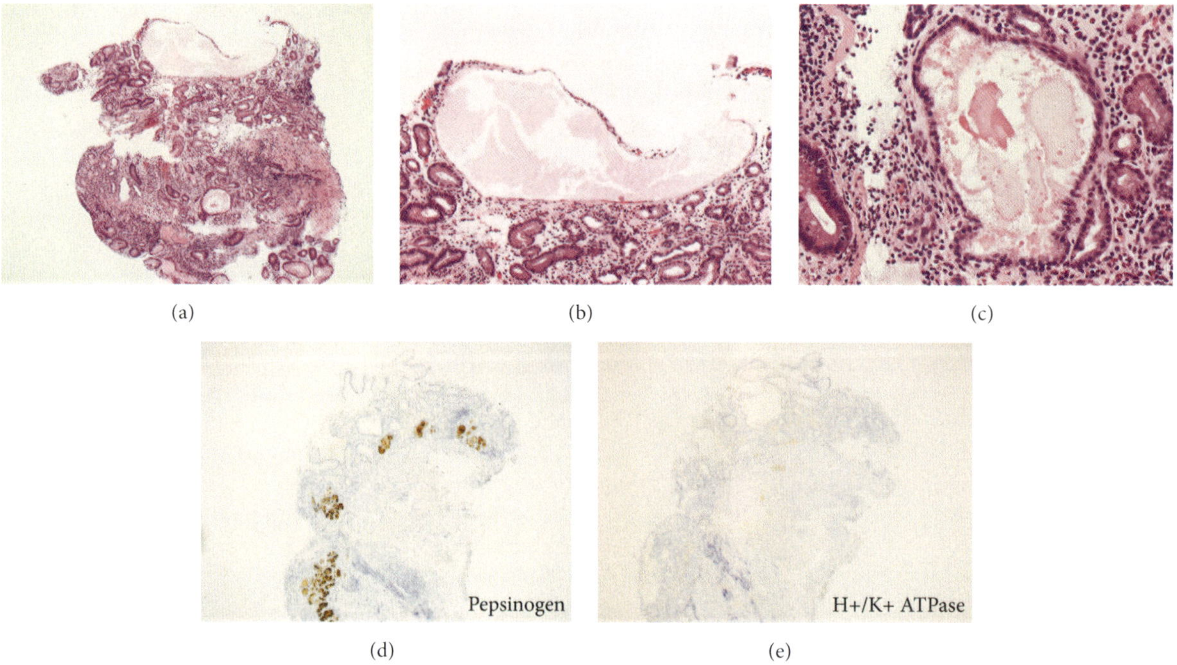

FIGURE 4: Pathology images of Case 2. Biopsy from the gastric mucosa shows cystically dilated glands (hematoxylin and eosin staining, (a): ×4.2, (b): ×10, (c): ×20). Immunohistochemical study shows that pepsinogen-positive cells ((d), ×4.2) are present, whereas H+/K+ ATPase-positive cells are absent ((e), ×4.2).

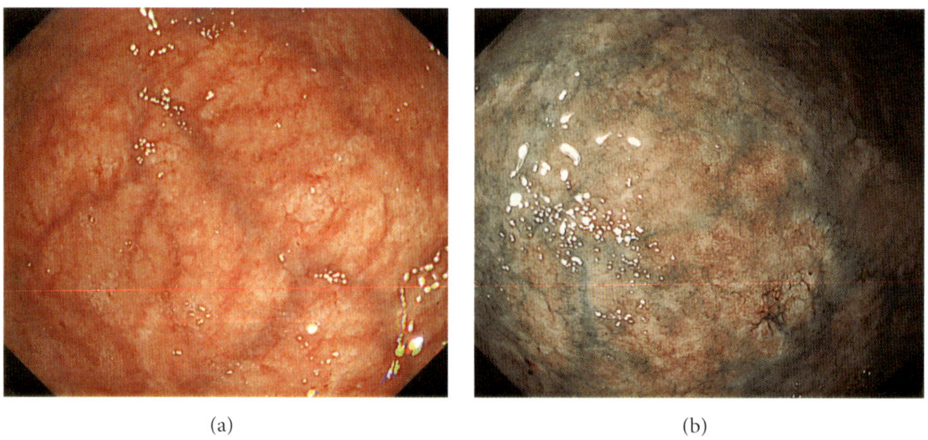

FIGURE 5: Esophagogastroduodenoscopy images of Case 2. Endoscopy performed 12 months later shows no white substances even in the gastric fornix ((a): white light, (b): narrow-band imaging).

not identified on repeat endoscopy performed 12 months later. Therefore, this feature may spontaneously disappear during the course.

As previously described, white globe appearance in the stomach has been reported as an endoscopic feature indicative of cancer [1–3]. However, our earlier report showed detailed endoscopic and pathological pictures of white globe appearance observed in the noncancerous gastric mucosa and they revealed that the pathological features are different between cases with and without cancer lesions [4]. Pathologically, biopsy specimens taken from the white globe appearance with a cancer lesion contain eosinophilic materials with necrotic epithelial fragments within the lumen of the dilated glands; they are called intraglandular necrotic debris [1, 2, 9]. Meanwhile, specimens taken from the white globe appearance without cancer had cystic dilatation of the gastric fundal glands but no eosinophilic materials or necrotic epithelial fragments were identified [4]. For the present patients, we speculated that the deposited material was mucus in Case 2 and degenerated epithelial cells and mucus in Case 1. This report revealed that the pathological features of white globe appearance in autoimmune atrophic gastritis are somewhat similar to those observed for noncancerous stomach. However, a crucial difference between the white globe appearance observed in noncancerous stomach and that of autoimmune atrophic gastritis is that the former shows pseudoparietal cell hyperplasia with tongue-like protrusions of parietal cell cytoplasm (parietal cell protrusion) [4], while the latter shows a decrease or elimination of parietal cells via the autoimmune response.

Given that the white globe appearance in noncancerous gastric mucosa and that of autoimmune atrophic gastritis show similar pathologic features, several possible mechanisms can be hypothesized for the pathogenesis. First, obstruction of outflow from the glands within the gastric mucosa might induce such features. In autoimmune atrophic gastritis, inflammatory response to the parietal cells leads to the destruction of oxyntic glands. It is likely that such damage induces narrowing or collapse of the ducts, finally resulting in intramucosal cyst formation of the dilated glands. As reported previously, white globe appearance in noncancerous stomach shows parietal cell protrusion, which might cause outflow obstructions as well [4]. Thus, alteration of the duct structure may be the primary cause of the white globe appearance observed in noncancerous gastric mucosa and that of autoimmune atrophic gastritis.

The second hypothesis is that elevated levels of gastrin could induce white globe appearance. In autoimmune gastritis, hypochlorhydria from the loss of parietal cell mass leads to stimulation of the patient's antral G cells, which in turn results in gastrin secretion and hypergastrinemia [10]. As described above, the two patients showed elevated levels of serum gastrin. Meanwhile, patients with white globe appearance in noncancerous stomach have been taking acid secretion inhibitors [4]. Although we did not measure gastrin levels in these patients, such medications most likely induced hypergastrinemia. Therefore, elevated gastrin levels may play a part in inducing white globe appearance. However, concrete mechanisms between hypergastrinemia and formation of white globe appearance have not been elucidated yet.

In conclusion, we present two cases with white globe appearance observed in the stomach with autoimmune atrophic gastritis. The pathogenesis of white globe appearance has not yet been described; hence, further investigations are warranted.

References

[1] H. Doyama, N. Yoshida, S. Tsuyama et al., "The "white globe appearance" (WGA): a novel marker for a correct diagnosis of early gastric cancer by magnifying endoscopy with narrow-band imaging (M-NBI)," *Endoscopy International Open*, vol. 03, no. 02, pp. E120–E124, 2015.

[2] N. Yoshida, H. Doyama, H. Nakanishi et al., "White globe appearance is a novel specific endoscopic marker for gastric cancer: A prospective study," *Digestive Endoscopy*, vol. 28, no. 1, pp. 59–66, 2016.

[3] H. Omura, N. Yoshida, T. Hayashi et al., "Interobserver agreement in detection of "white globe appearance" and the ability of educational lectures to improve the diagnosis of gastric lesions," *Gastric Cancer*, vol. 20, no. 4, pp. 620–628, 2017.

[4] M. Iwamuro, T. Tanaka, H. Sakai et al., "Two cases of white globe appearance in non-cancerous stomach," *Ecancermedicalscience*, vol. 12, 2018.

[5] M. E. Pittman, L. Voltaggio, F. Bhaijee, S. A. Robertson, and E. A. Montgomery, "Autoimmune metaplastic atrophic gastritis," *The American Journal of Surgical Pathology*, vol. 39, no. 12, pp. 1611–1620, 2015.

[6] A. Minalyan, J. N. Benhammou, A. Artashesyan, M. S. Lewis, and J. R. Pisegna, "Autoimmune atrophic gastritis: Current perspectives," *Clinical and Experimental Gastroenterology*, vol. 10, pp. 19–27, 2017.

[7] J. Y. Park, T. C. Cornish, D. Lam-Himlin, C. Shi, and E. Montgomery, "Gastric lesions in patients with autoimmune metaplastic atrophic gastritis (AMAG) in a tertiary care setting," *The American Journal of Surgical Pathology*, vol. 34, no. 11, pp. 1591–1598, 2010.

[8] E. Lahner, G. L. Norman, C. Severi et al., "Reassessment of intrinsic factor and parietal cell autoantibodies in atrophic gastritis with respect to cobalamin deficiency," *American Journal of Gastroenterology*, vol. 104, no. 8, pp. 2071–2079, 2009.

[9] Y. Watanabe, M. Shimizu, T. Itoh, and K. Nagashima, "Intraglandular necrotic debris in gastric biopsy and surgical specimens," *Annals of Diagnostic Pathology*, vol. 5, no. 3, pp. 141–147, 2001.

[10] M. D. Burkitt and D. M. Pritchard, "Review article: Pathogenesis and management of gastric carcinoid tumours," *Alimentary Pharmacology & Therapeutics*, vol. 24, no. 9, pp. 1305–1320, 2006.

43

Thromboelastometry Identified Alteration of Clot Stabilization and Factor XIII Supplementation Need in a Patient with Decompensated Liver Disease Undergoing Liver Biopsy

Tomaz Crochemore and Felicio Aragão Savioli

Hospital Leforte, Department of Critical Care, São Paulo, SP, Brazil

Correspondence should be addressed to Tomaz Crochemore; tomazcr@gmail.com

Academic Editor: Engin Altintas

Liver disease has been considered the prototype of hemorrhagic disease. Disorder in any component of coagulation system can lead to hemorrhage. Deficiency of factor XIII may impair clot strength and clot stabilization and can be accessed by thromboelastometry. We report a case of a patient with a rapid evolution of liver disease who underwent a liver biopsy. Thromboelastometry was performed, evidencing impairment of clot stability. This clotting disorder was corrected with factor XIII concentrate after unsuccessful administration of antifibrinolytic drugs and hepatic biopsy was performed without hemorrhagic complications. *Case Presentation*. We report the case of a previously healthy 38-year-old man, who presented to our emergency department with clinical signs of rapid progression of acute liver failure. The laboratory tests revealed platelets of $142x10^3$/mm3, plasma fibrinogen concentration of 221 mg/dl, increased international nationalized ratio (INR 1.9), total bilirubin of 3.9mg/dl, direct bilirubin of 2.3mg/dl, ALT 751U/l, and AST 540U/l without acute bleeding. A liver biopsy was indicated. Based on the results of the thromboelastometry, Tranexamic Acid was administered to correct hyperfibrinolysis followed by factor XIII concentrate to correct factor XIII deficiency. Thromboelastometry was normal despite conventional coagulation tests were still altered. So, liver biopsy was performed with no signs of bleeding and without need of further transfusion. *Conclusion*. Thromboelastometry may be considered a useful, feasible, and safe tool to monitor and manage coagulopathy in patients with liver disease, with the potential advantage of helping avoid unnecessary transfusion in such patients.

1. Introduction

Coagulopathy in liver disease has been considered as one of the major challenges in the area of thrombosis and hemostasis [1]. In recent years liver disease has been proven to be no longer an exclusively hemorrhagic disease; otherwise, clinical signs of thrombosis can be found [2]. The clinical manifestation depends on imbalance between pro- and anticoagulant drivers as well as pro- and antifibrinolytic components [1].

Traditionally, patients with decompensated liver disease who exhibit abnormal results of conventional coagulation tests (CCT) have been subjected to prophylactic transfusion of blood components before undergoing an invasive procedure. However, CCT are poor predictors of bleeding, and allogeneic blood components transfusion is associated with poor outcome.

Studies in patients with liver disease have suggested that thromboelastometry (ROTEM®) may be a better test in predicting risk of bleeding than coagulation conventional tests and platelet count [3]. Thromboelastometry accesses the entire process of clot formation including the initiation, maximum firmness, and stabilization of the clot [4]. Specific coagulation disorder as dysfibrinogenemia, hyperfibrinolysis, and factor XIII deficiency can be identified early [5].

Therefore, thromboelastometry used for identifying coagulopathy and guided hemostatic therapy could be considered in cases of patients with liver disease with risk of bleeding and need to undergo an invasive procedure such as liver biopsy. Consequently, our objective was to describe a case of a patient with fast onset liver disease with unknown cause whose hepatic biopsy procedure was successfully guided by thromboelastometry. Coagulopathy was corrected

TABLE 1: Sequential analysis of thromboelastometry (ROTEM®) parameters.

PARAMETERS	1ST ROTEM	2ND ROTEM	3RD ROTEM	4TH ROTEM
EXTEM CT (S)	80	64	83	64
EXTEM CFT (s)	105	105	133	122
EXTEM α-ANGLE(°)	70	69	66	68
EXTEM MCF (mm)	52	51	50	50
EXTEM ML (%)	37	24	21	15
FIBTEM MCF (mm)	13	11	10	12
APTEM MCF (mm)	53	51	51	51
APTEM ML (%)	20	20	19	15

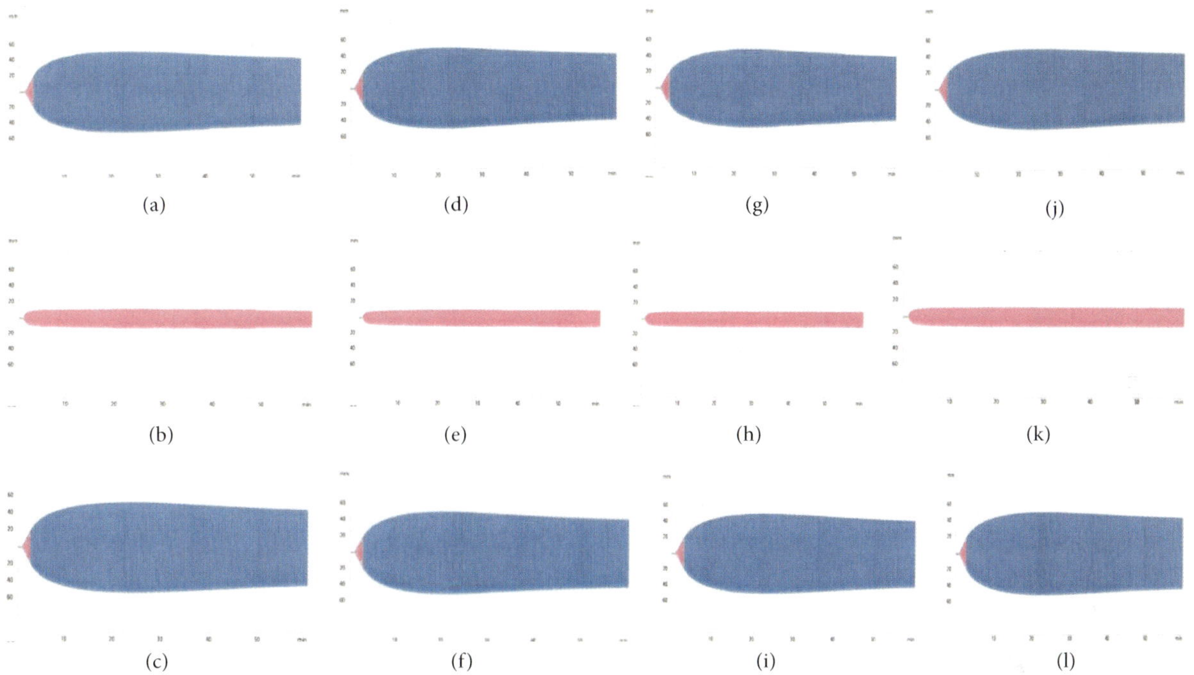

FIGURE 1: Sequential thromboelastometry (ROTEM). ((a), (b), and (c)) Thromboelastometry analysis at the hospital admission ((a) EXTEM, (b) FIBTEM, and (c) APTEM). ((d), (e), and (f)) Second thromboelastometry analysis performed after Tranexamic Acid administration ((d) EXTEM, (e) FIBTEM, and (f) APTEM). ((g), (h), and (i)) Third thromboelastometry analysis performed after additional administration of Tranexamic Acid ((g) EXTEM, (h) FIBTEM, and (i) APTEM). ((j), (k), and (l)) Thromboelastometry analysis performed after factor XIII concentrate (Fibrogammin® P, CSL Behring, Marburg, Germany) ((j) EXTEM, (k) FIBTEM, and (l) APTEM).

with coagulation factor concentrate and hemostatic drugs without transfusion of allogeneic blood component.

2. Case Presentation

We report the case of a previously healthy 38-year-old man, Afro-Brazilian, with no previous medical records. He presented to our emergency department with an acute onset of abdominal pain, jaundice, fever, nausea, weakness, and malaise. His arterial blood pressure was 90/50mmHg, heart rate was 90 bpm, axillary temperature was 35°C, and he was dehydrated. The laboratory examinations revealed serum creatinine of 0.8 mg/dl, platelets of 142 x 10^3/mm3, serum fibrinogen of 221 mg/dl, increased international nationalized ratio (INR 1.9), total bilirubin of 3.9mg/dl, direct bilirubin of 2.3mg/dl, ALT 751U/l, AST 540U/l, ceruloplasmin of 17 mg/dl, ferritin of 3200 ng/dl, iron of 276mcg/dl, TIBC (total iron-binding capacity) of 267mcg/dl, transferrin saturation of 103%, hemoglobin (Hb) of 14 g/dl, and hematocrit (Ht) of 41,3% without acute bleeding. US (ultrasound) showed signs of inflammation and liver fibrosis as well as iron overload. A liver biopsy was indicated. First ROTEM test showed in EXTEM CT 80s, CFT 105s, alfa-angle 70°, MCF 52 mm, and ML 37%; FIBTEM MCF 13 mm and APTEM MCF 53 mm and ML 20% (Table 1/Figures 1(a), 1(b), and 1(c)). Tranexamic Acid 1 g was administered to correct hyperfibrinolysis. Second ROTEM test presented improvement in the hyperfibrinolysis but not completely, so another 1 g of Tranexamic Acid was administered with EXTEM CT 64s, CFT 105s, alfa-angle 69°, MCF 51 mm, and ML 24%; FIBTEM MCF 11 mm, APTEM MCF 51 mm, and ML 20% (Table 1/Figures 1(d), 1(e), and 1(f)). The third ROTEM test showed persistence of maximum lysis above 15% with EXTEM CT 83s, CFT 133s, alfa-angle 66°, MCF 50 mm, and ML 21%; FIBTEM MCF

10 mm and APTEM MCF 51 mm and ML 19% (Table 1/Figures 1(g), 1(h), and 1(i)). This time 1500U of factor XIII concentrate was administrated to correct factor XIII deficiency and fourth ROTEM test was normal with EXTEM CT 64s, CFT 122s, alfa-angle 68°, MCF 50 mm, and ML 15%; FIBTEM MCF 12 mm and APTEM MCF 51 mm and ML 15% (Table 1/Figures 1(j), 1(k), and 1(l)). Thromboelastometry was normal despite CCT were still altered. So, liver biopsy was performed which succeeded with no signs of bleeding and without need of further transfusion. He was discharged from the hospital 5 days after admission.

3. Discussion

Liver disease is often associated with coagulation disorders. CCT are usually quite altered and therefore transfusion of blood components has been a frequent practice. Transfusion of allogeneic blood products is associated with a higher risk of infection, pulmonary failure, and mortality [6, 7]. However, CCT present late results and are punctual since they access only 5% of thrombin generation [8]. Thus, CCT are limited to predict bleeding or guide transfusion therapy with blood components.

In 2001, the concept of the cell-based coagulation model described by Monroe and Hoffman pointed out the role of the surface of cell membrane for the generation of thrombin. This complex process of clot formation is triggered from the release of the tissue factor by the endothelium. In this cellular model, the clot formation process goes through 3 stages: thrombin generation including initiation and amplification phases; maximum clot firmness or propagation phase; and last phase the clot stabilization [9]. Both the fibrinolytic system and factor XIII are considered the determinants of clot stabilization.

Rotational thromboelastometry is a laboratory method performed at the bedside that accesses the entire process of clot formation. First ROTEM identifies the initial process involving the coagulation factors of both the extrinsic and intrinsic pathway to generate thrombin. Subsequent phase consists in a fibrin clot formation from fibrinogen, platelets, and also factor XIII when clot reaches maximum firmness [4]. The final phase of stabilization involves the fibrinolytic system as well as factor XIII activated responsible for cross-linking of fibrin [10].

Discovered in 1940s, blood coagulation factor XIII (F XIII) is a transglutaminase that is present in plasma, activated by the combined action of thrombin and Ca2+. Its function includes cross-linking of fibrin monomers between themselves to generate a stable fibrin strand, but also cross-linking of fibrinogen with $\alpha2$ antiplasmin, a potent plasmin inhibitor, to protect the fibrin clot from fibrinolysis [11, 12]. Thus, factor XIII acts on the clot firmness but mainly on clot stabilization. FXIII deficiency is not detected by routine coagulation assays and needs to be searched by measuring FXIII levels with quantitative assay [4, 5]. Inherited FXIII deficiency with undetectable FXIII activity is associated with a severe bleeding tendency. FXIII levels below 50% are associated with a smaller α2AP incorporation and enhanced clot lysis [10, 13].

Thromboelastometry allows the evaluation of factor XIII deficiency in two different ways. First, factor XIII deficiency can be thought of if the maximum clot firmness (MCF) in FIBTEM remains reduced even after adequate replacement of fibrinogen. The other possibility is when the maximum lysis found in EXTEM is above 15%; however, the maximum lysis remains above 15% to APTEM, even after the administration of antifibrinolytic drugs [14]. In both situations, the quantitative measurement of factor XIII is not mandatory, since thromboelastometry accesses the quality of formation and stabilization of the clot. Sudden quantitative reduction in the measurement of factor XIII may compromise the stabilization of the clot, without critically low levels of factor XIII being detected necessarily.

In this reported case, traditionally the patient with acute liver disease and INR 1.9 would probably be transfused with fresh frozen plasma because of the high risk of bleeding during liver biopsy. However, thromboelastometry performed identified impairment in clot stabilization. According to the first ROTEM test, Tranexamic Acid 1 g was administered to correct hyperfibrinolysis defined by ML EXTEM > 15% (Figures 1(a), 1(b), and 1(c)). There was partial improvement in the second test that still showed hyperfibrinolysis parameters 8 h after the first test (Figures 1(d), 1(e), and 1(f)). An additional dose of 1 g Tranexamic Acid was administered, but without changing the ML in both EXTEM and APTEM. At this time, the third ROTEM test showed ML EXTEM above 15%; then 1500U of factor XIII concentrated was administered (Figures 1(g), 1(h), and 1(i)). The control ROTEM was normal and liver biopsy was undergone without any bleeding complication, confirming the usefulness of factor XIII infusion to increase clot stability confirmed by thromboelastometry in a situation where acquired factor XIII deficiency is expected (Figures 1(j), 1(k), and 1(l)).

4. Conclusion

This case reports the use of thromboelastometry for diagnosis of specific coagulation disorder in patients with liver disease with high risk of bleeding and need to undergo an invasive procedure such as liver biopsy.

Thromboelastometry identified factor XIII deficiency and guided the therapy with factor XIII concentrate correcting clotting disorder. Factor XIII replacement improved the clot stabilization and liver biopsy was performed without bleeding complications. No transfusion of allogeneic blood component was needed. Nevertheless, additional studies are needed to define the ability of thromboelastometry to identify factor XIII deficiency in liver disease patients, but also to define the role of factor XIII concentrate to improve clot stabilization.

Consent

Written informed consent was obtained from the patient for publication of this case report and any accompanying images.

Acknowledgments

We thank Carolina Martinez Savioli for proofreading this manuscript and Dr. João Carlos de Campos Guerra for providing laboratory data.

References

[1] A. Tripodi, M. Primignani, V. Chantarangkul et al., "An imbalance of pro- vs anti-coagulation factors in plasma from patients with cirrhosis," *Gastroenterology*, vol. 137, no. 6, pp. 2105–2111, 2009.

[2] A. Tripodi, "Hemostasis in Acute and Chronic Liver Disease," *Seminars in Liver Disease*, vol. 37, no. 1, pp. 28–32, 2017.

[3] T. Crochemore, F. M. De Toledo Piza, E. Silva, and T. D. Corrêa, "Thromboelastometry-guided hemostatic therapy: An efficacious approach to manage bleeding risk in acute fatty liver of pregnancy: A case report," *Journal of Medical Case Reports*, vol. 9, no. 1, 2015.

[4] T. Crochemore, F. M. Piza, R. d. Rodrigues, J. C. Guerra, L. J. Ferraz, and T. D. Corrêa, "A new era of thromboelastometry," *Einstein (São Paulo)*, vol. 15, no. 3, pp. 380–385, 2017.

[5] E. Abuelkasem, S. Lu, K. Tanaka, R. Planinsic, and T. Sakai, "Comparison between thrombelastography and thromboelastometry in hyperfibrinolysis detection during adult liver transplantation," *British Journal of Anaesthesia*, vol. 116, no. 4, pp. 507–512, 2016.

[6] B. Sarani, W. J. Dunkman, L. Dean, S. Sonnad, J. I. Rohrbach, and V. H. Gracias, "Transfusion of fresh frozen plasma in critically ill surgical patients is associated with an increased risk of infection," *Critical Care Medicine*, vol. 36, no. 4, pp. 1114–1118, 2008.

[7] C. C. Silliman and N. J. D. McLaughlin, "Transfusion-related acute lung injury," *Blood Reviews*, vol. 20, no. 3, pp. 139–159, 2006.

[8] K. G. Mann, "Thrombin Formation," *Chest*, vol. 124, no. 3, pp. 4S–10S, 2003.

[9] M. Hoffman and D. M. Monroe III, "A cell-based model of hemostasis," *Thrombosis and Haemostasis*, vol. 85, no. 6, pp. 958–965, 2001.

[10] D. C. Rijken and S. Uitte De Willige, "Inhibition of Fibrinolysis by Coagulation Factor XIII," *BioMed Research International*, vol. 2017, 2017.

[11] M. Martinuzzo, L. Barrera, D. Altuna et al., "Effects of Factor XIII Deficiency on Thromboelastography. Thromboelastography with Calcium and Streptokinase Addition is more Sensitive than Solubility Tests," *Mediterranean Journal of Hematology and Infectious Diseases*, vol. 8, no. 1, Article ID e2016037, 2016.

[12] S. R. Fraser, N. A. Booth, and N. J. Mutch, "The antifibrinolytic function of factor XIII is exclusively expressed through $\alpha 2$-antiplasmin cross-linking," *Blood*, vol. 117, no. 23, pp. 6371–6374, 2011.

[13] S. Kattula, J. R. Byrnes, S. M. Martin et al., "Factor XIII in plasma, but not in platelets, mediates red blood cell retention in clots and venous thrombus size in mice," *Blood Advances*, vol. 2, no. 1, pp. 25–35, 2018.

[14] O. M. Theusinger, W. Baulig, L. M. Asmis, B. Seifert, and D. R. Spahn, "In vitro factor XIII supplementation increases clot firmness in rotation thromboelastometry (ROTEM®)," *Thrombosis and Haemostasis*, vol. 104, no. 2, pp. 385–391, 2010.

44

An Unusual Case of Gastrointestinal Bleeding from Isolated Gallbladder Varices in a Patient with Pancreatic Cancer Complicated by Portal Biliopathy

Mahir Gachabayov,[1] Kubach Kubachev,[2] Elbrus Abdullaev,[1] Nonna Zarkua,[2] Abakar Abdullaev,[1] and Artur Fokin[2]

[1] *Department of Abdominal Surgery, Vladimir City Clinical Hospital of Emergency Medicine, Vladimir, Russia*
[2] *Department of Surgery Named after N. D. Monastyrskiy, North-Western State Medical Academy Named after I. I. Mechnikov, Saint Petersburg, Russia*

Correspondence should be addressed to Mahir Gachabayov; gachabayovmahir@gmail.com

Academic Editor: Olga I. Giouleme

Portal biliopathy is the complex of abnormalities of extrahepatic and intrahepatic bile ducts, cystic duct, and gallbladder, arising as a result of extrahepatic portal vein obstruction and noncirrhotic portal fibrosis, which can be caused by coagulopathies, tumors, inflammation, postoperative complications, dehydration, and neonatal umbilical vein catheterization. We report a case of a 55-year-old male patient with the history of pancreatic cancer and cholecystoenteric anastomosis presenting with gastrointestinal bleeding from gallbladder varices via the anastomosis.

1. Introduction

Portal biliopathy (PB) is the complex of abnormalities of extrahepatic and intrahepatic bile ducts, cystic duct, and gallbladder, arising as a result of extrahepatic portal vein obstruction (EHPVO) and noncirrhotic portal fibrosis, which can be caused by coagulopathies, tumors, inflammation, postoperative complications, dehydration, and neonatal umbilical vein catheterization [1–4]. Although jaundice and common bile duct (CBD) compression associated with portal hypertension were described by Fraser et al. in 1944, the term "portal biliopathy" was not used until the early 1990s [2, 5, 6]. The incidence of PB is unknown due to its rarity. However, ectopic varices were estimated to be encountered in 12–30% in the field of portal hypertension [7]. They are usually located in the gallbladder and bile ducts where they can coexist and are usually asymptomatic [8, 9]. Few reports have been published on this topic. We herein report an extremely rare case of gastrointestinal bleeding as a result of bleeding from gallbladder varices via cholecystoenteric anastomosis caused by pancreatic carcinoma.

2. Case Presentation

A 55-year-old male patient was admitted to ICU with a 9-hour history of melena, fatigue, and nausea. His past medical history was significant for unresectable Stage 3 pancreatic adenocarcinoma (T4N1M0) which was proven during explorative laparotomy 4 months prior to admission. At that laparotomy preventive cholecystoenteric anastomosis was formed. Nevertheless, the patient was reported to develop jaundice for which choledochal stent was placed a month later. He also had well-controlled hypertension and peptic ulcer disease. On admission, the patient was pale and hypotonic, with HR 96 bpm, BP 105/60 mmHg, Hb 8.0 g/dL, serum amylase 94 U/L, total bilirubin 0.8 mg/dL, and direct bilirubin 0.2 mg/dL. Fluid replacement therapy, PPIs, and hemostatic agents were started. Esophagogastroduodenoscopy was negative for both the source and signs of bleeding while colonoscopy after preparation with laxatives was positive for signs of gastrointestinal bleeding and negative for source. Contrast-enhanced CT was performed thereafter which revealed an extremely rare picture of isolated

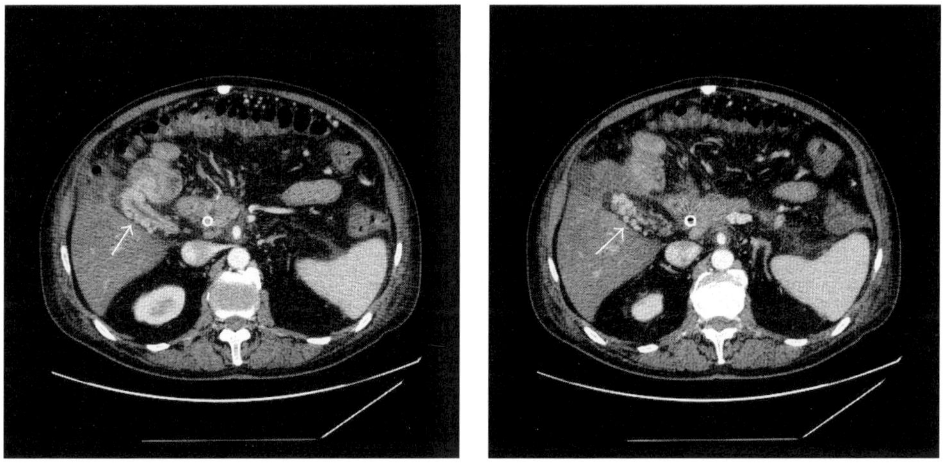

(a) (b)

FIGURE 1: Abdominal contrast-enhanced CT, axial plane, showing gallbladder varices (diffuse variceal dilation of veins in the gallbladder wall).

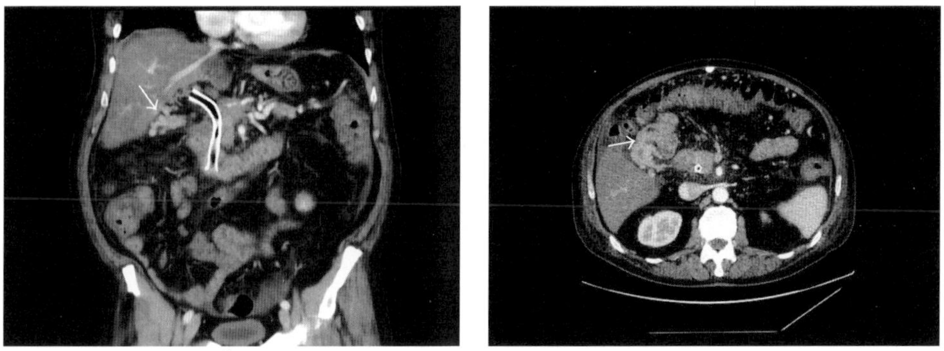

(a) (b)

FIGURE 2: Abdominal contrast-enhanced CT. (a) Oblique plane, showing gallbladder varices, and (b) axial plane, showing gallbladder varices and cholecystoenteric anastomosis.

gallbladder varices bleeding to the gastrointestinal tract via cholecystoenteric anastomosis (Figures 1 and 2). The patient underwent laparotomy with disconnection of cholecystoenteric anastomosis. The gallbladder seemed to be difficult to remove due to the carcinogenic infiltration of its neck, so the gallbladder wall was repaired. The etiology of portal biliopathy with isolated gallbladder varices was deemed to be combined: due to the infiltration (either inflammatory or carcinogenic) of small branches of portal vein and the minor compression of portal vein by the stented common bile duct (Figure 3). On the 3rd postoperative day the patient developed ileus which was resolved conservatively. On the 8th postoperative day surgical site infection without major septic consequences developed which was also resolved conservatively. The patient was discharged on 14th postoperative day. On the follow-up after 1 month the patient was relatively well without any episodes of recurrent bleeding and jaundice but with the progression of tumor intoxication.

3. Discussion

Ectopic varices are dilated mesoportal veins and/or portosystemic collateral that can occur along the entire gastrointestinal tract outside the common pathologic variceal sites. They represent 2–5% of gastrointestinal variceal bleeding; however, they are associated with a 4-fold increased risk of bleeding when compared with esophageal varices and can have a mortality rate as high as 40% [10]. Ectopic varices are commonly associated with portal hypertension in the context of liver cirrhosis or portal vein thrombosis [11]. Several cases of isolated varices of different sites including one-sided portal hypertension, isolated small bowel, large bowel, or duodenal varices have been reported [12–15].

The drainage vein of the gallbladder, the cystic vein, in some cases can be prominent, accompanying the cystic duct and ending in the right branch of the portal vein; in some cases they can drain blood from the gallbladder directly to the liver parenchyma [16]. The drainage veins of biliary ducts form epicholedochal and paracholedochal plexuses (Petren's plexus) running along the CBD [17, 18]. Portal vein thrombosis or compression can lead to the development of new collateral, thus, forming portal cavernoma and varicosity of cystic veins and epi- and paracholedochal plexuses [19]. Pancreatic cancer has been reported and is well-recognized to be one of the causes of PB [20].

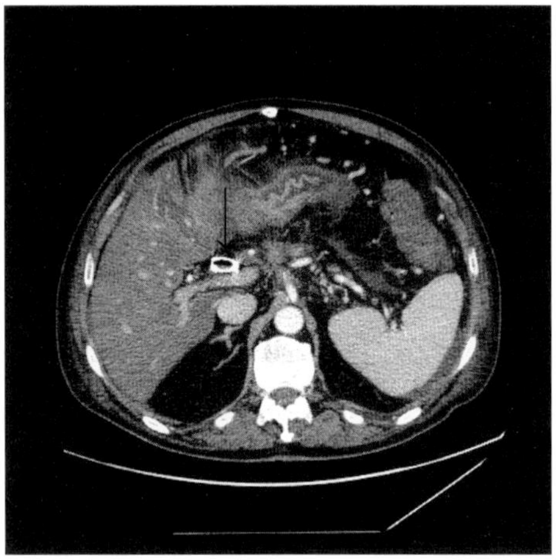

FIGURE 3: Abdominal contrast-enhanced CT, axial plane. Stented common bile duct is intimately close to the portal vein causing its minor compression.

Clinical presentation of PB is diverse varying from asymptomatic to obstructive jaundice and cholangitis. Symptomatic PB is rare, with estimates ranging between 5% and 38% of patients with portal vein thrombosis [17, 19, 21, 22]. In 2–4% of cases, patients with long-term obstruction or inadequate endoscopic or surgical management may develop secondary biliary cirrhosis [1]. Among complications of PB, obstructive syndrome with its consequences is more specific for CBD varices, while gallbladder varices can be complicated by bleeding and even rupture [23]. Bleeding from the gallbladder varices can occur either to the peritoneal cavity leading to a life-threatening hemoperitoneum or to the cavity of gallbladder itself leading to hemobilia and gastrointestinal bleeding [8, 9, 20, 24, 25]. In our case gallbladder varices were bleeding to the cavity of the gallbladder itself; however, the route of blood transmission emerged to be cholecystoenteric anastomosis instead of major duodenal papilla and hemobilia. To the best of our knowledge, our case is the second case of bleeding gallbladder varices via the anastomosis leading to major gastrointestinal bleeding [26].

Some authors support duplex scan and color flow Doppler sonography to be the gold standard for PB showing anechoic, serpentine areas in the wall or around the gallbladder with venous flow on Doppler imaging [27, 28]. Contrast-enhanced ultrasound has been shown to be more sensitive and accurate to distinguish between vascular structures and solid masses [3]. Although endoscopic ultrasonography has been shown to add to the differentiation between CBD varices, stones, and tumors in cases when other radiologic modalities failed, it is not routinely recommended in the workup of the patient with PB [29]. Contrast-enhanced CT is also helpful in the diagnosis of gallbladder varices being accurate in the imaging of vascular structures [30, 31]. MRCP features of PB have been shown to be biliary stenosis, wavy appearance of the bile ducts, angulation of the CBD, and upstream dilatation of the bile ducts [32].

Asymptomatic cases of PB do not require any treatment. Portosystemic shunt surgery seems to be the procedure of choice in patients with radiologic findings of PB who are otherwise asymptomatic and are being operated on for other complications of portal hypertension, such as variceal bleeding or symptomatic hypersplenism [33]. In emergency cases, especially in patients with life-threatening intra-abdominal or gastrointestinal bleeding, the vector shifts toward simplicity and minimal invasiveness [26].

To conclude, portal biliopathy is a rare but potentially life-threatening clinical entity which should be considered in differential diagnosis in patients with the history of pancreatic cancer. High index of clinical suspicion, multitechnique imaging approach, and prompt and adequate treatment are essential for the successful management of patients with portal biliopathy.

References

[1] R. Chandra, D. Kapoor, A. Tharakan, A. Chaudhary, and S. K. Sarin, "Portal biliopathy," *Journal of Gastroenterology and Hepatology*, vol. 16, no. 10, pp. 1086–1092, 2001.

[2] S. K. Sarin, V. Bhatia, and U. Makwane, "Portal biliopathy in extra hepatic portal vein obstruction," *Indian Journal of Gastroenterology*, vol. 11, supplement 1, p. A82, 1992.

[3] H. Nunoi, M. Hirooka, H. Ochi et al., "Portal biliopathy diagnosed using color Doppler and contrast-enhanced ultrasound," *Internal Medicine*, vol. 52, no. 10, pp. 1055–1059, 2013.

[4] S. S. Pargewar, S. N. Desai, S. Rajesh, V. P. Singh, A. Arora, and A. Mukund, "Imaging and radiological interventions in extra-hepatic portal vein obstruction," *World Journal of Radiology*, vol. 8, no. 6, pp. 556–570, 2016.

[5] J. Fraser and A. K. Broun, "A clinical syndrome associated with a rare anomaly of vena portal system," *Surgery, Gynecology & Obstetrics*, vol. 78, pp. 520–524, 1944.

[6] O. Baskan, C. Erol, and Y. Sahingoz, "Portal biliopathy, magnetic resonance imaging and magnetic resonance cholangiopancreatography findings: a case series," *Gastroenterology Report*, vol. 4, no. 1, pp. 68–72, 2016.

[7] Y. Chawla, J. B. Dilawari, and S. Katariya, "Gallbladder varices in portal vein thrombosis," *American Journal of Roentgenology*, vol. 162, no. 3, pp. 643–645, 1994.

[8] D. Kevans, R. MacNicholas, and S. Norris, "Gallbladder wall variceal haemorrhage with associated rupture: a rare cause of mortality in the cirrhotic patient," *European Journal of Gastroenterology and Hepatology*, vol. 21, no. 8, pp. 955–957, 2009.

[9] R. Vilallonga, O. González, S. Bergamini, J. M. Fort, and M. Armengol, "Gallbladder variceal bleeding in a patient with alcoholic cirrhosis: a rare entity," *Revista Española de Enfermedades Digestivas*, vol. 104, no. 3, pp. 153–154, 2012.

[10] W. E. A. Saad, A. Lippert, N. E. Saad, and S. Caldwell, "Ectopic varices: anatomical classification, hemodynamic classification, and hemodynamic-based management," *Techniques in Vascular and Interventional Radiology*, vol. 16, no. 2, pp. 158–175, 2013.

[11] Y. K. Chawla and V. Bodh, "Portal vein thrombosis," *Journal of Clinical and Experimental Hepatology*, vol. 5, no. 1, pp. 22–40, 2015.

[12] H. Thrainsdottir, V. Petursdottir, S. Blöndal, and E. S. Björnsson, "Pancreatic mass leading to left-sided portal hypertension, causing bleeding from isolated gastric varices," *Case Reports in Gastrointestinal Medicine*, vol. 2014, Article ID 956490, 3 pages, 2014.

[13] M. C. Garcia, G. Ahlenstiel, H. Mahajan, and D. Van Der Poorten, "Small bowel varices secondary to chronic superior mesenteric vein thrombosis in a patient with heterozygous Factor v Leiden mutation: a case report," *Journal of Medical Case Reports*, vol. 9, no. 1, article 210, 2015.

[14] J. D. Haddad and B. W. Lacey, "Isolated non-hemorrhagic cecal varices," *Gastroenterology Report*, vol. 2, no. 4, pp. 316–319, 2014.

[15] A. Podboy, P. Kamath, and J. Tabibian, "Isolated duodenal varices without cirrhosis," *The American Journal of Gastroenterology*, vol. 111, no. 4, p. 454, 2016.

[16] F. Arthur, "The cystic vein: the significance of a forgotten anatomic landmark," *JSLS: Journal of the Society of Laparoendoscopic Surgeons*, vol. 1, no. 3, pp. 263–266, 1997.

[17] E. M. Walser, B. R. Runyan, M. G. Heckman et al., "Extrahepatic portal biliopathy: proposed etiology on the basis of anatomic and clinical features," *Radiology*, vol. 258, no. 1, pp. 146–153, 2011.

[18] T. Petren, "Die extrahepatischen gallenwegsvenen and ihre: pathologischanatomische bedeutum," *Verhandlungen der Anatomischen Gesellschaft*, vol. 41, pp. 139–143, 1932.

[19] M. S. Khuroo, G. N. Yattoo, S. A. Zargar et al., "Biliary abnormalities associated with extrahepatic portal venous obstruction," *Hepatology*, vol. 17, no. 5, pp. 807–813, 1993.

[20] S. Y. Kim, J. H. Cho, E. J. Kim, S. J. Choi, and Y. S. Kim, "Successful hemostasis using a covered self-expandable metallic stent for spurting hemobilia in patients with advanced pancreatic cancer-induced portal biliopathy," *Gastrointestinal Endoscopy*, 2016.

[21] R. K. Dhiman, A. Behera, Y. K. Chawla, J. B. Dilawari, and S. Suri, "Portal hypertensive biliopathy," *Gut*, vol. 56, no. 7, pp. 1001–1008, 2007.

[22] J. B. Dilawari and Y. K. Chawla, "Pseudosclerosing cholangitis in extrahepatic portal venous obstruction," *Gut*, vol. 33, no. 2, pp. 272–276, 1992.

[23] U. Hellerich and S. Pollak, "Spontaneous gallbladder rupture caused by variceal hemorrhage: an unusual complication of portal vein thrombosis," *Beiträge zur Gerichtlichen Medizin*, vol. 49, pp. 319–323, 1991.

[24] R. Pravisani, W. Bugiantella, D. Lorenzin, V. Bresadola, and C. A. Leo, "Fatal hemoperitoneum due to bleeding from gallbladder varices in an end-stage cirrhotic patient A case report and review of the literature," *Annali Italiani di Chirurgia*, In press.

[25] E. C. Chu, W. Chick, D. J. Hillebrand, and K.-Q. Hu, "Fatal spontaneous gallbladder variceal bleeding in a patient with alcoholic cirrhosis," *Digestive Diseases and Sciences*, vol. 47, no. 12, pp. 2682–2685, 2002.

[26] S. Getzlaff, C. A. Benz, D. Schilling, and J. F. Riemann, "Enteroscopic cyanoacrylate sclerotherapy of jejunal and gallbladder varices in a patient with portal hypertension," *Endoscopy*, vol. 33, no. 5, pp. 462–464, 2001.

[27] I. Mishin, "Gallbladder varices—a case report," *Romanian Journal of Gastroenterology*, vol. 14, no. 2, pp. 165–168, 2005.

[28] P. W. Ralls, D. S. Mayekawa, K. P. Lee, P. M. Colletti, M. B. Johnson, and J. M. Halls, "Gallbladder wall varices: diagnosis with color flow Doppler sonography," *Journal of Clinical Ultrasound*, vol. 16, no. 8, pp. 595–598, 1988.

[29] L. Palazzo, P. Hochain, C. Helmer et al., "Biliary varices on endoscopic ultrasonography: clinical presentation and outcome," *Endoscopy*, vol. 32, no. 7, pp. 520–524, 2000.

[30] M. S. West, B. S. Garra, S. C. Horii et al., "Gallbladder varices: imaging findings in patients with portal hypertension," *Radiology*, vol. 179, no. 1, pp. 179–182, 1991.

[31] C. Besa, J. P. Cruz, A. Huete, and F. Cruz, "Portal biliopathy: a multitechnique imaging approach," *Abdominal Imaging*, vol. 37, no. 1, pp. 83–90, 2012.

[32] E. Özkavukcu, A. Erden, and I. Erden, "Imaging features of portal biliopathy: frequency of involvement patterns with emphasis on MRCP," *European Journal of Radiology*, vol. 71, no. 1, pp. 129–134, 2009.

[33] S. Chattopadhyay and S. Nundy, "Portal biliopathy," *World Journal of Gastroenterology*, vol. 18, no. 43, pp. 6177–6182, 2012.

A Rare Clinical Presentation of Cholangiocarcinoma

Elisa Gravito-Soares,[1,2] Marta Gravito-Soares,[1,2] Pedro Figueiredo,[1,2] and Luis Tomé[1,2]

[1] *Gastroenterology Department, Centro Hospitalar e Universitário de Coimbra, Coimbra, Portugal*
[2] *Faculty of Medicine, University of Coimbra, Coimbra, Portugal*

Correspondence should be addressed to Elisa Gravito-Soares; es18497@gmail.com

Academic Editor: Gregory Kouraklis

Cholangiocarcinoma is an uncommon tumor, often diagnosed in the context of obstructive jaundice. Brain metastasis rarely occurs with the cerebellum being a rare site of spread of this type of tumor. Few cases of cholangiocarcinoma have been reported in the literature and this type of tumor is associated with a very poor outcome. We present a very rare form of clinical presentation of cholangiocarcinoma with neurologic symptoms due to cerebellar metastases.

1. Introduction

Cholangiocarcinoma is a rare tumor of the bile duct, often diagnosed in the context of obstructive jaundice [1–3]. Usually, patients with cholangiocarcinoma have a locally advanced disease at the diagnosis with distant metastasis being uncommon [1]. Brain metastasis is rare and associated with poor prognosis [2].

Very few cases of brain metastasis due to primary cholangiocarcinoma [3–8] have been reported in the literature and there is only one case with neurologic symptoms at presentation [3]. In this work, we describe the case of a patient with headache, as initial symptom of an extrahepatic cholangiocarcinoma with cerebellar metastasis.

2. Case Report

An autonomous 66-year-old Caucasian man with past medical history of arterial hypertension and social alcohol consumption (15 g/day) was admitted with two weeks of nausea, vomiting, and jaundice. About 4 months earlier, the patient started daily occipital headache with frequent recurrence to the emergency department, misdiagnosed as uncontrolled arterial hypertension. There was no history of blood transfusions, recent trips, over-the-counter drugs, prior infectious diseases, or jaundice episodes. Physical examination was unremarkable except for mucocutaneous jaundice and mild discomfort in the upper right quadrant of the abdomen. Neurologic examination revealed no significant abnormalities, including cerebellar signs such as vertigo, ataxia, nystagmus, dysmetria, dysarthria, dysdiadochokinesia, or other signs. Laboratory analysis showed lactate dehydrogenase 268 U/L (125–220 U/L), aspartate aminotransferase 150 U/L (<31 U/L), alanine aminotransferase 316 U/L (<34 U/L), alkaline phosphatase 955 U/L (40–150 U/L), gamma-glutamyl transferase 1465 U/L (<38 U/L), total bilirubin 4.5 mg/dL (0.3–1.2 mg/dL), and direct bilirubin 3.2 mg/dL (0.1–0.5 mg/dL). Serum albumin, serum amylase, and prothrombin time were normal. Tumor marker CA 19-9 was elevated (299 U/mL; <37 U/mL) and alpha-fetoprotein and carcinoembryonic antigen (CEA) were normal. An extensive etiological workup was performed excluding liver diseases, infections, autoimmune conditions, and risk factors for cholangiocarcinoma. Abdominal ultrasound showed dilatation of the common bile duct (12 mm) and intrahepatic ducts and gallstones. Esophagogastroduodenoscopy was normal. Computed tomography scan (CT) of the brain revealed one mound-shaped lesion with biconvex dural contact in the right cerebellum with heterogeneous contrast enhancement (Figure 1). Other causes than neoplastic lesion were ruled out, including cryptococcosis, toxoplasmosis, syphilis, or human immunodeficiency virus infection. Subsequently, for a better characterization of the cerebellar lesion, brain magnetic resonance imaging (MRI) was performed revealing multiple bilateral lesions with strong and irregular contrast enhancement, central necrosis, and mass effect, suggesting cerebellar

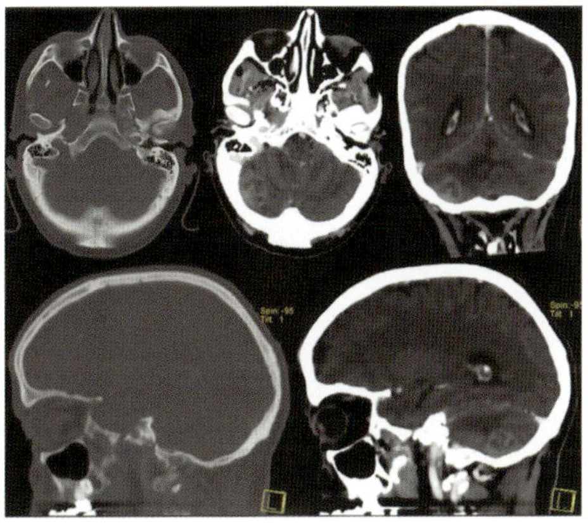

FIGURE 1: Brain computed tomography scan (bone and brain windows) showing one lesion in the right cerebellum with heterogeneous contrast enhancement.

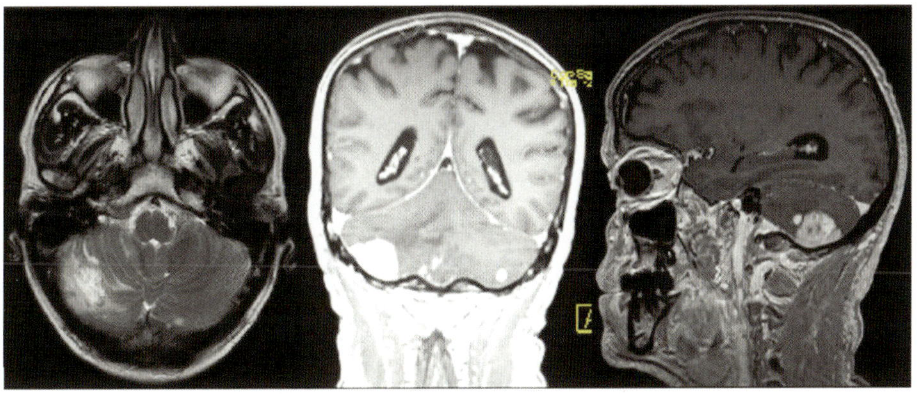

FIGURE 2: Magnetic resonance imaging showing multiple bilateral lesions in the cerebellum with strong and irregular contrast enhancement, central necrosis, and mass effect.

metastases (Figure 2). In order to find out the primary site of this tumor, a thorough examination of the cutaneous tegument was performed, excluding melanoma. Colonoscopy was normal. Cervical-thoracic-abdominal-pelvic CT confirmed dilatation of intrahepatic and extrahepatic bile ducts with progressive narrowing of the common bile duct at the prepancreatic level. The narrowed segment of the bile duct showed a parietal contrast enhancement without well-defined intraluminal mass (Figure 3). Thus, endoscopic retrograde cholangiopancreatography (ERCP) was attempted. However, this procedure revealed being impossible to perform due to edema and congestion of the duodenal mucosa with pearly-white appearance, resulting in luminal stricture. Biopsies showed a lymphovascular permeation of the duodenum due to a poorly differentiated adenocarcinoma with positive immunohistochemical staining for CK7 and CK19, consistent with a primary biliary neoplasm. Positron emission tomography scan (PET) with 18-fluorodeoxyglucose was performed revealing a hypermetabolic lesion at the common bile duct/duodenum topography with cerebellar metastasis and, additionally, other secondary lesions in the thoracic-abdominal lymph nodes, left suprarenal gland, and multiple bone sites (Figure 4).

The patient started systemic steroids with initial improvement of neurologic symptoms. However, subsequently neurological worsening was verified with gait ataxia and vertigo and therefore brain radiotherapy was started after a multidisciplinary therapeutic decision meeting. The patient died within six weeks of diagnosis, having performed only one session of whole-brain radiotherapy (WBRT).

3. Discussion

Cholangiocarcinoma is a rare tumor and the most common malignancy of the biliary tract. Its incidence has been continuously increasing and usually develops in the setting of progressive cholestasis and chronic inflammation [1, 2]. However, the patient did not present cholangiocarcinoma risk factors, including parasitic infections, primary sclerosing cholangitis, biliary-ducts cysts, hepatolithiasis, toxins, or other less-established risk factors such as inflammatory bowel disease, hepatitis C or B, liver cirrhosis, diabetes, obesity, significant alcoholism (>40 g/day), or smoking [1, 9]. Despite a mean age of 50 years for the onset of symptoms, diagnosis is usually made at the age of 65. Based on the anatomic site of origin, cholangiocarcinoma is classified as intrahepatic, perihilar, and extrahepatic with distinct tumor

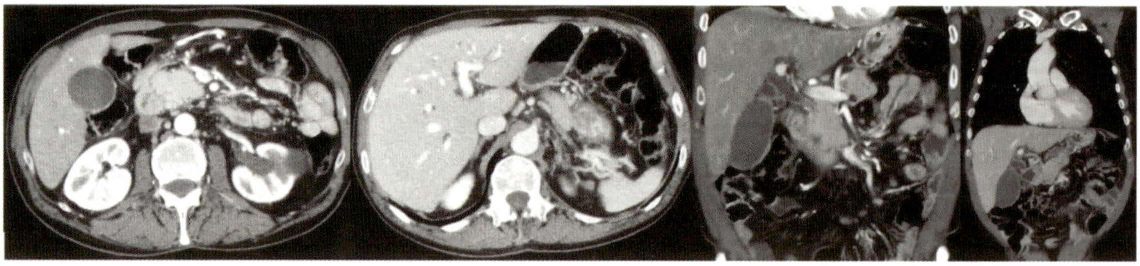

Figure 3: Cervical-thoracic-abdominal-pelvic computed tomography revealed parietal contrast enhancement without intraluminal well-defined mass at the distal common bile duct level with upstream dilatation of the extrahepatic and intrahepatic bile ducts.

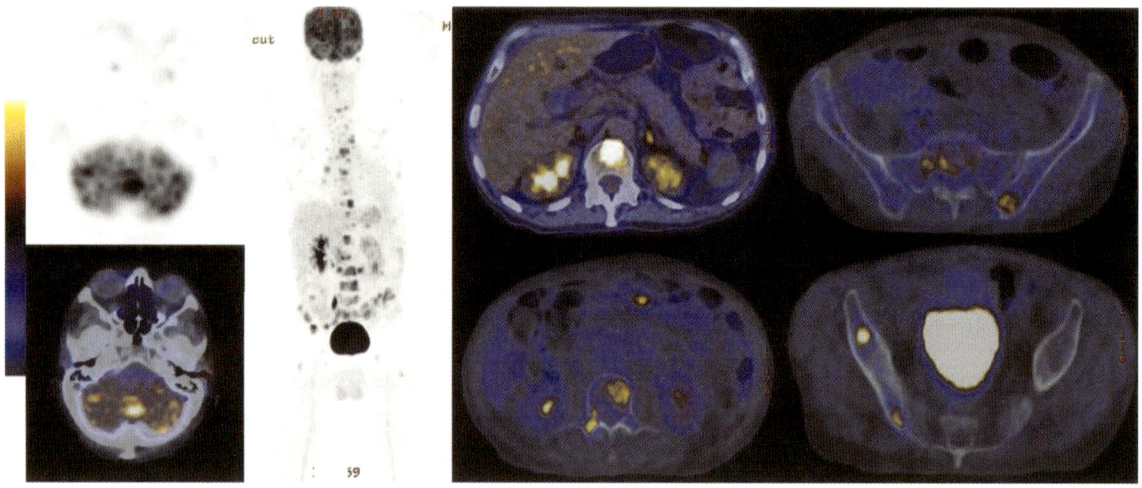

Figure 4: 18-Fluorodeoxyglucose positron emission tomography revealing a hypermetabolic lesion at the common bile duct/duodenum topography with cerebellar, thoracic-abdominal lymph nodes, left suprarenal gland, and bone metastasis.

biology, clinical presentation, and management. Extrahepatic cholangiocarcinoma is the second most common subtype (27–42%) with a mild male predominance. It can arise as mass-forming type, periductal infiltrating type, or intraductal growth type, usually with obstructive jaundice or associated complications, such as cholangitis and mass effect symptoms [1, 3]. CT and MRI present a high diagnostic accuracy (up to 93%). PET can be useful in cases of metastatic disease of unknown primary tumor [1]. ERCP provides additional diagnostic value in the assessment of strictures, cytological analysis, and stent-placement for biliary decompression [1]. Elevated CA 19-9 favors the diagnosis of cholangiocarcinoma, after other malignant, inflammatory, and infectious diseases of hepatobiliary-pancreatic system have been excluded [1]. A recent study that assessed the diagnostic and prognostic value of CA 19-9 and CEA in cholangiocarcinoma verified that more than 50% of patients with cholangiocarcinoma had normal CEA level and high CA 19-9 level (median of 103.0 U/L). This cut-off for CA 19-9 had prognostic value, being associated with a higher probability of metastasis and lower curative treatment rates [9].

In early stage of cholangiocarcinoma, Whipple surgery represents the main treatment. However, most patients present with advanced disease and therefore curative treatment is almost never feasible. Given the intrinsic resistance to radiation and chemotherapy, the prognosis remains dismal with a 5-year survival rate of 27–37% [1]. Thus, most patients only benefit from symptom-based supportive care.

Cholangiocarcinoma often spreads to the regional lymph nodes and adjacent organs. Distant metastasis is rare with bones, muscles, and thyroid gland being the most frequently involved sites. Brain metastasis is extremely rare with very few cases [3–7] and one case series reported in the literature that showed 0.15% of incidence [2]. Since brain imaging is not performed routinely, but only in the presence of symptoms related to space-occupying lesions (headache, motor weakness, gait disturbance, or altered mental status), the real prevalence of brain metastasis is not well established [2]. Furthermore, this tumor is poorly vascularized making hematogenous mechanism of spread unlikely. Regarding brain metastasis, the exclusive involvement of posterior fossa is also rare, reported only once [3, 7]. Usually, the distribution of brain metastases follows the relative weight of each area (80% in the cerebral hemispheres, 15% in the cerebellum, and 5% in the brainstem) [8]. The mechanism of cerebellar metastasis in cholangiocarcinoma is not yet known [3]. Published literature has only described that gastrointestinal tumors have an unknown predilection to metastasize to the posterior fossa, maybe related to spread via Batson's venous plexus [8].

Chindaprasirt et al. described the only existent case series of brain metastasis by cholangiocarcinoma. They showed that all eight cases were intrahepatic or perihilar tumors with the median age of 60 years. Diagnosis was based on neurologic symptoms in all patients, three of whom received WBRT and one underwent surgery. The median survival after diagnosis of brain metastasis was 9.5 weeks [2], being worse than other metastatic brain tumors [10, 11].

As far as we know, brain metastasis has never been reported in extrahepatic cholangiocarcinoma. In addition, this is the second reported case of initial neurologic symptoms and brain metastasis exclusively to the posterior fossa [3].

In conclusion, we report the case of an atypical presentation of extrahepatic cholangiocarcinoma with neurologic symptoms related to cerebellar metastasis, a rare site of spread. The prognosis was very poor, similar to other locations of cholangiocarcinoma. Therefore, clinicians should consider the possibility of brain spread in any type of cholangiocarcinoma, including extrahepatic location. Neurologic symptoms may precede hepatobiliary dysfunction.

Abbreviations

CEA: Carcinoembryonic antigen
CT: Computed tomography scan
MRI: Magnetic resonance imaging
ERCP: Endoscopic retrograde cholangiopancreatography
PET: Positron emission tomography scan
WBRT: Whole-brain radiotherapy.

Consent

Written informed consent was obtained for this case report publication.

Authors' Contributions

Elisa Gravito-Soares and Marta Gravito-Soares contributed equally to writing the manuscript and reviewing the literature. Elisa Gravito-Soares is the article guarantor. Pedro Figueiredo and Luis Tomé reviewed the manuscript.

References

[1] Y. Ghouri, I. Mian, and B. Blechacz, "Cancer review: Cholangiocarcinoma," *Journal of Carcinogenesis*, vol. 14, no. 1, 2015.

[2] J. Chindaprasirt, A. Sookprasert, K. Sawanyawisuth, P. Limpawattana, and S. Tiamkao, "Brain Metastases from Cholangiocarcinoma: a First Case Series in Thailand," *Asian Pacific Journal of Cancer Prevention*, vol. 13, no. 5, pp. 1995–1997, 2012.

[3] M. S. Gudesblatt, W. Sencer, M. Sacher, C. F. Lanzieri, and S. K. Song, "Cholangiocarcinoma presenting as a cerebellar metastasis: case report and review of the literature," *Journal of Computed Tomography*, vol. 8, no. 3, pp. 191–195, 1984.

[4] S. Shuangshotu, S. Rungruxsirivorn, and R. Panyathanya, "Intracranial metastasis of hepatic carcinomas: a study of 9 cases within 28 years," *Journal of the Medical Association of Thailand*, pp. 72–307, 1989.

[5] K. Mimatsu, T. Oida, A. Kawasaki et al., "Long-term survival after resection of mass-forming type intrahepatic cholangiocarcinoma directly infiltrating the transverse colon and sequential brain metastasis: report of a case," *Surgery Today*, vol. 41, no. 10, pp. 1410–1413, 2011.

[6] B. William and J. Grem, "Brain metastasis and leptomeningeal carcinomatosis in a patient with cholangiocarcinoma," *Gastrointest Cancer Research*, vol. 4, p. 144, 2011.

[7] A. E. Mirrakhimov, N. Nwankwo, T. Zdunek, and N. Bucher, "Cholangiocarcinoma and brain lesions: an extremely rare finding," *BMJ Case Reports*, vol. 2013, no. 1, pp. bcr2013009235–bcr2013009235, 2013.

[8] L. Nayak, E. Q. Lee, and P. Y. Wen, "Epidemiology of brain metastases," *Current Oncology Reports*, vol. 14, no. 1, pp. 48–54, 2012.

[9] R. Coelho, M. Silva, E. Rodrigues-Pinto et al., "CA 19-9 as a Marker of Survival and a Predictor of Metastization in Cholangiocarcinoma," *GE—Portuguese Journal of Gastroenterology*, vol. 24, no. 3, pp. 114–121, 2017.

[10] P. Sperduto, N. Kased, D. Roberge, Z. Xu, R. Shanley, and X. Luo, "Summary report on the graded prognostic assessment: an accurate and facile diagnosis-specific tool to estimate survival for patients with brain metastases," *Journal of Clinical Oncology*, pp. 30–419, 2012.

[11] T. K. Owonikoko, J. Arbiser, A. Zelnak et al., "Current approaches to the treatment of metastatic brain tumours," *Nature Reviews Clinical Oncology*, vol. 11, no. 4, pp. 203–222, 2014.

Hydrogen Peroxide Induced Colitis: A Case Report and Literature Review

Dushyant Pawar,[1] Anna Calara,[1] Roy Jacob,[2] Nancy Beck,[3] and Alan N. Peiris[4]

[1] *School of Medicine, Texas Tech University Health Sciences Center, Lubbock, TX, USA*
[2] *Department of Radiology, University Medical Center, Lubbock, TX, USA*
[3] *Department of Pediatrics, Texas Tech University Health Sciences Center, Lubbock, TX, USA*
[4] *Department of Internal Medicine, Texas Tech University Health Sciences Center, Lubbock, TX, USA*

Correspondence should be addressed to Dushyant Pawar; dushyant.s.pawar@ttuhsc.edu

Academic Editor: Tetsuo Hirata

Constipation is a common condition. Hydrogen peroxide enemas have rarely been reported as a home remedy for constipation in the pediatric age group. We present a case report and literature review of hydrogen peroxide induced colitis in pediatric siblings, aged 2 years and 9 years. The siblings presented with vomiting and bloody diarrhea an hour following the enema. Physical exam, vital signs, blood, and electrolyte counts were normal, but CT scans showed mucosal thickening of the rectum and colon. Their symptoms resolved after oral intake was curtailed and fluids were replaced intravenously. We discuss existing reports of complications from hydrogen peroxide enemas. Patients may present with abdominal pain and bloody diarrhea. Onset of symptoms varied from minutes to a day and bowel ulceration with necrosis and perforation has occurred, although fatality is rare. Diagnostic tests included computed tomography (CT) scan, sigmoidoscopy, or biopsy. Recovery period ranged from 3 days to 8 months. Public education regarding the dangers of hydrogen peroxide enemas is needed.

1. Introduction

Constipation is a common problem, reported in up to 30% of children. Home treatment for constipation includes eating foods high in fiber such as vegetables, citrus fruits, beans, and whole grains. A healthcare provider should be consulted before giving a laxative or enema to children. Internet searches for homemade remedies to treat constipation deliver hydrogen peroxide enema among the results. Hydrogen peroxide has been known to cause colitis and, in a few cases, bowel perforation. The earliest use of hydrogen peroxide enema in the pediatric population is documented by Olim and Ciuti to treat meconium ileus in the newborn [1].

Herein we present an unusual case of two siblings, aged 2 years and 9 years, presenting with bloody diarrhea and vomiting due to chemical colitis following hydrogen peroxide enema. We also present a systematic review of prior such cases. Few such cases have been reported in the pediatric population.

2. Case Presentation

Two siblings, a 2-year-old male and a 9-year-old female, had been constipated for 2 days. Patients did not have a family history of gastrointestinal issues and past medical history was unremarkable. The mother of the patients was providing both children with a regular but meat-free soy-based diet of her own volition. However, the children had rock-hard stools that could not be passed. Both patients were not given any prior conventional or homemade remedies. However, following an Internet search, both patients were then given an enema of hydrogen peroxide mixed with warm water. Concentration of hydrogen peroxide used is unknown. Following the enema, the patients passed stools but, an hour later, started vomiting and had bloody diarrhea.

Upon admission, vital signs were normal. Both patients had soft abdomens on exam, which were nontender to deep palpation, nondistended, and no guarding was noted. Physical exam did not raise concerns for perforations and the

Table 1

Author and year	Patient age	Presenting history	Complications	Iatrogenic	Concentration used	Symptom onset	Treatment/recovery period
Pumphrey (1951) [2]	50 years	Peptic ulcer. Constipation 6 d prior	Abdominal soreness, severe tenesmus, bloody mucus. Fever 103 F. Bowel mucosa covered with gray tenacious membrane, ulcerated, purulent exudate up to 24 cm from dentate line	Yes	2 : 1 hydrogen peroxide & water	Unknown	Granulation tissue cauterized with silver nitrate. Recovery: 8 m
Pumphrey (1951) [2]	76 years	Chronic constipation	Developed bloody mucus stools every 30–60 mins. Ulcerative proctosigmoiditis up to 24 cm	No (self)	Full strength hydrogen peroxide	30 mins	1 gm sulfasalazine qid, rectal instillations of warm oil, 1 teaspoon of psyllium seed oral bid. Recovery: 3 w
Olim and Ciuti (1954) [1]	2 days	Meconium ileus due to pancreatic cystic fibrosis	None: meconium evacuated	Yes	1 : 3 3% hydrogen peroxide & water, via enterotomy		
Ludington et al. (1958) [3]	62 years	Peptic ulcer	Abd pain, rebound tenderness, left lower quadrant mild rigidity, decreased sensation on right side. Fever 103 F 2 seromuscular tears along mesenteric borders of sigmoid and transverse colon	Yes	125 cc hydrogen peroxide in a liter of warm water, retained for 15 mins	Within hours	Laparotomy for seromuscular tears, gangrenous mucosa 4 cm dia. excised and repaired. Recovery: uneventful
Sheehan and Brynjolfsson (1960) [4]	41 years	Duodenal ulcer, constipation	Severe abd pain, rectal bleeding, vomiting, lost 500 ml of blood. Administered plasma. Died due to hemolytic reaction of unknown causes, followed by anuria, uremia, hemoglobinuric nephrosis	No	Unknown	Immediate	Plasma for blood loss. Died due to following complications
Meyer et al. (1981) [5]	22 years	Constipation	Small bloody bowel movements every half hour with tenesmus and lower abd pain. Friable necrotic mucosa to 15 cm. Rectal mucosa improved but erythematous post 5 d	No	10 ml 3% hydrogen peroxide + 30 ml water	30 mins	Parenteral fluids, antibiotics, and rectal steroids. Recovery: mucosa normal at 10 d, asymptomatic at 1 m
Meyer et al. (1981) [5]	47 years	Constipation	Lower abd cramps, tenesmus, rectal bleeding over 24 hours. Diffuse, granular, friable mucosa and discrete ulcerations w yellow/green pseudomembrane. Focal acute ulcerations with edema and congestion of lamina propria	No	Enema of methylene blue dye + 1 oz (29 ml) peroxide in 500 ml water	5 mins	100 units ACTH over 8 hrs and then 30 mg prednisone for 2 wks. Recovery: no bleeding at 3 d, normal mucosa at 21 d

Table 1: Continued.

Author and year	Patient age	Presenting history	Complications	Iatrogenic	Concentration used	Symptom onset	Treatment/recovery period
Meyer et al. (1981) [5]	28 years	Constipation	Onset of severe abd cramps, loose bloody bowel movements. Fever 102 F, BP 150/90, pulse 110, RR 14. Diffuse ulcerations at 10 cm; congestion and edema in lamina propria	No	Enema of 150 ml 3% hydrogen peroxide and 60 ml food coloring	Few minutes later	Parenteral ACTH 100 units for 5 days, prednisone 30 mg daily. Recovery: 7 d, asymptomatic at 5 w
Bollen et al. (1998) [6]	13 years	Chronic constipation after being sexually abused	Abd pain, rectal bleeding, no defecation. Hemorrhagic mucosal ulcerations from rectum to splenic angle. 48 hrs, sclerotic lamina propria. Mucosal glands focally destroyed, ischemia, microabscesses with polymorphonuclear leukocytes	Yes	1 : 1 water & 10% hydrogen peroxide	1 hr	No oral feeding for 48 hrs. Gradual complete recovery
Gan and Price (2003) [7]	67 years	Type 2 diabetes, prostate cancer	Profuse diarrhea, initially nonbloody. Later, bloody tenesmus, urgency, soft and nontender abdomen. Normal rectal examination, other than a diffusely hardened prostate. Friable, inflamed mucosa in rectum, several white patches in inflammation area extending to 15 cm. No fibrosis, scarring	No (self)	100 ml to 200 ml 3.5% hydrogen peroxide enema	24 hrs	Recovery: 10 d
Kirrane and Hoffman (2007) [8]	57 years	Abdominal pain, rectal bleeding, tachycardia	Lightheadedness, general weakness, abdominal pain. 12 hours later, multiple episodes of rectal bleeding. Tachycardia (heart rate 110 bpm). Distended abd, discomfort to palpation, no focal tenderness. Distended large bowel, thickened sigmoid colon consistent with colitis. No free air or gas embolization	No	30 ml 35% hydrogen peroxide + 750 ml water	Within minutes; bleeding post 12 hrs	Recovery: 3 d Treated with intravenous fluids and oral simethicone
Almalouf et al. (2008) [9]	19 years	2 week abdominal pain from chronic cholecystitis, constipation following hydrocodone administration	Post 1 hr, abd pain, rectal bleeding. Acute abd, friable mucosa, leukocytosis, free retroperitoneal air	Yes	Soap suds with hydrogen peroxide (500 ml, unknown conc)	1 hour	Ceftriaxone, metronidazole. NPO 3 d until white blood cell counts within normal range. Recovery: 7 d

Table 1: Continued.

Author and year	Patient age	Presenting history	Complications	Iatrogenic	Concentration used	Symptom onset	Treatment/recovery period
Desai and Orledge (2010) [10]	43 years	Left-sided abdominal pain, hematochezia	Hematochezia every 30 mins, bowel wall thickening from rectum to distal one-third of transverse colon	No	Commercial sodium phosphate/sodium biphosphate + hydrogen peroxide	Unknown	Recovery: 1 d
Kibria et al. (2010) [11]	61 years	Constipation unresponsive to milk of magnesia	Abd pain, bloody stools 1 hr later. Left lower quadrant tenderness. Rectosigmoid wall thickening, inflammation Friable mucosa, discrete ulcerations & yellow/green pseudomembranes up to 40 cm from anus. Focal acute ulcerations, congestion of lamina propria	Yes	Enema with 90 ml each of hydrogen peroxide, sodium phosphate, and docusate sodium	1 hr	Parenteral fluids, levofloxacin, and metronidazole. Recovery: 3 m
Volonte et al. (2010) [12]	31 years	Severe constipation following spinal trauma. 4000 ml/wk glycerol enema for defecation	Severe abdominal pain soon after enema. 3 hr later CT showed extensive gas in portal vein. Resolved 48 hr later	Yes	700 cc hypertonic solution of 5% glycerin and 300 cc of 3% hydrogen peroxide solution	Within hours	Recovery: 3 h
Lim et al. (2011) [13]	49 years	Abdominal pain	Lower abdominal pain with bloody stools	No	Unknown	2 hours	NPO, IV fluids, antibiotics. Recovery: 5 d
Love et al. (2012) [14]	59 years	Hypertension, coronary artery disease, diabetes, chronic kidney disease, constipation	Rectal bleeding, fecal incontinence over 12 hrs. Soft abd with diffuse tenderness on left lateral side. Rectal exam, presacral thickening, diminished anal tone. Colitis extending to 35 cm, edema & hemorrhage in lamina propria with "bubbly" appearance of goblet cells	No	120 ml hydrogen peroxide (1 : 1 3% hydrogen peroxide & water)	Minutes after	Antibiotic and mesalamine enema. Recovery: 2 d
Taş et al. (2011) [15]	27 years	Constipation over 2 yrs	Post 2 hrs, abd pain, bloody diarrhea. Mild lower quadrant abd tenderness, painful digital rectal exam. Friable, granular ulcerated rectal mucosa. Rectal histopath exam, mucosal congestion, hemorrhage, necrosis, lymphatic ductal ectasia	No	200 ml 3% hydrogen peroxide	2 hours	Enema with budesonide (2 mg). Recovery: 3 d

patients denied abdominal pain. Complete blood count and metabolic panel for both patients were within normal limits.

Abdominal CT for the patient of age 2 years showed mucosal thickening of the rectum and sigmoid colon with no free air. The patient aged 9 years had a more extensive mucosal thickening of the rectum, sigmoid, and descending colon but showed no perforation or free fluid. Both patients were admitted to the pediatric intensive care unit, had their oral intake withheld, and were given IV fluids. They showed clinical improvement the same day and were then transferred to the pediatric ward. Both patients were discharged 24 hours later with resolution of emesis and bloody stool. They were prescribed polyethylene glycol laxative, 17 grams, daily for constipation.

3. Discussion

We found 21 published cases related to hydrogen peroxide enema. Prior cases show the patient population as mostly older adults with constipation from secondary causes. To our knowledge, this is the first case of colitis due to hydrogen peroxide enema in siblings in the pediatric age group. The most recent case report was published in 2016 [16]. Cases related to oral ingestion of hydrogen peroxide as well as those associated with contamination during endoscopic examinations were excluded.

In 11 of the 21 cases, enema was self-administered; in the rest, enema was administered under physician supervision. The enema was administered to treat constipation, except for one case where the patient used it to treat prostate cancer. The enema concentrations varied and are listed in Table 1. Following the enema, patients were able to relieve their constipation but then presented with symptoms of abdominal pain/tenderness, bloody diarrhea, fever, tenesmus, leukocytosis, and/or tachycardia [17]. Endoscopy findings included mucosal friability, exudates, ulceration, necrosis, and/or perforation of the distal colon or rectum (Table 1) [17]. The onset of bloody diarrhea after administration of hydrogen peroxide enema varied from a few minutes to an entire day following the enema. Diagnostic tests varied with some combination of CT scan (4 cases), sigmoidoscopy (11 cases), or biopsy (4 cases). In our case, diagnosis was made solely using abdominal CT scan and patient history, without relying on additional sigmoidoscopy and biopsy findings because the temporal relationship of presenting symptoms following the enema favored the diagnosis of hydrogen peroxide induced colitis.

Recovery period ranged from 3 days to 8 months, with mostly uneventful gradual recovery. Recommended treatment included bowel rest, fluid resuscitation, and broad spectrum antibiotics, NSAIDs, or corticosteroids [17]. Depending on the extent of injury, most patients recovered after conservative medical therapy. However, serious consequences included death due to idiopathic hemolytic reaction following plasma transfusion to correct blood loss [4], portal vein embolism [12], and colonic rupture [3]. A summary comparing and contrasting diagnostic tests findings, medications prescribed, and complications of hydrogen peroxide induced colitis are documented in Table 1.

Hydrogen peroxide is available over the counter in concentrations of 3% and a "food grade" variety of 35%. Although it has a warning label stating "For external use only," a study by the National Survey of Consumers and Health Professionals found that only 7% of consumers read usage warnings. Hence, public education on the dangers of hydrogen peroxide enema may be needed. It may be effective since patients tend to follow the advice of a competent physician over information obtained from the Internet [18]. Hydrogen peroxide has also been used for other indications like enlarged prostate and cancer of prostate [7]. Therefore, patients with unexplained colitis or proctitis may be queried about use of hydrogen peroxide enema.

Finally, the siblings followed a meat-free soy-based diet, and although soy protein has been known to be an allergen, we did not find an association between soy protein and constipation.

Acknowledgments

The authors wish to acknowledge the contribution of the Texas Tech University Health Sciences Center Clinical Research Institute for their assistance with this research. Funding for article processing charges is provided by Texas Tech University Health Sciences Center Department of Internal Medicine.

References

[1] C. B. Olim and A. Ciuti, "Meconium ileus: a new method of relieving obstruction; report of two cases with successful management," *Annals of Surgery*, vol. 140, no. 5, pp. 736–740, 1954.

[2] R. E. Pumphrey, "Hydrogen peroxide proctitis," *The American Journal of Surgery*, vol. 81, no. 1, pp. 60–62, 1951.

[3] L. G. Ludington, S. W. Hartman, J. E. Keplinger, and F. S. Williams, "Incomplete Rupture of the Colon Following Hydrogen Peroxide Enema," *A.M.A Archives of Surgery*, vol. 76, no. 4, pp. 658–660, 1958.

[4] J. F. Sheehan and G. Brynjolfsson, "Ulcerative colitis following hydrogen peroxide enema: case report and experimental production with transient emphysema of colonic wall and gas embolism," *Laboratory Investigation; A Journal of Technical Methods And Pathology*, vol. 9, pp. 150–168, 1960.

[5] C. T. Meyer, M. Brand, V. A. DeLuca, and H. M. Spiro, "Hydrogen peroxide colitis: A report of lhree patients," *Journal of Clinical Gastroenterology*, vol. 3, no. 1, pp. 31–35, 1981.

[6] P. Bollen, A. Goossens, B. Hauser, and Y. Vandenplas, "Colonic ulcerations caused by an enema containing hydrogen peroxide," *Journal of Pediatric Gastroenterology and Nutrition*, vol. 26, no. 2, pp. 232-233, 1998.

[7] S. I. Gan and L. M. Price, "Waiting-list induced proctitis: The hydrogen peroxide enema," *Canadian Journal of Gastroenterology & Hepatology*, vol. 17, no. 12, pp. 727–729, 2003.

[8] B. M. Kirrane and R. S. Hoffman, "Abdominal pain and rectal bleeding after an enema," *Clinical Toxicology*, vol. 45, no. 8, p. 968, 2007.

[9] P. Almalouf, T. M. Shehab, A. M. R. Daniel, E. A. Robinson, and J. L. Barnett, "Therapeutic hydrogen peroxide enema causing severe acute colitis," *International Journal of Colorectal Disease*, vol. 23, no. 11, pp. 1139-1140, 2008.

[10] Y. Desai and J. Orledge, "Chemical colitis from a hydrogen peroxide enema.," *Journal of the Mississippi State Medical Association*, vol. 51, no. 11, pp. 314–316, 2010.

[11] R. Kibria, S. A. Ali, and C. J. Barde, "Gone but not forgotten. "bubble gum enema" containing hydrogen peroxide and causing life-threatening colitis," *Gastrointestinal Endoscopy*, vol. 72, no. 3, pp. 619-620, 2010.

[12] F. Volonte, P. Gervaz, P.-A. Poletti, and P. Morel, "Portal vein gas embolism following oxygen peroxide enema," *Colorectal Disease*, vol. 12, no. 10, pp. e335–e336, 2010.

[13] C. H. Lim, H. Y. Lee, W. C. Kim et al., "A case of chemical colitis caused by hydrogen peroxide enema," *The Korean Journal of Gastroenterology*, vol. 58, no. 2, p. 100, 2011.

[14] B. L. Love, D. Pharm, S. Siddiqui, B. J. Mccallum, and R. M. Helman, "Severe chemical colitis due to hydrogen peroxide enema," *Journal of Clinical Gastroenterology*, vol. 46, no. 1, p. 87, 2012.

[15] A. Taş, Y. Y. Aydin, M. Arhan, and S. Köklü, "Hydrogen peroxide exposure mimicking ulcerative proctitis," *Digestive and Liver Disease*, vol. 43, no. 4, pp. 331-332, 2011.

[16] J. S. Lee and J. K. Yoo, "Chemical colitis caused by hydrogen peroxide enema in a child: case report and literature review," *Journal of Toxicology and Environmental Health*, vol. 32, Article ID e2017002, 2016.

[17] S. Sheibani and L. B. Gerson, "Chemical colitis," *Journal of Clinical Gastroenterology*, vol. 42, no. 2, pp. 115–121, 2008.

[18] J. Laugesen, K. Hassanein, and Y. Yuan, "The impact of internet health information on patient compliance: a research model and an empirical study," *Journal of Medical Internet Research*, vol. 17, no. 6, article e143, 2015.

47

A Mysterious DRESS Case: Autoimmune Enteropathy Associated with DRESS Syndrome

Abimbola Adike,[1] Vaishnavi Boppana,[1] Dora Lam-Himlin,[2] Melissa Stanton,[2] Steven Nelson,[2] and Kevin C. Ruff[1]

[1] *Division of Gastroenterology and Hepatology, Mayo Clinic, Scottsdale, AZ, USA*
[2] *Department of Laboratory Medicine and Pathology, Mayo Clinic, Scottsdale, AZ, USA*

Correspondence should be addressed to Abimbola Adike; adike.abimbola@mayo.edu

Academic Editor: Hirotada Akiho

Drug Reaction with Eosinophilia and Systemic Symptoms (DRESS) is a rare but potentially life-threatening cutaneous hypersensitivity reaction characterized by extensive mucocutaneous eruption, fever, hematologic abnormalities, and extensive organ involvement. Here, we present a case of a young woman with DRESS syndrome following exposure to vancomycin with renal, cutaneous, and gastrointestinal involvement. To the best of our knowledge, this is the first case description in the literature of DRESS of the gastrointestinal tract with autoimmune enteropathy.

1. Introduction

Drug Reaction with Eosinophilia and Systemic Symptoms (DRESS) is an uncommon, potentially life-threatening adverse drug reaction. It is also known as drug-induced hypersensitivity reaction, drug-induced delayed multiorgan hypersensitivity syndrome, or drug rash with eosinophilia and systemic symptoms and was previously described in earlier literature as drug-induced pseudolymphoma [1] or anticonvulsant hypersensitivity syndrome as anticonvulsants are the most frequently implicated drugs. Many other drugs including allopurinol, sulfonamides, minocycline, olanzapine, vancomycin, and dapsone have been reported as causative drugs in DRESS [2, 3].

Cases of DRESS can be described as definite, probable, or possible, using the European Registry of Severe Cutaneous Adverse Reaction (RegiSCAR) scoring system which includes clinical features, organ involvement, and disease duration [4]. The most common organ involvement in DRESS is the liver and kidneys, but many other organs can also be involved including the gastrointestinal tract [4].

Case reports represent a major source of information on DRESS in the literature [4]. However, there is a relative paucity of reports on the gastrointestinal manifestations of DRESS. Our case report is the first to describe an evolvement of DRESS to autoimmune enterocolopathy.

2. Case Report

A 29-year-old woman with a history severe symptomatic pectus excavatum underwent a repair. She otherwise had no significant past medical history. The surgery was complicated by a *Staphylococcus caprae* right chest pocket infection which was treated with vancomycin. Three weeks following initiation of vancomycin, the patient presented with a diffuse, eruptive, exfoliative, and nonpruritic whole body rash with nonerosive mucositis. She also reported large volume, nonbloody, postprandial diarrhea with up to 4 to 5 loose stools a day. On presentation, the patient was found to have a temperature of 102 F and was hemodynamically stable.

Laboratory values showed white blood cell count 34.5×10^9 with 22% eosinophilia, hemoglobin 8.1 g/dl, creatinine of 2 mg/dl from a prior baseline of 0.7 mg/dl, and bicarbonate 16 mmol/L with a normal anion gap. Blood cultures, acute hepatitis panel, and a stool lactoferrin were negative, as was a complete panel of enteric infectious stool studies including bacterial, viral, and parasitic pathogens. Cytomegalovirus (CMV) DNA checked at weeks 1 and 3 following onset of

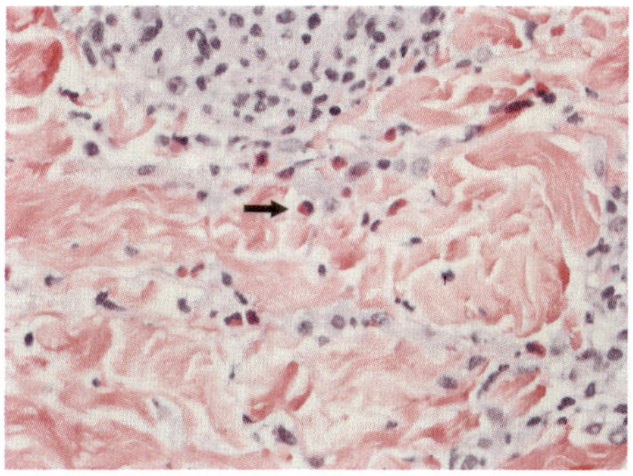

Figure 1: Skin biopsy demonstrating a perivascular and interstitial lymphohistiocytic infiltrate with numerous eosinophils (arrow). Hematoxylin-eosin stain, 400x.

diarrhea was undetectable and at week 4, CMV DNA was 13, 300 IU/mL. At week one following onset of diarrhea, the following viruses were also tested: human herpes virus 6 (HHV) DNA was positive, and Epstein Barr virus (EBV) DNA was <2000 IU/mL. Gastrin was 100 pg/ml. 24-hour urine 5-hydroxyindoleacetic acid and vasointestinal peptide were normal. Stool alpha-1-antitrypsin was normal. Celiac gene testing was positive for DQ8. Tissue transglutaminase A IgA level was <1.2 U/ml with an IgA of 292 mg/dl. A skin biopsy of the right upper extremity (Figure 1) showed prominent papillary dermal edema with spongiosis and a dense lymphohistiocytic infiltrate with eosinophils which were felt to be consistent with a drug reaction. Computed tomography of the abdomen with oral contrast showed diffuse mesenteric edema without obstruction.

Upper endoscopy showed a normal appearing esophagus and stomach with localized mildly scalloped mucosa in the 2nd portion of the duodenum (Figure 2). Colonoscopy showed granularity in the left colon and a white thin exudate in the entire examined colon (Figure 2). The terminal ileum was normal. Histopathological evaluation of the gastrointestinal tract revealed loss of parietal cells, mild glandular disarray, acute inflammation, and apoptotic activity in the stomach (Figure 3, hematoxylin and eosin, original magnification 200x) and patchy villous atrophy and absence of goblet cells and Paneth cells in the duodenum with crypt abscesses and apoptosis (Figure 3, hematoxylin and eosin, original magnification 200x); and in the terminal ileum, as in the duodenum, there was also an absence of goblet and Paneth cells, with crypt dropout (Figure 3, hematoxylin and eosin, original magnification 200x). Colon biopsies showed cryptitis and crypt abscess with minimal crypt distortion. Although the surface epithelium appeared attenuated, the deeper crypts had goblet cells present (Figure 3, hematoxylin and eosin, original magnification 200x). CMV immunohistochemical stains performed on upper and lower GI biopsies were negative.

The patient subsequently developed severe protein-calorie malnutrition requiring total parenteral nutrition. Vancomycin was felt to be the etiology of the drug reaction with peripheral eosinophilia and systemic symptoms (DRESS) with gastrointestinal, cutaneous, and renal involvement. Vancomycin was discontinued immediately on suspicion that this was a case of DRESS syndrome. The diarrhea responded to high dose intravenous steroids at 2 mg/kg. She was also treated with ganciclovir for CMV viremia.

At followup two months later, the patient was weaned off parenteral nutrition and intravenous corticosteroids, now at an oral dose of 1 mg/kg, and tolerating a regular diet with complete resolution of diarrhea. Repeat upper and lower endoscopy revealed duodenal mucosa was endoscopically normal. Histopathological evaluation overall (Figure 4) revealed less acute inflammation and fewer architectural changes when compared to her prior biopsies but was suggestive of an evolving autoimmune enterocolopathy with villous blunting of the duodenum and absence of goblet and Paneth cells in the colon. Anti-enterocyte IgA and IgG showed linear periapical staining of enterocytes consistent with the presence of anti-enterocyte antibodies.

3. Discussion

First coined in 1996, DRESS is a life-threatening adverse drug reaction [1, 2]. DRESS typically presents with fever, rash, lymphadenopathy, eosinophilia, and multiorgan involvement. It has a period of latency of about two to eight weeks from drug exposure [3], with one prospective series reporting a median time interval after drug exposure of 22 days [4]. DRESS typically has a relatively later onset of presentation than other drug eruptions [4]. Our patient presented three weeks after drug exposure to vancomycin with fever, a morbilliform exfoliative rash involving more than 50% of her total body surface area, and peripheral eosinophilia, with acute kidney injury and large volume nonbloody diarrhea. After exclusion of other potential causes including hepatitis, it was felt that this was a definite case of DRESS syndrome from vancomycin exposure, with a RegiSCAR score of 6 (fever, peripheral eosinophilia, skin rash involving more than 50% of the total body surface area, multiorgan involvement, and disease duration of more than 15 days) [4]. In recent years, there has been an increase in the number of DRESS attributed to vancomycin [5]. Despite prompt withdrawal of the culprit drug, DRESS can have a relapsing-remitting course [6]. Retrospective studies have reported a mortality rate of 5–10% [7].

The pathogenesis of DRESS is not well understood. Drug specific activation of T-cells and herpesvirus reactivation has been suggested to be the pathogenesis of DRESS with expansion of regulatory T-cells leading to virus reactivation [3]. It is also possible that antiviral T-cells cross react with the culprit drug [3]. HHV 6, CMV, EBV, and other herpesviruses have been implicated in the pathogenesis of DRESS. The presence of HHV 6 has been said to predict a relapsing course of DRESS with worse prognosis [8, 9].

In addition to a positive HHV 6, our patient had florid CMV viremia which was treated with antiviral therapy. CMV viremia was the unlikely culprit of our patient's symptoms for the following reasons: (1) initial CMV DNA was tested twice and were undetectable at the onset of symptoms. (2) CMV immunohistochemical stains on all upper/lower GI

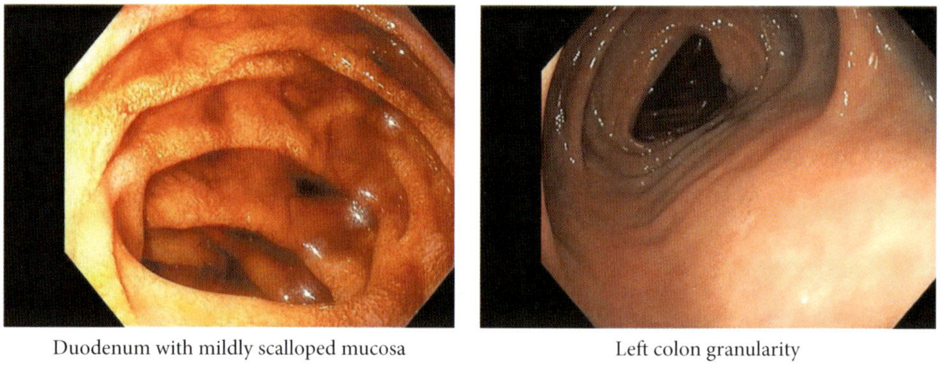

FIGURE 2: Localized mildly scalloped mucosa in the 2nd portion of the duodenum and granularity in the left colon.

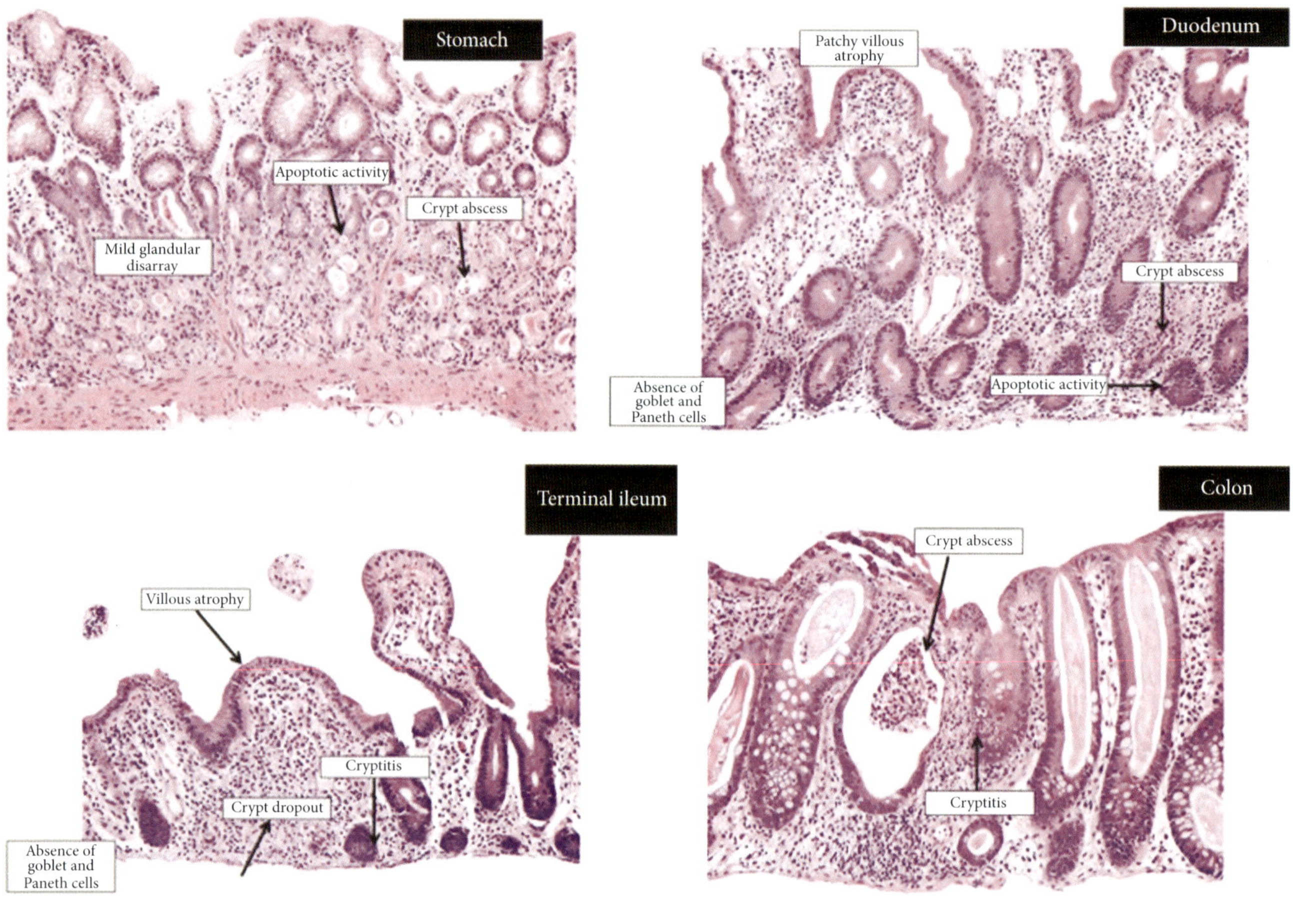

FIGURE 3: Biopsies of the stomach show loss of parietal cells, mild glandular disarray, acute inflammation, and apoptotic activity (hematoxylin and eosin, original magnification 200x); biopsies of the duodenum show absence of goblet cells and Paneth cells (hematoxylin and eosin, original magnification 200x); biopsies of the terminal ileum are similar to the duodenum. There is an absence of goblet cells and Paneth cells. This field shows crypt dropout as well (hematoxylin and eosin, original magnification 200x); biopsies of the colon show cryptitis and crypt abscess with minimal crypt distortion.

biopsies were negative prior to treatment of CMV viremia. (3) The histopathological features of her upper/lower GI biopsies were not felt to be consistent with CMV enteritis or colitis. (4) The patient's skin biopsies were consistent with a lymphohistiocytic infiltrate with eosinophils which were felt to be consistent with a drug reaction, and not related to a viral infection. For these reasons, we believe that viral reactivation eventually occurred during the course of illness in this patient and was not solely responsible for her constellation of symptoms. Antiviral agents are not routinely used to treat DRESS in the absence of evidence for viral reactivation [8].

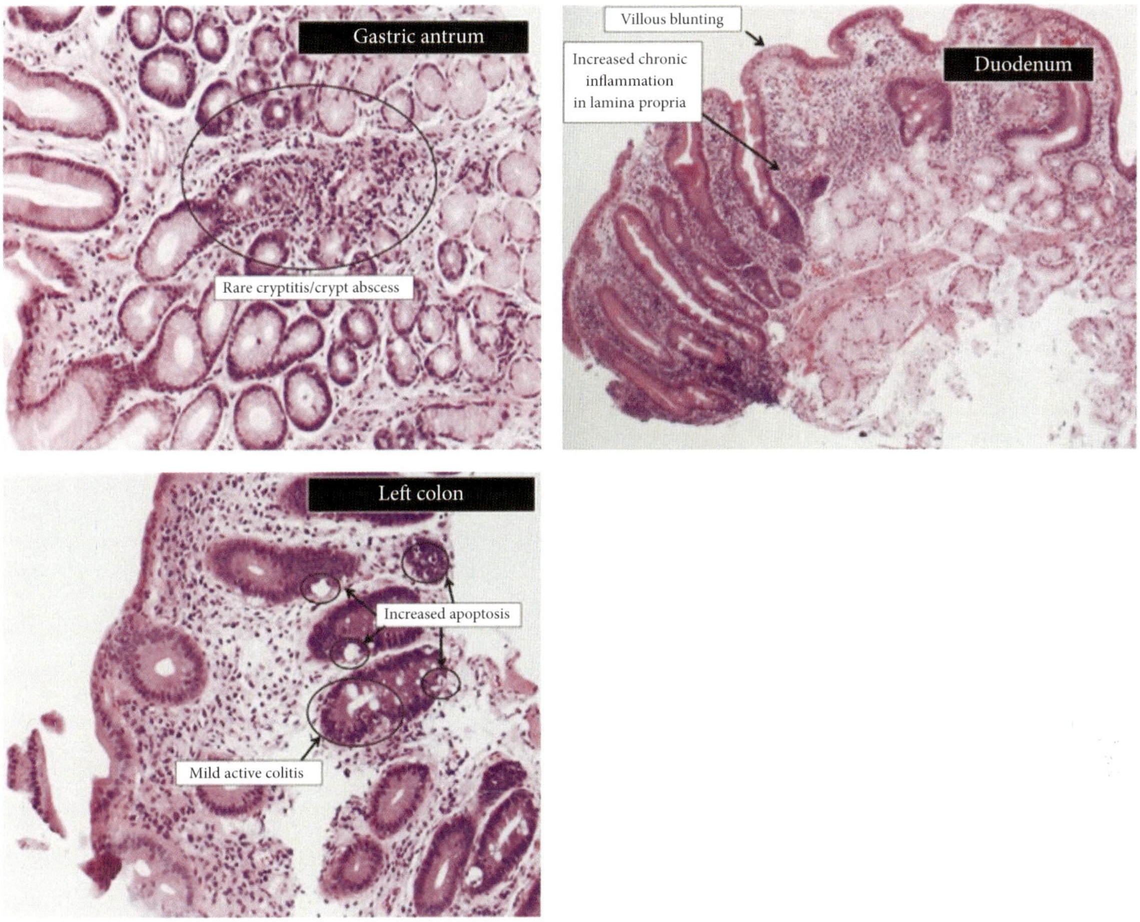

FIGURE 4: Overall acute inflammation and fewer architectural changes than that reported in this patient's prior biopsy. The gastric biopsies show increased lamina propria chronic inflammation with only rare crypts with cryptitis and crypt abscesses. Oxyntic glands are in abundance in the gastric body biopsies; The duodenum shows both goblet cells and Paneth cells and mild villous blunting, in contrast to the marked changes seen previously; The colon shows patchy active colitis, increased apoptosis, and marked loss of goblet cells.

Clinical manifestations of DRESS involving the GI tract can include nausea, vomiting, bloody, and nonbloody diarrhea [2]. Histopathological gastrointestinal manifestations of DRESS can range from active colitis with cryptitis, erosion, and ulceration, to eosinophilic infiltrate in the lamina propria, to chronic inflammation with architectural distortion [2]. Prompt withdrawal of the offending drug is the most critical part of management of DRESS [10]. Systemic steroids (0.5 mg/kg to 2 mg/kg) with supportive management are the mainstay of therapy in these patients with a gradual slow taper over a period of 3–6 months while monitoring clinical and laboratory data [10].

While most patients will have complete recovery from DRESS after withdrawal of the offending agent [10], long-term sequelae of DRESS have been reported [11]. In particular, autoimmune diseases have been reported in retrospective cohort studies, including Grave's disease, autoimmune hemolytic anemia, lupus, alopecia areata, and type one diabetes [11–13]. DRESS has also been associated with hemophagocytic lymphohistiocytosis (HLH) [2, 14]. Previously, Swanson et al. reported a fatal case report of a young woman who developed DRESS from antiepileptic drugs with subsequent HLH diagnosed about 5 months after her initial presentation; with endoscopy biopsies that revealed marked villous atrophy in the duodenum with absence of goblet and Paneth cells in the duodenum and colon [2]. Like this patient, our patient also had no eosinophils on initial or subsequent gastrointestinal biopsies. However, her histopathological evaluation of the small bowel showed villous atrophy, apoptotic bodies, and complete absence of goblet and Paneth cells; biopsies of the stomach showed an unusual pattern of injury with chronic inflammation, glandular abscesses, and parietal cell atrophy while in the colon, there was increased apoptosis and marked loss of goblet cells and Paneth cells. Taken together, these histopathological features are reminiscent of autoimmune enterocolopathy [15]. Autoimmune enteropathy is characterized by refractory diarrhea with malabsorption, histologic changes on small intestinal biopsy, and the need for immunosuppressive treatment [15]. The diagnostic criteria for autoimmune enteropathy include chronic diarrhea, malabsorption, small bowel villi blunting, deep crypt lymphocytosis, and increased apoptotic bodies with minimal intraepithelial lymphocytosis and exclusion of other causes of villous atrophy. Our patient met all of these criteria. Although our patient also had a positive anti-enterocyte antibody, anti-enterocyte or anti-goblet cell antibodies are supportive but are not necessarily diagnostic of autoimmune enteropathy [16]. Treatment includes budesonide, prednisone, and other immunosuppressants such as 6-mercaptopurine, azathioprine, mycophenolate mofetil, or cyclosporine [15]. There is very limited data on prognosis of autoimmune enteropathy [15]. To the best of our knowledge, this is the first case report in the literature that describes an evolving autoimmune enterocolopathy from DRESS syndrome.

In conclusion, DRESS is a poorly understood systemic drug eruption which can have significant mortality. While most patients completely recover from DRESS syndrome, a few patients can develop autoimmune diseases. This is the first case report described in the literature of autoimmune enterocolopathy associated with DRESS syndrome.

References

[1] H. Bocquet, M. Bagot, and J. C. Roujeau, "Drug-induced pseudolymphoma and drug hypersensitivity syndrome (Drug Rash with Eosinophilia and Systemic Symptoms: DRESS)," *Seminars in Cutaneous Medicine and Surgery*, vol. 15, no. 4, pp. 250–257, 1996.

[2] E. A. Swanson, L. Low, and B. V. Naini, "Severe enterocolitis associated with antiepileptic-induced drug reaction with eosinophilia and systemic symptoms," *Human Pathology*, vol. 45, no. 9, pp. 1973–1977, 2014.

[3] T. Shiohara, M. Inaoka, and Y. Kano, "Drug-induced hypersensitivity syndrome (DIHS): a reaction induced by a complex interplay among herpesviruses and antiviral and antidrug immune responses," *Allergology International*, vol. 55, no. 1, pp. 1–8, 2006.

[4] S. H. Kardaun, P. Sekula, L. Valeyrie-Allanore et al., "Drug reaction with eosinophilia and systemic symptoms (DRESS): an original multisystem adverse drug reaction. Results from the prospective RegiSCAR study," *British Journal of Dermatology*, vol. 169, no. 5, pp. 1071–1080, 2013.

[5] K. G. Blumenthal, S. U. Patil, and A. A. Long, "The importance of vancomycin in drug rash with eosinophilia and systemic symptoms (dress) syndrome," *Allergy and Asthma Proceedings*, vol. 33, no. 2, pp. 165–171, 2012.

[6] S. L. Fernando, "Drug-reaction eosinophilia and systemic symptoms and drug-induced hypersensitivity syndrome," *Australasian Journal of Dermatology*, vol. 55, no. 1, pp. 15–23, 2014.

[7] P. Cacoub, P. Musette, V. Descamps et al., "The DRESS syndrome: a literature review," *American Journal of Medicine*, vol. 124, no. 7, pp. 588–597, 2011.

[8] M. Eshki, L. Allanore, P. Musette et al., "Twelve-year analysis of severe cases of drug reaction with eosinophilia and systemic symptoms: a cause of unpredictable multiorgan failure," *JAMA Dermatology*, vol. 145, no. 1, pp. 67–72, 2009.

[9] M. Tohyama, K. Hashimoto, M. Yasukawa et al., "Association of human herpesvirus 6 reactivation with the flaring and severity of drug-induced hypersensitivity syndrome," *British Journal of Dermatology*, vol. 157, no. 5, pp. 934–940, 2007.

[10] Z. Husain, B. Y. Reddy, and R. A. Schwartz, "DRESS syndrome: Part II. Management and therapeutics," *Journal of the American Academy of Dermatology*, vol. 68, no. 5, pp. 709.e1–709.e9, 2013.

[11] Y. Kano, M. Tohyama, M. Aihara et al., "Sequelae in 145 patients with drug-induced hypersensitivity syndrome/drug reaction with eosinophilia and systemic symptoms: survey conducted by the Asian Research Committee on Severe Cutaneous Adverse Reactions (ASCAR)," *Journal of Dermatology*, vol. 42, no. 3, pp. 276–282, Mar 2015.

[12] Y.-C. Chen, C.-Y. Chang, Y.-T. Cho, H.-C. Chiu, and C.-Y. Chu, "Long-term sequelae of drug reaction with eosinophilia and systemic symptoms: a retrospective cohort study from Taiwan," *Journal of the American Academy of Dermatology*, vol. 68, no. 3, pp. 459–465, 2013.

[13] Y. Ushigome, Y. Kano, T. Ishida, K. Hirahara, and T. Shiohara, "Short- and long-term outcomes of 34 patients with drug-induced hypersensitivity syndrome in a single institution," *Journal of the American Academy of Dermatology*, vol. 68, no. 5, pp. 721–728, 2013.

[14] Y.-C. Yang, S.-T. Jou, Y.-H. Chang, J.-S. Liang, and W.-T. Lee, "Hemophagocytic syndrome associated with antiepileptic drug," *Pediatric Neurology*, vol. 30, no. 5, pp. 358–360, 2004.

[15] N. M. Gentile, J. A. Murray, and D. S. Pardi, "Autoimmune enteropathy: a review and update of clinical management," *Current Gastroenterology Reports*, vol. 14, no. 5, pp. 380–385, 2012.

[16] S. Akram, J. A. Murray, D. S. Pardi et al., "Adult autoimmune enteropathy: Mayo Clinic Rochester experience," *Clinical Gastroenterology Hepatology*, vol. 5, pp. 1282–1290, 2007, A relatively large experience with adult AIE.

48

Metastatic Renal Cell Cancer to Thyroid Diagnosed by Endoscopic Ultrasound Guided Fine Needle Aspiration Technique

Yousef Abdel-Aziz,[1] Tariq Hammad,[1] Mohamad Nawras,[1] Hayder Abdulwahid,[2] and Ali Nawras[1]

[1]*Department of Internal Medicine, Division of Gastroenterology, University of Toledo Medical Center, Toledo, OH, USA*
[2]*Department of Pathology, University of Toledo Medical Center, Toledo, OH, USA*

Correspondence should be addressed to Yousef Abdel-Aziz; yousefabdelaziz88@hotmail.com

Academic Editor: Jiro Watari

Medical literature about the role of endoscopic ultrasound (EUS) in identifying thyroid lesions is limited. We present a case of secondary thyroid cancer from renal cell carcinoma (RCC) metastasis, diagnosed by thyroid EUS-fine needle aspiration (FNA) approach that was done for staging of esophageal adenocarcinoma, in a patient with 11-year history of complete right nephrectomy for RCC. An 81-year-old female patient underwent EUS for the evaluation of a newly discovered distal esophageal cancer. A hypoechoic, round, and well-demarcated mass that measured 26.9 mm × 21.9 mm was noticed in the right lobe thyroid gland. Therefore FNA was performed. The cytological results were consistent with metastatic RCC. In conclusion, EUS-FNA of thyroid nodule is a feasible and safe technique that can be used to evaluate any suspicious thyroid nodule. This case emphasizes the importance of carefully examining the thyroid gland during routine upper esophageal EUS examinations in the presence of history of nonthyroidal cancer.

1. Introduction

Medical literature about the role of endoscopic ultrasound (EUS) in identifying thyroid lesions is limited. We present a case of secondary thyroid cancer from renal cell carcinoma (RCC) metastasis, diagnosed by thyroid EUS-fine needle aspiration (FNA) approach that was done for staging of esophageal adenocarcinoma, in a patient with 11-year history of complete right nephrectomy for RCC.

2. Case Presentation and Technique

An 81-year-old female patient presented to our facility with dysphagia to both solids and liquids. For the evaluation of her dysphagia, she underwent esophagogastroduodenoscopy (EGD). Initially, EGD examination of the esophagus revealed a distal esophageal mass of 5 cm in length extending 2 cm inside the gastric cardia, that was biopsied, and the histopathologic results revealed esophageal adenocarcinoma. For staging, the patient underwent computed tomography (CT) of the chest, which showed the lower esophageal mass with mediastinal lymphadenopathy. Next, the patient underwent upper gastrointestinal (GI) EUS for assessment of the esophageal adenocarcinoma and the mediastinal lymph nodes. The endosonographic examination of the esophageal mass was performed with the scope being positioned at the proximal border of the mass. The mass was hypoechoic and heterogeneous and involved three-quarters of the circumference of the esophageal lumen, involving all esophageal wall layers to the adventitia. The EUS-FNA examination of the mediastinal lymph nodes revealed no lymphatic spread. A diagnosis of esophageal adenocarcinoma with stage of T3N0M0 was made. Upon withdrawing the EUS scope, examination of the thyroid revealed hypoechoic, round, and well-demarcated mass that measured 26.9 mm × 21.9 mm in the right lobe (Figure 1(a)). The radial echoendoscope was

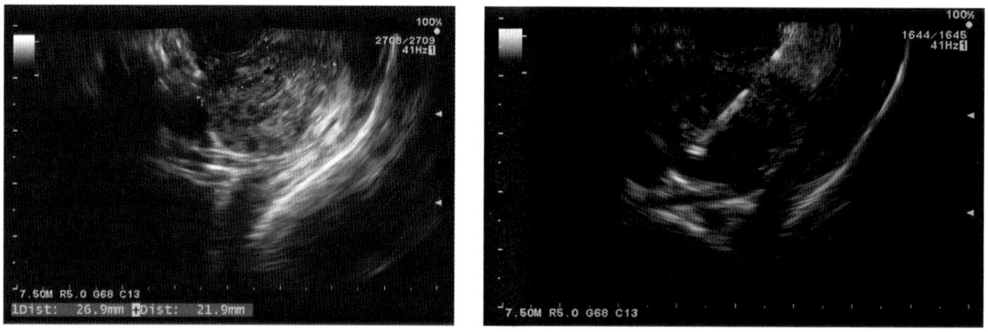

(a) (b)

Figure 1: (a) EUS examination of the thyroid revealed a hypoechoic, round, and well-demarcated mass that measured 26.9 mm × 21.9 mm in the right lobe. (b) Under echoendosonographic guidance, FNA with a 25-gauge needle (Expect EUS-FNA 25 G needle; Boston Scientific, Menomonie, WI, USA) was performed successfully.

then withdrawn and the Olympus video curvilinear array echoendoscope was advanced through the mouth into the proximal esophagus. Color Doppler US with a linear-array echoendoscope revealed no vascular flow within or vascular invasion by the nodule. Under echoendosonographic guidance, 2 passes of FNA with a 25-gauge needle (Expect EUS-FNA 25 G needle; Boston Scientific, Menomonie, WI, USA) were performed successfully close to the upper esophageal sphincter on the right side without adverse events (Figure 1(b)). Cytopathologist was present in the room and confirmed the adequacy of the sample. The linear echoendoscope was then withdrawn and the Olympus video GIF-180 gastroscope was advanced again into the esophagus and a 23 mm × 105 mm self-expandable partially covered metallic esophageal stent was then deployed across the stricture under fluoroscopic guidance. The patient tolerated the procedure well without complications. The thyroid FNA results showed renal cell carcinoma with positive immunohistochemical stains for PAX8 and CAIX and negative for thyroid transcription factor-1 (TTF-1), thyroglobulin, and chromogranin (Figures 2(a)–2(c)). A diagnosis of metastatic RCC was made. The patient had a history of right renal cell carcinoma (RCC) status after right nephrectomy 11 years ago (Figure 2(d)). The patient was referred for further oncology workup and management. Subsequent positron emission tomography (PET) scan is shown in Figure 3.

3. Discussion

Metastatic disease to the thyroid gland is rare, and adenocarcinomas from the kidney, lung, breast, and colon along with squamous cell carcinomas (mainly head and neck) represent the majority of primary sites [1]. Renal cell cancers can recur, with a recurrence rate of about 60% within 2 years, 70% within 3 years, 80% within 4 years, and most of the rest within 5 years [2]. Recurrences can, however, occur many years later, with some reported cases after 30 years [3].

The use of EUS for the diagnosis of thyroid disease was first described in 2001 by Ohshima et al. [4] followed by Koike et al. [5] in 2002, who both described the usefulness of EUS in the diagnosis of esophageal infiltration of thyroid cancer. However, neither of these studies described the use of EUS-FNA for evaluation of these malignancies. In 2004, Dewitt et al. [6] described the first EUS-FNA of the thyroid in a patient presenting with a superior mediastinal mass with a final cytopathologic diagnosis of benign nodular goiter. In 2014, Foppiani et al. [7] described RCC metastasis into a hot thyroid nodule that was diagnosed by conventional percutaneous FNA.

During an upper EUS examination, the thyroid gland is usually visualized close to the upper esophageal sphincter. However, EUS is limited in visualizing the upper portions of the thyroid glands [4, 5].

In 2015, a multi-institutional study of 62 cases of secondary thyroid cancer showed that FNA biopsy has a sensitivity and specificity of 80% and 93%, respectively [1]. In 2016, Song et al. [8] described the transcutaneous ultrasonographic features and the diagnostic role of core needle biopsy in 8 patients with metastatic RCC nodule. The ultrasonographic features of metastatic RCC showed solid, hypoechoic, noncalcified nodules in all cases. 88.9% of nodules had a well-defined smooth margin. In 100% of cases, there was increased vascularity with 55% showing extensive vascularity. In this study, one FNA (11%) was able to confirm metastatic RCC (under transcutaneous ultrasonographic guidance), whereas all six core needle biopsies confirmed metastatic RCC. Alkhatib et al. [9] described the first study that evaluated the endosonographic findings of the thyroid gland during a routine upper EUS in 100 cases. The results of the study showed thyroid lesions in 12 cases, out of which three previously undiagnosed thyroid cancers were visualized during EUS (two primary papillary thyroid cancers and one anaplastic thyroid cancer). However, there was not any described case of metastatic RCC to thyroid diagnosed by EUS-FNA approach. Transesophageal EUS-guided fine needle aspiration of thyroid lesions was feasible when the lesion was in the inferior portion of the thyroid gland, and the tip of the scope was at 18 cm or more from the incisors. EUS has the advantage of assessing esophagopharyngeal invasion by thyroid cancer which can affect the staging and operative planning [4, 5]. Additionally, the sensitivity, positive predictive value, and negative predictive value of EUS tend to be better than those

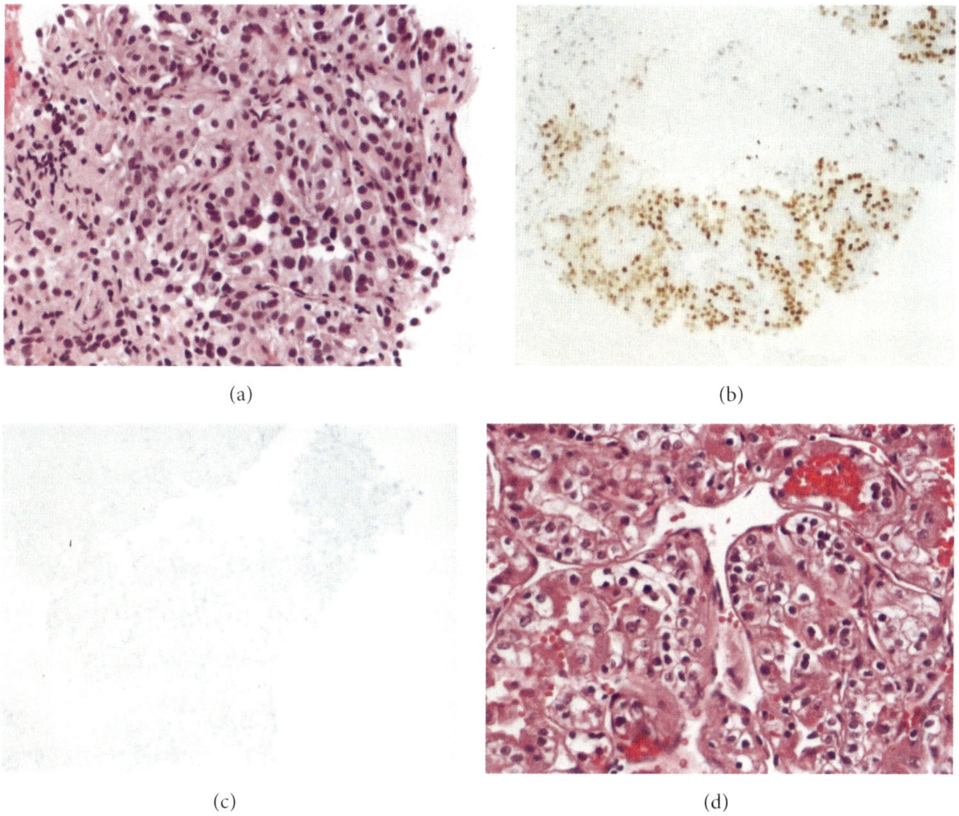

(a) (b) (c) (d)

FIGURE 2: (a) Cell block of thyroid nodule FNA is displaying multiple nests of clear cells, which have clear to eosinophilic cytoplasm. These nests are separated by delicate vascular network and surrounded by lymphocytic infiltrate (hematoxylin-eosin stain, original magnification ×400). (b) Staining of cell block with PAX-8 shows strong nuclear positivity (PAX-8 immunohistochemistry stain, original magnification ×200). (c) Staining the cell block with thyroid transcription factor-1 (TTF-1) shows negative staining (TTF-1 immunohistochemistry stain, original magnification ×200). (d) Kidney section is showing multiple nests of clear cells, which have clear to eosinophilic cytoplasm. These nests are separated by delicate vascular network (hematoxylin-eosin stain, original magnification ×400).

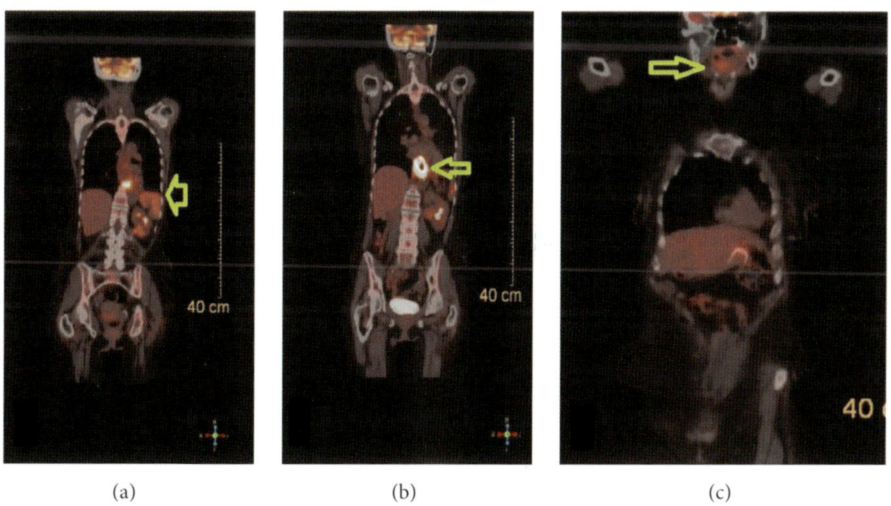

(a) (b) (c)

FIGURE 3: *PET scan image that was done one month after the diagnosis of thyroid RCC and esophageal adenocarcinoma.* Increased PET activity is appreciated within the lower esophagus. There was a lesion in the left adrenal gland which is PET avid that could represent adrenal metastasis (arrow). (b) A stent is present in the lower esophagus (arrow) crossing the GE junction into the stomach. Increased PET activity is appreciated within the lower esophagus, surrounding the esophageal stent. (c) Enlarging lesion in the right lobe of the thyroid (arrow) with increased PET activity compared to the remainder of the gland.

of magnetic resonance imaging (MRI) and esophagography [4]. Furthermore, EUS with FNA of thyroid lesions can be considered in case transcutaneous ultrasound and FNA are either unsuccessful (e.g., in case of a large retrosternal goiter) or contraindicated (e.g., because of interposing vessels). The true incidence for adverse events of EUS-FNA is not well reported. However, the risk of dissemination could occur with both transcutaneous and EUS-FNA. Because transcutaneous ultrasound with FNA is less invasive than EUS with FNA, it should continue to be the first-line evaluation in the routine diagnosis of and obtaining cytological specimens from thyroid gland lesions. However, in patients undergoing upper endoscopy or EUS for other indications, our case illustrated that EUS-FNA of thyroid lesions found during upper gastrointestinal EUS is feasible and safe.

Consent

Informed consent was obtained for this case.

Authors' Contributions

Yousef Abdel-Aziz did the literature review and wrote the manuscript. Tariq Hammad reviewed and edited the manuscript. Hayder Abdulwahid reviewed and provided the pathology slides. Mohamad Nawras edited the supplied images. Ali Nawras edited the manuscript and is the article guarantor.

References

[1] M. Pusztaszeri, H. Wang, E. S. Cibas et al., "Fine-needle aspiration biopsy of secondary neoplasms of the thyroid gland: A multi-institutional study of 62 cases," *Cancer Cytopathology*, vol. 123, no. 1, pp. 19–29, 2015.

[2] D. W. McNichols, J. W. Segura, and J. H. DeWeerd, "Renal Cell Carcinoma: Long-Term Survival and Late Recurrence," *The Journal of Urology*, vol. 126, no. 1, pp. 17–23, 1981.

[3] S. Yadav and N. Bennani-Baiti, "Renal cell carcinoma metastasis to the thyroid: How long is long enough?" *Acta Oncologica*, vol. 53, no. 9, pp. 1277-1278, 2014.

[4] A. Ohshima, H. Yamashita, S. Noguchi et al., "Usefulness of endoscopic ultrasonography (EUS) in diagnosing esophageal infiltration of thyroid cancer," *Journal of Endocrinological Investigation*, vol. 24, no. 8, pp. 564–569, 2001.

[5] E. Koike, H. Yamashita, S. Noguchi et al., "Endoscopic ultrasonography in patients with thyroid cancer: Its usefulness and limitations for evaluating esophagopharyngeal invasion," *Endoscopy*, vol. 34, no. 6, pp. 457–460, 2002.

[6] J. Dewitt, W. Youssef, J. LeBlanc et al., "EUS-guided FNA of a thyroid mass," *Gastrointestinal Endoscopy*, vol. 59, no. 2, pp. 307–310, 2004.

[7] L. Foppiani, M. Massollo, P. Del Monte, R. Bandelloni, A. Arlandini, and A. Piccardo, "Late-Onset Metastasis of Renal Cell Carcinoma into a Hot Thyroid Nodule: An Uncommon Finding Not to Be Overlooked," *Case Reports in Endocrinology*, vol. 2015, pp. 1–4, 2015.

[8] O. K. Song, J. S. Koo, J. Y. Kwak, H. J. Moon, J. H. Yoon, and E. Kim, "Metastatic renal cell carcinoma in the thyroid gland: ultrasonographic features and the diagnostic role of core needle biopsy," *Ultrasonography*, vol. 36, no. 3, pp. 252–259, 2016, https://www.ncbi.nlm.nih.gov/pubmed/27956733.

[9] A. A. Alkhatib, A. A. Mahayni, G. R. Chawki, L. Yoder, F. A. Elkhatib, and M. Al-Haddad, "Endosonographic examination of thyroid gland among patients with nonthyroid cancers," *Endoscopic Ultrasound*, vol. 5, no. 5, pp. 328–334, 2016.

Moderate Hypertriglyceridemia Causing Recurrent Pancreatitis: A Case Report and the Literature Review

Vijay Gayam,[1] Amrendra Kumar Mandal,[1] Pavani Garlapati,[1] Mazin Khalid,[1] Arshpal Gill,[1] and Khalid Mowyad[2]

[1] *Department of Medicine and Gastroenterology, Interfaith Medical Center, 1545 Atlantic Avenue, Brooklyn, NY, USA*
[2] *Department of Medicine, Wayne State University/Detroit Medical Center, Detroit, MI, USA*

Correspondence should be addressed to Vijay Gayam; vgayam@interfaithmedical.com

Academic Editor: Antonio Macrì

Recurrent acute pancreatitis secondary to hypertriglyceridemia (HTG) with levels below 1000 mg/dL has been rarely reported in the literature. HTG is the third most common cause of acute pancreatitis and has been established in the literature as a risk factor when levels are greater than 1000 mg/dL. A 43-year-old patient presented to the hospital with severe epigastric abdominal pain. Initial laboratory investigations were significant for a lipase level of 4143 U/L and a triglyceride level of 600 mg/dL. Computed tomography (CT) of the abdomen showed diffuse enlargement of the pancreas consistent with pancreatitis. A diagnosis of severe acute pancreatitis secondary to high triglycerides was made based on the revised Atlanta classification 2012. The patient was initially managed with intravenous boluses of normal saline followed by continuous insulin infusion. Diabetic Ketoacidosis (DKA) was ruled out due to a past medical history of diabetes. Her clinical course was complicated by acute respiratory distress syndrome requiring intubation and mechanical ventilation. During the course, she improved symptomatically and was extubated. She was started on nasogastric feeding initially and subsequently switched to oral diet as tolerated. After initial management of HTG with insulin infusion, oral gemfibrozil was started for long-term treatment of HTG. Emerging literature implicates HTG as an independent indicator of poor prognosis in acute pancreatitis (AP). Despite the paucity of data, the risk of developing AP must be considered even at triglyceride levels lower than 1000 mg/dL.

1. Introduction

Acute pancreatitis is the leading gastrointestinal cause of hospitalization in the United States [1]. The two most common causes of acute pancreatitis are gallstones and alcohol [2].

Hypertriglyceridemia is the third most common cause of acute pancreatitis and accounts for 1 to 4 percent of total cases [3]. It has been established in the literature as a risk factor when levels are higher than 1000 mg/dL [4]. Moderate hypertriglyceridemia is defined as triglyceride (TG) levels between 200 and 999 mg/dL [5]. Although hypertriglyceridemia is an established risk factor for acute pancreatitis, the precise relationship between acute pancreatitis and triglyceride levels remains unclear. In acute pancreatitis, there appears to be a process of triglyceride conversion into toxic free fatty acids (FFA) by pancreatic lipases resulting into lipotoxicity [6, 7]. The severity of acute pancreatitis in patients with HTG is dependent on both the inflammatory response caused by acute pancreatitis and the injury caused by lipotoxicity from triglyceride hydrolysis. We present a patient with recurrent acute pancreatitis secondary to elevated triglyceride levels that remained below 1000 mg/dL. Secondary causes were also considered, as other conditions can elevate triglycerides and can culminate in HTG induced acute pancreatitis [8]. In our patient, a workup of secondary causes of hypertriglyceridemia was unremarkable apart from a past medical history of diabetes.

2. Case Presentation

A morbidly obese 43-year-old female with a history of hypertension, dyslipidemia, and diabetes mellitus presented

TABLE 1: Showing trend of Triglycerides level during the hospital stay.

Lab parameters	Day 1	Day 3	Day 5	Day 11
Triglyceride level	600 mg/dL	393 mg/dL	247 mg/dL	165 mg/dL

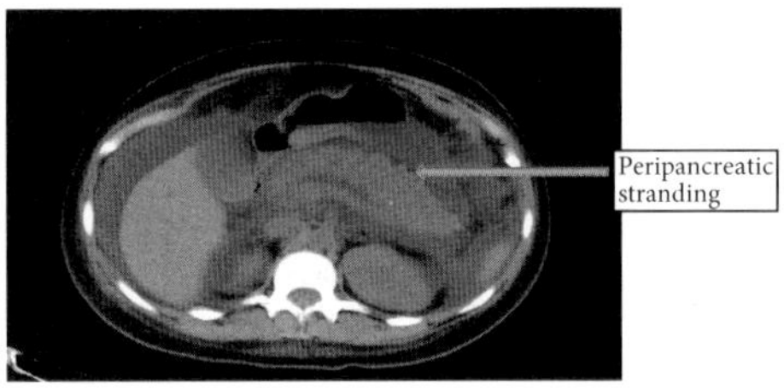

FIGURE 1: CT scan of the abdomen showing acute pancreatitis (arrow).

with severe abdominal pain. She had an episode of acute pancreatitis one year ago. She complained of right upper quadrant pain radiating to the back over 6-hour duration alongside six episodes of vomitus. A review of systems was only notable for a headache and dizziness. She reported no family history of dyslipidemia or acute pancreatitis. She denied tobacco, alcohol, or illicit substance use. There was no history of gallstones, appendectomy, new medications, procedures (including ERCP), or any complications related to her diabetes.

Admission vitals revealed afebrile patient with a heart rate of 103/min, respiratory rate of 20/min, BP 116/62 mmHg, and oxygen saturation of 96% on a nasal cannula at 5 liter/min. The patient was alert and orientated but was in moderate distress. The abdomen was obese and soft and with tenderness in the epigastric region. There was no guarding, rigidity, or Murphy's sign. Her body mass index (BMI) was 47.1. Other systemic signs of elevated triglycerides including xanthelasma, corneal arcus, and tendon xanthoma were absent.

Initial laboratory investigations showed an elevated white cell count of 16.9 μ/L (4.5 -11 μ/L), haemoglobin 12.2 g/dL (12-16 g/dL), platelet count 368000 mm^3 (130,000-400,000mm^3), sodium 129 mEq/L (136-144 mEq/L), potassium 3.8 mEq/L (3.5-5mEq/L), anion gap of 2 (8-16), BUN 45 mg/dL (7-20 mg/dL), creatinine 0.6 (0.4-1.3), glucose 206 mg/dL (74-117 mg/dL), and serum calcium 7.9 mg/dL (8.5-10.2 mg/dL). Liver function tests showed total bilirubin 0.5 mg/dL (0.1-1.2mg/dL), aspartate aminotransferase 16 IU/L (8-46 IU/L), alanine aminotransferase 11 U/L (7-55 IU/L), total protein 8.5 g/dL (6.1-7.9 g/dL), albumin 4 g/dL (3.5-5.5 g/dL), and PT 11.6 seconds (9.8-13.4 seconds). Initial arterial blood gas (ABG) analysis showed pH 7.5, pCO2 37.5, and pO2 67 at FiO_2 of 40%.

The patient had an elevated lipase of 4143 U/L (reference 22-51 U/L), total cholesterol of 694 mg/dL (100-199 mg/dL), and a triglyceride level of 600 mg/dL (reference 0-149 mg/dL). Computed tomography (CT) of the abdomen showed diffuse enlargement of the pancreas consistent with pancreatitis (Figure 1). There was no evidence of gallstones or biliary sludge which was also confirmed by an ultrasound abdomen. Other competing etiologies including alcohol, autoimmune pancreatitis, abdominal trauma, pancreatic divisum, sphincter of Oddi dysfunction (SOD), viral infection, drugs, and toxins were all ruled out, making the most likely diagnosis hypertriglyceridemia-induced AP (HTG AP).

The patient was treated with boluses of intravenous (IV) normal saline and supportive care. On the second day of admission, the patient developed hypotension and had persistent tachycardia. She likely developed acute respiratory distress syndrome (ARDS) from complications of acute pancreatitis. Fluid overload was ruled out with a sonogram of the inferior vena cava (diameter of 1.5 cm), a central venous pressure of 6 cm of H2O, and echocardiography indicating left ventricular ejection fraction of 55% with no left ventricular diastolic dysfunction. The patient was subsequently transferred to the intensive care unit for hypovolemic shock and respiratory distress requiring intubation and mechanical ventilation. As per revised Atlanta classification, she was categorized as severe acute pancreatitis based on Marshall scoring system for organ failure with a score of 3, with a score of 1 from respiratory failure (PaO_2/FiO_2 of 240) and two from cardiovascular (systolic BP <90, not fluid responsive). Patient's fasting blood glucose was 288 mg/dL (74-117 mg/dl), and diabetic ketoacidosis (DKA) was ruled out with the absence of serum or urine ketones, no elevated anion gap, and no acidosis. ABG analysis showed pH of 7.5, bicarbonate of 23, and an anion gap of 2.

Following the patients decline into shock, an ABG indicated an acidic pH of 6.99, PCO_2 9.4, PO_2 134, and HCO_3 of 5.4. The serum bicarbonate level was low at 15 mmol/L and the calculated anion gap was elevated at 22 (normal 8–16). Lactic acid level was 3.8 mmol/L (0.5-1.9 mmol/L).

Repeat abdominal contrast-enhanced CT on the third day showed marked pancreatic and peripancreatic infiltration consistent with AP and no signs of necrosis. Continuous insulin infusion was started for HTG from day 1, lowering her triglyceride levels down to 247 mg/dL over five days as shown in Table 1. She was also started on a liquid diet via nasogastric tube from day 5. After nine days in the ICU, the patient was successfully extubated and was switched to oral diet on day 11, which was gradually advanced as tolerated. She was downgraded to the floor on the same day and discharged on day 17. The patient required nasal oxygen to maintain saturation as she was recovering from ARDS. She was discharged on gemfibrozil 600mg twice daily to prevent further episodes of HTG AP. Patient has been followed upon discharge and remains compliant with gemfibrozil, leading to a controlled triglyceride level of 123 mg/dL and no further episodes of AP.

3. Discussion

Acute pancreatitis has several etiologies, but alcohol and gallstones make up the majority of the cases [9]. The exact mechanism of acute pancreatitis (AP) remains unclear and has been hypothesized as an imbalance between proinflammatory and anti-inflammatory cytokines [10]. Hypertriglyceridemia (HTG) is the third most common cause in literature and is classically considered a risk factor with levels higher than 1000mg/dL [4]. Our patient had a triglyceride (TGs) of 597 mg/dL one year ago during her first episode of AP. In the present case, TGs were 600 mg/dL. Our findings were consistent with those of Zhang et al. who observed hypertriglyceridemia-related acute pancreatitis in 102 patients with TG between 500mg/dL and 1000mg/dL. The same cohort of patients also had a high AP recurrence rate of 14.71%. However, the period between recurrent episodes of AP was not established [11].

There is emerging literature implicating HTG as an independent indicator of poor prognosis in AP [12]. Elevated serum TGs in patients with AP are independently and proportionally correlated with persistent organ failure regardless of etiology. However, severe or very severe HTG plus high lipase levels (>3 times the upper limit of normal) are associated with elevated free fatty acid (FFA) levels and can further be complicated by systemic inflammation from acute pancreatitis [12].

A prior meta-analysis concluded that HTG AP is associated with worse outcomes including higher mortality and the higher rates of systemic inflammatory response syndrome (SIRS) as compared to non-HTG AP [13]. Sue et al. studied 2519 patients and observed that patients were more likely to develop persistent organ failure when triglycerides levels were elevated [14]. They also noted even a modest HTG of >200mg/dL could be a statistically significant risk factor for ICU admission. This highlights the need to consider elevated triglycerides and obtain these labs in patients with presumed HG AP to determine etiology and to serve as a prognostic factor as in our patient who required ICU admission.

Management is important in HTG AP due to a high risk of complications. Insulin infusion has been used in literature successfully [15, 16]. However, selected patients with severe HTG AP might benefit from plasmapheresis, but evidence to support its use needs to be validated from various trials [17, 18]. Our patient was started on insulin infusion followed by fibrate to control triglycerides levels and prevent further episodes of HTG AP. Further studies are needed to establish HTG AP in patients with triglyceride levels below 1000mg/dL. Meanwhile, clinicians should be aware of the possibility of developing acute pancreatitis with a triglyceride level lower than 1000 mg/dL. Insulin infusion should be considered in these rapidly reduced triglyceride levels.

Consent

Informed consent was obtained from the patient.

References

[1] A. F. Peery, E. S. Dellon, J. Lund et al., "Burden of gastrointestinal disease in the United States: 2012 update," *Gastroenterology*, vol. 143, no. 5, pp. 1179.e3–1187.e3, 2012.

[2] C. E. Forsmark and J. Baillie, "AGA Institute Technical Review on Acute Pancreatitis," *Gastroenterology*, vol. 132, no. 5, pp. 2022–2044, 2007.

[3] J. Scherer, V. P. Singh, C. S. Pitchumoni, and D. Yadav, "Issues in hypertriglyceridemic pancreatitis: an update," *Journal of Clinical Gastroenterology*, vol. 48, no. 3, pp. 195–203, 2014.

[4] R. Khan, W. Jehangir, K. Regeti, and A. Yousif, "Hypertriglyceridemia-Induced Pancreatitis: Choice of Treatment," *Gastroenterology Research*, vol. 8, no. 3-4, pp. 234–236, 2015.

[5] L. Berglund, J. D. Brunzell, A. C. Goldberg et al., "Evaluation and treatment of hypertriglyceridemia: an endocrine society clinical practice guideline," *The Journal of Clinical Endocrinology & Metabolism*, vol. 97, no. 9, pp. 2969–2989, 2012.

[6] S. Navina, C. Acharya, J. P. DeLany et al., "Lipotoxicity causes multisystem organ failure and exacerbates acute pancreatitis in obesity," *Science Translational Medicine*, vol. 3, no. 107, Article ID 107ra110, 2011.

[7] F. Yang, Y. Wang, L. Sternfeld et al., "The role of free fatty acids, pancreatic lipase and Ca2+ signalling in injury of isolated acinar cells and pancreatitis model in lipoprotein lipase-deficient mice," *Acta Physiologica*, vol. 195, no. 1, pp. 13–28, 2009.

[8] W. Tsuang, U. Navaneethan, L. Ruiz, J. B. Palascak, and A. Gelrud, "Hypertriglyceridemic pancreatitis: presentation and management," *American Journal of Gastroenterology*, vol. 104, no. 4, pp. 984–991, 2009.

[9] D. B. Kim, W. C. Chung, J. M. Lee, K.-M. Lee, J. H. Oh, and E. J. Jeon, "Analysis of factors associated with the severity of acute pancreatitis according to etiology," *Gastroenterology Research and Practice*, vol. 2017, 2017.

[10] M. Manohar, A. K. Verma, S. U. Venkateshaiah, N. L. Sanders, and A. Mishra, "Pathogenic mechanisms of pancreatitis," *World Journal of Gastrointestinal Pharmacology and Therapeutics*, vol. 8, no. 1, p. 10, 2017.

[11] X.-L. Zhang, F. Li, Y.-M. Zhen, A. Li, and Y. Fang, "Clinical study of 224 patients with hypertriglyceridemia pancreatitis," *Chinese Medical Journal*, vol. 128, no. 15, pp. 2044–2049, 2015.

[12] H. Nawaz, E. Koutroumpakis, J. Easler et al., "Elevated serum triglycerides are independently associated with persistent organ failure in acute pancreatitis," *American Journal of Gastroenterology*, vol. 110, no. 10, pp. 1497–1503, 2015.

[13] G.-J. Wang, C.-F. Gao, D. Wei, C. Wang, and S.-Q. Ding, "Acute pancreatitis: Etiology and common pathogenesis," *World Journal of Gastroenterology*, vol. 15, no. 12, pp. 1427–1430, 2009.

[14] L. Y. Sue, M. Batech, D. Yadav et al., "Effect of Serum Triglycerides on Clinical Outcomes in Acute Pancreatitis: Findings from a Regional Integrated Health Care System," *Pancreas*, vol. 46, no. 7, pp. 874–879, 2017.

[15] M. S. Kuchay, K. J. Farooqui, T. Bano, M. Khandelwal, H. Gill, and A. Mithal, "Heparin and insulin in the management of hypertriglyceridemia-associated pancreatitis: Case series and literature review," *Archives of Endocrinology and Metabolism*, vol. 61, no. 2, pp. 198–201, 2017.

[16] A. Coskun, N. Erkan, S. Yakan et al., "Treatment of hypertriglyceridemia-induced acute pancreatitis with insulin," *Przegląd Gastroenterologiczny*, vol. 10, no. 1, pp. 18–22, 2015.

[17] T. Furuya, M. Komatsu, K. Takahashi et al., "Plasma exchange for hypertriglyceridemic acute necrotizing pancreatitis: report of two cases," *Therapeutic Apheresis*, vol. 6, no. 6, pp. 454–458, 2002.

[18] C. Stefanutti, S. Di Giacomo, and G. Labbadia, "Timing clinical events in the treatment of pancreatitis and hypertriglyceridemia with therapeutic plasmapheresis," *Transfusion and Apheresis Science*, vol. 45, no. 1, pp. 3–7, 2011.

50

Rare Case of an Epithelial Cyst in an Intrapancreatic Accessory Spleen Treated by Robot-Assisted Spleen Preserving Distal Pancreatectomy

Willemijn P. M. van Dijck,[1] Vincent P. Groot,[1] Lodewijk A. A. Brosens,[2] Jeroen Hagendoorn,[1] Inne H. M. Borel Rinkes,[1] Maarten S. van Leeuwen,[3] and I. Quintus Molenaar[1]

[1]*Department of Surgery, UMC Utrecht Cancer Center, University Medical Center Utrecht, Utrecht, Netherlands*
[2]*Department of Pathology, UMC Utrecht Cancer Center, University Medical Center Utrecht, Utrecht, Netherlands*
[3]*Department of Radiology, UMC Utrecht Cancer Center, University Medical Center Utrecht, Utrecht, Netherlands*

Correspondence should be addressed to I. Quintus Molenaar; i.q.molenaar@umcutrecht.nl

Academic Editor: Hideto Kawaratani

Epithelial cyst in an intrapancreatic accessory spleen (ECIPAS) is exceedingly rare with only 57 cases reported since the first publication in 1980. Comprehensive clinical and diagnostic features remain to be clarified. We present a case of ECIPAS in a 21-year-old Philippine woman who was admitted with right upper quadrant abdominal pain. A cystic lesion in the pancreatic tail was discovered and evaluated by computed tomography and magnetic resonance images. Based on clinical and radiological features a solid pseudopapillary neoplasm was suspected. The patient underwent robot-assisted spleen preserving distal pancreatectomy. Pathological evaluation revealed a 26 mm intrapancreatic accessory spleen with a 16 mm cyst, lined by multilayered epithelium in the tail of the pancreas. The postoperative course was uneventful. Differentiating ECIPAS from (pre)malignant cystic pancreatic neoplasms based on clinical and radiological features remains difficult. When typical radiological signs can be combined with scintigraphy using Technetium-99m labelled colloid or Technetium-99m labelled erythrocytes, which can identify the solid component of the lesion as splenic tissue, it should be possible to make the right diagnosis noninvasively. When pancreatectomy is inevitable due to symptoms or patient preference, minimally invasive laparoscopic or robot-assisted spleen preserving distal pancreatectomy should be considered.

1. Introduction

Accessory spleens exist in up to 10% of the general population, with a fifth arising within the pancreatic tail [1]. However, presence of an epithelial cyst in an intrapancreatic accessory spleen (ECIPAS) is remarkably rare, with only 42 published reports covering 57 cases in the English literature since Davidson et al. reported the first case in 1980 [2–42]. ECIPAS is often misdiagnosed as a cystic neuroendocrine tumor or solid pseudopapillary tumor, resulting in unnecessary surgical resection. Since ECIPAS is a nonneoplastic lesion, surgery is not indicated. Clearly, a correct preoperative diagnosis is a key and can avoid unnecessary surgery. Currently, however, comprehensive clinical and imaging features remain to be clarified.

Here we present the first case of an epithelial cyst in an intrapancreatic accessory spleen treated with robot-assisted minimally invasive spleen preserving distal pancreatectomy, using the da Vinci surgical system. Although standard protocol for cystic lesions of the pancreas was followed, including CT and MRI evaluation and presentation in a multidisciplinary meeting, the correct diagnosis was not reached. Clinical, radiological, and pathological features are discussed to contribute to a better understanding of these rare lesions, thereby aiming at a reduction of performing unnecessary surgery.

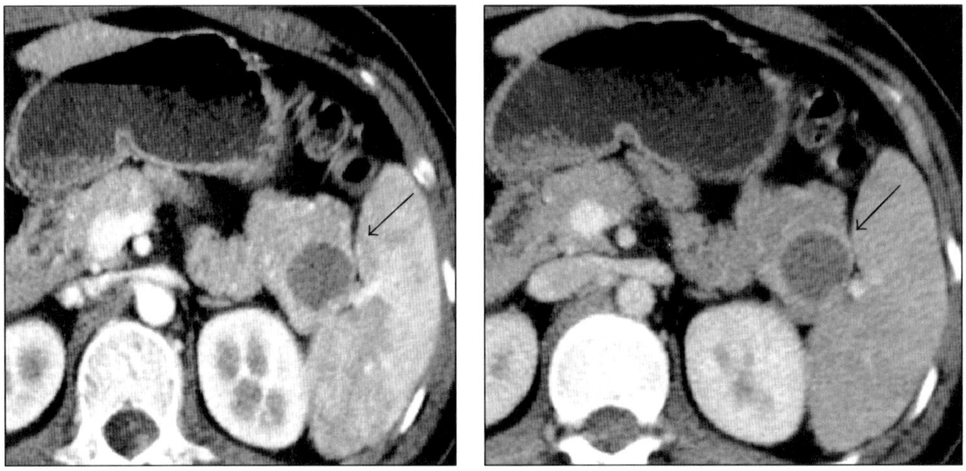

(a) (b)

FIGURE 1: (a) Arterial and (b) portal-venous phase CT, confirming cystic lesion in pancreatic tail without soft-tissue component.

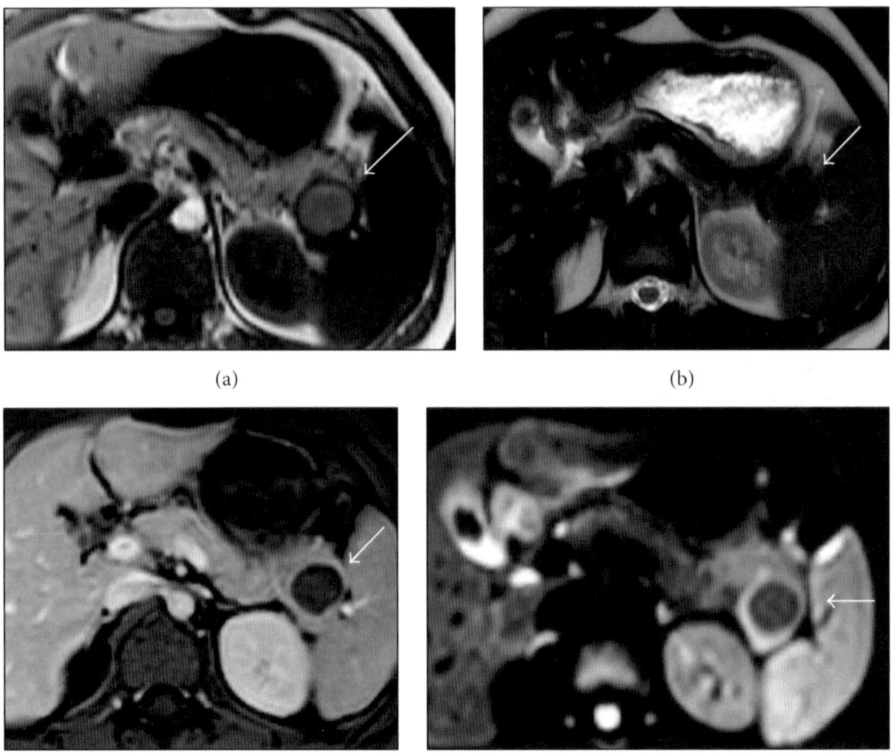

(a) (b) (c) (d)

FIGURE 2: MRI exam showing (a) T1-weighted image, (b) T2-weighted image, (c) Gd-enhanced image, and (d) DWI image of the lesion. Note how DWI best demarcates soft-tissue rim surrounding cystic component, with equivalent signal intensity to spleen.

2. Case Report

A 21-year-old Philippine woman was referred to the University Medical Center Utrecht with right upper quadrant abdominal pain since one year. An initial abdominal ultrasound showed cholecystolithiasis. Incidentally, a cystic lesion was detected in the tail of the pancreas. Additional CT imaging exposed a 24 mm cystic lesion in the pancreatic tail, in close proximity to the spleen (Figure 1). The caudal wall of the cyst appeared to be thickened and enhanced. Following our protocol for cystic lesions of the pancreas, a subsequent MRI was performed and revealed a 31 mm cystic lesion with hyperintensity on T1-weighted images, indicative of previous haemorrhage (Figure 2(a)). Enhancement of the cystic wall was seen in the venous phase, with some gadolinium enhancing of the center of the lesion during the arterial

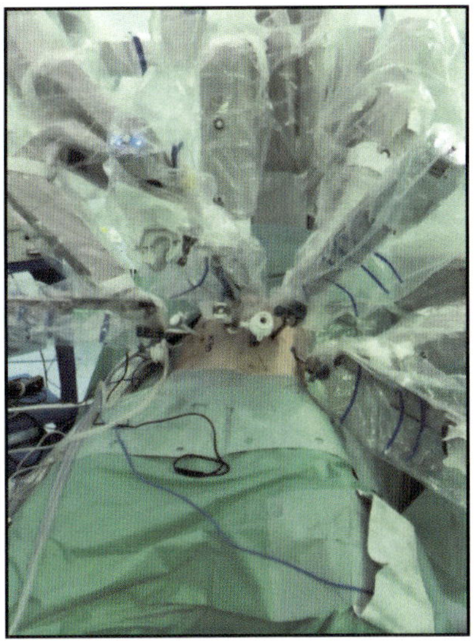

FIGURE 3: Port positioning for robot-assisted spleen preserving distal pancreatectomy.

phase (Figure 2(c)). The rim of the lesion showed some diffusion restriction on diffusion-weighted imaging (DWI) (Figure 2(d)).

The patient had no medical history and additional physical examination and laboratory tests were normal. The patient case was further discussed in a multidisciplinary meeting and a solid pseudopapillary neoplasm (Hamoudi or Frantz tumor) with past haemorrhage was considered as the most likely diagnosis based on clinical and radiological findings. Owing to the low malignant potential of the suspected solid pseudopapillary neoplasm in the tail of the pancreas, a robot-assisted spleen preserving distal pancreatectomy was advised. In addition, a cystic neuroendocrine tumor and mucinous cystadenoma were in the differential diagnosis. Due to questionable sensitivity, endoscopic ultrasound is not part of standard work-up for pancreatic (cystic) lesions at our institution [43]. Following this, we decided not to perform additional endoscopic ultrasound since the indication for resection of the hypervascular cystic lesion was already established.

Robot-assisted minimally invasive spleen preserving distal pancreatectomy was performed using the da Vinci system (Intuitive Surgical Inc, Sunnyvale, CA) (Figure 3). The patient, under general anaesthesia, was placed in lithotomy position tilted to the left side. Pneumoperitoneum was established and the camera was placed in the right pararectal line. First, the gastrocolic ligament was divided while preserving the gastroepiploic artery. Mobilisation began at the neck of the pancreas in order to achieve control of the proximal splenic artery. The duodenum was exposed, and the superior mesenteric vein was identified at the root of the mesentery. Both the splenic artery and the vein were isolated and left intact. Taking sufficient margin, the pancreatic tail was transected with a stapler device and extracted from the abdominal cavity in an endobag. The total operation time was 2 hours and 4 minutes, with a total blood loss of 20 mL.

Macroscopically, the specimen showed a well-demarcated and encapsulated dark-red lesion with a diameter of 26 mm harbouring a 16 mm cyst (Figure 4(a)). Microscopically, the lesion consisted of normal splenic tissue with alternating red and white pulp surrounded by a thin fibrous capsule (Figure 4(b)). A cystic space lined by stratified squamous epithelium without atypia was present within the splenic tissue. Immunohistochemical staining demonstrated that the epithelial lining was positive for Cytokeratin AE1/AE3 and Cytokeratin 5 but negative for Calretinin D2-40 and CD34, showing that this was indeed epithelial lining and not mesothelial lining, a lymphangioma, or a hemangioma (Figure 4(c)). No papillary or pseudopapillary structures were observed. Based on these findings, ECIPAS was established as the final pathological diagnosis. The postoperative course was uneventful and the patient was discharged from hospital after five days.

3. Discussion

In a report on 2700 necropsies, approximately 10% was found to have an accessory spleen [1]. These accessory spleens were typically located in the splenic hilum (80%) or the pancreatic tail (17%). An epithelial cyst arising in such an intrapancreatic accessory spleen remains a rare entity. However, the increasing use of abdominal CT-scans and other imaging seems to lead to an increasing number of detected cases [30, 33]. This case report shows that, although protocols with respect to cystic lesions of the pancreas were followed and the patient was evaluated in a multidisciplinary meeting, diagnosing ECIPAS may be quite challenging. Presently, there are no accurate criteria to differentiate preoperatively between a (pre)malignant cystic neoplasm of the pancreas and ECIPAS.

When reviewing our own case and all other documented cases ($n = 57$) [2–42], we found that ECIPAS occurs slightly more frequent in woman than men (32 : 25) and is diagnosed mostly at middle age, with a median age of 45 years (range 12–75 years). Interestingly, the majority of patients ($n = 44$), including our patient, are from Asian descent, suggesting that racial factors and genetic background might play a role in the genesis of this lesion. Most often ECIPAS is an incidental finding as most patients (32 of 57) are asymptomatic. However, some patients reported nonspecific complaints such as abdominal pain, weight loss, nausea, and vomiting. When documented, serum CA 19-9 was elevated in 24 patients and was normal in 18 patients. It is argued that high CA 19-9 originates directly from the squamous epithelial lining and high serum levels are caused by trauma or increased intracystic pressure [8]. The median maximum diameter of the cystic lesions was 34 mm (range 14–150 mm) and all lesions were located in the tail of the pancreas. Cysts were described as multilocular in 26 patients and unilocular in 31 patients. Every patient underwent either open ($n = 46$) or laparoscopic ($n = 10$) distal pancreatectomy. Although improved surgical techniques have resulted in lower morbidity and better cosmetic results, laparoscopic and open distal pancreatectomy still result in mortality rates of 0.4% and 1.2%, respectively [44]. Correct diagnosis would therefore

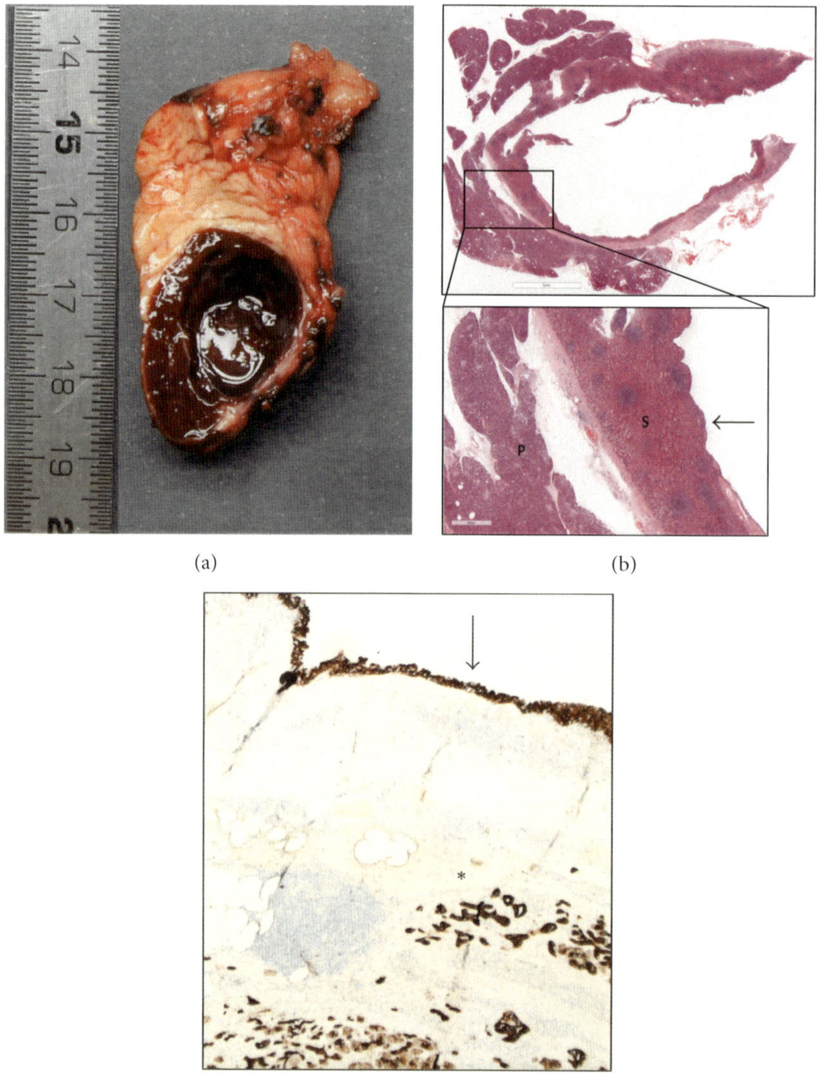

(a) (b)

(c)

Figure 4: (a) Photograph of the cut gross specimen showing well-defined splenic tissue with a unilocular cyst. (b) Hematoxylin-eosin staining showing pancreatic parenchyma (P) and adjacent splenic parenchyma (S) and the cyst wall lined by multilayered epithelium without atypia (arrow). (c) Cytokeratin 5 staining showing positivity in the cyst lining (arrow) and in surrounding pancreatic parenchyma (asterisk) indicating epithelial lining.

save patients from unnecessary surgery and its associated risks.

The presented patient was the first to undergo robot-assisted minimally invasive spleen preserving distal pancreatectomy for ECIPAS. By performing this procedure robotically, surgeons experience more freedom of movement of the surgical instruments, elimination of tremor, and a three-dimensional vision of the operative field. These advantages lead to improved precision in operation technique and may lead to a higher success rate of spleen preservation when performing distal pancreatectomy. Documented advantages of robot-assisted surgery over laparoscopic and open distal pancreatectomy include reduced blood loss, fewer complications, less postoperative pain, faster recovery, and thus a shorter hospital stay [45]. However, robot-assisted surgery also has some important limitations; robotic arm-interference makes it difficult to operate in multiple quadrants of the abdomen, the operation time is generally longer, and associated costs are higher.

Since 1980, a correct preoperative diagnosis of ECIPAS has been reported in only five cases [15, 21, 26, 32]. These accurate diagnoses were partly based on the smoothness of the cystic inner wall and solid component, a differentiating morphological feature suggestive of a benign tumor [26]. Additionally, epithelial cysts commonly show low signal intensity on T1-weighted images and high signal on T2-weighted images [21]. Lastly and most importantly, the density of tumor's solid component was recognized to match splenic tissue on postcontrast CT and MRI. On MRI, the ectopic splenic tissue shows a spleen-like signal on DWI (See Figure 2(d)). The presence of a relatively large amount of splenic tissue surrounding the cyst could thus make a correct diagnosis more likely with careful examination. However, if the amount of splenic tissue is small, accurate diagnosis before surgery remains challenging. When the presence of intrapancreatic splenic tissue is suggested on initial imaging, several techniques could be used to identify the ectopic splenic tissue, including Technetium-99m sulfur colloid scintigraphy and Technetium-99m heat-damaged red blood cell scintigraphy [46]. Splenic tissue traps up to 90% of the injected blood cells. When subsequent single-photon emission computed tomography (SPECT) imaging shows focal uptake in the pancreatic tail, a finding that is consistent with intrapancreatic splenic tissue, the correct diagnosis of an intrapancreatic spleen could be feasible [47]. However, compared to the normal spleen, uptake will be lower in an intrapancreatic spleen as it contains only a small amount of functioning splenic tissue. As yet, no malignant development of ECIPAS has been reported. When this benign lesion is correctly diagnosed, the patient can be discharged from follow-up.

In conclusion, ECIPAS is a rare entity with undefined criteria for preoperative diagnosis. However, we propose that, especially in middle-aged Asian patients, ECIPAS should be included in the differential diagnosis when considering cystic lesions of the pancreatic tail. In case of radiological signs of a smooth cystic wall, homogenous enhancement, and matching density of the solid component of the cyst and the adjacent spleen, the diagnosis of ECIPAS should be taken into consideration and Technetium-99m scintigraphy or SPECT-imaging should be performed. Further understanding of clinical and imaging features might lead to better diagnoses and might prevent unnecessary surgery for this benign lesion. When pancreatectomy is inevitable due to symptoms or patient preference, minimally invasive laparoscopic or robot-assisted spleen preserving distal pancreatectomy should be considered.

Consent

The patient involved in this study gave her written informed consent authorizing use and disclosure of her protected health information.

Competing Interests

None of the authors has competing interests.

Authors' Contributions

Willemijn P. M. van Dijck and Vincent P. Groot contributed equally to this work.

References

[1] B. Halpert and Z. A. Alden, "Accessory spleens in or at the tail of the pancreas. A survey of 2,700 additional necropsies," *Archives of Pathology*, vol. 77, pp. 652–654, 1964.

[2] E. D. Davidson, W. G. Campbell, and T. Hersh, "Epidermoid splenic cyst occurring in an intrapancreatic accessory spleen," *Digestive Diseases and Sciences*, vol. 25, no. 12, pp. 964–967, 1980.

[3] M. Hanada, M. Kimura, M. Kitada, T. Nakajima, K. Yamada, and M. Yoshii, "Epidermoid cyst of accessory spleen," *Acta Pathologica Japonica*, vol. 31, no. 5, pp. 863–872, 1981.

[4] T. Morohoshi, T. Hamamoto, T. Kunimura et al., "Epidermoid cyst derived from an accessory spleen in the pancreas. A case report with literature survey," *Acta Pathologica Japonica*, vol. 41, no. 12, pp. 916–921, 1991.

[5] Y. Nakae, T. Hayakawa, T. Kondo et al., "Epidermoid cyst occurring in a pancreatic accessory spleen: to the editor," *Journal of Clinical Gastroenterology*, vol. 13, no. 3, pp. 362–364, 1991.

[6] X. Tang, Y. Tanaka, and Y. Tsutsumi, "Epithelial inclusion cysts in an intrapancreatic accessory spleen," *Pathology International*, vol. 44, no. 8, pp. 652–654, 1994.

[7] H. Furukawa, T. Kosuge, Y. Kanai, and K. Mukai, "Epidermoid cyst in an intrapancreatic accessory spleen: CT and pathologic findings," *American Journal of Roentgenology*, vol. 171, no. 1, p. 271, 1998.

[8] K. Higaki, A. Jimi, J. Watanabe, A. Kusaba, and M. Kojiro, "Epidermoid cyst of the spleen with CA19-9 or carcinoembryonic antigen productions: report of three cases," *The American Journal of Surgical Pathology*, vol. 22, no. 6, pp. 704–708, 1998.

[9] H. Tateyama, T. Tada, T. Murase, S. Fujitake, and T. Eimoto, "Lymphoepithelial cyst and epidermoid cyst of the accessory spleen in the pancreas," *Modern Pathology*, vol. 11, no. 12, pp. 1171–1177, 1998.

[10] S. Sasou, S.-I. Nakamura, and M. Inomata, "Epithelial splenic cysts in an intrapancreatic accessory spleen and spleen," *Pathology International*, vol. 49, no. 12, pp. 1078–1083, 1999.

[11] S. K. Choi, S. I. Ahn, K. C. Hong et al., "A case of epidermoid cyst of the intrapancreatic accessory spleen," *Journal of Korean Medical Science*, vol. 15, no. 5, pp. 589–592, 2000.

[12] S. Tsutsumi, T. Kojima, Y. Fukai et al., "Epidermoid cyst of an intrapancreatic accessory spleen—a case report," *Hepato-Gastroenterology*, vol. 47, no. 35, pp. 1462–1464, 2000.

[13] Y. Horibe, M. Murakami, K. Yamao, Y. Imaeda, K. Tashiro, and M. Kasahara, "Epithelial inclusion cyst (epidermoid cyst) formation with epithelioid cell granuloma in an intrapancreatic accessory spleen," *Pathology International*, vol. 51, no. 1, pp. 50–54, 2001.

[14] A. M. Fink, S. Kulkarni, P. Crowley, and J. A. Crameri, "Epidermoid cyst in a pancreatic accessory spleen mimicking an infected abdominal cyst in a child," *American Journal of Roentgenology*, vol. 179, no. 1, pp. 206–208, 2002.

[15] H. Yokomizo, M. Hifumi, T. Yamane et al., "Epidermoid cyst of an accessory spleen at the pancreatic tail: diagnostic value of MRI," *Abdominal Imaging*, vol. 27, no. 5, pp. 557–559, 2002.

[16] T. Sonomura, S. Kataoka, T. Chikugo et al., "Epidermoid cyst originating from an intrapancreatic accessory spleen," *Abdominal Imaging*, vol. 27, no. 5, pp. 560–562, 2002.

[17] H. Watanabe, Y. Yamaguchi, K. Ohtsubo et al., "Epidermoid cyst of the intrapancreatic accessory spleen producing CA19-9," *Digestive Endoscopy*, vol. 16, no. 3, pp. 244–248, 2004.

[18] H. Kanazawa, J. Kamiya, M. Nagino et al., "Epidermoid cyst in an intrapancreatic accessory spleen: a case report," *Journal of Hepato-Biliary-Pancreatic Surgery*, vol. 11, no. 1, pp. 61–63, 2004.

[19] K. Ru, A. Kalra, and A. Ucci, "Epidermoid cyst of intrapancreatic accessory spleen," *Digestive Diseases and Sciences*, vol. 52, no. 5, pp. 1229–1232, 2007.

[20] V. Lépilliez, M. Chemaly, T. Ponchon, B. Napoleon, and J. Saurin, "Endoscopic resection of sporadic duodenal adenomas: an efficient technique with a substantial risk of delayed bleeding," *Endoscopy*, vol. 40, no. 10, pp. 806–810, 2008.

[21] O. Itano, N. Shiraga, E. Kouta et al., "Epidermoid cyst originating from an intrapancreatic accessory spleen," *Journal of Hepato-Biliary-Pancreatic Surgery*, vol. 15, no. 4, pp. 436–439, 2008.

[22] E. L. Servais, I. S. Sarkaria, G. J. Solomon, P. Gumpeni, and M. D. Lieberman, "Giant epidermoid cyst within an intrapancreatic accessory spleen mimicking a cystic neoplasm of the pancreas: case report and review of the literature," *Pancreas*, vol. 36, no. 1, pp. 98–100, 2008.

[23] Z. Zhang and J. C. Wang, "An epithelial splenic cyst in an intrapancreatic accessory spleen. A case report," *Journal of the Pancreas*, vol. 10, pp. 664–666, 2009.

[24] G. Reiss, J. Z. Sickel, K. See-Tho, and S. Ramrakhiani, "Intrapancreatic splenic cyst mimicking pancreatic cystic neoplasm diagnosed by EUS-FNA," *Gastrointestinal Endoscopy*, vol. 70, no. 3, pp. 557–558, 2009.

[25] K. Kadota, Y. Kushida, Y. Miyai et al., "Epidermoid cyst in an intrapancreatic accessory spleen: three case reports and review of the literatures," *Pathology and Oncology Research*, vol. 16, no. 3, pp. 435–442, 2010.

[26] O. Itano, N. Chiba, T. Wada et al., "Laparoscopic resection of an epidermoid cyst originating from an intrapancreatic accessory spleen: report of a case," *Surgery Today*, vol. 40, no. 1, pp. 72–75, 2010.

[27] M. A. Khashab, M. I. Canto, V. K. Singh, R. H. Hruban, M. A. Makary, and S. Giday, "Endosonographic and elastographic features of a rare epidermoid cyst of an intrapancreatic accessory spleen," *Endoscopy*, vol. 43, supplement 2, pp. E193–E194, 2011.

[28] A. J. Horn and S. M. Lele, "Epidermoid cyst occurring within an intrapancreatic accessory spleen. A case report and review of the literature," *Journal of the Pancreas*, vol. 12, no. 3, pp. 279–282, 2011.

[29] H. Yamanishi, T. Kumagi, T. Yokota et al., "Epithelial cyst arising in an intrapancreatic accessory spleen: a diagnostic dilemma," *Internal Medicine*, vol. 50, no. 18, pp. 1947–1952, 2011.

[30] H. S. Hwang, S. S. Lee, S. C. Kim, D. W. Seo, and J. Kim, "Intrapancreatic accessory spleen: clinicopathologic analysis of 12 cases," *Pancreas*, vol. 40, no. 6, pp. 956–965, 2011.

[31] Y. Iwasaki, N. Tagaya, A. Nakagawa et al., "Laparoscopic resection of epidermoid cyst arising from an intrapancreatic accessory spleen: a case report with a review of the literature," *Surgical Laparoscopy, Endoscopy and Percutaneous Techniques*, vol. 21, no. 5, pp. e275–e279, 2011.

[32] A. Urakami, K. Yoshida, Y. Hirabayashi et al., "Laparoscopy-assisted spleen-preserving pancreatic resection for epidermoid cyst in an intrapancreatic accessory spleen," *Asian Journal of Endoscopic Surgery*, vol. 4, no. 4, pp. 185–188, 2011.

[33] S. Hu, L. Zhu, Q. Song, and K. Chen, "Epidermoid cyst in intrapancreatic accessory spleen: computed tomography findings and clinical manifestation," *Abdominal Imaging*, vol. 37, no. 5, pp. 828–833, 2012.

[34] N. Panagiotopoulos, M. Acharya, R. Ahmad, D. Bansi, and L. Jiao, "Epithelial inclusion cyst arising within an intra-pancreatic splenunculus," *International Journal of Surgery Case Reports*, vol. 3, no. 3, pp. 118–120, 2012.

[35] A. C. Harris, M. A. Chaudry, D. Menzies, and P. C. Conn, "Laparoscopic resection of an epidermoid cyst within an intrapancreatic accessory spleen: a case report and review article," *Surgical Laparoscopy, Endoscopy and Percutaneous Techniques*, vol. 22, no. 4, pp. e246–e249, 2012.

[36] R. Hong, N. Choi, K. Sun, S. Lim, and Y. Han, "Epidermoid cyst arising from an intrapancreatic accessory spleen: a case report and review of the literature," *Oncology Letters*, vol. 5, no. 2, pp. 469–472, 2013.

[37] A. Hamidian Jahromi, M. K. Fallahzadeh, N. Dela Cruz, and Q. Chu, "Intrapancreatic accessory spleen causing mass: a case report and review of the literature," *Eurorad*, vol. 165, pp. 153–156, 2013.

[38] C.-L. L. Lee, Y. Di, Y.-J. Jiang, C. Jin, and D.-L. Fu, "Epidermoid cyst of intrapancreatic accessory spleen: a case report and literature review," *World Journal of Surgical Procedures*, vol. 3, no. 3, pp. 54–59, 2013.

[39] M. Wakasugi, M. Tori, H. Akamatsu et al., "Laparoscopic distal pancreatectomy for multiple epithelial cysts in an intrapancreatic accessory spleen. A case report and review of literature," *Journal of the Pancreas*, vol. 14, no. 6, pp. 636–641, 2013.

[40] N. Zavras, N. Machairas, P. Foukas, A. Lazaris, P. Patapis, and A. Machairas, "Epidermoid cyst of an intrapancreatic accessory spleen: a case report and literature review," *World Journal of Surgical Oncology*, vol. 12, no. 1, article 92, 2014.

[41] M. K. Kwak, N. K. Lee, S. Kim et al., "A case of epidermoid cyst in an intrapancreatic accessory spleen mimicking pancreas neoplasms: MRI with DWI," *Clinical Imaging*, vol. 40, no. 1, pp. 164–166, 2016.

[42] M. Narita, K. Hanada, K. Moriyoshi, R. Matsusue, H. Hata, and T. Yamaguchi, "Laparoscopic resection of an epidermoid cyst arising from intrapancreatic accessary spleen," *Journal of the Pancreas*, no. 1, pp. 138–141, 2016.

[43] S. D. Mansfield, J. Scott, K. Oppong et al., "Comparison of multislice computed tomography and endoscopic ultrasonography with operative and histological findings in suspected pancreatic and periampullary malignancy," *British Journal of Surgery*, vol. 95, no. 12, pp. 1512–1520, 2008.

[44] R. Venkat, B. H. Edil, R. D. Schulick, A. O. Lidor, M. A. Makary, and C. L. Wolfgang, "Laparoscopic distal pancreatectomy is associated with significantly less overall morbidity compared to the open technique: A systematic review and meta-analysis," *Annals of Surgery*, vol. 255, no. 6, pp. 1048–1059, 2012.

[45] M. Strijker, H. C. van Santvoort, M. G. Besselink et al., "Robot-assisted pancreatic surgery: a systematic review of the literature," *HPB*, vol. 15, no. 1, pp. 1–10, 2013.

[46] S. J. Lehtinen, C. M. Schammel, M. Devane, and S. D. Trocha, "Intrapancreatic accessory spleen presenting as a pancreatic mass," *Journal of Gastrointestinal Oncology*, vol. 4, pp. E23–E26, 2013.

[47] G. Low, A. Panu, N. Millo, and E. Leen, "Multimodality imaging of neoplastic and nonneoplastic solid lesions of the pancreas," *Radiographics*, vol. 31, no. 4, pp. 993–1015, 2011.

A Case of Thermal Esophageal Injury Induced by Sodium Picosulfate with Magnesium Citrate

Dong-Hyuk Yang, Byoung Wook Bang, Kye Sook Kwon, Hyung Kil Kim, and Yong Woon Shin

Division of Gastroenterology, Department of Internal Medicine, Inha University School of Medicine, Incheon, Republic of Korea

Correspondence should be addressed to Byoung Wook Bang; bangbu@inha.ac.kr

Academic Editor: R. J. L. F. Loffeld

Although thermal esophageal injuries caused by hot food or tea have been reported, thermal esophageal injury due to sodium picosulfate with magnesium citrate (PSMC) used for bowel preparation is rarely reported. We report the case of a 56-year-old man who presented with esophageal injury after ingestion of PSMC. Instead of dissolving the PSMC in water before ingestion, he drank water immediately after swallowing PSMC powder. As soon as he drank water, he developed severe chest pain and hematemesis. Upper endoscopy revealed severe hemorrhagic, ulcerative mucosal change from upper to mid-esophagus. He was hospitalized for nine days, received conservative treatment (fasting and parenteral nutrition), and recovered without complications. When PSMC is used as a colonic cleansing agent, patients should be educated to take it after dissolving it sufficiently in 150 mL of water to avoid esophageal thermal injury.

1. Introduction

Colonoscopic examination is increasing in Korea as a screen for colorectal cancer [1]. Bowel cleansing agents are very important for successful colonoscopy. Polyethylene glycol and PSMC are widely used bowel cleansers. Polyethylene glycol is the most commonly used laxative. However, it may cause adverse effects such as nausea, vomiting, and abdominal discomfort. In addition, it may be rejected due to its unpleasant odor and taste [2]. PSMC, which has a similar bowel cleansing effect, is used for easier administration. PSMC is a dual-action laxative that has an orange scent. The active components include sodium picosulfate, magnesium oxide, and citric acid. When PSMC is dissolved in water, magnesium oxide and citric acid combine to form magnesium citrate, which acts as osmotic laxative [2], and sodium picosulfate, a stimulant laxative [3]. Due to its dual action, PSMC is a powerful laxative and patients comply well because of the pleasant fragrance. However, inappropriate use of PSMC can cause serious side effects [2, 3]. When it contacts water, an exothermic reaction occurs; therefore it should be dissolved in water and cooled before taking it. Here, we report a case of thermal injury of esophagus with acute bleeding caused by incorrect use of the PSMC.

2. Case Report

A 56-year-old man visited our hospital with severe chest pain and hematemesis. He was scheduled to receive colonoscopy in a local hospital. He did not sufficiently dissolve the PSMC powder in 150 mL of water as described in the drug instructions. Instead, he swallowed the PSMC powder and immediately drank water. Instantly after drinking water, he felt severe chest pain and shortly thereafter vomited about a cup of blood. On arrival at the emergency room, he was hemodynamically stable and alert. His blood pressure was 137/67 mmHg, pulse rate was 97 beats/minute, and body temperature was 36.8°C. His initial hemoglobin level was 15.7 g/dL. Other results of laboratory tests were within normal ranges, including electrolyte level, coagulation test, and cardiac enzyme level. The chest radiograph showed no active lung lesions. We found no evidence of arrhythmic change or ischemic heart disease on the electrocardiogram. The patient underwent upper endoscopy (Figure 1) and we

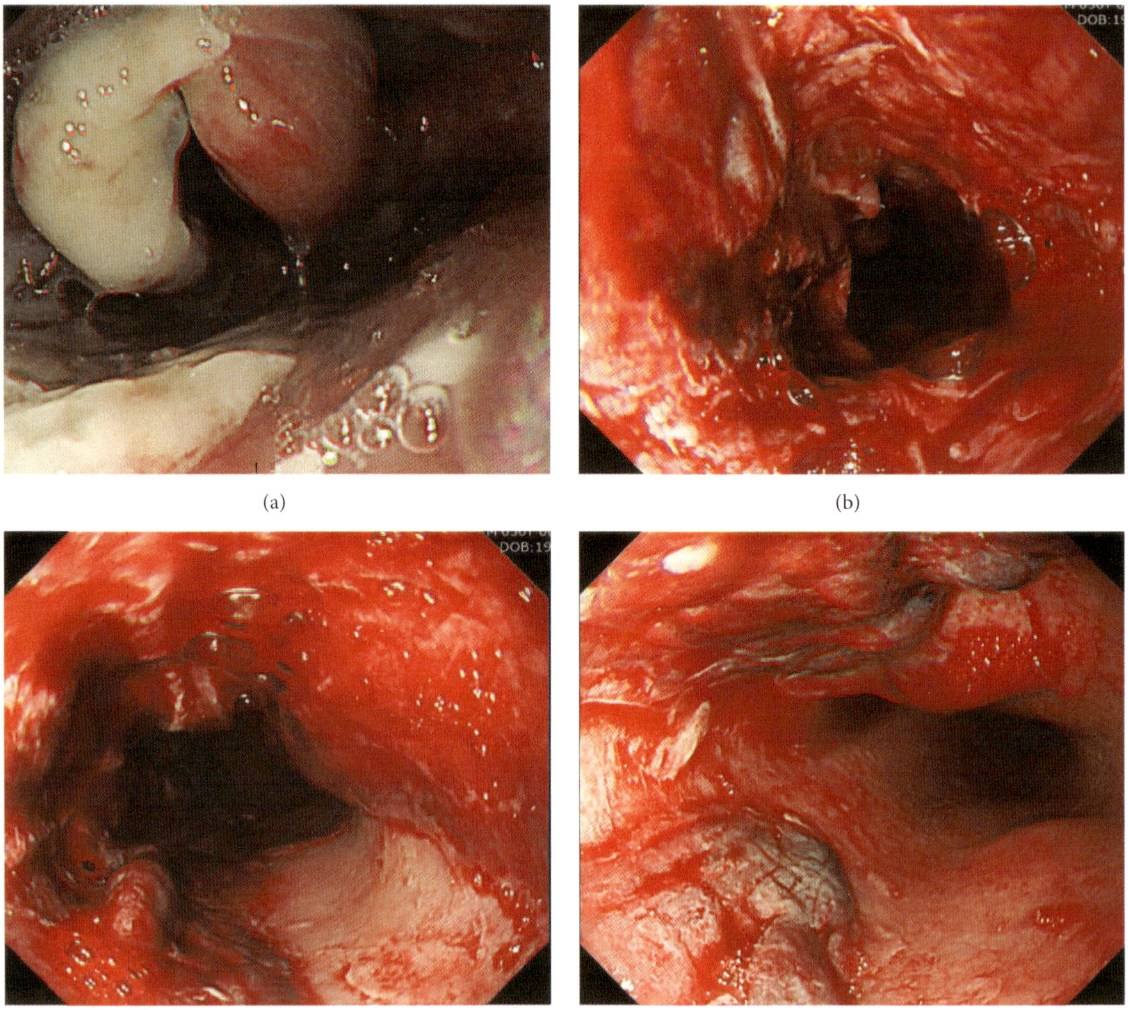

(a) (b) (c) (d)

FIGURE 1: Upper endoscopy at admission. The epiglottis appeared swollen with moderate mucosal injury (a). Diffuse edematous and friable mucosa with deep ulceration and hemorrhage from the upper (b) to mid-esophagus ((c) and (d)).

detected diffuse edematous and friable mucosa with deep ulceration and oozing bleeding from the upper (Figure 1(b)) to mid-esophagus (Figures 1(c) and 1(d)). The epiglottis appeared swollen, although he did not complain of dyspnea (Figure 1(a)). Chest CT revealed diffuse mild esophageal wall thickening (Figure 2). Esophageal perforation or mediastinitis was not detected. The patient was diagnosed with acute thermal injury of esophagus by PSMC powder. During his hospital stay, he was treated conservatively, including fasting, empirical antibiotics, and parenteral nutritional support. Seven days after admission, endoscopy revealed that diffuse ulcerative lesions were improved with no more bleeding (Figures 3(a) and 3(b)). He started on a liquid diet and was discharged without any symptoms. Endoscopy one month later showed mild scarring without stricture (Figures 3(c) and 3(d)), and he was free of symptoms.

3. Discussion

Acute thermal injuries of the esophagus can be caused by ingestion of hot solid or liquid materials [4–10]. The esophageal thermal injury caused by ingestion of hot liquid materials is characterized by a candy-cane appearance of alternating bands of whitish pseudomembrane and linear erythema [4–6]. On the other hand, esophageal injuries resulting from eating solid foods such as hot jelly roll [7], hamburger [8], and hot steamed eggs [9] appeared as a localized ulcer [7–9]. The reason for the different endoscopic findings from liquid and solid materials is that the candy-cane esophagus is caused by the transient rapid flow of hot liquids, whereas localized ulcers are caused by the pressure effect of hot solids. Therefore, the appearance of thermal injury of the esophagus varies depending on the type of ingested substance. In this case, not only localized deep ulcers but also linear erythema was observed in the esophagus. The reason for these atypical endoscopic findings was that the patient swallowed PSMC powder and drank water, resulting in slow movement of the semiliquid material from the pharynx to the upper esophagus.

PSMC is a low volume bowel cleansing agent that was introduced to the Korean market in 2011, although it has been

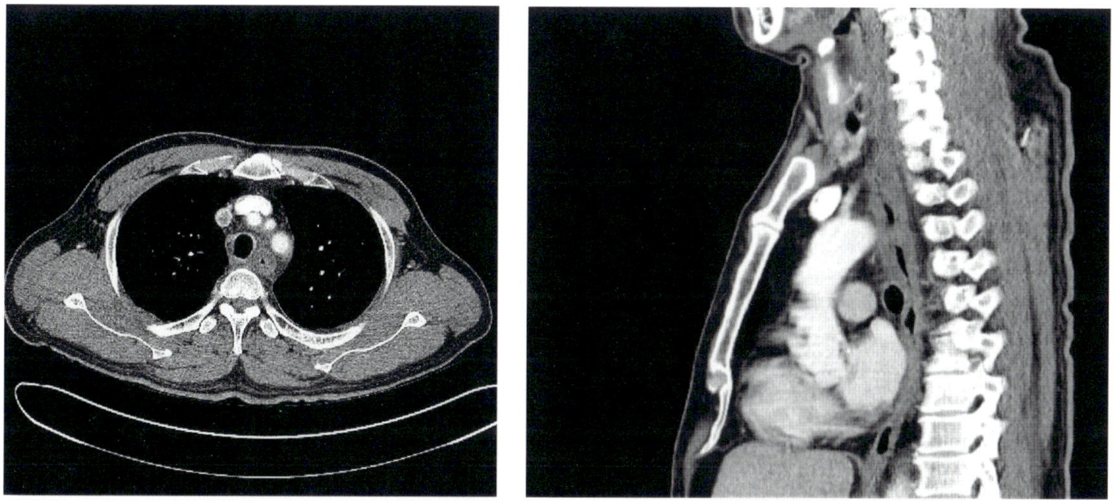

(a) (b)

Figure 2: Chest computed tomography (CT). Transverse plain (a) and sagittal plain (b) images of the chest CT showed diffuse esophageal wall edema and thickening. However, esophageal perforation or mediastinitis was not detected.

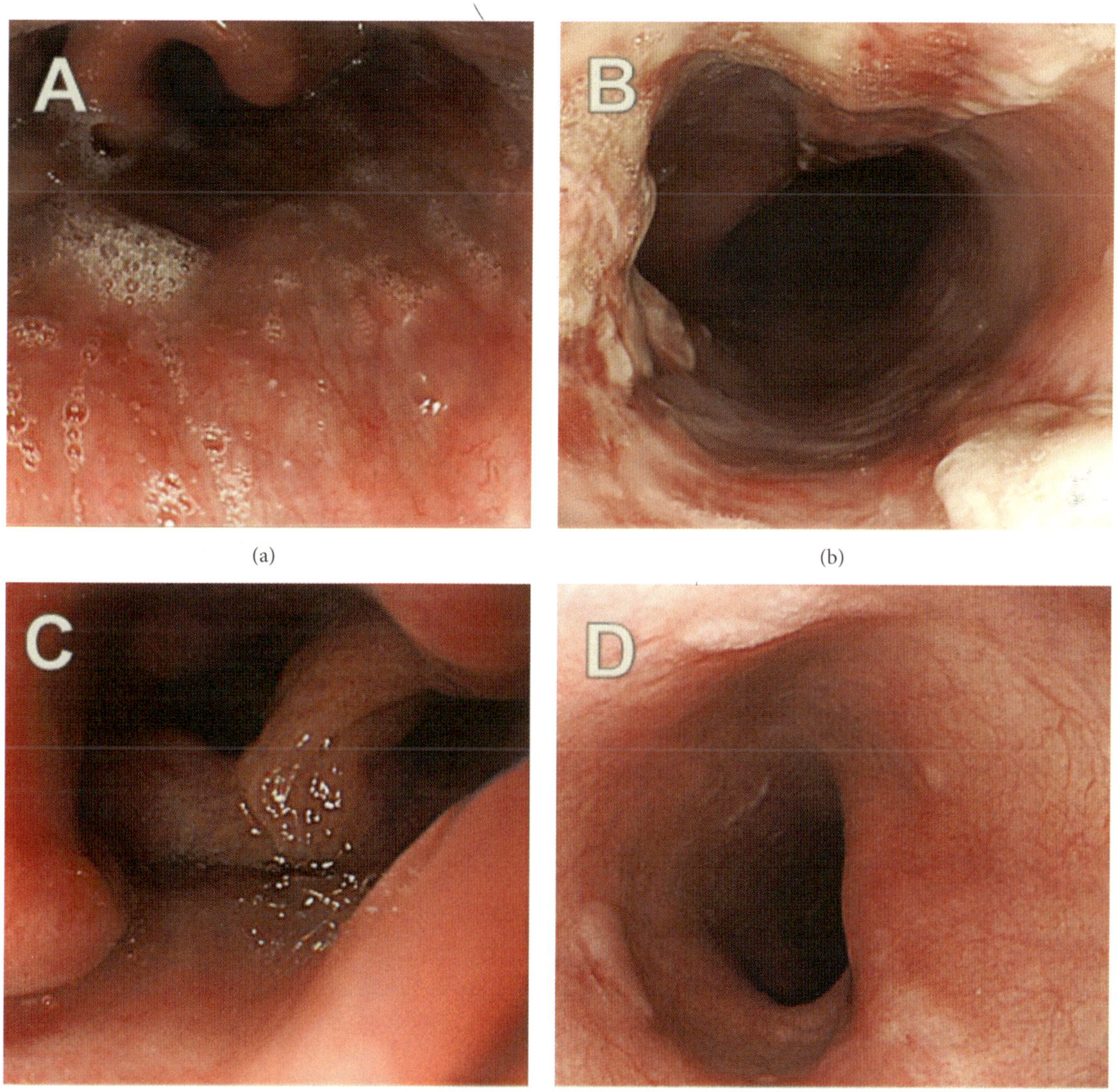

(a) (b)

(c) (d)

Figure 3: Upper endoscopy after conservative treatment. Endoscopic finding one week after thermal injury ((a) and (b)). The epiglottis was nearly healed and diffuse ulcerative lesions of the esophagus were improving without more bleeding. Endoscopic finding one month after thermal injury ((c) and (d)). The epiglottis was completely healed and whitish scars were seen in the esophagus.

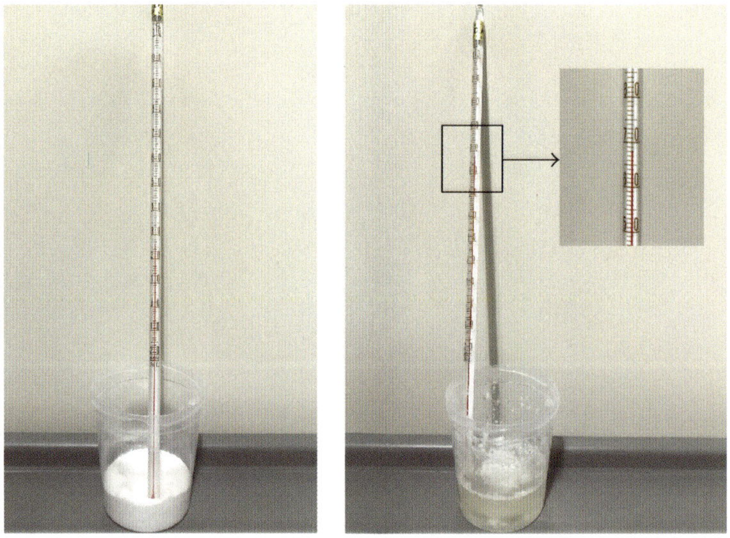

(a) (b)

Figure 4: Exothermic reaction of Picolight® powder. (a) A pack of Picolight powder in a plastic container. The temperature of the powder was 25°C. (b) The temperature was measured immediately after mixing the Picolight powder with 30 cc of water. The temperature rose to 68°C.

used widely for more than 20 years in European countries [11]. A pack of picosulfate with magnesium citrate (Picolight powder, Pharmbio, Seoul, Korea) consists of 10 mg of sodium picosulfate, 3.5 g of magnesium oxide, and 12 g of anhydrous citric acid. An exothermic reaction occurs when magnesium oxide reacts with anhydrous citric acid to form magnesium citrate ($MgO + C_6H_8O_7 + H_2O \rightarrow C_6H_6MgO_7 + 2H_2O$). To confirm the exothermic reaction, the authors measured the temperature change after dissolving a pack of PSMC powder in water. When a pack of PSMC powder was poured into 30 mL of water and stirred, it boiled and the temperature rose to 68°C (Figure 4). Third-degree burn of skin can occur when hot water at 69°C contacts the skin for several seconds [12]. Thus, drinking water after swallowing PSMC powder will cause a severe thermal injury to the esophagus. In addition, when PSMC powder is dissolved in a small amount of water, it produces a strong acidic liquid, leading to corrosive esophagitis [13]. Therefore, although PSMC powder is considered safe, incorrect usage may lead to severe side events such as thermal injury of esophagus or stomach. It is recommended that PSMC should be completely dissolved in sufficient quantity of water and cooled before drinking. According to drug instructions, the PSMC powder should be dissolved in 150 mL of water before drinking.

To date, four cases of PSMC-related thermal injuries have been reported in Korea, including our case. The thermal injury occurred in the upper esophagus in our case, and in other cases it occurred in the esophagus and stomach [11, 14] and stomach [15]. Fortunately, all cases recovered with conservative management without complications such as esophageal stricture or perforation. However, considering the fact that PSMC is widely used as a colon cleansing agent and the fact that many cases of thermal injury may not have been reported, clinicians should educate the patients about exactly how to use this medicine to prevent these thermal injuries.

Treatment of esophageal thermal injury is conservative, including fasting, hydration, administration of proton pump inhibitor, and empirical antibiotics. The prognosis is generally favorable [4–10]. No esophageal stricture or perforation has been reported as a complication of esophageal thermal injury.

In conclusion, we report a case of esophageal thermal injury caused by the incorrect use of PSMC. Although acute thermal injury of esophagus has a favorable prognosis, appropriate management and careful observation are needed to prevent further damage. Endoscopists and dispensing pharmacists should educate patients to not swallow PSMC powder for bowel preparation.

Acknowledgments

This research was supported by the Inha University Research Grant.

References

[1] K. S. Choi, J. K. Jun, H.-Y. Lee, M.-I. Hahm, J. H. Oh, and E.-C. Park, "Increasing uptake of colorectal cancer screening in Korea: a population-based study," *BMC Public Health*, vol. 10, article no. 265, 2010.

[2] J. Love, E.-J. Bernard, A. Cockeram et al., "A multicentre, observational study of sodium picosulfate and magnesium citrate as a precolonoscopy bowel preparation," *Canadian Journal of Gastroenterology*, vol. 23, no. 10, pp. 706–710, 2009.

[3] S. M. Hoy, L. J. Scott, and A. J. Wagstaff, "Sodium picosulfate/magnesium citrate: a review of its use as a colorectal cleanser," *Drugs*, vol. 69, no. 1, pp. 123–136, 2009.

[4] S. K. Dutta, K. Y. Chung, and B. S. Bhagavan, "Thermal injury of the esophagus," *New England Journal of Medicine*, vol. 339, no. 7, pp. 480-481, 1998.

[5] M. E. Cohen and J. G. Kegel, "Candy cocaine esophagus," *Chest*, vol. 121, no. 5, pp. 1701–1703, 2002.

[6] E. K. Choi, H. L. Gin, H.-Y. Jung et al., "The healing course of thermal esophageal injury: a case report," *Gastrointestinal Endoscopy*, vol. 62, no. 1, pp. 158–160, 2005.

[7] D. A. Lieberman and E. B. Keeffe, "Esophageal burn and the microwave oven.," *Annals of Internal Medicine*, vol. 97, no. 1, p. 137, 1982.

[8] R. Eliakim, "Thermal injury from a hamburger: a rare cause of odynophagia," *Gastrointestinal Endoscopy*, vol. 50, no. 2, pp. 282-283, 1999.

[9] S. M. Kim, S. H. Jung, and Y. M. Kim, "Esophageal ulcer by thermal injury from steamed egg," *Korean Journal of Gastrointestinal Endoscopy*, vol. 32, no. 3, pp. 190–193, 2006.

[10] J. H. Lee, H. J. Kim, and T. H. Kim, "A case of epoxy resin induced thermal injury in upper gastrointestinal tract," *Korean Journal of Gastrointestinal Endoscopy*, vol. 30, no. 6, pp. 325–329, 2005.

[11] J. P. Suh, Y. S. Choi, and S. H. Lee, "Education and Imaging. Gastroenterology: acute mucosal injury of esophagus and stomach induced by sodium picosulfate/magnesium citrate for bowel preparation," *Journal of Gastroenterology and Hepatology (Australia)*, vol. 29, no. 8, p. 1571, 2014.

[12] A. R. Moritz and F. C. Henriques, "Studies of thermal injury: II. The relative importance of time and surface temperature in the causation of cutaneous curns," *The American Journal of Pathology*, vol. 23, no. 5, pp. 695–720, 1947.

[13] K. Ramasamy and V. V. Gumaste, "Corrosive ingestion in adults," *Journal of Clinical Gastroenterology*, vol. 37, no. 2, pp. 119–124, 2003.

[14] J. Y. Seo, K. J. Kang, H. S. Kang et al., "Corrosive esophagitis caused by ingestion of picosulfate," *Clinical Endoscopy*, vol. 48, no. 1, pp. 66–69, 2015.

[15] D. S. Lee, H. S. Kim, S. H. Lee, J. H. Jeon, and Y. K. Lee, "A case of PICOLIGHT powder induced thermal injury of the gastric mucosa," *The Korean Journal of Helicobacter and Upper Gastrointestinal Research*, vol. 14, no. 1, pp. 58–60, 2014.

52

Combined Approach of Cryoablation and Stent-In-Stent Technique for Removal of an Embedded Esophageal Stent

Madhuri Chandnani, Jonah Cohen, and Tyler M. Berzin

Center for Advanced Endoscopy, Division of Gastroenterology, Beth Israel Deaconess Medical Center and Harvard Medical School, Boston, MA, USA

Correspondence should be addressed to Madhuri Chandnani; mchandna@bidmc.harvard.edu

Academic Editor: Hirotada Akiho

Self-expanding removable stents are used for the treatment of esophageal strictures. Partially covered metal stents become embedded in the esophageal wall due to mucosal tissue reaction providing good anchorage. This can also lead to extreme difficulty in the removal of such stents. Several different individual techniques have been used in literature for removal of these esophageal stents. Ours is the first case using a combination of cryoablation and stent-in-stent technique for removal of an extremely difficult case of embedded esophageal stent.

1. Introduction

Self-expanding removable esophageal stents have been used in a variety of conditions including refractory or recurrent benign esophageal strictures, malignant obstructions, tracheoesophageal fistula, perforations, or leaks [1]. Self-expanding plastic stents (SEPS) were initially thought to be very successful in treating benign esophageal conditions, but newer studies have shown self-expanding metal stents (SEMS) being more effective than SEPS in treating both benign and malignant cases of dysphagia due to the higher rate of stent migration, recurrence of symptoms, and technical difficulties with SEPS [1, 2].

Fully covered SEMS (FC-SEMS) are appropriate for benign disease because the complete stent coating prevents tissue ingrowth and allows for reliable endoscopic removal of the stent. Partially covered SEMS (PC-SEMS) with its proximal and distal exposed bare metal flares and uncovered SEMS typically develop reactive mucosal tissue hypertrophy causing tissue ingrowth into the stent interstices, which can help lower migration rates, but render such stents often unremovable [1–3]; thus these stents should typically only be used for patients with malignancy. Various techniques have been described for the retrieval of PC-SEMS, once they have become embedded, including a 'stent-in-stent' technique, whereby a fully covered stent is deployed inside the embedded stent, causing pressure necrosis of the ingrown tissue, potentially allowing removal of both stents later. Here, we report the use of a combination of cryoablation and 'stent-in-stent' technique for retrieval of a fully embedded esophageal PC-SEMS.

2. Case

A 72-year-old man with history of localized esophageal carcinoma with a history of neoadjuvant chemoradiation and esophagectomy presented to a local hospital with dysphagia four months after the surgery. Endoscopy revealed a benign-appearing esophageal stricture at the site of the anastomosis, and biopsies confirmed benign tissue. He was treated with a series of esophageal dilations and temporary placement of a FC-SEMS by his surgeon. This stent was removed after 3 months of placement; however, the patient developed recurrent symptoms after several weeks. Given no evidence of cancer recurrence, a 100 mm × 23 mm Wallflex PC-SEMS (Boston Scientific, Natick, MA) was placed by his surgeon as an attempt for a permanent solution to the patient's dysphagia.

The patient developed recurrent dysphagia after 3 months. A CT chest with oral contrast demonstrated the

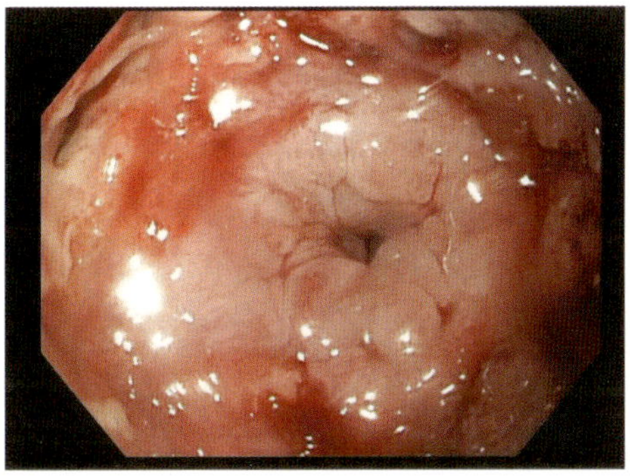

Figure 1: Embedded stent with tissue ingrowth.

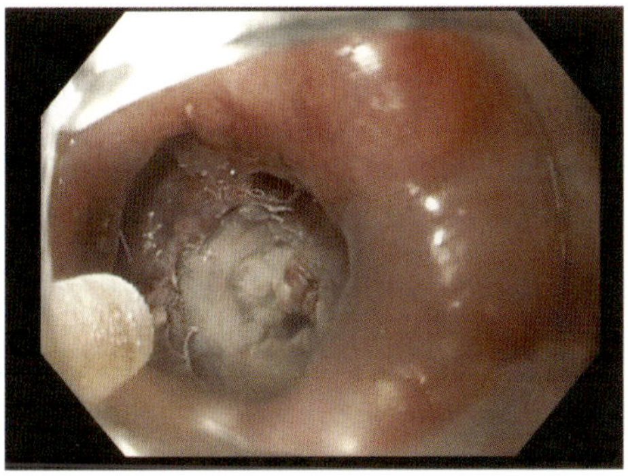

Figure 2: Cryoablation of tissue ingrowth of stent.

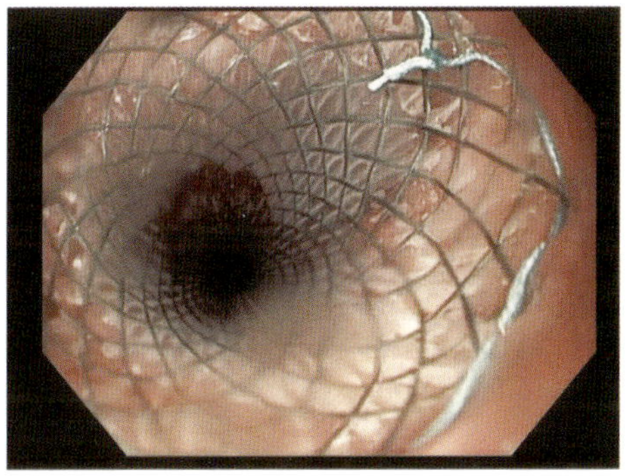

Figure 3: New fully covered stent-in-stent placement.

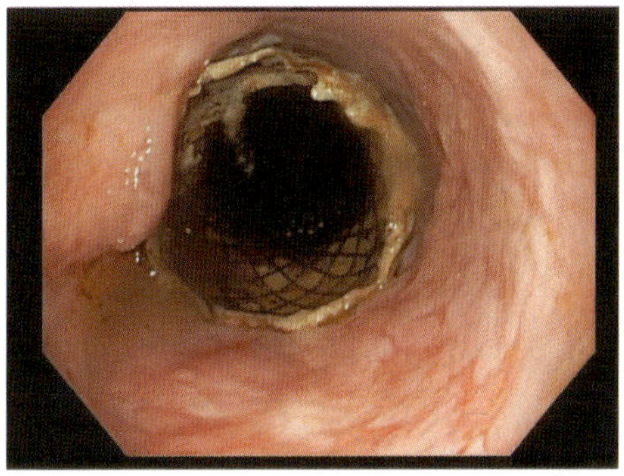

Figure 4: Fully covered esophageal stent.

PC-SEMS in appropriate position at the anastomosis but demonstrated evidence of circumferential soft tissue extending approximately 2 cm in length and 7 mm in depth nearly occluding the proximal side of the stent. An upper endoscopy confirmed the above finding, and biopsies which concluded this represent benign and hypertrophic tissue.

This patient was then referred to our institution for further management and consideration of stent removal. At the time of referral, the PC-SEMS had been in place for almost 5 months. Repeat endoscopy demonstrated a benign-appearing stricture in midesophagus, beyond which the standard 9.8 mm endoscope could not pass. An ultraSlim 5.5 mm gastroscope was then advanced through the stricture, and the stent was identified beneath the tissue ingrowth and extending across the anastomosis. The proximal edges of the stent were not visible and fully covered by tissue ingrowth (Figure 1). Cryoablation of the tissue ingrowth was performed using the CryoSpray (TruFreeze, Lexington, MA) Ablation (Figure 2) for 20 seconds, followed by placement of a 125 mm × 23 mm Wallflex FC-SEMS (Boston Scientific, Natick, MA) within the previously placed PC-SEMS (Figure 3) in order to promote tissue necrosis and permit subsequent removal of both stents. This rescue FC-SEMS was removed after 2 weeks on repeat endoscopy, with less tissue ingrowth visible on the proximal end and with no stricture evident. An attempt was made to remove the PC-SEMS but was unsuccessful. Thus, a 125 mm × 23 mm Wallflex FC-SEMS was again placed within the embedded PC-SEMS. Endoscopy was repeated after 4 months with successful removal of the rescue FC-SEMS. Less hypertrophic tissue was seen at the proximal end of the PC-SEMS and the PC-SEMS was now able to be pulled away from the embedded stent's proximal margin mucosa. Given the distal end of the stent which was still embedded, the stent was unable to be removed safely. Thus, another 125 mm × 23 mm Wallflex FC-SEMS was placed within the PC-SEMS. A repeat endoscopy was performed at 6 months with successful retrieval of both the FC-SEMS (Figure 4) and PC-SEMS (Figures 5 and 6) with minimal resistance with the help of rat-tooth forceps under fluoroscopic guidance. The patient was symptom-free and was started on high dose oral proton pump inhibitor with slow taper to a low daily dose.

3. Discussion

Various techniques have been described in the literature for PC-SEMS retrieval such as using rat-tooth forceps, argon plasma coagulation (APC) [4, 5], piecemeal extraction [6], and 'stent-in-stent' technique. In this case, cryoablation was initially used to facilitate reduction of the amount of granulation tissue ingrowth allowing the reopening of the esophageal diameter and passage of endoscope to place a "rescue" FC-SEMS inside the previously placed PC-SEMS, which subsequently helped to regress the esophageal wall tissue hypertrophy with pressure necrosis allowing for eventual retrieval of the embedded PC-SEMS.

Cryoablation has been used for the treatment of benign, dysplastic, and neoplastic lesions of the esophagus [7–9]. The

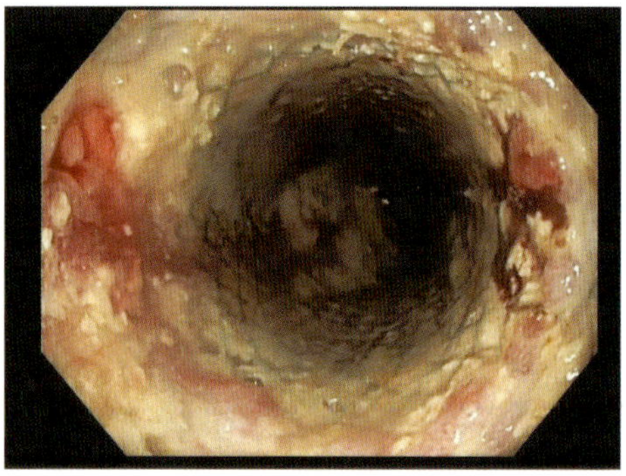

FIGURE 5: Partially covered esophageal stent after removal of the fully covered stent.

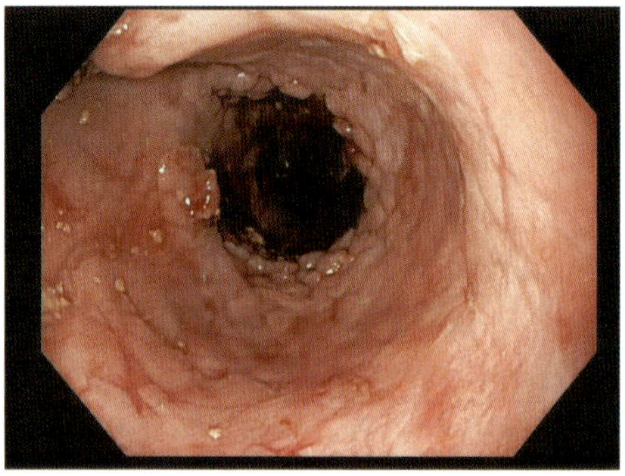

FIGURE 6: After removal of partially covered stent.

major advantages of cryoablation over other forms of ablation are that it does not require tissue contact for application, so a small probe can be used for narrow lumen esophagus; it causes less pain and does not typically necessitate use of prophylactic pain meds; and it is shown to have less rate of stricture formation after the procedure [7, 10]. It is our belief that for treatment of extensive tissue ingrowth, cryoablation may also be safer than prolonged use of various cautery methods for treating tissue adjacent to a metal stent, which may transmit heat to surrounding tissue, or may even melt when APC is used in certain settings.

Hirdes et al. [11] reported the safety and efficacy of 'stent-in-stent' technique using FC-SEMS or SEPS for safe removal of embedded PC-SEMS. In 2 of the 23 cases, persistent tissue hyperplasia was seen after removal of the rescue fully covered stent, and the 'stent-in-stent' technique had to be repeated once more before successful retrieval of embedded stents. There was severe bleeding noted in 1 case requiring treatment with argon plasma coagulation and blood transfusion. On review of literature, no other major complications have been reported using this technique. Stent-in-stent technique is known to be a safe and feasible method for the removal of an embedded esophageal stent [12–14]. The rescue stents are generally fully covered and are long enough to cover the entire stenotic area with diameter at least same as or bigger than the embedded PC-SEMS. It has also been used for retrieval of an embedded stent in colon wall in one case report [15].

Low and Kozarek [16] have proposed other methods of stent retrieval based on stent designs such as removing a Z-stent by invaginating the proximal edge of the stent and grasping it with a polyp snare or using rat-tooth forceps to grasp and pull the distal edge of an Ultraflex PC-SEMS off the esophageal wall, resulting in invagination of the distal stent on itself. The distal invagination technique is more suitable for the more flexible stents.

Chandrasekhar et al. [17] describe the use of 'double-step invagination technique' wherein the embedded PC-SEMS stent is retrieved in 2 steps, after pressure necrosis has been achieved with stent-in-stent technique. First, traction is applied to the distal edge of the stent with alligator forceps resulting in invagination of the distal edge of the PC-SEMS on itself, occluding the lumen of the stent. The second step is to grasp the in-folded distal edge with alligator forceps and apply gentle traction resulting in further invagination of the remaining portion of PC-SEMS within itself with successful extraction of the stent.

In cases like ours with tissue embedding at both the proximal and distal ends, stripping of the stent using forceps or invagination techniques was difficult with a significant risk of complications. Reducing the tissue burden with a combination of cryoablation and stent-in-stent technique provided greater chances of successful stent retraction and should be considered a valid clinical option for removal of embedded esophageal stents.

References

[1] P. Sharma, R. Kozarek, and J. M. Inadomi, "Role of esophageal stents in benign and malignant diseases," *American Journal of Gastroenterology*, vol. 105, no. 2, pp. 258–273, 2010.

[2] P. Hindy, J. Hong, Y. Lam-Tsai, and F. Gress, "A Comprehensive Review of Esophageal Stents. Gastroenterol Hepatol," *Gastroenterol Hepatol*, vol. 8, no. 8, pp. 526–534, 2012.

[3] N. Vakil, U. Gross, and N. Bethge, "Human tissue responses to metal stents," *Gastrointestinal Endoscopy Clinics of North America*, vol. 9, no. 3, pp. 359–365, 1999.

[4] P. Eisendrath, M. Cremer, J. Himpens, G. B. Cadière, O. le Moine, and J. Devière, "Endotherapy including temporary stenting of fistulas of the upper gastrointestinal tract after laparoscopic bariatric surgery," *Endoscopy*, vol. 39, no. 7, pp. 625–630, 2007.

[5] F. Fiocca, F. Cereatti, P. Antypas, and G. Donatelli, "Argon plasma coagulation: A less-expensive alternative to the "stent-in-stent" technique for removal of embedded partially covered esophageal stents," *Gastrointestinal Endoscopy*, vol. 83, no. 2, p. 453, 2016.

[6] P. D. Siersema, M. Y. V. Homs, J. Haringsma, H. W. Tilanus, and E. J. Kuipers, "Use of large-diameter metallic stents to seal traumatic nonmalignant perforations of the esophagus," *Gastrointestinal Endoscopy*, vol. 58, no. 3, pp. 356–361, 2003.

[7] G. B. Smallfield, "Endoscopic cryotherapy for Barrett esophagus," *Journal of Gastroenterology and Hepatology*, vol. 11, no. 11, pp. 770–772, 2015.

[8] N. J. Shaheen, B. D. Greenwald, A. F. Peery et al., "Safety and efficacy of endoscopic spray cryotherapy for Barrett's esophagus with high-grade dysplasia," *Gastrointestinal Endoscopy*, vol. 71, no. 4, pp. 680–685, 2010.

[9] A. M. Chen and P. J. Pasricha, "Cryotherapy for Barrett's Esophagus: Who, How, and Why?" *Gastrointestinal Endoscopy Clinics of North America*, vol. 21, no. 1, pp. 111–118, 2011.

[10] A. Overwater and B. L. A. M. Weusten, "Cryoablation in the management of Barrett's esophagus," *Current Opinion in Gastroenterology*, vol. 33, no. 4, pp. 261–269, 2017.

[11] M. M. C. Hirdes, P. D. Siersema, M. H. M. G. Houben, B. L. A. M. Weusten, and F. P. Vleggaar, "Stent-in-stent technique for removal of embedded esophageal self-expanding metal stents," *American Journal of Gastroenterology*, vol. 106, no. 2, pp. 286–293, 2011.

[12] A. Aiolfi, D. Bona, C. Ceriani, M. Porro, and L. Bonavina, "Stent-in-stent, a safe and effective technique to remove fully embedded esophageal metal stents: case series and literature review," *Endoscopy International Open*, vol. 03, no. 04, pp. E296–E299, 2015.

[13] M. C. W. Spaander, T. H. Baron, P. D. Siersema et al., "Esophageal stenting for benign and malignant disease: European Society of Gastrointestinal Endoscopy (ESGE) Clinical Guideline," *Endoscopy*, vol. 48, no. 10, pp. 939–948, 2016.

[14] G. Vasilikostas, N. Sanmugalingam, O. Khan, M. Reddy, C. Groves, and A. Wan, "'Stent in a stent' - An alternative technique for removing partially covered stents following sleeve gastrectomy complications," *Obesity Surgery*, vol. 24, no. 3, pp. 430–432, 2014.

[15] J. B. Gornals, T. Golda, and A. Soriano, "Stent-in-stent technique for removal of a metal stent embedded in the colon wall by using a fully covered, self-expandable metal esophageal stent (with video)," *Gastrointestinal Endoscopy*, vol. 76, no. 3, pp. 695-696, 2012.

[16] D. E. Low and R. A. Kozarek, "Removal of esophageal expandable metal stents: Description of technique and review of potential applications," *Surgical Endoscopy*, vol. 17, no. 6, pp. 990–996, 2003.

[17] T. S. Chandrasekar, R. Y. Kalamegam, G. B. Janakan, S. Suriyanarayanan, P. S. Menta, and V. T. Chandrasekar, "Double-step invagination technique—A novel approach to retrieve embedded esophageal self-expanding metal stent," *Indian Journal of Gastroenterology*, vol. 36, no. 5, pp. 424–428, 2017.

53

Pyogenic Liver Abscess with No Predisposing Risk Factors

Matthew Chadwick,[1] Leonid Shamban,[2] and Michael Neumann[2]

[1]*Department of Internal Medicine, Genesys Regional Medical Center, 1 Genesys Pkwy, Grand Blanc, MI 48439, USA*
[2]*Department of Gastroenterology, Genesys Regional Medical Center, 1 Genesys Pkwy, Grand Blanc, MI 48439, USA*

Correspondence should be addressed to Matthew Chadwick; Matthew.Chadwick@ascension.org

Academic Editor: Yoshihiro Moriwaki

Pyogenic liver abscesses (PLA) are an uncommon cause of hospitalization in the United States. The majority of such cases are polymicrobial and are most commonly caused by seeding of infection from the biliary system. PLA is frequently associated with specific comorbidities such as diabetes mellitus, history of liver transplant, underlying hepatobiliary, or pancreatic disease. Herein, we describe a 47-year-old healthy male with no known risk factors associated with PLA who presented to the hospital with acute fever, abdominal pain, and dark colored urine. Initially the patient had a negative right upper quadrant ultrasound. However, the patient continued to have persistent fevers and abnormal liver biochemistries with negative liver serology that led to checking a magnetic resonance cholangiopancreatography which suggested multiple liver abscesses. Computer tomography guided aspiration revealed a monobacterial *Streptococcus* species within the abscess, which is commonly associated with arterial bacteremia as a source of PLA. Arterial bacteremia is one of most rare causes of PLA. The patient's septic workup was negative for any source of infection. This case demonstrates a patient with no risk factors who was diagnosed with PLA caused by apparent arterial bacteremia with no clear source of infection.

1. Introduction

Commonly the identifiable causes of pyogenic liver abscesses (PLA) have been attributed to hematogenous seeding, biliary, or contiguous spread [1]. Previous reports suggest that biliary spread has been associated with *E. coli*, portal vein seeding has been associated with *Streptococcus anginosus*, and cryptogenic causes have been associated with *Klebsiella* [2]. Certain risk factors including diabetes, underlying hepatobiliary or pancreatic disease, history of liver transplant, and chronic use of proton-pump inhibitors (PPI) are typically present in patients with pyogenic hepatic abscesses [3]. Herein we describe a case of cryptogenic streptococcus pyogenic liver abscess in an otherwise healthy male with no risk factors.

2. Case Presentation

A 43-year-old Caucasian male with a past medical history significant for depression which was well controlled with Prozac presented to the Emergency Department with nausea, vomiting, myalgias, and dark colored urine. He admitted to recent travel to Virginia Beach but denied any history of travel outside of the United States. He denied any high risk sexual behavior, previous blood transfusions, or intravenous (IV) drug use. He worked as a police officer with limited field work exposure. He denied any new medications including antibiotics; acetaminophen containing products; nonsteroidal medications; or over-the-counter herbal medications, vitamins, or supplements. He had no previous surgical history or dental procedures and family history was unremarkable for chronic liver disease or gastrointestinal (GI) pathology. His review of systems was negative except for subjective fevers, abdominal pain, diarrhea, and the aforementioned symptoms.

He was evaluated in the Emergency Department and was found to be tachycardic, tachypneic, and febrile with a maximum temperature of 103.1°F. Physical exam revealed a well appearing Caucasian male in no distress who was alert and oriented to place, person, and time. He was noted to have scleral icterus. Cardiovascular exam revealed tachycardia

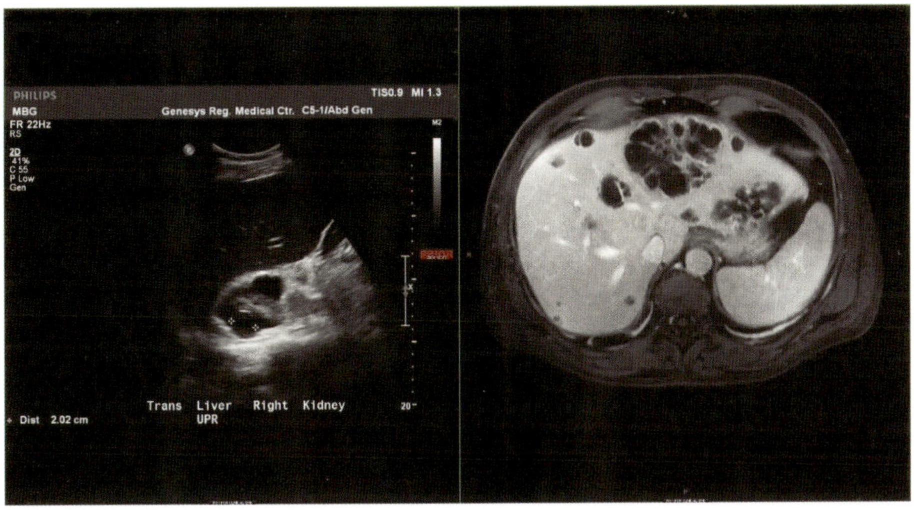

FIGURE 1: Transverse imaging showing initial negative ultrasound (left) and follow-up MRCP showing liver abscesses (right).

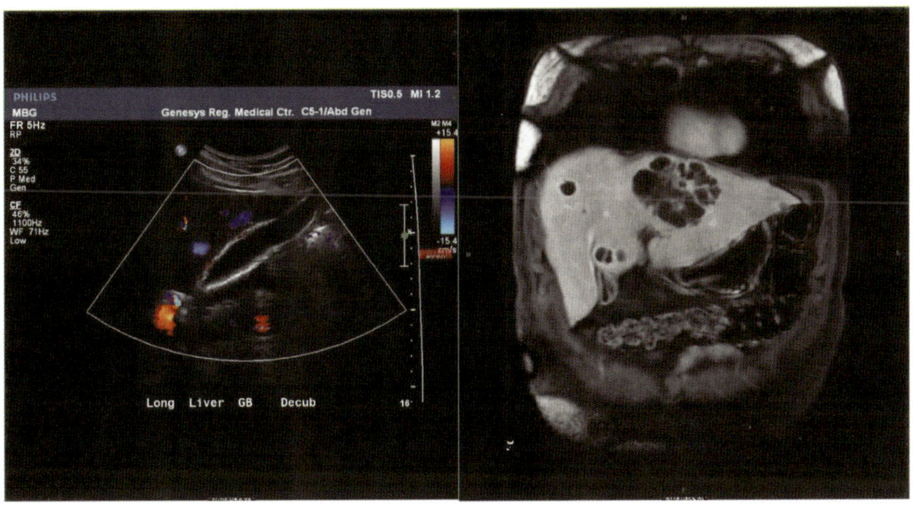

FIGURE 2: Long imaging showing initial negative ultrasound (left) and follow-up coronal MRCP showing liver abscesses (right).

with no murmurs, rubs, or gallops. Pulmonary exam was clear to auscultation without any rales, rhonchi, or wheezing. Abdominal exam revealed a soft, nontender, nondistended abdomen with positive bowel sounds without palpable ascites or organomegaly. Dermatological exam revealed jaundice but no erythema or wounds. Examination of the extremities revealed no evidence of edema, nail splinter hemorrhages, palmar Janeway lesions, or palmar Osler nodes. Initial laboratory evaluation revealed elevated liver biochemistries with an AST of 45 U/L, ALT of 93 U/L, alkaline phosphatase of 139 U/L, total bilirubin of 5.4 mg/dL, direct bilirubin of 2.7 mg/dL, white blood cell count of 15.1 K/cmm, hemoglobin of 14.1 g/dL, platelets of 240 K/cmm, and an INR of 1.50. The patient's alkaline phosphatase was only mildly elevated; therefore the decision was made not to order a gamma-glutamyltransferase. Patient was started on empiric ceftriaxone and admitted to the hospital.

Follow-up evaluation included a viral hepatitis panel (Table 1). A right upper quadrant abdominal ultrasound with Doppler flow was performed which showed a normal appearing liver without suspicious mass or biliary duct dilation, an unremarkable gallbladder, a 4 mm common bile duct, and an unremarkable liver Doppler interrogation (Figures 1 and 2).

The patient continued to have persistent symptoms of myalgias, fevers, and jaundice; therefore the gastroenterology service was consulted to evaluate the patient. Additional liver serology revealed an acetaminophen level of <5 mcg/mL, salicylate level <0.3 mg/dL, and a ceruloplasmin of 41 mg/dL, and iron studies revealed an iron level of 16 μg/dl, total iron binding capacity of 171 μg/dl, iron saturation of 9.4%, and a ferritin of 1914.0 ng/mL, which were consistent with inflammatory process. His autoimmune workup revealed negative smooth muscle and antimitochondrial antibodies with an ANA of <1:40.

At the same time the Infectious Disease (ID) service was consulted and a full septic workup was pursued including the workup noted in Table 1. Doxycycline was added to the regimen until chlamydia was ruled out. The patient continued

Table 1: Infectious disease workup.

Test	Results
Hepatitis A IgM	Nonreactive
Hepatitis B Surface Antigen	Nonreactive
Hepatitis B Core Antibody IgM	Nonreactive
Hepatitis C Antibody	Nonreactive
Hepatitis C Viral RNA	<30 IU/mL
Influenza A	Negative
Influenza B	Negative
Urine Culture	No growth
Epstein Barr Viral Antibody IgG	137.0 U/ml
Epstein Barr Viral Antibody IgM	<10.0 U/ml
Cytomegalovirus Antibody IgG	1.50 U/ml
Cytomegalovirus Antibody IgM	<8.0 AU/mL
N. Gonorrhea PCR	Not detected
C. trachomatis PCR	Not detected
RPR	Non-reactive
Giardia Lamblia	Negative
Cryptosporidium	Negative

to have persistent fevers and elevated liver biochemistries with an AST of 51 U/L, ALT of 61 U/L, alkaline phosphatase of 136 U/L, total bilirubin of 3.5 mg/dl, and an INR of 1.36 and therefore on his fourth day in the hospital a magnetic resonance cholangiopancreatography (MRCP) was performed which showed abnormal liver lesions concerning for multiple abscesses given the rapid change from the recent ultrasound.

Interventional radiology was consulted and using computerized tomography (CT) the largest abscess was able to be drained and produced foul-smelling turbid yellow fluid. The cultures revealed streptococcus, not group D, although the lab noted that they were not able to provide susceptibility due to the fastidious nature of the organism. Two sets of blood cultures were obtained and were negative at 120 hours. Due to the negative blood cultures and lack of physical exam findings consistent with endocarditis the ID service determined that echocardiogram was not necessary. The patient began to improve clinically, a PICC line was inserted, and the patient was discharged home on ceftriaxone. Two months later the patient had a follow-up CT of the abdomen and pelvis with and without IV contrast which showed improvement in the liver abscesses and an otherwise unremarkable liver, gallbladder, and biliary tree. Four months later the patient had a colonoscopy performed which showed no evidence of diverticular disease.

3. Discussion

PLA is estimated to have an annual incidence of 2.3 cases per 100,000 in the general population with a predominance of cases in males, with male: female ratio 1.3:1 [4, 5]. It is even more common amongst hospitalized patients, with one review showing an incidence of 8-22 cases per 100,000 hospital admissions [6]. PLA is the most common visceral abscess in the United States and accounts for nearly 48% of all visceral abscesses [7]. It is important to identify and treat these cases early as untreated PLA has been found to be unvaryingly fatal [8]. Even with treatment studies have found PLA to be fatal in 7.8 to 28.6% of cases [6].

Due to its fatality it is important to identify patients who may be at higher risk for developing PLA in order to aid in making a diagnosis. Several concomitant comorbid conditions have been associated with PLA including diabetes mellitus, biliary disease, hypertension, intra-abdominal infection, immunosuppression, pancreatic disease, liver transplant, malignant stricture, and inflammation of the GI tract [1, 7, 9, 10]. In the described case the patient did not have a history of hypertension, diabetes mellitus, liver transplant, or immunosuppression. The patient was only 43 years of age at the time of diagnosis, far younger than the mean age of 64 [2]. He also had extensive abdominal imaging including ultrasound, MRCP, and CT scan which did not reveal any evidence of biliary disease, pancreatic disease, malignant stricture, or inflammation in the GI tract. Studies have also shown an increased risk of PLA with PPI use [3]; however the patient had not been prescribed or taking over-the-counter PPI prior to his hospitalization.

The patient originally presented with nausea, vomiting, myalgia, and dark colored urine to the Emergency Department. The classic triad associated with PLA is compromised of fever, jaundice, and right upper quadrant abdominal pain although studies have shown that only 10% of patients with PLA present with all three symptoms [7]. More recently studies have shown that fever, chills, and abdominal pain are the three most common presenting symptoms of PLA [6, 11]. This patient did not demonstrate signs of abdominal discomfort or jaundice, although he did have persistent fevers throughout his hospital course.

In addition to these presenting symptoms the patient also had dark colored urine. While not classically associated with PLA there have been case reports of patients presenting with dark colored urine in a patient with PLA caused by *Klebsiella pneumonia* [4], while our patient's cultures were consistent with *Streptococcus*. To our knowledge there have been no reported cases of dark colored urine presenting from a patient with PLA caused by a *Streptococcus* species. The patient did also present with mildly elevated liver transaminases, which correlates with previous reports that streptococcus anginosus group often has less pronounced liver transaminases compared to other causes of PLA [12].

Previously appendicitis was the most common cause of PLA; however due to improved detection and treatment of appendicitis this is no longer a common cause of PLA [8]. The most common causes of PLA are biliary tract disease, portal bacteremia, contiguous spread of infection from intra-abdominal pathology, and intestinal disease [1, 3, 13]. Of these sources biliary tract disease has been found to be the most common cause of PLA in the United States, causing an estimated 50-60% of all cases [1, 8]. Portal bacteremia is the second most common cause of PLA accounting for 10-20% of all cases of PLA [1]. The most common cause of portal bacteremia is complicated sigmoid diverticulitis, with less common causes being supra-infected GI tumors and inflammatory bowel disease [1]. After biliary disease, perforated bowel has been found to be the next most common intra-abdominal cause of PLA formation [1, 14, 15]. Again, despite these being the most common cause of PLA our patient's lab work and imaging showed no evidence of biliary or other intra-abdominal pathology. It is noted however that abdominal ultrasound depends on the experience of the operator and may miss a slight dilation of the bile duct or small calculi in the bile duct in its retropancreatic portion. He also had blood cultures that were negative.

Another cause of PLA is arterial hematogenous spread, although this has been found to be a very rare cause [8, 9, 14]. The most common cause of arterial bacteremia leading to PLA formation is endocarditis, pyelonephritis, lung infections, peripheral suppurative thrombophlebitis in IV drug users, and oral infections [1, 8, 9]. These cases are usually found in patients with concomitant diabetes mellitus, leukemia, immunosuppression, or chronic granulomatous disease [1, 8]. There were no clinical signs of pulmonary, oral, or genitourinary infection during the patient's hospitalization. The patient denied any history of IV drug abuse and no clinical signs of thrombophlebitis were noted during his hospital stay. The patient did also have negative blood cultures and was determined by the ID team to be at minimal risk for infective endocarditis. In addition, there was no clinical evidence to suggest that the patient had diabetes mellitus, leukemia, immunosuppression, or chronic granulomatous disease.

The majority of cases of PLA are polymicrobial [3, 7, 14]. Monomicrobial PLA is more commonly associated with hematogenous spread, especially arterial origin [1, 7]. Studies have found that the majority of PLA from arterial bacteremia have positive blood cultures. Also 66% of PLA patients have positive blood cultures regardless of its origin [1, 6]. The three most common bacteria to cause PLA are *E. coli*, *Klebsiella pneumonia*, and *Streptococcus* species [7]. The patient in the above described case had a single organism, streptococcus not group D, cultured from his abscess. Monobacterial PLA, especially from *Streptococcus* species, is highly indicative of hematogenous spread [8]. Our patient had no evidence of bacteremia, no identifiable sources for bacteremia, and no evidence of concomitant comorbidities associated with arterial bacteremia known to cause PLA.

References

[1] S. Lardière-Deguelte, E. Ragot, K. Amroun et al., "Hepatic abscess: Diagnosis and management," *Journal of Visceral Surgery*, vol. 152, no. 4, pp. 231–243, 2015.

[2] T. C. Y. Pang, T. Fung, J. Samra, T. J. Hugh, and R. C. Smith, "Pyogenic liver abscess: An audit of 10 years' experience," *World Journal of Gastroenterology*, vol. 17, no. 12, pp. 1622–1630, 2011.

[3] H.-F. Lin, K.-F. Liao, C.-M. Chang, C.-L. Lin, and S.-W. Lai, "Correlation between proton pump inhibitors and risk of pyogenic liver abscess," *European Journal of Clinical Pharmacology*, vol. 73, no. 8, pp. 1019–1025, 2017.

[4] L. Deng, R. Jia, W. Li et al., "A Klebsiella pneumoniae liver abscess presenting with myasthenia and tea-colored urine: A case report and review of 77 cases of bacterial rhabdomyolysis," *Medicine (Baltimore)*, vol. 96, no. 51, Article ID e9458, 2017.

[5] A. H. Mohsen, S. T. Green, R. C. Read, and M. W. McKendrick, "Liver abscess in adults: Ten years experience in a UK centre," *QJM: Monthly Journal of the Association of Physicians*, vol. 95, no. 12, pp. 797–802, 2002.

[6] N.-P. Foo, K.-T. Chen, H.-J. Lin, and H.-R. Guo, "Characteristics of pyogenic liver abscess patients with and without diabetes mellitus," *American Journal of Gastroenterology*, vol. 105, no. 2, pp. 328–335, 2010.

[7] M. Barakat, S. Hernandez, J. Benoit, S. Pourshahid, Y. Mamoon, and G. T. Martin, "Clostridium tertium: An Unusual Cause of Pyogenic Liver Abscess," *ACG Case Reports Journal*, vol. 5, 2018.

[8] H. M. Heneghan, N. A. Healy, S. T. Martin et al., "Modern management of pyogenic hepatic abscess: a case series and review of the literature," *BMC Research Notes*, vol. 4, no. 1, p. 80, 2011.

[9] H. A. Terzi, T. Demiray, M. Koroglu et al., "Intra-abdominal abscess and primary peritonitis caused by streptococcus anginosus," *Jundishapur Journal of Microbiology*, vol. 9, no. 6, Article ID e33863, 2016.

[10] J. Rahimian, T. Wilson, V. Oram, and R. S. Holzman, "Pyogenic liver abscess: Recent trends in etiology and mortality," *Clinical Infectious Diseases*, vol. 39, no. 11, pp. 1654–1659, 2004.

[11] C.-J. Huang, H. A. Pitt, P. A. Lipsett et al., "Pyogenic hepatic abscess: Changing trends over 42 years," *Annals of Surgery*, vol. 223, no. 5, pp. 600–607, 1996.

[12] K. Morii, S. Fujiwara, S. Nakamura, and H. Okushin, "Streptococcus Anginosus Group-associated Pyogenic Liver Abscess," *Internal Medicine*, vol. 57, no. 15, pp. 2271-2272, 2018.

[13] C. Serraino, C. Elia, C. Bracco et al., "Characteristics and management of pyogenic liver abscess," *Medicine (Baltimore)*, vol. 97, no. 19, Article ID e0628, 2018.

[14] J. Cherian, R. Singh, M. Varma, S. Vidyasagar, and C. Mukhopadhyay, "Community-acquired methicillin-resistant pyogenic liver abscess," *Journal of Investigative Medicine High Impact Case Reports*, vol. 4, no. 3, Article ID 232470961666057, 2016.

[15] F. Bonenfant, E. Rousseau, and P. Farand, "Streptococcus anginosus Pyogenic Liver Abscess following a Screening Colonoscopy," *Canadian Journal of Infectious Diseases & Medical Microbiology*, vol. 24, Article ID 802545, 2 pages, 2013.

Gastrointestinal Bleeding Secondary to Portal Hypertensive Duodenopathy in a Patient with Decompensated Liver Cirrhosis

Rohini Krishna,[1] Samuel O. Igbinedion,[1] Richie Diaz,[2] Nazneen Hussain,[3] and Moheb Boktor[3]

[1]*Department of Internal Medicine, Louisiana State University Health Sciences Center, Shreveport, LA, USA*
[2]*School of Medicine, Louisiana State University Health Sciences Center, Shreveport, LA, USA*
[3]*Department of Gastroenterology and Hepatology, Louisiana State University Health Sciences Center, Shreveport, LA, USA*

Correspondence should be addressed to Samuel O. Igbinedion; sigbi1@lsuhsc.edu

Academic Editor: Yoshiro Kawahara

With alcoholic cirrhosis and nonalcoholic fatty liver disease continuously on the rise in the United States, there is also a corresponding rise in portal hypertension. Portal hypertensive duodenopathy (PHD) is a complication of portal hypertension not commonly seen in cirrhotic patients. We present a case of a 46-year-old man who presented with decompensated liver cirrhosis secondary to gastrointestinal bleed. The patient underwent esophagogastroduodenoscopy (EGD) with findings indicative of PHD. Patient subsequently underwent transjugular intrahepatic portosystemic shunt (TIPS) with resolution of gastrointestinal bleed. We highlight TIPS as a management strategy in patients with PHD for whom less invasive measures are not effective.

1. Introduction

Portal hypertension is a common complication of chronic liver disease and is primary responsible for most clinical presentations of cirrhosis [1]. In the United States, portal hypertension often occurs secondary to cirrhosis. Noncirrhotic portal hypertension accounts for a minor number of cases [1]. Known complications of portal hypertension include esophageal varices, ascites, portal hypertensive gastropathy, spontaneous bacterial peritonitis, and hepatorenal syndrome, among many others [1]. Portal hypertensive duodenopathy (PHD) is a less common finding of portal hypertension syndrome in cirrhotic patients [2]. It is estimated to occur in 14 to 25% of cirrhotic patients [3]. A recent European retrospective study estimates its prevalence to be 8.4% when duodenal erosions/ulcers are excluded from the definition, due to the inability to rule out a peptic origin in a majority of the patients [2].

Defining features of PHD on endoscopy include erythema, scattered petechiae, friable mucosa, erosions, ulcers, edema, lesions, and duodenal polyps. There have been several reports detailing these varying endoscopic findings in the duodenum consistent with PHD [3–6]. These findings can be responsible for overt or occult signs of gastrointestinal bleeding and thus need to be highlighted for clinical benefit [7]. We report a case of gastrointestinal bleed secondary to portal hypertensive duodenopathy in a patient with decompensated liver cirrhosis. We intend to highlight PHD as a cause of acute gastrointestinal bleed in cirrhotic patients.

2. Case Report

A 46-year-old male with a history of alcoholic liver cirrhosis complicated by small esophageal varices after banding and moderate ascites was awaiting liver transplant (MELD 24, Child-Pugh class B). He presented with a 3-day history of abdominal pain. He described the pain as sharp and located around the periumbilical area with notable suprapubic discomfort. He also reported associated symptoms of nausea, hematochezia, and general malaise. On further review of systems, he reported chills, increased fatigue, shortness of breath, lightheadedness, and decreased appetite 4 days prior to presentation. He reported compliance at home with

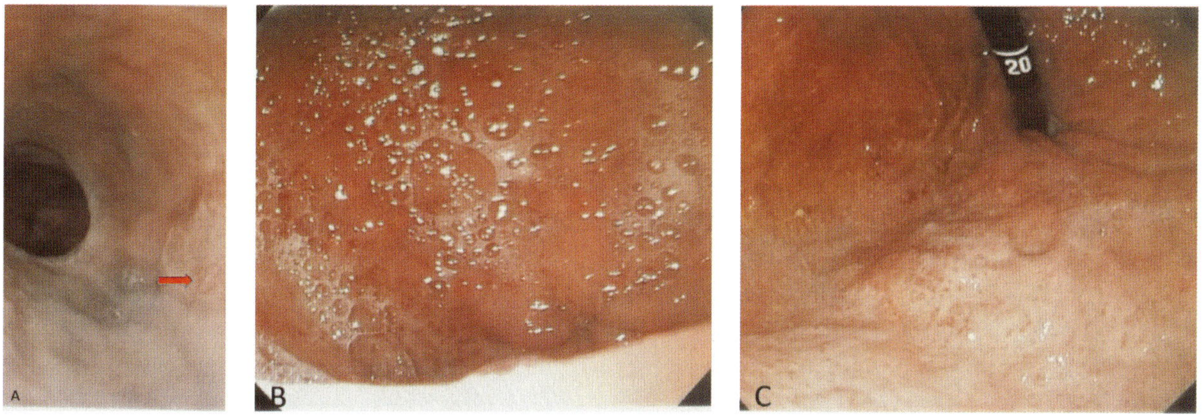

(a) (b) (c)

FIGURE 1: Endoscopy findings of ulcerations in the distal esophagus (arrow) from prior banding of small esophageal varices and diffuse portal hypertensive gastropathy.

a sodium-restricted diet and medications. Physical exam was significant for abdominal distension with positive fluid wave, generalized abdominal tenderness, and splenomegaly. Scant blood was noted on the rectal exam. Laboratory studies revealed stable hemoglobin of 12.4 g/dL, hematocrit of 36.8%, platelet of 83 K/UL, leukocytosis of 15.4 K/UL with 78% neutrophils and 16% bands, sodium of 130 mmol/L, ammonia of 83 Umol/L, ALT of 40 U/L, AST of 42 U/L, and alkaline phosphatase of 127 U/L. International normalized ratio (INR) was 2.02. Diagnostic paracentesis revealed serosanguinous fluid and ascitic fluid polymorphonuclear neutrophils (PMN) count of 686 cells/mm^3, consistent with culture negative neutrocytic ascites. Blood cultures revealed no growth of organisms. The patient was started on intravenous (IV) ceftriaxone, IV pantoprazole infusion, and an IV bolus of octreotide followed by continuous infusion. He completed a 5-day course of IV ceftriaxone therapy.

The patient underwent an esophagogastroduodenoscopy (EGD) which showed ulcerations in the distal esophagus from prior banding of small esophageal varices and diffuse portal hypertensive gastropathy (Figure 1). Mucosal edema and erythema with an area of oozing of blood were identified in the duodenum bulb and between proximally located duodenal folds with no specific identifiable lesion. These findings correlated with a diagnosis of portal hypertensive duodenopathy (Figure 2). Colonoscopy was performed, and it showed no active bleeding. However, there were old blood clots in the terminal ileum in addition to mild inflammation in the terminal ileum near the ileocecal valve. Video capsule endoscopy was also performed, and it revealed no active bleeding. Because of the concern of the possible failure of the patient on medical therapy for portal hypertension while awaiting liver transplant, the patient was referred for evaluation by a transjugular intrahepatic portosystemic shunt (TIPS). The patient successfully underwent the TIPS procedure. Follow-up occurred one month later in clinic. At this time, the patient reported resolution of the hematochezia.

3. Discussion

Portal hypertensive duodenopathy is a clinical condition that describes the mucosal and histopathologic abnormalities in the duodenum in patients with portal hypertension [7, 8]. Some reports consider this condition in a different category, portal hypertensive enteropathy [8]. Mucosal erythema, mucosal edema, mucosal breaks (erosions or ulcers), and vascular lesions are findings that characterize PHD as a condition [7]. Duodenal polyps have been identified in newer reports as another finding secondary to PHD [5, 6]. These findings are only observed and categorized under patient evaluation with EGD, video capsule endoscopy, or deep enteroscopy [8]. Clinical manifestation of these findings can range from asymptomatic presentation to fatal gastrointestinal bleeding [8]. In a 2007 descriptive study on portal hypertensive patients by Barakat et al., 51.4% were found to have endoscopic features of PHD, with PHD identified as the source of GI bleed in close to 10% of the patients [7]. Histopathologic evidence of duodenopathy, including intestinal vasculopathy, was prevalent in 85% of the patients, with no difference in prevalence between patients with and without endoscopic duodenopathy [7]. This highlighted that the histopathologic evidence of duodenopathy does not always indicate endoscopic duodenopathy, hence lending no clinical utility.

Our patient presented with endoscopic features concerning PHD. The patient also had evidence of diffuse portal hypertensive gastropathy on endoscopy. Predisposing risk factors for PHD are difficult to pinpoint. On analysis of PHD versus other endoscopic findings in patients with portal hypertension, Barakat et al. (2007) revealed the absence of correlation between PHD and the size of esophageal varices and/or presence of variceal bleed. There was, however, a relation to the extent and severity of gastric lesions [7]. Further studies seem to suggest a relationship between PHD development and the degree of portal hypertension as demonstrated by large esophageal varices, severe portal hypertensive

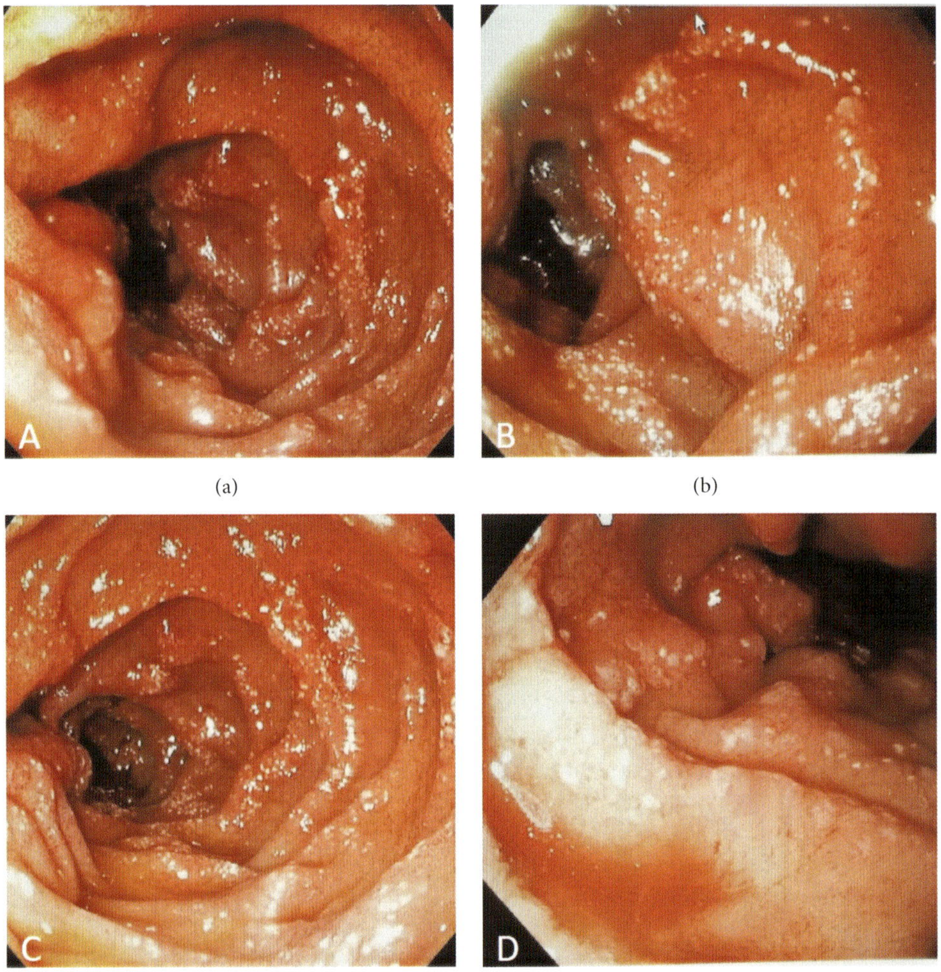

(a) (b) (c) (d)

Figure 2: Endoscopic findings of erosions, mucosal erythema, and edema in the duodenum with minor oozing of blood noted.

gastropathy, and high hepatic venous pressure gradients [2, 9]. However, other reports have diminished its relationship to the portal pressure, instead identifying the point at which the pressure causes congestive changes to be the culprit in PHD development [7, 10].

The association of PHD in patients with prior variceal band ligation is very significant, and this relationship is well documented [2, 11]. One such study showed an increase in the number of patients with PHD from 6.6% to 46.7% after variceal band ligation ($p < 0.001$) [12]. This study linked the development of PHD with an increase in VEGF expression in gastric and intestinal cells after variceal obliteration [12]. Our patient had other evidence of portal hypertension prior to development of PHD, but the history of prior endoscopic band ligation was significant in his development of PHD. He was found to have PHD on subsequent endoscopy with evidence of overt GI bleed. Our case highlights the importance of identifying PHD in patients with decompensated liver cirrhosis, as this could possibly lead to a devastating gastrointestinal bleed.

Treatment of PHD is not established, and recommendations are based on strategies documented in case reports [5, 11, 13]. Medical therapy which includes prophylaxis with beta blocker has been notably effective [13]. Endoscopic therapy, which includes polypectomy, endoclip use, and argon plasma coagulation, has been reported to be successful [8, 13]. However, liver transplant is the optimal treatment strategy in patients who are surgical candidates, and PHD resolves in these patients afterwards [2]. This is likely due to the resolution of the portal hypertension syndrome. In some cases like this reported, PHD can be the cause of either self-limited bleeding and erythematous lesions or even massive hemorrhage requiring emergent shunting procedures [7]. We report a rare case of gastrointestinal bleeding secondary to PHD. Further prospective studies are needed to better understand the pathophysiology of PHD. Clinicians should also consider TIPS as a management strategy in patients with PHD for whom less invasive measures are not effective.

Consent

An informed consent was obtained from this patient for this case report.

Acknowledgments

This is to acknowledge that this case was presented as a poster in the ACP 2018 Annual Louisiana Associates Meeting.

References

[1] A. Berzigotti, S. Seijo, E. Reverter, and J. Bosch, "Assessing portal hypertension in liver diseases," *Expert Review of Gastroenterology & Hepatology*, vol. 7, no. 2, pp. 141–155, 2013.

[2] L. Menchen, C. Ripoll, I. Marin-Jimenez et al., "Prevalence of portal hypertensive duodenopathy in cirrhosis: clinical and haemodynamic features," *European Journal of Gastroenterology & Hepatology*, vol. 18, no. 6, pp. 649–653, 2006.

[3] R. Gupta, V. A. Saraswat, M. Kumar, S. R. Naik, and R. Pandey, "Frequency and factors influencing portal hypertensive gastropathy and duodenopathy in cirrhotic portal hypertension," *Journal of Gastroenterology and Hepatology*, vol. 11, no. 8, pp. 728–733, 1996.

[4] A. Gurung, P. E. Jaffe, and X. Zhang, "Duodenal polyposis secondary to portal hypertensive duodenopathy," *World Journal of Gastrointestinal Endoscopy*, vol. 7, no. 17, pp. 1257–1261, 2015.

[5] J.-D. Zeitoun, A. Chryssostalis, B. Terris, F. Prat, M. Gaudric, and S. Chaussade, "Portal hypertensive duodenal polyp: a case report," *World Journal of Gastroenterology*, vol. 13, no. 9, pp. 1451-1452, 2007.

[6] S. B. Pillai, V. R. Ram Ganesh, A. Mohanakrishnan, and V. Nirmala, "Portal duodenopathy presenting as polyposis," *Indian Journal of Pathology & Microbiology*, vol. 53, no. 3, pp. 558-559, 2010.

[7] M. Barakat, M. Mostafa, Z. Mahran, and A.-G. Soliman, "Portal hypertensive duodenopathy: Clinical, endoscopic, and histopathologic profiles," *American Journal of Gastroenterology*, vol. 102, no. 12, pp. 2793–2802, 2007.

[8] P. Mekaroonkamol, R. Cohen, and S. Chawla, "Portal hypertensive enteropathy," *World Journal of Hepatology*, vol. 7, no. 2, pp. 127–138, 2015.

[9] R. Shudo, Y. Yazaki, S. Sakurai, H. Uenishi, H. Yamada, and K. Sugawara, "Duodenal erosions, a common and distinctive feature of portal hypertensive duodenopathy," *American Journal of Gastroenterology*, vol. 97, no. 4, pp. 867–873, 2002.

[10] M. Rabinovitz, R. R. Schade, V. Dindzans, D. H. Van Thiel, and J. S. Gavaler, "Prevalence of duodenal ulcer in cirrhotic males referred for liver transplantation - Does the etiology of cirrhosis make a difference?" *Digestive Diseases and Sciences*, vol. 35, no. 3, pp. 321–326, 1990.

[11] A. Oluyemi and A. Amole, "Portal hypertensive duodenopathy manifesting as kissing duodenal ulcers in a Nigerian with alcoholic cirrhosis: A case report and brief review of the literature," *Case Reports in Medicine*, vol. 2012, Article ID 618729, 4 pages, 2012.

[12] H. R. El-Khayat, A. El Khattib, M. Nosseir, M. A. Ezz, H. El-Amin, and Y. M. Fouad, "Portal hypertensive enteropathy before and after variceal obliteration: an endoscopic, histopathologic and immunohistochemical study," *Journal of Gastrointestinal and Liver Diseases*, vol. 19, no. 2, pp. 175–179, 2010.

[13] N. H. Urrunaga and D. C. Rockey, "Portal hypertensive gastropathy and colopathy," *Clinics in Liver Disease*, vol. 18, no. 2, pp. 389–406, 2014.

A Rare Encounter with an Expanding Pseudocyst of the Spleen

Ashish Lal Shrestha and Pradita Shrestha

Department of General Surgery, United Mission Hospital, Tansen, Palpa, Nepal

Correspondence should be addressed to Ashish Lal Shrestha; butchgrunty@yahoo.com

Academic Editor: Olga I. Giouleme

Background. Splenic Pseudocyst (SP) is a diagnostic rarity, with cystic lesions of spleen themselves being uncommon. Establishing a preoperative diagnosis could help in specific management but this is rather challenging. Here we present a common presentation of an uncommon diagnosis. *Case Presentation.* A 47-year-old lady, previously well, presented to the outpatient clinic with intermittent left hypochondrial pain radiating towards left shoulder for 2 months not associated with fever, jaundice, or weight loss. Abdominal examination revealed nontender hepatosplenomegaly. The initial abdominal ultrasonogram (USG) was suggestive of a hydatid cyst, for which she received a course of antihelminthics. At follow-up, after finding no clinical improvement and radiological worsening, she underwent an exploratory laparotomy. A cyst replacing entire lower pole and a significant portion of splenic hilum was found. Total splenectomy was performed. The specimen was reported to be a SP. *Conclusion.* SP is a unique entity, usually misdiagnosed as a parasitic lesion and often treated with antihelminthic medicines. The natural course of disease, however, follows a subsequent failure of symptom resolution and radiological worsening that ultimately demands surgical attention. Based on size, location, and intraoperative findings, either total or partial splenectomy is required. The final histopathological report often presents a diagnostic surprise.

1. Introduction

Cysts in the spleen are uncommon, and amongst these one rare kind is SP [1, 2]. Previous blunt abdominal trauma is implicated in at least 75% of cases [1, 3].

We report an interesting case of a rare and expanding SP without history of previous abdominal trauma. The clinical presentations, investigative findings, and management are discussed with relevant literature review.

The rarity of this case lies in the fact that it is often misdiagnosed and wrongly treated and eventually requires surgical exploration [4]. Unless a high degree of clinical suspicion is maintained, it is likely to be missed and may result in complications that may be fatal at times.

The peroperative findings and final histopathological report usually take the surgeon by surprise.

2. Case Presentation

A 47-year-old lady without significant past medical or surgical history presented to the outpatient clinic with intermittent episodes of left hypochondrial pain radiating towards the left shoulder for 2 months. She did not have associated fever, jaundice, or altered bowel habits. Some loss of appetite was noted without loss of weight. She could not recall any abdominal trauma in the recent past. Physical examination was unremarkable except for a nontender hepatosplenomegaly.

Hematological and biochemical tests were normal. Abdominal radiographs were unremarkable. Abdominal USG revealed a complex cystic lesion in the spleen measuring $4 \times 8 \times 6$ cm with poorly defined double wall and multiple internal septations suggesting a likely hydatidosis along with enlarged fatty liver.

She was given a course of antihelminthics, vaccinated against capsulated organisms predicting possibility of a subsequent splenectomy, and asked to return a month later.

At follow-up, her symptoms persisted and repeated abdominal USG showed expanding splenic cyst measuring $9 \times 8 \times 8$ cm. CECT scan of the abdomen showed a nonenhancing cystic lesion arising from lower pole and hilum of spleen measuring $10 \times 9 \times 9$ cm with multiple internal septations and abutting the tail of pancreas as shown in Figure 1.

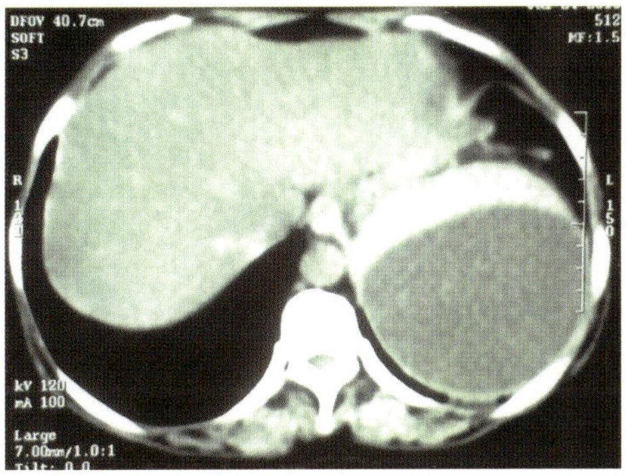

FIGURE 1: CECT scan of the abdomen showing a nonenhancing cystic lesion arising from lower pole and hilum of spleen measuring 10 × 9 × 9 cm with multiple internal septations and abutting the tail of pancreas.

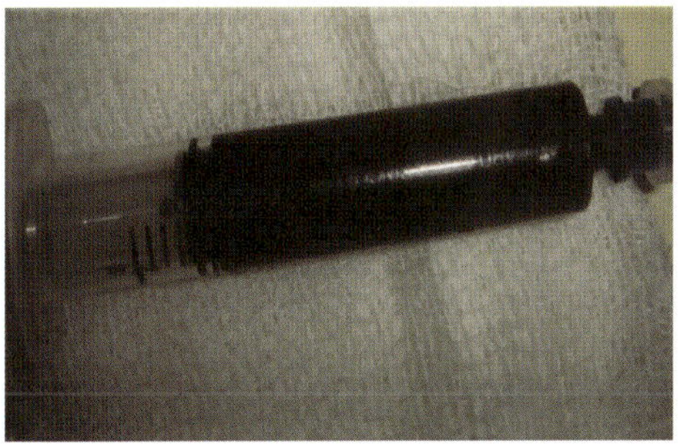

FIGURE 2: The brownish translucent fluid aspirated from the expanding splenic cyst, the routine bacterial culture of which was later reported to be sterile.

A list of differentials was considered that included a splenic hydatid cyst, pancreatic tail pseudocyst, and a mesenteric cyst. In view of clinical and radiological worsening, she was taken for an elective exploration through a left subcostal incision.

At laparotomy, a huge splenic cyst was found occupying entire lower pole and significant portion of hilum and measuring 9 × 9 × 8 cm. The aspiration of this revealed a brownish translucent fluid as shown in Figure 2, the routine bacterial culture of which was later reported to be sterile.

The cyst was causing pressure atrophy of the residual splenic parenchyma and also had multiple dense perisplenic and pericystic adhesions. Total splenectomy was done. During intraoperative manipulation, the cyst wall got inadvertently ruptured. The image of splenectomy specimen is shown in Figure 3.

She had an uneventful postoperative recovery and was discharged on the 7th postoperative day. At 2-week and one-year follow-up, she remained symptom-free.

Histopathologically, gross examination confirmed the operative findings and showed a unilocular already cut-open cyst measuring 9 × 5 cm with wall thickness measuring 2–5 mm.

Microscopic section showed a cyst wall that was composed of hyalinized fibrous tissue without epithelial lining. Also noted were plenty of extravasated red blood cells and hemosiderin laden macrophages over the cyst wall. There was

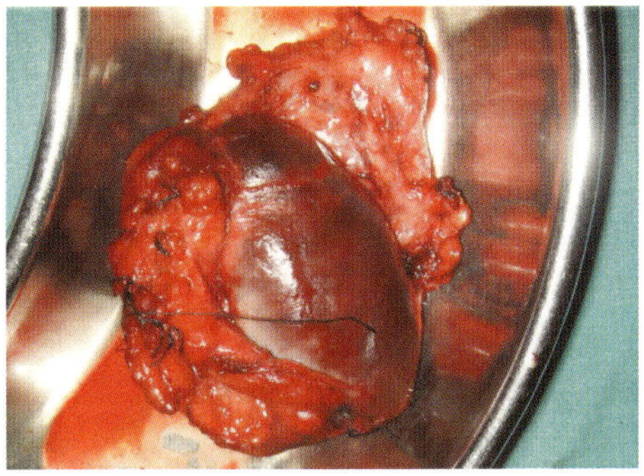

FIGURE 3: The intraoperative image of the splenic cyst causing pressure atrophy of the residual splenic parenchyma. During intraoperative manipulation, the cyst wall was inadvertently ruptured.

no evidence of cellular atypia. The microscopic image of the SP is shown in Figure 4.

The features confirmed a SP.

3. Discussion

Splenic cysts have been a matter of curiosity, with a reported incidence of only around 800 globally [1, 5–7]. Since their recognition in 1829 by Andral and first splenectomy in 1867 by Pean for this condition, there have been infrequent reports in the literature [8]. The earlier system classified these lesions into type 1 (true cysts with lining epithelium) and type 2 (false cysts without lining epithelium) [9–12]. A consecutive modification divided these into parasitic and nonparasitic varieties, further categorizing nonparasitic ones into primary (epithelial/true) and secondary (false/pseudo) types [13]. Parasitic ones follow a geographical distribution and account for more than 2/3rds of cases in the endemic areas [8]. Of these, the commonest etiology is *Echinococcus granulosus* [8]. This holds true even in the clinical context of Nepal [14]. More recently, a pathological classification was suggested dividing nonparasitic cysts into congenital, traumatic, neoplastic, and degenerative types [10, 11].

Of all the cysts, SPs constitute 70–80%, particularly affecting women, children, and young adults [1, 4, 8, 15]. The incidence can be expected to rise further with nonoperative management of blunt abdominal trauma becoming more popular.

In symptomatic 2/3rds, symptoms include left hypochondrial pain radiating to the left shoulder or chest [5, 8, 16]. Other symptoms include early satiety, vomiting, dysphagia, and infrequently ipsilateral atelectasis and lower lobe pneumonia depending upon the location and organ of compression [1, 17]. Symptoms also depend on the size of the SP which forms the basis for operative treatment and predicting complications. While SP larger than 5 cm usually dictates operative management, the risk of complications, like sudden increase in size due to intracystic bleed, secondary infections, and even fatality due to spontaneous intraperitoneal rupture, has been noted in larger SP [1, 5, 18]. SP may sometimes attain great dimensions with those exceeding 15 cm entitled giant pseudocysts [4, 11, 19, 20].

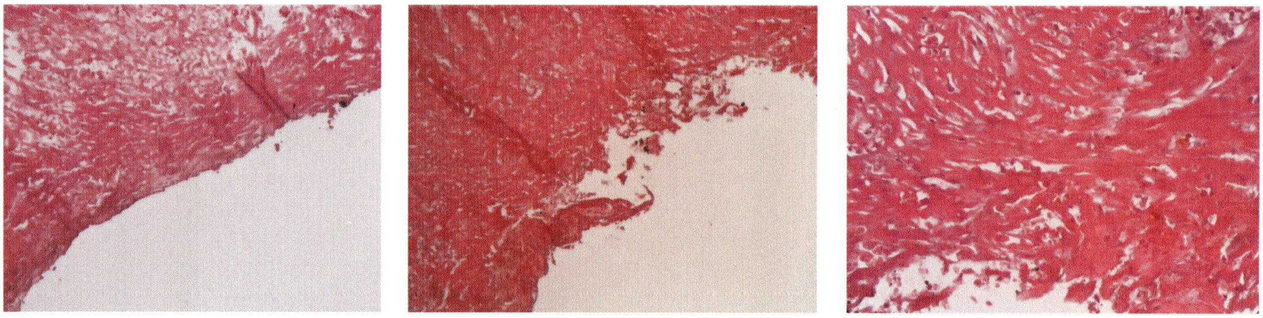

(a) (b) (c)

FIGURE 4: Microscopic appearance of the Splenic Pseudocyst (stained with Eosin/Hematoxylin stain) at (a) 10x magnification, (b) 25x magnification, (c) 40x magnification.

SP may also be incidental sonological finding or detected due to calcification on radiographs [17]. USG, CECT, MRI, and MRA can all help to delineate cystic nature of the lesion [4, 8]. However, the precise preoperative radiological diagnosis remains challenging, although it could be a great aid to efficient and specific management.

Most often, misdiagnosed as parasitic lesions, these cysts are often treated with antihelminthics only to find unsatisfactory response and radiological deterioration at follow-up. Our patient had a similar treatment course.

Etiologically, SP represents a resolved hematoma in the parenchymal or subcapsular location due to a preceeding blunt injury [1, 2, 4]. Suggested alternate etiologies include infections and degenerative diseases [4, 21].

In gross appearance, majority of these are unilocular and smooth walled while microscopic findings consist of fibrous wall tissue without an epithelial lining [4, 5, 7, 8, 19].

Traditional approach to SP larger than 5 cm has been total splenectomy. However, with growing knowledge about protective role of spleen as an organ of reticuloendothelial and hematopoietic importance, more specifically in terms of OPSI, the current approach has been of splenic conservation [4, 7, 22]. In this regard, partial splenectomy, cyst aspiration, deroofing, marsupialisation, decapsulation, and cystectomy have all been described by both open and laparoscopic routes [4, 20, 22, 23]. Laparoscopic unroofing and drainage have been found to have a recurrence rate of 20–40%, and hence to avoid this, marsupialisation or decapsulation has been the recommended technique [18, 24].

Certain characteristics of SP like hilar location, large size with near complete replacement of parenchyma, associated hypersplenism, and doubtful diagnosis are the few important situations where total splenectomy may not be avoidable [7, 22, 25].

In our patient, the likelihood of hydatid etiology was considered earlier in view of endemicity of infestation and hence was managed in similar lines. There was no way to prove or disprove this diagnosis, and the much talked about "Casoni's intradermal test" was also unavailable in a rural set-up like ours.

At follow-up, since no clinical improvement was found predicting a possibility of life threatening complication like rupture or hemorrhage in future, elective exploration was considered. This was supported with evidence of expanding cyst dimensions and hilar location that made the decision of total splenectomy rather simple. Following this, the patient had an uneventful recovery and remained symptom-free at 1-year follow-up.

4. Conclusions

In conclusion, SP is uncommon pathology that is capable of mimicking commoner conditions like hydatidosis. The clinical and radiological pictures may be frequently misleading with consequent mismanagement. A high degree of clinical suspicion is, therefore, as essential as the understanding of potential complications to avoid clinical mishaps.

Definitive diagnosis is possible only on histopathology and usually poses a diagnostic surprise. However, once treated adequately, SP has a good outcome. Hence, awareness of its clinical presentation and good pathological expertise are important adjuncts in the diagnosis.

Abbreviations

SP: Splenic Pseudocyst
USG: Ultrasonogram
CECT: Contrast enhanced computed tomography
MRI: Magnetic resonance imaging
MRA: Magnetic resonance arteriogram
OPSI: Overwhelming postsplenectomy infections.

Consent

Written informed consent was obtained from the patient for publication of this case report and accompanying images.

Authors' Contributions

Ashish Lal Shrestha participated in the conception and design of the report and wrote the paper, and Pradita Shrestha analyzed the report. Both have been involved in the diagnosis, surgical management, and follow-up of the patient. Both authors read and approved the final paper. Both the authors were involved in planning, analyzing the case, and writing the paper.

Acknowledgments

The authors would like to thank the ward staff of the hospital for providing support and helping in management of the patient.

References

[1] G. J. Gibeily and B. L. Eisenberg, "Splenic pseudocysts—diagnosis and management," *Western Journal of Medicine*, vol. 148, no. 4, pp. 464–466, 1988.

[2] G. Galyfos, Z. Touloumis, K. Palogos et al., "Oversized pseudocysts of the spleen: report of two cases," *International Journal of Surgery Case Reports*, vol. 5, no. 2, pp. 104–107, 2014.

[3] R. Kostka and Z. Vernerová, "Post-traumatic pseudocyst of the spleen," *Rozhl V Chir Mesicnik Ceskoslovenske Chir Spolecnosti*, vol. 89, no. 9, pp. 464–468, 2010.

[4] K. Kalinova, "Giant pseudocyst of the spleen: a case report and review of the literature," *Journal of Indian Association of Pediatric Surgeons*, vol. 10, no. 3, pp. 176–178, 2005.

[5] A. Verma, A. Yadav, S. Sharma et al., "A rare splenic pseudocyst," *Journal of Surgical Case Reports*, vol. 2013, no. 9, article rjt086, 2013.

[6] F. Roberson, "Solitary cysts of the spleen," *Annals of Surgery*, vol. 111, no. 5, pp. 848–850, 1940.

[7] F. Altintoprak, E. Dikicier, T. Kivilcim, T. Ergonenc, and O. N. Dilek, "An uncommon clinical entity, although common theoretically: pseudocyst of spleen—two case reports and review of the literature," *European Journal of General Medicine*, vol. 9, no. 12, Article ID 5000114746, 2012.

[8] M. J. Zinner, *Maingot's Abdominal Operations*, McGraw-Hill Professional, New York, NY, USA, 11th edition, 2006.

[9] J. W. Martin, "Congenital splenic cysts," *The American Journal of Surgery*, vol. 96, no. 2, pp. 302–308, 1958.

[10] S. B. Ingle, C. R. Hinge, and S. Patrike, "Epithelial cysts of the spleen: a minireview," *World Journal of Gastroenterology*, vol. 20, no. 38, pp. 13899–13903, 2014.

[11] L. Morgenstern, "Nonparasitic splenic cysts: pathogenesis, classification, and treatment," *Journal of the American College of Surgeons*, vol. 194, no. 3, pp. 306–314, 2002.

[12] R. H. Fowler, "Nonparasitic benign cystic tumors of the spleen," *International Abstracts of Surgery*, vol. 96, no. 3, pp. 209–227, 1953.

[13] S. B. Ingle, C. R. Hinge, and S. N. Jatal, "An interesting case of primary epithelial cyst of spleen," *Indian Journal of Pathology and Microbiology*, vol. 56, no. 2, pp. 181-182, 2013.

[14] B. Devleesschauwer, A. Ale, P. Torgerson et al., "The burden of parasitic zoonoses in nepal: a systematic review," *PLOS Neglected Tropical Diseases*, vol. 8, no. 1, 2014.

[15] P. Mirilas, A. Mentessidou, and J. E. Skandalakis, "Splenic cysts: are there so many types?" *Journal of the American College of Surgeons*, vol. 204, no. 3, pp. 459–465, 2007.

[16] A. H. Sarmast, H. I. Showkat, F. Q. Parray, and R. Lone, "Non parasitic splenic cyst: a case report," *Acta Medica Iranica*, vol. 50, no. 12, pp. 849–851, 2012.

[17] R. J. Williams and G. Glazer, "Splenic cysts: changes in diagnosis, treatment and aetiological concepts," *Annals of The Royal College of Surgeons of England*, vol. 75, no. 2, pp. 87–89, Mar 1993.

[18] E. H. Chin, R. Shapiro, D. Hazzan, L. B. Katz, and B. Salky, "A ten-year experience with laparoscopic treatment of splenic cysts," *JSLS: Journal of the Society of Laparoendoscopic Surgeons/Society of Laparoendoscopic Surgeons*, vol. 11, no. 1, pp. 20–23, 2007.

[19] M. Cisse, I. Konate, O. Ka, M. Dieng, A. Dia, and C. T. Toure, "Giant splenic pseudocyst, a rare aetiology of abdominal tumor: a case report," *Cases Journal*, vol. 3, no. 1, article no. 16, 2010.

[20] R. Sierra, W. C. Brunner, J. T. Murphy, J. B. Dunne, and D. J. Scott, "Laparoscopic marsupialization of a giant posttraumatic splenic cyst," *JSLS: Journal of the Society of Laparoendoscopic Surgeons/Society of Laparoendoscopic Surgeons*, vol. 8, no. 4, pp. 384–388, 2004.

[21] K. Chakradhar, S. Prasad, S. Kumar, and M. Valiathan, "A rare presentation of splenic tuberculosis with a pseudocyst," *BMJ Case Reports*, vol. 2014, 2014.

[22] V. K. Kundal, M. Gajdhar, R. Kundal, C. Sharma, D. Agarwal, and A. Meena, "Giant epithelial non-parasitic splenic cyst," *Journal of Case Reports*, vol. 3, no. 1, pp. 106–109, 2013.

[23] A. H. Khan, A. L. Bensoussan, A. Ouimet, H. Blanchard, A. Grignon, and M. Ndoye, "Partial splenectomy for benign cystic lesions of the spleen," *Journal of Pediatric Surgery*, vol. 21, no. 9, pp. 749–752, 1986.

[24] C. Palanivelu, M. Rangarajan, M. V. Madankumar, and S. J. John, "Laparoscopic internal marsupializaton for large nonparasitic splenic cysts: effective organ-preserving technique," *World Journal of Surgery*, vol. 32, no. 1, pp. 20–25, 2008.

[25] M. Abd Ellatif, "Giant Splenic Cyst with Hypersplenism: laparoscopic Splenectomy," *Journal of Gastroenterology and Hepatology Research*, vol. 2, no. 4, pp. 549–551, 2013.

Permissions

All chapters in this book were first published in CRGM, by Hindawi Publishing Corporation; hereby published with permission under the Creative Commons Attribution License or equivalent. Every chapter published in this book has been scrutinized by our experts. Their significance has been extensively debated. The topics covered herein carry significant findings which will fuel the growth of the discipline. They may even be implemented as practical applications or may be referred to as a beginning point for another development.

The contributors of this book come from diverse backgrounds, making this book a truly international effort. This book will bring forth new frontiers with its revolutionizing research information and detailed analysis of the nascent developments around the world.

We would like to thank all the contributing authors for lending their expertise to make the book truly unique. They have played a crucial role in the development of this book. Without their invaluable contributions this book wouldn't have been possible. They have made vital efforts to compile up to date information on the varied aspects of this subject to make this book a valuable addition to the collection of many professionals and students.

This book was conceptualized with the vision of imparting up-to-date information and advanced data in this field. To ensure the same, a matchless editorial board was set up. Every individual on the board went through rigorous rounds of assessment to prove their worth. After which they invested a large part of their time researching and compiling the most relevant data for our readers.

The editorial board has been involved in producing this book since its inception. They have spent rigorous hours researching and exploring the diverse topics which have resulted in the successful publishing of this book. They have passed on their knowledge of decades through this book. To expedite this challenging task, the publisher supported the team at every step. A small team of assistant editors was also appointed to further simplify the editing procedure and attain best results for the readers.

Apart from the editorial board, the designing team has also invested a significant amount of their time in understanding the subject and creating the most relevant covers. They scrutinized every image to scout for the most suitable representation of the subject and create an appropriate cover for the book.

The publishing team has been an ardent support to the editorial, designing and production team. Their endless efforts to recruit the best for this project, has resulted in the accomplishment of this book. They are a veteran in the field of academics and their pool of knowledge is as vast as their experience in printing. Their expertise and guidance has proved useful at every step. Their uncompromising quality standards have made this book an exceptional effort. Their encouragement from time to time has been an inspiration for everyone.

The publisher and the editorial board hope that this book will prove to be a valuable piece of knowledge for researchers, students, practitioners and scholars across the globe.

List of Contributors

Turan Calhan and Barış Soydaş
Department of Gastroenterology, Mehmet Akif ˙Inan Training and Research Hospital, Şanlıurfa, Turkey

Abdurrahman Sahin and Resul Kahraman
Department of Gastroenterology, Umraniye Training and Research Hospital, Istanbul, Turkey

Ali Tosun
Department of Radiology, Mehmet Akif ˙Inan Training and Research Hospital, Şanlıurfa, Turkey

Egemen Cebeci
Department of Nephrology, Okmeydanı Training and Research Hospital, Istanbul, Turkey

Youssef Botros and Mary Mathews
Department of Internal Medicine, St. Joseph's Regional Medical Center, New York Medical College, Paterson, NJ 07503, USA

Hiren Patel and Walid Baddoura
Department of Gastroenterology, St. Joseph's Regional Medical Center, New York Medical College, Paterson, NJ 07503, USA

Nihar Shah
Department of Gastroenterology, Joan C. Edwards School of Medicine, Marshall University, Huntington, WV 25755, USA

Andrew de la Torre
Department of General and Hepatobiliary Surgery, St. Joseph's Regional Medical Center, Paterson, NJ 07503, USA

Sandra Sánchez Prudencio, Daniel Domingo Senra, Daniel Martín Rodríguez, Belén Botella Mateu, Carlos Esteban Jiménez-Zarza, Felipe de la Morena López and Beatriz de Cuenca Morón
Gastroenterology Department, Hospital Infanta Cristina, Avenida 9 de Junio, No. 2, 28981 Parla, Madrid, Spain

José Jiménez Reyes
Dermatology Department, Hospital Infanta Cristina, Avenida 9 de Junio, No. 2, 28981 Parla, Madrid, Spain

Manuel Nevado Santos
Pathology Department, Hospital Infanta Cristina, Avenida 9 de Junio, No. 2, 28981 Parla, Madrid, Spain

Patrick Schoeters
Department of Gastroenterology, AZ Herentals, 2200 Herentals, Belgium

Karl De Pooter
Department of Gastrointestinal Surgery, AZ Herentals, 2200 Herentals, Belgium

Dong Seok Lee
Department of Internal Medicine, Gangneung Asan Medical Center, University of Ulsan College of Medicine, Gangneung, Republic of Korea

Sang Jin Lee
Department of Internal Medicine, Gangneung Asan Medical Center, University of Ulsan College of Medicine, Gangneung, Republic of Korea
Department of Internal Medicine, Gangneung Asan Medical Center, Sacheon-myeon, Gangneung, Gangwon-do 210-711, Republic of Korea

Dario Raimondo and Francesca Rossi
Gastroenterology and Endoscopy Unit, Fondazione Istituto San Raffaele-G. Giglio, Contrada Pietra Pollastra Pisciotto, 90015 Cefalù, Italy

Emanuele Sinagra
Gastroenterology and Endoscopy Unit, Fondazione Istituto San Raffaele-G. Giglio, Contrada Pietra Pollastra Pisciotto, 90015 Cefalù, Italy
Ph.D. Course in Surgical Biotechnology and Regenerative Medicine, University of Palermo, Piazza delle Cliniche 2, 90100 Palermo, Italy
Euro-Mediterranean Institute of Science and Technology (IEMEST), Via Emerico Amari 123, 90100 Palermo, Italy

Giovanni Tomasello
Euro-Mediterranean Institute of Science and Technology (IEMEST), Via Emerico Amari 123, 90100 Palermo, Italy
Department of Surgical and Oncological Disciplines, University of Palermo, Piazza delle Cliniche 2, 90100 Palermo, Italy

Guido Martorana, Pier Enrico Marchesa and Tiziana Facella
Surgery Unit, Fondazione Istituto San Raffaele-G. Giglio, Contrada Pietra Pollastra Pisciotto, 90015 Cefalù, Italy

Marco Messina and Massimiliano Spada
Oncology Unit, Fondazione Istituto San Raffaele-G. Giglio, Contrada Pietra Pollastra Pisciotto, 90015 Cefalù, Italy

Rosario Squatrito
Internal Medicine Unit, Fondazione Istituto San Raffaele-G. Giglio, Contrada Pietra Pollastra Pisciotto, 90015 Cefalù, Italy

Ennio La Rocca
Internal Medicine Unit, Fondazione Istituto San Raffaele-G. Giglio, Contrada Pietra Pollastra Pisciotto, 90015 Cefalù, Italy
Unità Operativa di Medicina Interna e Trapiantologia, Ospedale San Raffaele, Via Olgettina 60, Milano, Italy

Attilio Ignazio Lo Monte
Department of Surgical and Oncological Disciplines, University of Palermo, Piazza delle Cliniche 2, 90100 Palermo, Italy

Giancarlo Pompei
Pathology Unit, Fondazione Istituto San Raffaele-G. Giglio, Contrada Pietra Pollastra Pisciotto, 90015 Cefalù, Italy

Kamel A. Gharaibeh and Arnaldo Lopez-Ruiz
Department of Internal Medicine, University of Mississippi Medical Center, 2500 North State Street, Jackson, MS 39216, USA

Tauqeer Yousuf
Department of Internal Medicine, University of Mississippi Medical Center, 2500 North State Street, Jackson, MS 39216, USA
Division of Hospital Medicine, Department of Medicine, University of Mississippi Medical Center, 2500 North State Street, Jackson, MS 39216, USA

Murad Baba and Amer Syed
Department of Internal Medicine, Jersey City Medical Center, 355 Grand Street, Jersey City, NJ 07302, USA

Jordan Fakhoury
New York Institute of Technology College of Osteopathic Medicine, Old Westbury Northern Boulevard, Old Westbury, NY 11568, USA

Ramin Niknam
Gastroenterohepatology Research Center, Shiraz University of Medical Sciences, Shiraz, Iran

Kamran Bagheri Lankarani
Health Policy Research Center, Shiraz University of Medical Sciences, Shiraz, Iran

Bita Geramizadeh
Department of Pathology, Transplant Research Center, Shiraz University of Medical Sciences, Shiraz, Iran

Sanjeev Singhal, Rahul Tugnait, Pankaj Kumar Arora, Bishwanath Tiwari, PawanMalik, Lav Gupta, Amit Bimal, Abhishek Gupta, Rahul Gupta, Pushkar Chouhan and ChandraKant Singh
Department of Surgery, Northern Railway Central Hospital, Basant Lane, New Delhi 110055, India

Anu Singhal
Department of Radiology, ESI PGIMSR, Basaidarapur, Ring Road, New Delhi 110015, India

Sanjay Singh Negi
GI and HPB Surgery, Dr. BL Kapoor Memorial Hospital, Pusa Road, New Delhi 110005, India

M. T. Branham, E. Campoy and M. Roqué
Institute of Histology and Embryology (IHEM-CCT-CONICET) and School of Medical Sciences, National University of Cuyo, M5502JMA Mendoza, Argentina

M. Pellicer
Pathology Laboratory, J5402EQC San Juan, Argentina

M. Palma
Surgery Unit, San Martin Hospital, E3100 Entre Rìos, Argentina

A. Correa
Surgery Unit, Español Hospital, M5501 Mendoza, Argentina

Ramy Mansour and Justin Miller
Genesys Regional Medical Center Gastroenterology, 1 Genesys Parkway, ATTN: Medical Education, Grand Blanc, MI 48439, USA

Matthias Peter Hilty and MarcoMaggiorini
Medical Intensive Care Unit, University Hospital of Zurich, Rämistrasse 100, 8091 Zurich, Switzerland

Marcel Halama and Andreas Geier
Department of Gastroenterology and Hepatology, University Hospital of Zurich, Rämistrasse 100, 8091 Zurich, Switzerland

Anne-Katrin Zimmermann
Department of Pathology, University Hospital of Zurich, R¨amistrasse 100, 8091 Zurich, Switzerland

Daniel Paramythiotis, Konstantinia Kofina, Vassileios N. Papadopoulos and AntoniosMichalopoulos
1st Propedeutic Surgical Clinic, Aristotle's University of Thessaloniki, AHEPA University Hospital, Stilponos Kyriakidi 1, 54636Thessaloniki, Greece

Firmin Ankouane and Mathurin Kowo
Department of Internal Medicine and Specialties, Faculty of Medicine and Biomedical Sciences, University of Yaounde 1, Yaounde University Teaching Hospital, Yaound´e, Cameroon

Bernadette Ngo Nonga
Department of Surgery and Specialties, Faculty of Medicine and Biomedical Sciences, University of Yaounde 1, Yaounde University Teaching Hospital, Yaound´e, Cameroon

Eric Magny and Edith HellMedjo
Department of Radiology and Imaging, Faculty of Medicine and Biomedical Sciences, University of Yaounde 1, Yaoundé, Cameroon

Elie Claude Ndjitoyap Ndam
Department of Internal Medicine and Specialties, Faculty of Medicine and Biomedical Sciences, University of Yaounde 1, Yaounde General Hospital, Yaoundé, Cameroon

Joel R. Brockmeyer
Minimally Invasive Bariatric Surgery and Advanced Laparoscopy Fellowship, Gundersen Medical Foundation, 1900 South Avenue, La Crosse, WI 54601, USA

Erin E. Connolly and Shanu N. Kothari
Department of General and Vascular Surgery, Gundersen Health System, 1900 South Avenue, La Crosse, WI 54601, USA

Richard J. Wittchow
Department of Pathology, Gundersen Health System, 1900 South Avenue, La Crosse, WI 54601, USA

Chelsea Kennedy-Snodgrass
NYUWinthrop Hospital, Department of Internal Medicine, 259 1st Ave, Mineola, NY 11501, USA

Vivian Keenan
NYUWinthrop Hospital, Department of Pulmonary and Critical Care, 259 1st Ave, Mineola, NY 11501, USA

Douglas S. Katz
NYUWinthrop Hospital, Department of Radiology, 259 1st Ave, Mineola, NY 11501, USA

Abhinav Tiwari and Himani Sharma
Department of Internal Medicine, University of Toledo Medical Center, Toledo, OH, USA

Khola Qamar, Yaseen Alastal, Thomas Sodeman and Ali Nawras
Department of Gastroenterology, University of Toledo Medical Center, Toledo, OH, USA

Shunsuke Sakuraba, Hajime Orita, Shuhei Ueda, Satoshi Tokuda, Tomoaki Ito, Tomoyuki Kushida, Mutsumi Sakurada, Hiroshi Maekawa and Koichi Sato
Department of Surgery, Juntendo Shizuoka Hospital, Shizuoka, Japan

Ryo Wada
Department of Pathology, Juntendo Shizuoka Hospital, Shizuoka, Japan

Thamer Kassim
Department of Medicine, Division of General Internal Medicine, Creighton University, Omaha, NE, USA

Joy-Marie Hermes
Creighton University School of Medicine, Omaha, NE, USA

Subhash Chandra and Abdullah Abdussalam
Department of Medicine, Division of Gastroenterology, Creighton University, Omaha, NE, USA

Ahmed Aly
Department of Radiology, Creighton University, Omaha, NE, USA

Jian Guan and Alvina Munaf
Department of Internal Medicine, Graduate Medical Education, Florida Hospital, 2501 N. Orange Suite 235, Orlando, FL 32804, USA

Alric V. Simmonds
Department of General Surgery, Graduate Medical Education, Florida Hospital, 2415 N. Orange Ave., Suite 400, Orlando, FL 32804, USA

Irteza Inayat
Central Florida Hepatology and Gastroenterology, Florida Hospital, 2415 N. Orange Ave., Suite 200, Orlando, FL 32804, USA

Julia Hermes-Laufer and Lola Del Puppo
Department of Internal Medicine, Hôpital de La Tour, Avenue J.-D.-Maillard 3, 1217 Geneva, Switzerland

Omar Kherad
Department of Internal Medicine, Hôpital de La Tour, Avenue J.-D.-Maillard 3, 1217 Geneva, Switzerland
Faculty of Medicine, University of Geneva, Geneva, Switzerland

Ihsan Inan
Department of Visceral Surgery, Clinique Générale Beaulieu, Chemin de Beau Soleil 20, 1206 Geneva, Switzerland

François-Xavier Troillet
Department of Gastroenterology, Hôpital de La Tour, Avenue J.-D.-Maillard 3, 1217 Geneva, Switzerland

Bharat Rao, Abhishek Gulati and Shyam Thakkar
Department of Gastroenterology, Allegheny Health Network, Pittsburgh, PA, USA
Allegheny Center for Digestive Health, 1307 Federal Street, Suite 301, Pittsburgh, PA 15212, USA

Blair Jobe
Department of Surgery, Allegheny Health Network, Pittsburgh, PA, USA
Esophageal and Lung Institute, 4815 Liberty Avenue, Mellon Pavilion, Suite 158, Pittsburgh, PA 15224, USA

Oluwaseun Shogbesan, Abdullateef Abdulkareem and Anthony Donato
Department of Internal Medicine, Reading Health System, Sixth Avenue and Spruce Street, West Reading, PA 19611, USA

Asad Jehangir and Sunila Byreddy
Hospitalist Services, Reading Health System, Sixth Avenue and Spruce Street, West Reading, PA 19611, USA

Sharon Swierczynski
Department of Pathology, Reading Health System, Sixth Avenue and Spruce Street, West Reading, PA 19611, USA

O. Phillips
St. George's University School of Medicine, West Indies, Grenada

A. Higdon and R. Colaco
Department of Surgery, Trinitas Regional Medical Center, Elizabeth, NJ, USA

H. Fish
Division of Surgical Pathology, Trinitas Regional Medical Center, Elizabeth, NJ, USA

Zhi-jun Yan, Jia-xinWang, You-yi Liu, Ping Gan, Xiao Han, Li-kun Luan and You-guo Dai
Department of Abdominal Surgery, Third Affiliated Hospital of Kunming Medical University, Kunming, Yunnan 650118, China

Zhen-hui Li
Department of Radiology, Third Affiliated Hospital of Kunming Medical University, Kunming, Yunnan 650118, China

Li-juan Zhang
Department of Pathology, Third Affiliated Hospital of Kunming Medical University, Kunming, Yunnan 650118, China

Tara Chen, Qiu Tong and Alexander Kurchin
Department of Surgery, Rochester General Hospital, Rochester, NY, USA

Lina Abdul Karim, Dong Hyang Kwon and Metin Ozdemirli
Medstar Georgetown University Hospital, Washington, DC, USA

John Gubatan, Nathan Raines and Hasan Khosravi
Department of Medicine, Beth Israel Deaconess Medical Center, Harvard Medical School, Boston, MA, USA

Tracy L. Challies
Department of Pathology, Beth Israel Deaconess Medical Center, Harvard Medical School, Boston, MA, USA

Tyler M. Berzin
Division of Gastroenterology and Hepatology, Beth Israel Deaconess Medical Center, Harvard Medical School, Boston, MA, USA

Sakiko Hiraoka, Masayasu Ohmori and Hiroyuki Okada
Department of Gastroenterology and Hepatology, Okayama University Graduate School of Medicine, Dentistry and Pharmaceutical Sciences, 2-5-1 Shikata-cho, Kita-ku, Okayama 700-8558, Japan

Masaya Iwamuro
Department of Gastroenterology and Hepatology, Okayama University Graduate School of Medicine, Dentistry and Pharmaceutical Sciences, 2-5-1 Shikata-cho, Kita-ku, Okayama 700-8558, Japan
Department of General Medicine, Okayama University Graduate School of Medicine, Dentistry and Pharmaceutical Sciences, 2-5-1 Shikata-cho, Kita-ku, Okayama 700-8558, Japan

Haruo Urata
Central Research Laboratory, Okayama University Medical School, 2-5-1 Shikata-cho, Kita-ku, Okayama 700-8558, Japan

Yoshitaka Kondo
Department of Gastroenterological Surgery, Okayama University Graduate School of Medicine, Dentistry and Pharmaceutical Sciences, 2-5-1 Shikata-cho, Kita-ku, Okayama 700-8558, Japan

Yoshiro Kawahara
Department of Endoscopy, Okayama University Hospital, 2-5-1 Shikata-cho, Kita-ku, Okayama 700-8558, Japan

Igor Dumic
Department of Hospital Medicine, Mayo Clinic Health System, Eau Claire, WI, USA

Mayo Clinic College of Medicine and Science, Rochester, MN, USA

Scott Martin
Department of Pathology, Mayo Clinic Health System, Eau Claire, WI, USA

Nadim Salfiti
Department of Gastroenterology and Hepatology, Mayo Clinic Health System, Eau Claire, WI, USA

Robert Watson
Department of Family Medicine, Mayo Clinic Health System, Eau Claire, WI, USA

Tamara Alempijevic
Department of Gastroenterology and Hepatology, Clinical Center of Serbia, Belgrade, Serbia
School of Medicine, Belgrade University, Belgrade, Serbia

Keerthana Kesavarapu and Mitchell Kang
Department of Internal Medicine, Drexel University Hospital, Philadelphia, PA, USA

Jaewook James Shin
Drexel School of Medicine, Philadelphia, PA, USA

Kenneth Rothstein
Department of Gastroenterology, Drexel University Hospital, Philadelphia, PA, USA
Department of Hepatology, Drexel University Hospital, Philadelphia, PA, USA

Timo Rath, Raja Atreya, Andreas Nägel and Markus F. Neurath
Department of Medicine 1, Friedrich-Alexander University Erlangen-Nuremberg, Division of Gastroenterology, Endocrinology and Pneumology, Ludwig Demling Endoscopy Center of Excellence, Ulmenweg 18, 91054 Erlangen, Germany

Walter Geißdörfer and Roland Lang
Institute of Clinical Microbiology, Immunology and Hygiene, University Hospital of Erlangen, Friedrich-Alexander University Erlangen-Nuremberg, Wasserturmstrasse 3-5, 91054 Erlangen, Germany

KoMatsuura, Shinsuke Hiramatsu, Rika Taketani, Kohei Ishibashi, Masanao Uraoka, Shinichi Baba, Akihiro Nakamura, Hiroshi Takihara, Chie Ueda and Taro Inoue
Department of Gastroenterology, Kishiwada Tokushukai Hospital, 4-27-1 Kamori-cho, Kishiwada, Osaka 596-0042, Japan

Muhammad Chowdhry, Christina Spyratou, Bruno Lorenzi, Sritharan Kadirkamanathan and Alexandros Charalabopoulos
Department of Upper Gastrointestinal Surgery, Broomfield Hospital, Mid Essex Hospital Services NHS Trust, Essex, UK

Seifeldin Hakim, Mihajlo Gjeorgjievski, Lohit Garg and Molly Orosey
Department of Internal Medicine, William Beaumont Hospital, Royal Oak, MI 48073, USA

Tusar Desai
Department of Gastroenterology, William Beaumont Hospital, Royal Oak, MI 48073, USA
Oakland University William Beaumont School of Medicine, Royal Oak, MI 48073, USA

Lekui Xiao, Winnie Mar and Karen L. Xie
Department of Radiology, University of Illinois at Chicago, USA

Ali Kord Valeshabad
Department of Radiology, University of Illinois at Chicago, USA
Division of Interventional Radiology, University of Illinois at Chicago, USA

Jennifer Acostamadiedo
Department of Medicine, Mercy Hospital and Medical Center, Chicago, IL, USA

CláudioMartins, Cristina Teixeira, Suzane Ribeiro, Daniel Trabulo, Cláudia Cardoso, JoãoMangualde, Ricardo Freire, Ana Luísa Alves, Élia Gamito, Isabelle Cremers and Ana Paula Oliveira
Department of Gastroenterology, Setúbal Hospital Center, São Bernardo Hospital, Setúbal, Portugal

Ailee Ikeda, Masaya Iwamuro, Toshihiro Inokuchi, Asuka Nakarai, Sakiko Hiraoka and Hiroyuki Okada
Department of Gastroenterology and Hepatology, Okayama University Graduate School of Medicine, Dentistry and Pharmaceutical Sciences, Okayama 700-8558, Japan

Takehiro Tanaka
Department of Diagnostic Pathology, Okayama University Hospital, Okayama 700-8558, Japan

Yuusaku Sugihara
Department of General Medicine, Okayama University Graduate School of Medicine, Dentistry and Pharmaceutical Sciences, Okayama 700-8558, Japan

Keita Harada and Yoshiro Kawahara
Department of Endoscopy, Okayama University Hospital, Okayama 700-8558, Japan

Aaron Fisher
Internal Medicine Resident, Beaumont Health, Royal Oak, MI, USA

Alexandra Halalau
General Internal Medicine Section Head, Beaumont Health, Royal Oak, MI, USA
Associate Professor, Oakland University William Beaumont School of Medicine, Rochester, MI, USA

Megan Murphy
Department of Internal Medicine, Thomas Jefferson University Hospital, Philadelphia, PA 19107, USA

Christina Tofani, Kunjal Gandhi and Anthony Infantolino
Department of Gastroenterology and Hepatology, Thomas Jefferson University Hospital, Philadelphia, PA 19107, USA

Masaya Iwamuro, Hiromitsu Kanzaki, Seiji Kawano and Hiroyuki Okada
Department of Gastroenterology and Hepatology, Okayama University Graduate School of Medicine, Dentistry and Pharmaceutical Sciences, 2-5-1 Shikata-cho, Kita-ku, Okayama 700-8558, Japan

Takehiro Tanaka
Department of Pathology, Okayama University Hospital, Okayama 700-8558, Japan

Yoshiro Kawahara
Department of Endoscopy, Okayama University Hospital, Okayama 700-8558, Japan

Tomaz Crochemore and Felicio Aragão Savioli
Hospital Leforte, Department of Critical Care, São Paulo, SP, Brazil

Mahir Gachabayov, Elbrus Abdullaev and Abakar Abdullaev
Department of Abdominal Surgery, Vladimir City Clinical Hospital of Emergency Medicine, Vladimir, Russia

Kubach Kubachev, Nonna Zarkua and Artur Fokin
Department of Surgery Named after N. D. Monastyrskiy, North-Western State Medical Academy Named after I. I. Mechnikov, Saint Petersburg, Russia

Elisa Gravito-Soares, Marta Gravito-Soares, Pedro Figueiredo and Luis Tomé
Gastroenterology Department, Centro Hospitalar e Universitário de Coimbra, Coimbra, Portugal
Faculty of Medicine, University of Coimbra, Coimbra, Portugal

Dushyant Pawar and Anna Calara
School of Medicine, Texas Tech University Health Sciences Center, Lubbock, TX, USA

Roy Jacob
Department of Radiology, University Medical Center, Lubbock, TX, USA

Nancy Beck
Department of Pediatrics, Texas Tech University Health Sciences Center, Lubbock, TX, USA

Alan N. Peiris
Department of Internal Medicine, Texas Tech University Health Sciences Center, Lubbock, TX, USA

Abimbola Adike, Vaishnavi Boppana and Kevin C. Ruff
Division of Gastroenterology and Hepatology, Mayo Clinic, Scottsdale, AZ, USA

Dora Lam-Himlin, Melissa Stanton and Steven Nelson
Department of Laboratory Medicine and Pathology, Mayo Clinic, Scottsdale, AZ, USA

Yousef Abdel-Aziz, Tariq Hammad, Mohamad Nawras and Ali Nawras
Department of Internal Medicine, Division of Gastroenterology, University of Toledo Medical Center, Toledo, OH, USA

Hayder Abdulwahid
Department of Pathology, University of Toledo Medical Center, Toledo, OH, USA

Vijay Gayam, Amrendra KumarMandal, Pavani Garlapati, Mazin Khalid and Arshpal Gill
Department of Medicine and Gastroenterology, Interfaith Medical Center, 1545 Atlantic Avenue, Brooklyn, NY, USA

Khalid Mowyad
Department of Medicine, Wayne State University/ Detroit Medical Center, Detroit, MI, USA

Willemijn P. M. van Dijck, Vincent P. Groot, Jeroen Hagendoorn, Inne H. M. Borel Rinkes and I. Quintus Molenaar
Department of Surgery, UMC Utrecht Cancer Center, University Medical Center Utrecht, Utrecht, Netherlands

Lodewijk A. A. Brosens
Department of Pathology, UMC Utrecht Cancer Center, University Medical Center Utrecht, Utrecht, Netherlands

Maarten S. van Leeuwen
Department of Radiology, UMC Utrecht Cancer Center, University Medical Center Utrecht, Utrecht, Netherlands

Dong-Hyuk Yang, Byoung Wook Bang, Kye Sook Kwon, Hyung Kil Kim and Yong Woon Shin
Division of Gastroenterology, Department of Internal Medicine, Inha University School of Medicine, Incheon, Republic of Korea

Madhuri Chandnani, Jonah Cohen and Tyler M. Berzin
Center for Advanced Endoscopy, Division of Gastroenterology, Beth Israel Deaconess Medical Center and Harvard Medical School, Boston, MA, USA

Matthew Chadwick
Department of Internal Medicine, Genesys Regional Medical Center, 1 Genesys Pkwy, Grand Blanc, MI 48439, USA

Leonid Shamban and Michael Neumann
Department of Gastroenterology, Genesys Regional Medical Center, 1 Genesys Pkwy, Grand Blanc, MI 48439, USA

Rohini Krishna and Samuel O. Igbinedion
Department of Internal Medicine, Louisiana State University Health Sciences Center, Shreveport, LA, USA

Richie Diaz
School of Medicine, Louisiana State University Health Sciences Center, Shreveport, LA, USA

Nazneen Hussain and Moheb Boktor
Department of Gastroenterology and Hepatology, Louisiana State University Health Sciences Center, Shreveport, LA, USA

Ashish Lal Shrestha and Pradita Shrestha
Department of General Surgery, United Mission Hospital, Tansen, Palpa, Nepal

Index

A

Abdominal Trauma, 1, 3, 68, 228, 254-255

Adenocarcinoma, 18, 24-26, 29-30, 32-33, 73-74, 115-116, 120-121, 144, 158, 191, 193-194, 204, 209, 223, 225

Amanita, 57, 59-60

Amatoxin Poisoning, 57, 60

Aminosalicylic Acid, 5

Amyand's Hernia, 42, 44-47

Anticoagulation Therapy, 34, 65, 70

Argon Plasma Coagulation, 1-2, 4, 244

Arterial Mediolysis, 84, 87

Atrial Fibrillation, 18, 20, 23, 82, 88, 122

Atrial Fibrillation Gut Syndrome, 20

Autoimmune Disease, 9-10, 95, 132, 142, 144

Azathioprine, 5-8, 11, 178, 181

B

Bleeding Rectal Ulcer, 80, 82

Bowel Ischemia, 35, 84-85, 94-95

Bowel Perforation, 93, 95-96, 212

C

Cannabinoid Hyperemesis Syndrome, 97, 99-100

Cannabis Use, 97-99

Colectomy, 13-14, 16, 63, 94

Crohn's Disease, 5, 7-8, 136, 139, 141, 147, 154, 157, 178

Cyclic Severe Hyperemesis, 97

D

Diarrhea, 13-15, 17, 57-59, 80-83, 98, 136-137, 142, 144, 178-181, 187-188, 190, 212, 215-216, 218-219, 221, 246

Dropped Gallstones, 75-79

Duodenal Intramural Hematoma, 1, 3

Duodenum, 2-4, 19, 29-30, 32-33, 38, 75-78, 81, 105-107, 131, 133-134, 144, 179, 181, 209-210, 219-221, 233, 250-252

Dysphagia, 9-12, 29-31, 40, 72-73, 93, 101, 103, 163-164, 166, 169, 223, 242, 255

E

Endoscopic Therapy, 1, 4, 27-28, 193, 252

Epinephrine Sclerotherapy, 1, 3

Esophageal Cicatricial Pemphigoid, 12

Esophageal Granular Cell Tumor, 38, 40

Esophageal Lichen Planus, 101, 103-104

Esophageal Stenosis, 10-11

F

Flexi-seal Device, 80-82

Fundic Gland Polyposis, 71, 74

G

Gastric Cancer, 24, 26, 52, 115-121, 158, 161-162, 195, 199

Gastric Hypomotility, 19-20, 23

Gastric Leiomyoma, 48-52

Gastroesophageal Junction, 72, 121, 126, 128, 194

Gastrointestinal Involvement, 96, 105, 218

Gastroparesis, 18-21, 23

Gastroscopy, 14, 19, 84-85

H

Helicobacter Pylori Infection, 98

Hemobilia, 53, 55-56, 84-85, 206-207

Hepatic Cytolysis, 66

Hepatocellular Carcinoma, 5-8

Hypertension, 1, 43, 53, 68, 75, 88, 111, 131, 134, 178-180, 190, 204-208, 215, 227, 248, 250-253

I

Ileoscopy, 14, 179

Infected Renal Cyst, 75-78

Inferior Vena Cava, 34, 81, 107, 148, 228

Inguinal Hernia, 42-47

L

Lanreotide Autogel, 13-15, 17

Laparoscopic Cholecystectomy, 30, 75-79, 98

Laparoscopic Magnetic Sphincter Augmentation, 71

Lichen Planus, 101, 103-104

Lumbar Abscess, 61-62, 64

M

Malignant Metastasis, 29

Mucosal Gastric Hematoma, 84

Mucosal Melanoma, 110, 112-114

Muscle Infiltration, 29

Mycophenolate Mofetil, 9, 12, 222

N

Necrotizing Acute Pancreatitis, 65, 70

O

Odynophagia, 29, 31, 163, 241

P

Percutaneous Liver Biopsy, 53, 55-56

Pneumatosis Intestinalis, 93-95

Portal Vein Thrombosis, 34-37, 66, 69-70, 205-207
Portosplenomesenteric Venous Thrombosis, 65, 70
Prothrombin Gene Mutation, 34
Proton Pump Inhibitor, 73-74, 132, 134, 167-168, 243
Pyelonephritis, 76, 78, 249

R
Radiofrequency Catheter Ablation, 18

S
S Deficiency, 65, 68-69, 144, 147-148
Segmental Arterial Mediolysis, 84, 87
Segmental Mediolytic Arteritis, 87
Sleeve Gastrectomy, 27, 34-37
Stricturing Disease, 101
Systemic Sclerosis, 93-96

T
Testicular Germ Cell Tumor, 105, 108

U
Ulcerating Ileocolitis, 57, 59